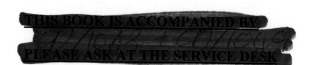

Assistive Technologies

Principles and Practice

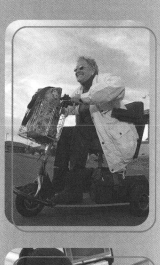

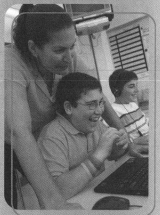

THIRD EDITION

COOK & HUSSEY'S
Assistive Technologies
Principles and Practice

Albert M. Cook, PhD, PE

Professor and Dean
Faculty of Rehabilitation Medicine
University of Alberta
Edmonton, Alberta

**Jan Miller Polgar, PhD, OT Reg. (Ont.)
FCAOT**

Associate Professor, School of
    Occupational Therapy
Chair, Graduate Program in Health
    and Rehabilitation Sciences
Faculty of Health Sciences
The University of Western Ontario
London, Ontario

**Author Emerita
Susan M. Hussey, MS, OTR/L**

Professor and Coordinator
Science and Allied Health Division
Sacramento City College
Sacramento, California

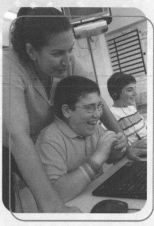

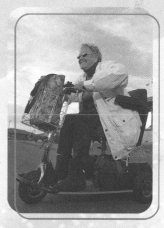

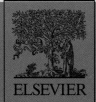

MOSBY
ELSEVIER

11830 Westline Industrial Drive
St. Louis, Missouri 63146

COOK & HUSSEY'S ASSISTIVE TECHNOLOGIES: PRINCIPLES
AND PRACTICE, THIRD EDITION
Copyright © 2008, 2002, 1995 by Mosby, Inc., an affiliate of Elsevier Inc.

ISBN: 978-0-323-03907-9

Notice

Neither the Publisher nor the Authors assume any responsibility for any loss or injury and/or damage to
persons or property arising out of or related to any use of the material contained in this book. It is the
responsibility of the treating practitioner, relying on independent expertise and knowledge of the patient,
to determine the best treatment and method of application for the patient.

The Publisher

Library of Congress Control Number: 2007928477

Publishing Director: Linda Duncan
Senior Editor: Kathy Falk
Senior Developmental Editor: Melissa Kuster Deutsch
Publishing Services Manager: Patricia Tannian
Project Manager: Claire Kramer
Designer: Andrea Lutes

Printed in China

Last digit is the print number: 9 8 7 6 5 4 3 2 1

For giving us the reason and the direction for this work,

we dedicate this book to all our students

and to consumers of assistive technologies, especially

Elizabeth Cook, Brian Cook, Beatrice Miller, and Geraldine Kraft

CONTRIBUTORS

Kim Adams, MSc in EE, PEng ATP
Assistant Professor
Faculty of Rehabilitation Medicine
University of Alberta
Edmonton, Alberta
Research Affiliate
Glenrose Rehabilitation Hospital
Edmonton, Alberta

Roger Calixto, Eng MSc
Graduate student
Biomedical Engineering Department
University of Alberta
Edmonton, Alberta

Lui Shi Gan, BSc
Master's candidate
Department of Biomedical Engineering
University of Alberta
Edmonton, Alberta

Andrew Ganton, BSc(Eng)
Research Associate
Department of Biomedical Engineering and Centre
    for Neuroscience
University of Alberta
Edmonton, Alberta

J. Andrew Rees, BSc (Mech. Eng)
Edmonton, Alberta

Tyler Simpson, BEng
Graduate student
Biomedical Engineering Department
University of Alberta
Edmonton, Alberta

Rebecca Watchorn
Graduate student
Psychology Department
University of Alberta
Edmonton, Alberta

EDITORIAL REVIEW BOARD

PREFACE

"Writing is no trouble: you just jot down ideas as they occur to you. The jotting is simplicity itself—it is the occurring which is difficult."

—Stephen Leacock

The use of assistive technologies by persons with disabilities to pursue self-care, educational, vocational, and recreational activities continues to increase in both quantity and quality. The number of academic programs, clinical centers, schools, and hospitals applying these assistive technologies has increased dramatically.

BACKGROUND

When we wrote the first edition nearly 15 years ago, there was a lack of carefully articulated *principles* and *practices* in the emerging assistive technology field, despite the growth in interest, application, and training. The common approach had been to focus on available devices with little synthesis of principles and practices. Some books focused on specialized areas (e.g., augmentative communication devices or seating systems), whereas others covered a broader range of devices. The first edition of this text was written to provide a framework for assistive technology application that was both *broad in scope* and *specific in content*. This approach was continued in the second edition with the addition of chapters describing the role of assistive technologies meeting educational and vocational needs of persons with disabilities. We are grateful for the extremely positive response to the first two editions from an international audience of professionals, educators, and students. In this third edition, Jan Polgar has taken over for Sue Hussey.

ORGANIZATION

Given the passage of time since the first edition and the rapid pace of technological change, it is not surprising that this edition has been significantly revised and expanded. The book is organized into five main parts. Part One presents information on the assistive technology industry, including a historical perspective, relevant legislation, and issues of professional practices (Chapter 1). In Chapter 2, the fundamental framework for the text, the Human Activity Assistive Technology (HAAT) model description, is developed. We have revised the HAAT model into a three-dimensional format and more closely related it to practice in rehabilitation, particularly occupational therapy. The HAAT model, the fundamental unifying concept in the text, is a framework that describes the consumer participating in activities together with the assistive technologies and their contexts of use. This model embodies the most fundamental of the concepts in the text (i.e., that assistive technologies represent someone [consumer with a disability] doing something [e.g., communicating, moving, manipulating] somewhere with someone [e.g., at home, at work, with peers, with strangers] through the use of assistive technologies). We use this model to develop principles for assistive technology application, which address everything from needs identification through system implementation to measurement of outcomes. The book also provides the basis for discussion of current practices in this field and of the major technologies now in use across a wide range of specific application areas. Chapter 3 discusses the human operator in terms of the skills and abilities that are brought to assistive technology use.

Part Two focuses on service delivery in assistive technologies. In Chapter 4 we focus on the service delivery system through which the consumer obtains assistive technologies. This chapter also includes a discussion of outcome measurement for assistive technologies. In Chapter 5, in which assistive technology funding is described, U.S. funding has been completely revised, and we have expanded the chapter to included Australian and Canadian funding programs. In making these revisions we received major assistance from Lew Golinker (United States), Trevor Jones (Australia), and Deb Finn (Canada).

Part Three is devoted to general purpose assistive technologies, which apply across a wide range of areas. In Chapter 6 we develop basic concepts underlying seating and positioning. The goals of seating and positioning include tissue integrity, positioning for postural control, and the achievement of comfort through proper positioning. The chapter is reorganized to identify principles of seating technologies that apply to each of these goals. The actual technologies are presented to highlight the applications to each of these areas, demonstrating the potential of each to meet one or more of the major goals of seating and positioning.

The most significant changes have occurred in those areas involving assistive technology in computer applications. In earlier editions, we separated computer use into a separate chapter. As time has passed, computer use has become much more common, and much of the information in previous editions regarding general computer use was no longer relevant. Our approach has been to treat the motor and sensory disabilities in separate chapters. In Chapter 7 we have combined computer access for individuals with motor disabilities with our discussion of control interfaces for all applications. Chapter 7 also discusses the development of principles of selection and effective application for control interfaces. Material related to input acceleration (e.g., prediction, abbreviations) has also been moved to this chapter. In Chapter 8 and Chapter 9, we have combined information regarding computer access for individuals with visual and auditory disabilities, respectively, with other assistive technologies that meet the needs of these populations. Chapter 8 also includes a discussion of World Wide Web access for persons with disabilities. In revising these chapters we received help from Gary Moulton and Annuska Perkins from the Accessibility Technology Group at Microsoft.

In Part Four our emphasis shifts to a discussion of specific areas of application for assistive technologies. Chapter 10 is completely new for this edition and addresses the emerging area of assistive technology applications for individuals who have cognitive disabilities. The augmentative communication chapter is now Chapter 11 and has been significantly revised with major assistance from Sarah Blackstone. The former chapter on mobility has been divided into two chapters to describe personal mobility (i.e., manual and electrically powered wheelchairs) and transportation. Chapter 12 describes structure and controls of manual and electrically powered wheelchairs. It identifies principles to guide recommendation of these technologies and introduces new advances in these areas. Chapter 13 has two main components: (1) technology for safe transportation when traveling in a vehicle, while seated either in the vehicle seat or in a wheelchair, and (2) technology for driving. A section that describes proper selection of a child restraint system and systems specific to children with physical disabilities is added in this edition.

In Chapter 14 we discuss the use of assistive technologies to replace or augment manipulative ability. Also included are a wide variety of technologies, which range from simple, low-technology aids (e.g., enlarged forks) to specialized electro-mechanical devices (e.g., feeders, electronic aids to daily living, robots).

In Part Five we consider two particularly significant contexts for assistive technology application. In Chapter 15 we describe educational applications and in Chapter 16, vocational applications. These two chapters bring together concepts, technologies, and strategies from the previous 14 chapters and show how they are interrelated in these major areas of application.

■ NEW TO THIS EDITION

Case examples and illustrations of devices in use foster the understanding of how assistive technologies are *used* and how they *function*. For this third edition, these have been expanded. The glossary of terms has also been expanded and incorporates a list of resources that includes major conferences, professional associations, and manufacturers' associations with Internet sites.

Many assistive technologies, especially those that are electronically based, have features that are best understood by seeing or experiencing them, in addition to reading about them. A major addition to this edition of the text is a CD with demonstrations of assistive technologies, interactive exercises with assistive technology characteristics, video case studies, and demonstrations of devices in use and Web links for obtaining more information. There is also an Evolve Web site for the text (http://evolve.elsevier.com/Cook/assistive/) that contains additional links and resources. Resources for instructors include a test bank and instructor's manual.

■ WHO WILL BENEFIT FROM THIS BOOK?

The primary audience for this book remains undergraduate and graduate university students. The first and second editions, however, also proved useful to assistive technology practitioners and assistive technology suppliers, many of whom used this text for RESNA (Rehabilitation Engineering & Assistive Technology Society of North America) certification examination review. These individuals represent a secondary audience: professionals who are practicing in this area even though they have had no formal training in this field while in school. Our intended audience is a transdisciplinary professional population including occupational therapists, speech-language pathologists, physical therapists, special educators, rehabilitation engineers, and vocational rehabilitation counselors.

■ CONCEPTUAL APPROACH

The strength of our approach is that concepts are unified through the use of the HAAT model and reinforced as each specific application is presented. For each specific technology application, we discuss assessment and training of the consumer, devices that are available, strategies for their use, and evaluation of outcomes. Learning objectives, key terms, study questions, and references are included for each chapter. Case studies have been added throughout the text. It is assumed that the reader will have a general understanding of normal human anatomy and physiology and disabilities.

It is our hope that those individuals familiar with assistive technologies will find something *new* in this text and that those readers who are new to this subject will develop *familiarity* with assistive technologies and appreciate their potential.

Albert M. Cook
Janice M. Polgar

ACKNOWLEDGMENTS

I am indebted to Sue Hussey for her work on the first and second editions of this book. She and I worked well together and found many ways to support, as well as challenge, each other to have the best result that we could. We are grateful for the strong support that those two editions generated. When Sue decided that she could not continue with the third edition, I immediately contacted my friend and colleague, Jan Polgar. I had known Jan through other projects and knew that she was thoughtful, critical, and highly productive—all qualities I wanted in a co-author. I also knew that she was fun and had a great attitude. While Jan may have questioned the wisdom of her decision to join me in developing this third edition, I have had no regrets. Working with Jan has been a delight from start to finish. Always thoughtful, always critical, and most important, always kind, she has made many major improvements in the text. Thank you, Jan, for all of the effort and for the quality product that resulted.

Book writing is a solitary pursuit, and I am indebted to a number of friends who have supported me over the course of this revision. Cheryl Kolbuc, Jeff Kolbuc, Linda Lawrence, and Ron Hazelaar have been remarkably supportive of me and my work. My friend Claire Redpath has helped me to understand much about myself and to place my work in perspective. Norma and Cheryl Harbottle and Dave Polvere provided technical support for this edition.

A book of this type, focusing on technology, requires a great deal of time for revision. This time is often stolen from family. I cannot express the gratitude I have for the continuing support, love, and understanding of my wife, Nancy, and the support of my daughters, Barbara and Jennifer. Finally, my son, Brian, continues to inspire me to understand the ways in which technology can ameliorate the problems faced by individuals who have disabilities.

Al Cook

When Al Cook asked me whether I would be interested in becoming his co-author for the third edition of this book, I thought it would be fun and exciting. And now, 2 years later, it is still mostly fun and exciting. I could not have asked for a better co-author than Al, who has been encouraging and supportive and who has been a wonderful teacher throughout.

During those times when this occupation became overwhelming, Al would offer wise advice or take more of this work into his busy schedule. Al, I value your friendship.

Many other people have supported me through this process. My colleagues in the School of Occupational Therapy at The University of Western Ontario maintained interest in the project and helped me to strategize approaches to different topics. I am grateful for my many friends in the seating and mobility field who shared their resources and expertise. My running and triathlon training partners, particularly the KIN boys, tolerated my tales of early morning writing sessions and the never-ending details of the process. In particular, I thank Jill Jacobson, my research associate, who helped with many elements of the preparation of this book and kept me organized. My parents, Charles and Evelyn Miller, gave me the confidence and perseverance to undertake a task of this size. Most important, I want to thank my family: my husband, Roger; my daughter, Andrea; and my son, Alex, for giving me the time to work on this book. I can't do what I do without you.

Jan Miller Polgar

There are many individuals who helped us with the preparation of this edition of our textbook, and we would like to acknowledge their valuable contributions. Chris Beliveau of the Glenrose Rehabilitation Hospital I CAN Centre in Edmonton provided pictures of devices in use, whereas Kathy Howrey provided much of the framework for Chapter 15. Rob Hussey provided some of the original artwork used in all three editions, and Gaëtan LaBelle provided the original artwork portraying the HAAT model in Chapter 2 of this edition. We are grateful for their creativity. Kathy Falk, senior editor; Melissa Kuster, senior developmental editor; Claire Kramer, project manager; and the editorial assistants at Elsevier provided highly professional support and assistance in the production of this text. A new feature of this edition is the accompanying CD. Melissa and Satyen Vora, producer, developed this CD from our content. Thanks to all of the Elsevier staff for making this project successful.

When the second edition was being developed, the editors obtained a series of pictures from an on-line source. Sue and I quickly agreed that the picture of a man in a wheelchair, obviously enjoying life to the fullest with the use of assistive technology, was our choice. We didn't know who the man was until we received an e-mail during the preparation of this third edition. His OT, Teresa Valois, identified Gary Miller as our "cover man." Teresa also informed us that Gary had passed away. We want to acknowledge the contribution Gary made to the second edition by bringing his sense of joy to our cover.

As Teresa noted, "It is sad to have Gary no longer coming into our Assistive Technology lab and clinic, but to know him was special and he was truly a great user of AT."

Jan Miller Polgar
Al Cook

CONTENTS

COOK & HUSSEY'S

Assistive Technologies

Principles and Practice

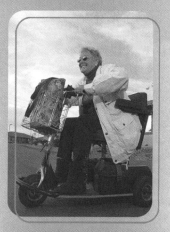

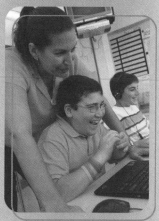

PART 1

Introduction and Framework

Introduction and Overview

Learning Objectives

On completing this chapter, you will be able to do the following:

1. Define assistive technology
2. Delineate the characteristics of assistive technologies
3. Describe the history of assistive technology practice
4. List the major legislative initiatives that have affected the application of assistive technologies
5. Describe the components of the assistive technology industry
6. Explain the roles of the consumer
7. Identify several distinguishing features of service delivery programs

8.   Identify the professionals who may work as assistive technology practitioners
9.   Understand the transdisciplinary approach to assistive technology service delivery
10. Discuss the major professional issues in assistive technology practice

Key Terms

Activity
Alpha Testing
Assistive Technology
Assistive Technology
 Practitioner (ATP)
Assistive Technology Service

Assistive Technology Supplier
Beta Testing
Consumer of Assistive Technologies
Device
Direct Consumer Services
Participation

Prototype
Quality Assurance
Reasonable Accommodation
Telerehabilitation
Transdisciplinary Team Approach
Universal Design

In the last 25 to 30 years there has been major growth in the application of technology in ameliorating the problems of persons with disabilities. Until the publication of the first edition of this book in 1994, there was no unified set of principles for this application of technology. This chapter begins by providing an overview of assistive technologies and the industry that supports their development and distribution. A brief historical perspective and a summary of the major United States federal legislation that provides the mandate for assistive technologies are also presented.

ASSISTIVE TECHNOLOGIES: A WORKING DEFINITION

The document *International Classification of Functioning, Disability, and Health* (ICF) describes a system developed by the World Health Organization (WHO) that is designed to describe and classify health and health-related states. These two domains are described by body factors (body structures and functions) and individual and societal elements (activities and participation) (WHO, 2001). It is a revision of the previous classification system, described in the *International Classification of Impairments, Disabilities, and Handicaps* (ICIDH) (WHO, 1980). Two primary shifts in philosophy discriminate between the ICIDH and the ICF classification systems: the recognition of the importance of the environment as a mediating factor in the performance of daily function and the use of more positive language (i.e., the construct of function replaces that of disability).

Body structures and function refer to the structural and physiological functions of the body. For example, the classification relating to vision lists the anatomical structures of the eye and the sensory and motor and perceptual elements of vision. **Activity** and **participation** are considered to be a single classification. There is much debate on whether it is

possible to differentiate between an activity and participation. Something that may be considered participation at one stage in life becomes an activity at a later stage. The ICF defines activities as the "execution of tasks" and participation as "involvement in life situations" (WHO, 2001, p. 10). Examples of the different components of activity and participation include learning and applying knowledge, communication, mobility, self-care, and community, social, and civic life.

The ICF recognizes two contextual factors that modify health and health-related states: environment and personal factors (WHO, 2001). The latter are not classified but merely identified and include age, sex, race, lifestyle habits, and social and cultural backgrounds, among other factors. The inclusion of these factors in the ICF recognizes their ability to influence differentially the outcome of the same impairment in two individuals.

The ICF does classify environmental elements. Assistive technologies are located in this classification, most prominently in the products and technology chapter. They are specifically mentioned related to activities of daily living, mobility, communication, religion, and spirituality and in specific contexts such as education, employment and culture, recreation, and sport (WHO, 2001). Many of the remaining environmental chapters have implications to assistive technology, although it is not mentioned explicitly. These chapters include access to public and private buildings, the natural and built outdoor environments, people and animals that provide physical and emotional support (personal care attendants and health care professionals are identified here; service animals are not), attitudes of individuals and others and services, systems, and policies, that include legislation (WHO, 2001). Scherer and Glueckauf (2005) reviewed the ICF and discussed the implications to provision of assistive technologies. They concluded that the revised classification system puts the onus on the assistive technology provider to demonstrate positive outcomes for assistive technology recommendations and use.

Definition of Assistive Technology Devices and Services

Dictionaries provide the following definition of technology: (1) the science or study of the practical or industrial arts, (2) applied science, and (3) a method, process, and so forth for handling a specific technical problem (Guralnik, 1979; McKechnie, 1983).

Surprisingly, none of these definitions says anything about a "device"; instead the emphasis is on the application of knowledge. This is an important concept, and the term **assistive technology** will be used to refer to a broad range of **devices,** services, strategies, and practices that are conceived and applied to ameliorate the problems faced by individuals who have disabilities.

Within this framework there are many ways to define assistive technologies. One widely used definition is that provided in Public Law (PL) 108-364 the Assistive Technology Act of 1998, as amended (2004). The definition of an assistive technology device in this law is as follows:

> Any item, piece of equipment or product system whether acquired commercially off the shelf, modified, or customized that is used to increase, maintain or improve functional capabilities of individuals with disabilities.

This definition has several important components, and because it will be used as a working definition throughout this book, these components will be examined in some detail. First, the definition includes commercial, modified, and customized devices. By including all types of devices, the statute encompasses an extremely wide range of applications. Second, this definition emphasizes *functional* capabilities of *individuals* with disabilities. Functional outcomes are the only real measure of the success of assistive technology devices, and throughout this text the importance of providing technologies that result in increased functional capability is stressed. Finally, the emphasis on individual persons with disabilities underscores the importance of treating each application of technology as a unique circumstance. No two applications are exactly the same in terms of the needs and skills of the person being served, the activities to be accomplished, and the context in which the application takes place.

PL 108-364 also defines an **assistive technology service** as any service that directly assists an individual with a disability in the selection, acquisition, or use of an assistive technology device. The law includes several specific examples that further clarify this definition: (1) evaluating needs and skills for assistive technology, (2) acquiring assistive technologies, (3) selecting, designing, repairing, and fabricating assistive technology systems, (4) coordinating services with other therapies, and (5) training both individuals with disabilities and those working with them to use the technologies effectively. This definition demonstrates the broad spectrum of services inherent in the delivery of assistive technologies.

Characterization of Assistive Technologies

In this section a characterization of assistive technologies is presented from several points of view. Each of these is a logical outgrowth of the definitions presented earlier, and each is useful in the process of applying assistive technologies. Box 1-1 shows several classifications used to distinguish different types of assistive technologies.

Assistive Versus Rehabilitative or Educational Technologies.   Technology can serve two major purposes: helping and teaching (Smith, 1991). Technology that helps an individual to carry out a functional activity is termed *assistive technology*. Our emphasis in this text is on assistive technologies that serve a variety of functional needs. Technology can also be used as part of an educational or rehabilitative process. In this case the technology is usually used as one modality in an overall education or rehabilitation plan. Technology in this sense is used as a tool for remediation or rehabilitation rather than being a part of the person's daily life and functional activities, and it will be referred to it as *rehabilitative* or *educational* technology, depending on the setting. Often rehabilitative or educational technology (e.g., cognitive retraining software) is used to develop skills for the use of assistive technologies, and some of these applications are discussed in later chapters. A benefit of characterizing assistive technologies is that

---

BOX 1-1   Characterizations of Assistive Technologies

Assistive versus rehabilitative or educational technologies
Low to high technology
Hard technologies and soft technologies
Appliances versus tools
Minimal to maximal technology
General versus specific technologies
Commercial to custom technology

Data from Odor P: Hard and soft technology for education and communication for disabled people, *Proc Int Comp Conf,* Perth, Australia, 1984; Rizer B, Ourand P, Rein J: *How adapted microcomputer technology contributes to successful educational and vocational outcomes.* Presented at Closing the Gap Conference, October 1990, Minneapolis; Smith RO: Technological approaches to performance enhancement. In Christiansen C, Baum C, editors: *Occupational therapy: overcoming human performance deficits,* Thoroughfare, NJ, 1991, Slack; Vanderheiden GC: Service delivery mechanisms in rehabilitation technology, *Am J Occup Ther* 41:703-710, 1987.

funding programs have targeted goals that require technology to meet specific purposes and items that can be described in a manner consistent with those purposes will be approved for funding.

Low to High Technology.   The next of these distinctions is between low- and high-technology devices. Although this distinction is imprecise, inexpensive devices that are simple to make and easy to obtain are often described as "low" technology and devices that are expensive, more difficult to make, and harder to obtain as "high" technology. According to this distinction, examples of low-technology devices are simple pencil and paper communication boards, modified eating utensils, and simple splints. Wheelchairs, electronic communication devices, and computers are examples of high-technology devices.

Hard and Soft Technologies.   The PL 108-364 definition of an assistive technology device applies primarily to hard technologies as they are defined here. The main distinguishing feature of hard technologies is that they are tangible. Odor (1984) has distinguished between *hard technologies* and *soft technologies*. Hard technologies are readily available components that can be purchased and assembled into assistive technology systems. This includes everything from simple mouth sticks to computers and software. On the other hand, soft technologies are the human areas of decision making, strategies, training, concept formation, and service delivery as described earlier in this chapter. Soft technologies are generally captured in one of three forms: (1) people, (2) written, and (3) computer (Bailey, 1996). These aspects of technology, without which the hard technology cannot be successful, are much harder to obtain. Assistive technology services as defined in PL 108-364 are basically soft technologies. Soft technologies are difficult to acquire because they are highly dependent on human knowledge rather than on tangible objects. This knowledge is obtained slowly through formal training, experience, and textbooks such as this one. The development of effective strategies of use also

has a major effect on assistive technology system success. Initially the formulation of these strategies may rely heavily on the knowledge, experience, and ingenuity of the assistive technology practitioner. With growing experience, the assistive technology user originates strategies that facilitate successful device use. The roles of both hard and soft technologies as integral portions of assistive technology systems are discussed in the section on activities in Chapter 2.

Appliances Versus Tools.   An appliance is a device that "provides benefits to the individual independent of the individual's skill level" (Vanderheiden, 1987, p. 705). Tools, on the other hand, require the development of skill for their use. Household appliances such as refrigerators do not require any skill to operate, whereas tools such as a hammer or saw do require skill. This same criterion applies to assistive technologies. The determining factor in distinguishing a tool from an appliance is that the quality of the result obtained using a tool depends on the skill of the user. For example, eyeglasses, splints, a seating system, or a keyguard for a computer are all appliances because the quality of the functional outcome does not depend on the skill of the user. On the other hand, success in maneuvering a powered wheelchair does depend on the skill of the user; therefore the wheelchair is classified as a tool. Examples of assistive technology tools and appliances are shown in Table 1-1.

In some instances the device may be a tool or an appliance, depending on how it is set up to be used. For example, an electronic aid to daily living (formerly called an environmental control system) that controls lights or appliances (see Chapter 14) requires a relatively complex set of electronic circuits that most would agree are high tech. However, this system can be set up so that the only skill required to operate it is to turn it on or off, in which case it may be considered an appliance. In other instances this system may require the user to learn a sophisticated method of scanning to operate it; the system would then be considered a tool. It is important to note that an appliance that requires user skill because it is poorly designed is not considered a tool.

TABLE 1-1	Examples of Assistive Technology Tools and Appliances	
Topic (Chapter No.)	Appliances	Tools
Control interfaces (7)	Keyguards	Joystick
Computer access (7)	Enlarging lens	Enlarged keyboard
Augmentative communication (11)	—	Alphabet board
Manipulation (14)	Environmental control*	Electric feeder
Mobility (12)	Wheelchair armrest	Manual wheelchair push rims
Sensory (8)	Eyeglasses	Long cane

*See text; classification depends on electronic aid for daily living and its functions.

As Vanderheiden (1987) points out, the successful use of assistive technology tools requires training, strategies, and special skills. These are soft technologies. For example, learning aids that facilitate the use of an assistive device are tools that are used only until the user gains sufficient skill to use the device independently. However, the use of the learning aid requires skill, and this aid is therefore a tool. Strategies for the use of an assistive device require skill and are therefore properly categorized as tools. Both appliances and tools require careful assessment, recommendation, and fitting (see Chapter 4), but only the tool also requires skill development (Vanderheiden, 1987). If training of care providers is included, as well as the consumer of the technology, then training also may be necessary for appliances. For example, when a new seating system is provided (Chapter 6), the care staff must be trained in how to position the person in the seating system. By including soft technologies in our concept of a tool, the importance of developing these skills together with the acquisition of the basic hard technology tool or appliance is emphasized.

Another important point raised by Vanderheiden (1987) is that the tools used by persons with disabilities are often different from those used by the general population, which means that, to develop skill, the assistive technology user often cannot observe someone using the same device. People routinely use observation, such as watching someone using a hammer, as a means of learning how to use a tool. When the person with a disability is the only one in that environment who is using the tool, he or she must rely more heavily on personal experience and formal training to learn to use it effectively. Increasingly, people with disabilities who are expert users of a particular type of assistive technology are serving as mentors to novice users.

Minimal to Maximal Technology. Assistive technologies are specified and designed to meet a continuum of needs. At one extreme are devices that provide some assistance or that augment the individual's ability to perform a task. For example, an individual with cerebral palsy may be able to speak, but on occasion his or her speech may be difficult to understand. In those instances the individual may clarify speech by using a letter board to spell out words not understood. Or a person with respiratory problems may be able to ambulate inside the house but, because of low endurance, may require a powered wheelchair to be able to do grocery shopping independently. In fact, many grocery stores now provide powered carts for individuals who need this type of augmented mobility. At the other extreme are maximal assistive technologies that replace significant amounts of ability to generate functional outcomes. For example, some individuals have no verbal communication ability and may require a device to be able to communicate.

Likewise, some individuals are totally dependent on a manual or powered wheelchair for personal mobility.

Minimal technologies generally *augment* rather than replace function. Classically, devices that augment have been termed *orthoses* or orthotic devices. Although this term originally referred to orthopedic braces of various types, it has been broadened to include all devices that assist or augment function. The term *prosthetics* or prosthetic device originally was used to describe devices that replaced a body part both structurally and functionally. Now this term has also been broadened to include all devices that provide a *functional* replacement.

General Versus Specific Technologies. Assistive technologies are differentiated according to whether they are used in many different applications or whether they are intended for a specific application. *General-purpose* assistive technologies include (1) seating and positioning systems, (2) control interfaces, and (3) computers. These are classified as general purpose because they are used across a wide range of applications. Body position affects the way an individual uses the assistive technology. Frequently, external support systems, an assistive technology, are necessary to achieve a body position that facilitates functional activities. Control interfaces are the means by which the user interacts with any assistive technology. Examples include the joystick on a powered wheelchair, the keyboard on a computer, or the handle that operates the closing mechanism on a reacher. Virtually every electronic assistive technology has a computer incorporated into it. Computers enhance the flexibility and the breadth of application of these devices. Thus computers are also included as general-purpose technologies.

Specific-purpose assistive technologies facilitate performance in one unique application area. Examples include devices for communication, manual and powered wheelchairs, feeding devices, hearing aids, and mobility aids for persons with visual impairments. Because these devices are intended for a specific use, it is possible to design them to maximize their capabilities to meet a particular need.

Commercial to Custom Technology. Another distinction shown in Box 1-1 is between commercially available devices and those that are custom made for an individual. There is actually a continuum from commercial devices (designed for the general public and designed for persons with disabilities), to modification of a commercial device, and finally to making a completely customized device.

Figure 1-1 illustrates the progression from commercially available devices to those that are completely customized for an individual. The term *commercially available* is used to refer to devices that are mass produced. These include commercial devices designed for the general population *(standard commercially available devices)* and assistive technologies

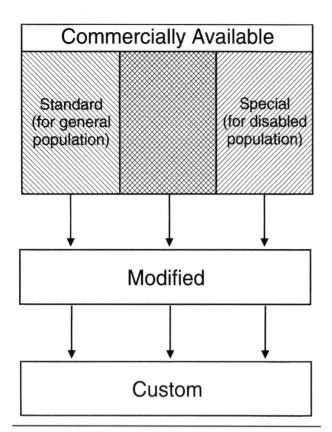

Figure 1-1   The progression from commercially available devices for the general population and commercially available devices for special populations to modified devices and custom devices.

(special commercially available devices), which are mass-produced devices designed for individuals with disabilities. For example, standard personal computers designed for the general population are often used by persons with disabilities. Increasingly, commercial products are being designed according to the principles of **universal design**: the design of products and environments to be usable by all people, to the greatest extent possible, without the need for adaptation or specialized design (North Carolina State University Center for Universal Design, 2001). In this approach, features that make a product more useful to persons who have disabilities (e.g., larger knobs; a variety of display options—visual, tactile, auditory; alternatives to reading text—icons, pictures) are built into the product. This approach is much less expensive than modifying a product after production to meet the needs of a person with a disability. In some cases (e.g., telecommunications equipment) this universal design approach is mandated by federal regulations. In some countries, universal design is known as "design for all." The North Carolina State University Center for Universal Design, in conjunction with advocates of universal design, has compiled a set of principles of universal design, shown in Box 1-2. This center also maintains a Web site on universal design (*www.design.ncsu.edu/cud*).

When an individual's needs for assistive technology cannot be met with a commercial device, special devices that are mass produced and commercially available for persons with disabilities can be attempted. Examples include wheelchairs, augmentative communication systems, and many aids to daily living. In some cases a combination of standard and special-purpose technologies are used; this is represented by the cross-hatched area of Figure 1-1. For example, a standard general-purpose computer may be used with special-purpose software to create an augmentative communication device (see Chapter 11).

If commercially available devices cannot meet an individual's needs, one may be modified to fit. This modification can vary from simple to very complex. For example, if an individual has difficulty using the keys on a computer keyboard, software that facilitates its use can be purchased. In this case the most expensive and complex part of the system (the computer) is a standard commercial product, and the software is the simplest and least expensive portion of the system. However, the software may have a cost that is much higher than expected relative to its simplicity because it is a special product and all the costs of development must be recovered from the small production run. A special commercially available device may be modified as well. For example, a commercially available augmentative communication device may require modification so that it can be mounted on a user's wheelchair.

When no commercial device or modification is appropriate, it is necessary to design one specifically for the task at hand. This approach results in a *custom* device. Because they are mass produced, commercial devices have a lower per unit cost than do custom devices. For example, seating and positioning systems for persons with severe disabilities may be individually contoured to achieve the necessary functional result, which can increase the cost (see Chapter 6).

Another important difference between modified or custom devices and commercial devices is the level of technical support that is available with each. A commercially produced device generally has written documentation and operator's manuals available. Although the quality of these written materials varies widely, some documentation is better than none, and modified or custom devices often have none. The manufacturer or supplier of commercial equipment provides technical support and repair. Because modified or custom devices are one of a kind, technical support may be hard to obtain, especially if the original designer and builder is no longer available (e.g., if the user moves to a new area).

Summary

Assistive technology can be characterized in many ways. It is useful to realize, however, that yesterday's high tech is tomorrow's low tech, custom devices become commercial if more than a few people need them, and appliances often enable the use of tools. Thus no good categorization is perfect or static. As the field advances, there will be new considerations that will further stretch our concepts and force new ways of categorizing and describing assistive technologies.

▰ HISTORICAL PERSPECTIVE ON ASSISTIVE TECHNOLOGY DEVICES AND SERVICES

(Very) Early Developments in Assistive Technologies

Although it is tempting to view assistive technologies and the assistive technology industry as innovations that have occurred over the past 30 years, to really investigate the origins of this field, it is necessary to go back much further in time. Imagine that we are in the Stone Age. Our friend Borg has broken his leg on a hunting expedition. Because there is no plaster yet available, his leg is not placed in a plaster

cast, and when it heals he has a decided limp. Determined to continue providing for his clan, he reaches for the nearest stick to assist his walking. Thus one of the first assistive technology devices is conceived, fabricated, and put into use. At that time this custom device is referred to as "high tech" because of its advanced design and its use of state-of-the-art materials. As time moves on, Borg's descendants begin to realize that assistive technologies can help meet other needs. His great-granddaughter, Myra, now in her later years, discovers that an empty animal horn can be used to make voices louder and help compensate for her fading hearing. One of the first uses of the wheel, a new invention that will be reinvented many times over the years, is to transport people. This key component of the current wheelchair is surprisingly similar to its predecessor. Most important, each version emphasizes function rather than form or style. Borg's walking stick also bears a strong resemblance to present-day canes and crutches. However, Myra's animal horn is only functionally related to the modern-day hearing aid. There is little structural relationship between these two devices, which brings us to the next major point in the history of assistive technologies.

Evolution of State-of-the-Art Assistive Technology

Assistive technologies have always been based on the materials and state-of-the-art technology available to the practitioners. In assistive technologies functional outcomes are emphasized above all other considerations. For this reason, some applications have had little change for many years. Borg's cane is one example; although the structure has remained the same, the materials have changed. However, other applications have only been possible as technologies have advanced.

During the Civil War in the United States, great strides were made in the development of prostheses, especially for the lower limb. Sockets were improved, creating a better fit and more functional outcome. A socket developed by Parmelee in 1863 featured the first suction attachment of a lower limb prosthesis (Murphy, Cook, and Harvey, 1982). This type of socket, still used in modern prostheses, eliminated discomfort caused by pelvic attachment bands and reduced alignment problems and the risk of breakage at the joint. The materials used in 1863, however, bear little resemblance to those used today. Current prostheses use composite metals and plastics, whereas Parmelee's device was made of wood and leather.

Miniature electronic circuits only available in the past 35 years have replaced Myra's horn. However, hearing aids were first patented in the 1890s, and the major function of amplifying sound has not changed over the years. What has changed is the *structure* of these aids. Now they fit into the ear, amplify a wider range of sounds, and are generally more effective (see Chapter 9). In the 1890s these aids were bulky and produced much lower fidelity. It was a long time between Myra's horn and the first hearing aids in the 1890s, but in the last 100 years the state of the art in this field has changed dramatically.

In some cases, current assistive technology applications were not possible as few as 15 years ago. The well-documented revolution in electronics is the reason for most of these gains, and computers are the vehicle by which the advancements have been made. The single most important change in computer design and construction was the reduction in complexity brought about by the development of the microprocessor electronic circuit "chip." This innovation, the *microprocessor,* resulted in reduced size (from a room full of electronics to a typewriter-sized device), reduced cost (affordable by an individual), and greatly increased functional capabilities. Although computers are usually thought of as stand-alone personal systems, microprocessors are built into a large number of devices, from computer printers to microwave ovens and other household appliances. These chips also make possible such important innovations as synthesized speech (see Chapters 8, 10, and 11), robotic aids (see Chapter 14, and computer graphics, all of which play major roles in assistive technology applications. It is difficult to find assistive technology applications in any functional performance area that have not been affected by microcomputer advances. Even in the area of seating and positioning, computer technology is being used for the design and manufacture of custom seat cushions (see Chapter 6). Throughout the remainder of this book the most important of these applications are described.)

U.S. Federal Legislation Affecting the Application of Assistive Technologies

Although industrial advancements and competition have driven the recent development of assistive technology devices, the development of assistive technology services and service delivery in the United States has been affected significantly by federal legislation. In this section only the recent legislation that has most directly affected the development and application of assistive technologies is discussed. Each of the major pieces of legislation that is discussed is summarized in Table 1-2. For the complete text of any federal law, refer to the Library of Congress's "Thomas" Web site at *www.thomas.loc.gov/.* Specific information on U.S. legislation related to assistive technologies is available on the Rehabilitation Engineering and Assistive Technology Society of North America (RESNA) Web site at *www.resna.org.*

In the United States, as shown in Table 1-3, statutes can be organized into two groups. The first group is statutes that provide structure to society by prohibiting discrimination and thereby facilitate access to or use of assistive technologies. This group includes Section 504 of the Rehabilitation Act of 1973 and the Americans With Disabilities Act. The second group includes those statutes that provide actual services that may include assistive technologies. This group includes the Individuals With Disabilities Education Act and health programs such as Medicaid and Medicare. Some statues appear in both categories.

Rehabilitation Act of 1973 (Amended). The Rehabilitation Act of 1973 established several important principles on which subsequent legislation has been based. The most far-reaching of these principles are nondiscrimination and **reasonable accommodation.** Section 504 of the Rehabilitation Act prohibits any activity receiving federal funds from discriminating solely on the basis of disability. To remedy discrimination, federally funded activities and programs must offer reasonable accommodations to facilities, programs, and benefits to ensure that people with disabilities have equal access and equal opportunity to derive benefits. As a result of the wide reach of federal funding, the nondiscrimination provisions of the Rehabilitation Act of 1973 compelled universities—recipients of many different types of federal funding—and local and state governments, and others to make architectural changes to campuses, public buildings, sidewalks, and museums to reduce barriers. Elevators were added to buildings, ramps and curb cuts were made to accommodate wheelchair users, and voice and Braille labels were added to signs (including elevators) to provide access for visually impaired persons. State and local programs that provide medical, social, recreational, and other services also had to make changes to ensure that people with disabilities had equal access to the programs and their benefits. The Rehabilitation Act's nondiscrimination provisions also extend to the activities of the federal government itself. Many of these efforts to accommodate individuals with disabilities involved the use of assistive technologies.

The Rehabilitation Act amendments of 1998, which are contained in the Workforce Investment Act of 1998 (PL 105-220), are the most recent amendments to the Rehabilitation Act. This act was also amended in 1986 (PL 99-506), 1992 (PL 102-569), and 1993 (PL 103-73). Together they include several provisions involving assistive technology. First the amendments require that each state include within its vocational rehabilitation plan a provision for assistive technology (referred to in PL 99-506 as *rehabilitation engineering or technology* and in PL 105-220 as *rehabilitation technology*). PL 99-506 defined rehabilitation engineering as the systematic application of technologies, engineering methods, or scientific principles to meet the needs of and address the barriers confronted by individuals with disabilities in areas that include education, rehabilitation, employment, transportation, independent living, and recreation. The term includes rehabilitation engineering, assistive technology devices, and assistive technology services (29 U.S.C. § 705[30]).

Because this plan is the basis by which states receive federal funding for vocational rehabilitation, there is a strong incentive to provide these technology-related services.

TABLE 1-2   Recent Major U.S. Federal Legislation Affecting Assistive Technologies

Legislation	Major Assistive Technology Impact
Rehabilitation Act of 1973, as amended	Mandated reasonable accommodation in all federally funded programs; requires both assistive technology devices and services be included in state vocational rehabilitation services plans and IPE for each client; Section 508 mandates equal access to electronic office equipment for all federal employees; defines rehabilitation technology as rehabilitation engineering and assistive technology devices and services; mandates rehabilitation technology as primary benefit to be included in IPE
Individuals with Disabilities Education Act Amendments of 1997	Recognized the right of every child to a free and appropriate education; included concept that children with disabilities are to be educated with their peers; extended reasonable accommodation, least restrictive environment, and assistive technology devices and services to age 3-21 years; mandated IEP for each child, to include consideration of assistive technologies; also included mandated services for children from birth to 2 years and expanded emphasis on educationally related assistive technologies
Assistive Technology Act of 1998, as amended (replaced Technology Related Assistance for Individuals With Disabilities Act of 1988)	First legislation to specifically address expansion of assistive technology devices and services; mandates consumer-driven assistive technology services, capacity building, advocacy activities, and statewide system change; supports grants to expand and administer alternative financing of assistive technology systems
Developmental Disabilities Assistance and Bill of Rights Act	Provides grants to states for developmental disabilities councils, university-affiliated programs, and protection and advocacy activities for persons with developmental disabilities; provides training and technical assistance to improve access to assistive technology services for individuals with developmental disabilities
Americans With Disabilities Act of 1990	Prohibits discrimination on the basis of disability in employment, state and local government, public accommodations, commercial facilities, transportation, and telecommunications, all of which affect the application of assistive technology; use of assistive technology affects requirement that Title II entities must communicate effectively with people who have hearing, vision, or speech disabilities; addresses telephone and television access for people with hearing and speech disabilities
Medicaid	Income-based ("means-tested") program; eligibility and services differ from state to state; federal government sets general program requirements and provides financial assistance to the states by matching state expenditures; largest funding source for assistive technology benefits among all funding programs; benefits may vary from state to state for adults; assistive technology for adults must be included in state's Medicaid plan or waiver program
Medicare	Major funding source for assistive technology (durable medical equipment); includes individuals aged 65 years or more and those who are permanently and totally disabled; federally administered with consistent rules for all states

The Rehabilitation Act also requires that provision for acquiring appropriate and necessary assistive technology devices and services be included in Individualized Written Rehabilitation Programs (IWRPs), renamed in the 1998 amendments as "Individualized Plans for Employment" (IPE), which are written for individuals with disabilities.

A third Rehabilitation Act provision with important assistive technology implications is Section 508. First added in the 1986 amendments and later strengthened in the 1998 amendments, this section was developed to ensure access to "electronic office equipment" by persons with disabilities who work for the federal government. Although limitation

TABLE 1-3   Groups of U.S. Legislation Related to Assistive Technologies

Category	Legislation
Statutes that facilitate access to or use of assistive technologies by providing structure to society by prohibiting discrimination	Section 504 of the Rehabilitation Act of 1973 Section 508 of the Rehabilitation Act of 1973 Americans With Disabilities Act The Developmental Disabilities Assistance and Bill of Rights Act
Statutes that provide services that may include assistive technologies	Sections of the Rehabilitation Act of 1973 Individuals With Disabilities Education Act Medicaid and Medicare The Developmental Disabilities Assistance and Bill of Rights Act

to the federal government may seem to be so restrictive as to severely reduce the impact of the law, the federal government is such a large purchaser of computers and other office technology that any purchasing specifications it makes take on the role of informal standards. This legislation has had a significant influence on the design and manufacture of computers and their accessibility to persons with disabilities. Persons who are blind or have low vision and those with difficulty in accessing the keyboard have benefited from standards derived as a result of Section 508, and several manufacturers have included technology that increases access in the basic designs of their computer systems. Many of these features are discussed further in Chapters 7 and 8.

The major intent of Section 508 is that electronic and information technology developed, procured, maintained, or used by the federal government be accessible to people with disabilities. Section 508 applies to federal departments and agencies. It covers access to electronic office equipment and electronic information services provided to the public by the federal government. This provision includes ensuring that end users with disabilities (1) have access to the same databases and application programs as other end users, (2) are supported in manipulating data and related information resources to attain equivalent end results as other end users, and (3) can transmit and receive messages using the same telecommunication systems as other end users. The U.S. Architectural and Transportation Barriers Compliance Board is now developing standards for Section 508. The guidelines accompanying Section 508 also detail the functional performance specifications for electronic office equipment accessibility. Because of provisions in the former Technology Act, now the Assistive Technology (AT) Act of 1998 (see p. 14), states and territories that receive AT Act funding and all subrecipients must comply with Section 508.

Americans With Disabilities Act (ADA) of 1990.

The Americans with Disabilities Act (ADA, PL 101-336) prohibits discrimination on the basis of disability in employment, state and local government, public accommodations, commercial facilities, transportation, and telecommunications. It also applies to the U.S. Congress. To be protected by the ADA, an individual must meet the following ADA definitions of disability: a person who has a physical or mental impairment that substantially limits one or more major life activities, a person who has a history or record of such an impairment, or a person who is perceived by others as having such an impairment. The ADA does not specifically name all the impairments that are covered. The ADA has four main titles: Title I (employment), Title II (state and local government agencies and public transportation), Title III (public accommodations), and Title IV (telecommunications), all of which affect the application of assistive technology.

The prohibition of employment discrimination on the basis of disability stated in Title I of the ADA requires employers with 15 or more employees, including religious entities with 15 or more employees, to provide qualified individuals with disabilities an equal opportunity to benefit from the full range of employment-related opportunities available to others. For example, it prohibits discrimination in recruitment, hiring, promotions, training, pay, fringe benefits, and other privileges of employment. It restricts questions that can be asked about an applicant's disability before a job offer is made. Many issues of employment involve the use and application of assistive technology because Title I of the ADA requires that employers make reasonable accommodation to the known physical or mental limitations of otherwise qualified individuals with disabilities unless it results in undue hardship. The application of Title I to employee fringe benefits protects employees with disabilities or family members with disabilities from discrimination in the provision of health insurance benefits, which is an important funding source for assistive technologies.

Title II covers all activities of state and local governments regardless of the government entity's size or receipt of federal funding. Title II requires that state and local governments give people with disabilities an equal opportunity to benefit from all their programs, services, and activities (e.g., public education, employment, transportation, recreation, health care, social services, courts, voting, and town meetings).

State and local governments are required to follow specific architectural standards in the new construction and alteration of their buildings. They also must relocate programs or otherwise provide access in inaccessible older buildings. In addition, the use of assistive technology such as specialized computer software affects the requirement that Title II entities must communicate effectively with people who have hearing, vision, or speech disabilities, which includes screen readers, enlarged computer screens, and augmentative and alternative communication devices. Public entities are not required to take actions that would result in undue financial and administrative burdens. They are required to make reasonable modifications to policies, practices, and procedures where necessary to avoid discrimination unless they can demonstrate that doing so would fundamentally alter the nature of the service, program, or activity being provided.

The transportation provisions of Title II cover public transportation services, such as city buses and public rail transit (e.g., subways, commuter rails, Amtrak). Public transportation authorities may not discriminate against people with disabilities in the provision of their services. They must comply with requirements for accessibility in newly purchased vehicles, make good faith efforts to purchase or lease accessible used buses, remanufacture buses in an accessible manner, and, unless it would result in an undue burden, provide paratransit where they operate fixed-route bus or rail systems. Paratransit is a service in which individuals who are unable to independently use the regular transit system (because of a physical or mental impairment) are picked up and dropped off at their destinations.

Title III covers businesses and nonprofit service providers that are public accommodations, privately operated entities offering certain types of courses and examinations, and privately operated transportation and commercial facilities. Public accommodations are private entities that own, lease, lease to, or operate facilities such as restaurants, retail stores, hotels, and movie theaters; private schools; convention centers; physicians' offices; homeless shelters; transportation depots; zoos; funeral homes; day care centers; and recreation facilities, including sports stadiums and fitness clubs. Transportation services provided by private entities are also covered by Title III.

Public accommodations must comply with basic nondiscrimination requirements that prohibit exclusion, segregation, and unequal treatment. They also must comply with specific requirements related to architectural standards for new and altered buildings and reasonable modifications to policies, practices, and procedures. In addition, public accommodations must use assistive technology for their requirement to offer effective communication for people with hearing, vision, or speech disabilities as well as other access requirements. Additionally, public accommodations must remove barriers in existing buildings where it is easy to do so without much difficulty or expense, given the public accommodation's resources.

Courses and examinations related to professional, educational, or trade-related applications, licensing, certifications, or credentialing must be provided in a place and manner accessible to people with disabilities, or alternative accessible arrangements must be offered. For example, courses and examinations given by computer should use appropriate computer assistive technology for people with vision, hearing, or cognitive disabilities.

Title IV addresses telephone and television access for people with hearing and speech disabilities, which has wide assistive technology implications, especially because emerging and developing technologies in the telecommunications and television fields are changing at a rapid pace. Title IV requires common carriers (telephone companies) to establish interstate and intrastate telecommunications relay services (TRS) 24 hours a day, 7 days a week. TRS enables callers with hearing and speech disabilities who use text telephones (TTYs) and callers who use voice telephones to communicate with each other through a third-party communications assistant. The Federal Communications Commission (FCC) has set minimum standards for TRS services. Title IV also requires closed captioning of federally funded public service announcements.

Widely hailed as a major civil rights bill for the disabled, the ADA has the potential of removing many of the barriers that have kept individuals with disabilities from engaging in all aspects of society. Assistive technologies surely play a major role in this process.

Individuals With Disabilities Education Act Amendments of 1997 and 2004. The Education for All Handicapped Children Act (EAHCA) of 1975, PL 94-142, later amended by the Individuals with Disabilities Education (IDEA) Act of 1990 and the IDEA Amendments of 1997 (IDEA 97), PL 105-17, establish the right of every child with a disability to receive a "free and appropriate public education" (FAPE). Before this law, more than 1 million children with disabilities were excluded from American public schools. Currently there are approximately 6 million children being served under IDEA.

The centerpiece of the IDEA is an individualized education plan (IEP) that describes each student's current educational performance and outlines the program of specially designed instruction (special education) and supplemental (related) services each child with a disability is to receive as part of his or her FAPE. IEPs also state specific educational goals to be achieved by the student, both short and long term (by the end of the school year). Assistive devices, and training in their use, have long been recognized as components of an FAPE. Indeed, students' need for and ability to benefit from these devices and services, and schools' obligations to provide these devices and services as special education or related services, predate the formal inclusion of definitions of assistive technology devices and services in the act. Definitions of those terms, copied from the Technology Act definitions, PL 100-407, were not formally added to the special education lexicon until 1990. A federal policy interpretation makes that clear. It was issued August 10, 1990, and stated that assistive technology devices and services had to be provided when they were necessary for students to receive an FAPE (Goodman, 1990). This policy letter was issued *before* the Individuals with Disabilities Education Act of 1990 became law. A much earlier policy letter (Desch, 1986) describes the implications of PL 94-142 regarding acquisition of assistive technologies by students with disabilities. In the 1997 IDEA Amendments PL 105-117, schools were directed to consider the assistive technology needs when formulating every IEP for students with disabilities. This provision is retained in the 2004 amendments.

Other important provisions of the EAHCA and IDEA are the requirement that children with disabilities are educated with their nondisabled peers to "the maximum extent appropriate." This is known as the "least restrictive environment" principle. Children with disabilities are to be removed from the regular class environment "only when the nature or severity of the disability is such that education in regular classes cannot be achieved satisfactorily."

The influence of this law has been far reaching. Devices ranging from sensory aids (visual and auditory) to augmentative communication devices to specialized computers have been used to provide access to educational programs for children with disabilities. Lack of local services or lack of funds is not a sufficient reason to deny services or devices justified in the IEP. If the IEP goals are not met, or if there are differences over what should be included in the IEP, there is a fair hearing process that may be pursued. The IDEA also mandates that schools begin to plan for the transition of students with disabilities to a wide range of possible post-high-school or adult activities, beginning many years before the student's anticipated departure from the education programs. When planning for transition, schools are expected to work closely with state vocational rehabilitation programs. Transition planning and programming is an important point for the discussion and provision of assistive technologies.

The focus of IDEA 97 is on improving results for children with disabilities. One major portion of the original act invited states to expand and improve services to infants and toddlers with disabilities and their families (Part H, the Infants and Toddlers with Disabilities Program). In 1997, Part H became Part C of IDEA 97.

Part C of IDEA 97 provides for services to infants and toddlers (birth through age 2 years). More than 177,000 children receive services under Part C, and of those, nearly 10,000 receive assistive technology devices and services. State AT Act projects have been active in promoting the use of assistive technology for the very young and have contributed to building the capacity to provide AT services under Part C. Technology provided includes battery-operated toys with easy-access switches, seating and positioning systems, mobility devices, computers and alternative access aids, communications software, and others. Adapted toys help the child learn the basic concept of cause and effect. Seating and positioning systems provide support and guide the growth of a child's body. Mobility devices also allow the child to move about in his or her environment. Computers and alternate access aids, such as large keypads and touch screens, can help children use software that develops communication, perceptual skills, fine motor skills, and many other skills. Through annual grants beginning in 1987, financial support is provided to develop, establish, and maintain a statewide system that offers early intervention services to all eligible children. Although participation in Part H (now Part C) was always voluntary, each state has chosen to develop a statewide system and, as of October 1, 1994, has committed to seeing that services are available to every eligible child and his or her family. The U.S. Department of Education, through the Office of Special Education Programs (OSEP), distributes funds under Part C to the states to help them carry out collaborative systems planning, policy development, and implementation of needed services for infants and toddlers who have disabilities.

The number of very young children using assistive technology has increased dramatically over the past 4 years. Besides assistive technology devices and services, states provide a variety of other services to children from birth to 2 years old, such as special education; physical and occupational therapy; nutrition services; audiology; nursing services; speech-language pathology; family training, counseling, and home visits; and vision services. The services to be provided to the child with a disability and the family are documented in an Individualized Family Service Plan (IFSP). Development of the IFSP, as with the IEP, is based on assessments of a child's capabilities, skills, and needs and is constructed through a team approach that includes family members.

Elementary and Secondary Education Act (2001 Reauthorization). This act (Public Law 107-110), also known as "*No Child Left Behind*" (NCLB), requires schools to test at least 95% of students with disabilities. These scores must be reported with other students' scores and are used in determining whether the school is making adequate yearly progress. School districts must also report the progress of students who receive special education separately as a part of determining adequate yearly progress. Assistive technologies can play an important role in achieving curriculum goals (see Chapter 15) and may assist schools in achieving adequate yearly progress. Some states are developing standards for technology used in education and these are directly related to NCLB as well (Edyburn, Higgins, and Boone, 2005).

Assistive Technology Act of 1998, as Amended (2004). Designated as PL 108-364, the Assistive Technology Act replaced the Technology-Related Assistance for Individuals with Disabilities Act of 1988 (PL 100-407) and the amendments to that law (PL 103-218) enacted in 1994. The 1986 Vocational Rehabilitation (VR) Amendments predated the Technology Act and it introduced numerous assistive technology provisions into the VR program. The Assistive Technology Act extends funding to the 50 states, the District of Columbia, Puerto Rico, and outlying areas (Guam, American Samoa, U.S. Virgin Islands, and the Commonwealth of the Northern Mariana Islands) that received federal funding under the Technology Act. The purposes of the Assistive Technology Act include the following:

1. Support states in their provision of assistive technology to individuals of all ages with disabilities through statewide programs.
2. Provide financial assistance to states to support their programs that provide access to assistive technology and assistive technology services.

The Assistive Technology Act is divided into three parts: Title I, State Grant Programs; Title II, National Activities; and Title III, Alternative Financing Mechanisms.

Title I provides grants to states to support capacity building and advocacy activities designed to assist the states in maintaining permanent, comprehensive, consumer-responsive, statewide programs of technology-related assistance. These include public awareness, interagency coordination, technical assistance, and training to promote access to assistive technology, and support to community-based organizations that provide assistive technology devices and services or assist individuals in using assistive technology. Title I also provides legal protection and advocacy services; funding for technical assistance, including a national public Internet site; and technical assistance to the states.

Title II provides for increased coordination of federal efforts related to assistive technology and universal design. It authorized funding for multiple grant programs from fiscal years 1999 through 2000, including grants for universal design research, Small Business Innovative Research grants related to assistive technology, grants to commercial or other organizations for research and development related to universal design concepts, grants or other mechanisms to address the unique assistive technology needs of urban and rural areas and of children and the elderly, and grants or other mechanisms to improve training of rehabilitation engineers and technicians.

Title III requires the Secretary of Education to award grants to states and outlying areas to pay for the federal share of the cost of the establishment and administration of, or the expansion and administration of, specified types of alternative financing systems for assistive technology for people with disabilities. These alternative-funding mechanisms may include a low-interest loan fund, an interest buy-down program, a revolving loan fund, a loan guarantee or insurance program, and others (RESNA Technical Assistance Project, 1999).

The primary changes in the 2004 amendment include the repeal of the provision that allows the law to expire on an annual basis. The law is now in force for 6 years. It includes the provision of assistive technology for individuals of all ages and attempts to make the provision of assistive technology and access to assistive technology services more consistent across the states and other U.S. jurisdictions (Association of Assistive Technology Act Programs, 2005).

Developmental Disabilities Assistance and Bill of Rights Act.

The developmental disabilities program was originally enacted as Title I of the Mental Retardation Facilities and Construction Act of 1963 (PL 88-164) and has been amended eight times since then. This program provides grants to states for developmental disabilities councils (DD councils), university-affiliated programs (UAPs), and protection and advocacy activities for persons with developmental disabilities (PADD). Grants to UAPs include grants for training projects with respect to assistive technology services for the purpose of assisting university-affiliated programs in providing training to personnel who provide, or will provide, assistive technology services and devices to individuals with developmental disabilities and their families. Such projects may provide training and technical assistance to improve access to assistive technology services for individuals with developmental disabilities and may include stipends and tuition assistance for training project participants.

Medicaid.

Medicaid is a federal program created in 1965 and codified as Title XIX of the Social Security Act (42 U.S.C. §§1396. et. seq.). It is an income, or "means-tested," program, so eligibility depends on a person's income level. Medicaid is an example of a program of joint federal and state responsibilities, called "cooperative federalism." These programs are noted by joint or shared responsibilities for financing and administration. The federal government guarantees no less than 50% funding for state outlays for their Medicaid programs, with the amounts increasing as the relative wealth of the state's population decreases. States with the poorest populations in the nation receive federal payments of as much as 80% of their total Medicaid outlays. The federal government, through the Centers for Medicare and Medicaid Services (CMS, formerly the Health Care Financing Administration [HCFA]) also establishes a broad outline of the people who must be eligible for Medicaid, the services Medicaid programs must offer, and the way those services must be delivered, but states then have many choices about who is eligible, which services are offered, and how they are delivered. States also are responsible for day-to-day program administration.

Medicaid is not a federally mandated program. Instead, states must elect to participate and express their desire to do so by submitting a "state plan for medical assistance" to CMS. Every state participates in Medicaid. The state plan is an acknowledgement that the state will follow all federally established Medicaid requirements and identifies all the choices the states will make regarding individual eligibility and covered services. The Medicaid program neither provides services directly nor pays cash assistance directly to individuals who need medical care. Rather, the program provides payment to providers (e.g., physicians, pharmacies, hospitals, therapists) for covered supplies and services rendered to qualified recipients.

Medicaid programs are the largest funding source for assistive technologies—both devices and services—in the United States. However, its program vocabulary was established decades before the phrase *assistive technology* was coined, so reference to assistive technology in Medicaid means access to items of durable medical equipment, or prosthetic devices. Reference to services means access to occupational, physical, or speech-language pathology or audiology services. An individual who seeks Medicaid funding for any of these items or services must generally meet a three-part test: (1) the individual must be eligible for Medicaid, (2) the specific device or service requested must be one that is covered by the Medicaid program, and (3) the individual must establish that the device or service requested is medically necessary.

Among Medicaid services, the broadest, in terms of total benefits covered, is known as Early and Periodic Diagnosis, Screening, and Treatment, or EPSDT. EPSDT is a benefit available to every Medicaid-eligible individual who is younger than age 21 years. Its scope includes every Medicaid service listed in the Medicaid Act, both those that are required by the statute and all the optional services the states are able to elect to include in their state plans. For children, all these services must be available. EPSDT's primary goal is early identification of health conditions, which is accomplished by mandatory periodic health screenings, and to minimize or eliminate disability by providing access to the broadest possible range of treatment. Any health condition identified in an EPSDT screening that requires treatment is to be treated as long as the intervention can possibly be covered by Medicaid. For children who require assistive technologies, EPSDT ensures access to Medicaid funding for their necessary devices and services (42 U.S.C. §1396[a][4][B]; 42 C.F.R. §§441.50-441.62).

The EPSDT benefit is available only to Medicaid recipients who are younger than 21 years. For those who are 21 years or older, a different set of Medicaid benefits may be offered. For adults, Medicaid programs are required to offer a small number of services identified in the federal statute, but then they are given the choice to add to their state plan any combination of approximately three dozen "optional" services. States typically have included approximately two dozen or more of these optional services, some of which are important funding sources for assistive technologies.

The flexibility of the Medicaid program also includes a state option to seek waivers of Medicaid program requirements for specifically identified populations with special needs (e.g., technology-dependent children). "Waivers" are an opportunity for states to extend Medicaid eligibility or expand the scope of Medicaid services in a targeted way to populations that are at risk of institutional care. By extending Medicaid eligibility, waivers provide access to the health services these individuals need to remain in their homes. Or, by providing access to items that do not "fit" within the state's definition of "durable medical equipment" or "prosthetic devices," institutional care can be avoided.

As shown in Box 1-3, there are 11 separate Medicaid service categories that have been identified for funding assistive technology or durable medical equipment. Some are mandatory services, meaning they must be included in the state's plan for medical assistance, whereas others are optional, meaning they can be provided to adults in the state at the option of the state. Each service category is more specifically defined in the federal regulations. For example, 42 C.F.R. §§440.70(b)(3) defines medical supplies, equipment, and appliances as mandatory items under home health services; 440.110 defines physical therapy, occupational therapy, and speech, hearing, and language therapy; 440.120(c), prosthetic devices; 440.130(c), preventive services; and 440.130(d), rehabilitation services.

Persons with disabilities who are seeking to use Medicaid as a source of funding for assistive technology must navigate an often cumbersome process that usually requires both their specific conditions and needs to be expressed in language designed to fit program criteria. With very few exceptions, the Medicaid law and its implementing regulations do not identify specific types of treatment or devices that are

---

BOX 1-3   Categories of Medicaid Funding for Assistive Technologies

MANDATORY SERVICE CATEGORIES FOR AT FUNDING
Home health care services (medical supplies, equipment, and appliances)
Early periodic screening, diagnosis, and treatment (for children)

OPTIONAL SERVICE CATEGORIES FOR AT FUNDING
Home health care (home health aide and personal care services)
Intermediate care facilities
Occupational therapy
Physical therapy
Preventive services
Private duty nursing
Prosthetic devices
Rehabilitation services
Speech, hearing, and language therapy

---

covered, only broad categories of health care. This situation imposes an interpretive obligation on state program administrators who must decide whether the specific item or service requested "fits" or is "covered" by one of the state's Medicaid services. Although access to many assistive technologies—both devices and services—is readily provided, these interpretive duties have proved a breeding ground for dispute about coverage and medical need. Many states have sought to avoid these disputes by adopting item- or service-specific clinical or coverage criteria. The most common items that are the subject of these criteria are communication devices and wheelchairs. In general, Medicaid coverage of assistive technologies is so broad because of the total number of people Medicaid serves, its special focus on needs identification and treatment of children, and its general purposes, which are outlined in the federal statute. The primary goal of Medicaid is to provide medical assistance to persons in need and to furnish them with rehabilitation and other services to help them "attain or retain capability for independence or self-care" (42 U.S.C. §1396). The federal regulations provide further that "each service must be sufficient in amount, duration and scope to reasonably achieve its purpose" (42 C.F.R. §440.230[b]).

Medicare.   The Medicaid and Medicare programs, created together in 1965, are codified as Title XVIII of the Social Security Act. Although Medicaid is focused on the needs of those who lack the financial means to meet the costs of necessary health care, Medicare initially was focused on the needs of the elderly, defined as individuals aged 65 years and older. It was believed that this population was less wealthy and less healthy and had access to less health insurance than did younger individuals and therefore needed assistance meeting the costs of their health care needs. Medicare subsequently was expanded to serve individuals with disabilities who are younger than age 65 years. Medicare is administered by the federal government, and the rules are the same for every state in the nation. Medicare is another major funding source for assistive technology. Like Medicaid, however, its program vocabulary characterizes devices as either *durable medical equipment* or prosthetic devices. It also covers occupational and physical therapy and speech-language pathology services. Medicare is a health insurance program for four groups: (1) individuals aged 65 years or older, (2) people of all ages who meet the standards of disability under the Social Security Act; (3) the disabled children of persons who had been working and who became disabled themselves, died, or retired at age 65 years; and (4) people with end-stage renal disease. It is divided into two parts. Part A, known as "hospital insurance," covers inpatient services, posthospital care in skilled nursing homes, hospice care, and home health care. Home health care includes durable medical equipment, occupational and physical therapy, and speech-language pathology services. Part B, known as "supplemental medical insurance," covers physician's services; laboratory services; durable medical equipment; medical supplies; prosthetic devices; rehabilitation therapy services, including speech-language pathology services; and home health care for beneficiaries not covered by Part A. Access to assistive technologies for Medicare recipients is overwhelmingly through the Part B benefit.

The Medicare program operates like a federally subsidized insurance program. Beneficiary contributions include cash deductions and coinsurance requirements under Parts A and B and monthly premiums for Part B. For individuals who are eligible for Medicare and who are also poor, state Medicaid programs can assume the Medicare cost-sharing requirements for those individuals who qualify for both Medicare and Medicaid. Also, like many insurers, Medicare is a cost reimbursement program, meaning that Medicare recipients must first obtain an item or service, then seek Medicare reimbursement for their outlays.

Some assistive technology devices are covered by Medicare as items of durable medical equipment or as prosthetic devices. Medicare defines durable medical equipment as equipment that (1) can withstand repeated use, (2) is primarily and customarily used to serve a medical purpose, (3) generally is not useful to a person in the absence of illness or injury, and (4) is appropriate for use in the home. Medicare also has a unique limitation among benefits and funding programs that applies to mobility aids. It claims that Congress has directed that it consider only a person's mobility related activities of daily living that arise in the person's home, as opposed to all typical mobility needs regardless of environment, which is the generally accepted and longstanding professional standard for mobility aid assessment.

Medicare reimbursement for items or services will be based on the same three factors as were stated for Medicaid: individual eligibility, coverage, and medical necessity. Medicare uses the phrase "reasonable and necessary" as a synonym of medical necessity. To be eligible for Medicare reimbursement, a covered item or service must be reasonable and necessary for the treatment of an illness or injury or to improve the functioning of a malformed body member. Medicare guidance further describes the concept of "reasonableness": although an item may be medically necessary, it may not be reimbursed by Medicare if (1) the cost of the item is disproportionate to the therapeutic benefits derived from its use, (2) the item is more expensive than an appropriate alternative, or (3) the item serves the same purpose as equipment already available to the beneficiary.

Like most insurance policies, Medicare excludes many items for coverage, including hearing aids and eyeglasses. Other exclusions apply to items or services deemed related to "convenience," "personal comfort," or "custodial care." Because these terms are subjective and the general acceptance of certain medical procedures changes over time, Medicare has established procedures for re-examining these conclusions. In 2001, for example, Medicare replaced guidance that called augmentative communication devices "convenience items" with new guidance that recognizes them as covered items of durable medical equipment. Medicare has since become the single largest payer of "speech-generating devices," a term Medicare staff coined, among all funding programs. (See discussion of history of Medicare policy reform for speech-generating devices at *www.aacfundinghelp.com.*)

■ ASSISTIVE TECHNOLOGY INDUSTRY TODAY

Now that assistive technology has been defined and historical and legislative factors affecting the delivery of assistive technology have been reviewed, the structure of the assistive technology industry can be described. Figure 1-2 depicts the components of the assistive technology industry and how they are interrelated. It is important to be aware of the function of each component, its contribution to the industry and the necessary interaction among these components.

Consumer and Direct Consumer Services

Without a consumer who uses the assistive technology devices and services, all the components in Figure 1-2 are unnecessary. Likewise, without a delivery system that actually provides the technology to the consumer, the supporting components in Figure 1-2 are ineffective. For this reason, the consumer and direct consumer services are shown at the center of the figure. However, it is important to note that the consumer may be involved in all aspects of the industry.

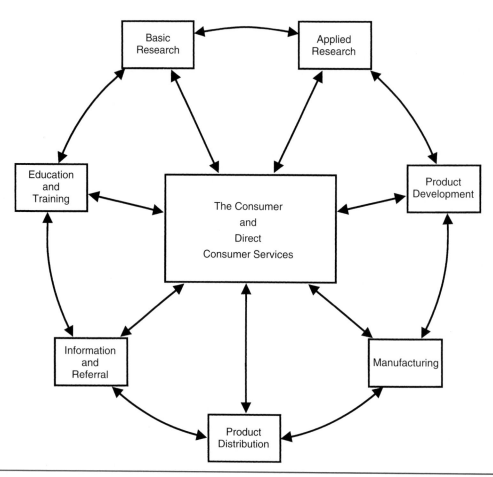

Figure 1-2   The assistive technology industry. The components center around the delivery of devices and services to consumers through direct services. The other industry components are arranged to illustrate their relationships to each other. (Modified from Smith RO: Models of service delivery in rehabilitation technology. In Perlman LG, Enders A, editors: *Rehabilitation service delivery: a practical guide,* Washington, DC, 1987, RESNA.)

Direct consumer services is the component in which a consumer's need for assistive technology is identified, an evaluation is completed, recommendations are made, and the system is implemented. The steps in providing these services are described in Chapter 4.

The Consumer.   The **consumer of assistive technologies** is viewed primarily as the recipient, or end user, of assistive technology. With this in mind, the industry components should be responsive to the consumer, his or her needs, and recommendations based on utilization of assistive technology services and products. As assistive technology systems are applied in the "real world," information from the consumer (and direct service providers) flows out to the other components so that changes in products and services can be made. Likewise, the other components interact among themselves and ultimately affect the consumer and the direct consumer service providers through research, new product development, and dissemination of information.

The consumer should not, however, be viewed solely as the recipient of the technology. The consumer must be considered an active participant in the other industry components as well if the application of assistive technologies is to be effective and the industry is to grow. A number of sources recognize the many roles of the consumer in the assistive technology industry. Corthell (1986) used the term *consumer as codeveloper* to describe a philosophy where the consumer is involved in all aspects of the assistive technology industry. The National Institute on Disability and Rehabilitation Research (NIDRR) furthers this concept by stressing the importance of *participatory research* in assistive technology. As Graves (1993) points out, it is people with disabilities, their families, and the professionals serving them who are the customers of NIDRR. It is imperative that the research activities be responsive to the needs of these individuals. Therefore projects funded by NIDRR must be participatory in nature and involve individuals who will benefit from the research (e.g., persons with disabilities) in all phases of the project, which includes involvement in designing and conducting, as well as disseminating, the research.

Consumers can also be effective in training others in how to use a particular device and in assistive technology education. For example, the Empowering End Users through Assistive Technology (EUSTAT) project in Europe has developed guidelines for trainers, a set of critical factors for assistive technology training and descriptive information on programs that provide assistive technology training for consumers *(http://portale.siva.it/bancadati/biblioteca/SchedaBiblioteca.asp?IDBiblioteca=1)*. One of the documents developed by EUSTAT is written for consumers of assistive technology services and gives practical guidance regarding how to access these services. Keep in mind, as you read about each component of the assistive technology industry, that there are many ways in which consumers can be and are involved.

Characteristics of Direct Consumer Service Programs. Assistive technology systems and services are delivered to the consumer through a variety of models and in different types of settings. There are several attributes that set direct consumer service programs apart from one another. The primary distinguishing factor, and the one most commonly used, is the type of administrative setting in which the service delivery program exists (Smith, 1987). On the basis of Smith's classification, Box 1-4 describes models of service delivery programs according to their administrative settings.

Smith (1987) also identifies several distinguishing features of service delivery programs. The *purpose and mission* may differ among service delivery programs. The purpose of some programs may be only to provide one-time evaluations, whereas other programs may provide comprehensive

---

BOX 1-4   Direct Consumer Service Delivery Settings

REHABILITATION SETTING
- Assistive technology services are part of a comprehensive rehabilitation program; may be a part of one of the therapy departments or its own department.
- The primary purpose is to support the other services of the rehabilitation setting; therefore there is usually multidisciplinary team involvement.
- Typical populations served are persons with spinal cord injuries, head injuries, cerebral vascular accidents, and amputations.
- Services are usually billed to third-party health insurance payers.

UNIVERSITY BASED
- Programs in this setting have largely evolved from a research component and may provide direct consumer services as well as education and training.
- Staff usually consists of personnel capable of performing clinical, research, and educational duties. The types of professionals involved in the team depend on the functional areas addressed by the setting.
- Those settings conducting research provide a national service. The direct consumer service component is usually regionally oriented.
- Funding is largely grant and contract related (particularly for the research component), although portions of the direct consumer services may be billed to third-party payers.

STATE AGENCY PROGRAM BASED
- State agency–based programs are usually a part of vocational rehabilitation departments or special education departments.
- Those programs based in vocational rehabilitation departments are statewide programs developed for the purpose of providing assistive technology services to individuals who need it for attaining or sustaining employment.
- The purpose of programs within special education departments is to facilitate the education of school-aged children. In some instances, school districts have their own

multidisciplinary team. In other cases there may be a team that covers the entire state.
- Administration of these programs varies and may be statewide or on a local level.
- Funding is usually mandated at the state or federal level and designated for these agencies.

PRIVATE PRACTICE
- A small number of assistive technology providers have gone into private practice. They may provide consultation to state agencies or rehabilitation centers.
- The population and functional service area varies and depends on the professional backgrounds of those involved in the business.
- Operated as a for-profit, small-business venture with fees for service charged. Usually based in one local area.

DURABLE MEDICAL EQUIPMENT SUPPLIER
- Usually these suppliers are for-profit agencies that address a range of equipment needs. Typically they provide walking aids, bathing and toileting aids, wheelchairs, and seating systems. Some suppliers may provide communication and environmental control equipment.
- These suppliers are reimbursed by third-party payers.
- These suppliers are known for their technical resources and ability to provide repair and maintenance services.
- There are some durable medical equipment suppliers that operate on a nationwide basis; others are local operations.

VETERANS ADMINISTRATION
- Assistive technology services are provided at many of the Veterans Administration hospitals. There is usually a multidisciplinary team approach.
- Research in the field of assistive technology is a large component of the services provided by the Veterans Administration, and significant contributions have been made in this area.
- The population served is restricted to veterans with service-related disabilities. Veterans with spinal cord injury have been a major group served by the Veterans Administration.

Continued

BOX 1-4 Direct Consumer Service Delivery Settings—cont'd

LOCAL AFFILIATE OF A NATIONAL NONPROFIT DISABILITY ORGANIZATION

- National organizations such as the United Cerebral Palsy Association, Easter Seal Society, Muscular Dystrophy Association, Association for Retarded Citizens, and American Foundation for the Blind provide assistive technology services through their local affiliates.
- The purpose of these organizations is often to serve individuals with a particular disability; therefore the populations served and the functional areas are geared primarily toward that disability group.
- Programs of the local chapters are usually administered at the local level, and assistive technology services vary among affiliates. Some local chapters may have a complete assistive technology team to provide services, whereas other chapters may only loan equipment.

- Funding for these agencies is through grants, contracts, donations, and fundraising events.

VOLUNTEER PROGRAMS

- Volunteer organizations in the United States that provide assistive technology services include groups such as the Telephone Pioneers of America, the Volunteers for Medical Engineering, and Rehabilitation Volunteer Network.
- Most of these groups have developed out of private industry and have as their purpose the provision of a philanthropic service.
- These groups usually provide services on a local or regional basis.
- The functional areas served depend on the expertise of the volunteers involved.

Data from Hobson DA, Shaw CG: Program development and implementation. In *Rehabilitation technology service delivery: a practical guide,* Washington, DC, 1987, RESNA Press; and Smith RO: Models of service delivery in rehabilitation technology. In *Rehabilitation technology service delivery: a practical guide,* Washington, DC, 1987, RESNA Press.

---

assistive technology services. The *functional areas,* or types of services, provided by assistive technology service delivery programs are other variables. Augmentative communication, seating and mobility, orthotics and prosthetics, sensory aids, computer access, robotics, and driving are some of the functional areas in which services are rendered. One program is unlikely to provide services in all these areas. Programs usually focus on a few of these functional areas.

The *type of population* served by an assistive technology program may be another distinguishing feature. For example, the United Cerebral Palsy Association (UCPA) supports a number of programs involving assistive technology that serve children and adults with cerebral palsy. The requirement for a military service–connected disability distinguishes the population served by the Department of Veterans Affairs. Service delivery programs also differ depending on the *geographical area* that they serve. Some programs are community based in that they are set up strictly to serve individuals in the community. Other programs provide specialized evaluation services to a large geographical region. On a larger scale, there are also providers such as national equipment distributors that have offices throughout the nation. Whether the program is in a rural or an urban area is another geographical factor reflected in the types of services provided. For example, programs in rural service delivery areas need to be able to provide services to farmers who have work-related injuries and require adaptation of their farm machinery to continue their livelihood.

To serve consumers who do not live in urban areas, some assistive technology service delivery occurs through

telerehabilitation programs. *Telerehabilitation* refers to the use of telecommunications technologies to capture and transmit visual and audio information, biomedical data (e.g., electroencephalograms, x-ray films, ultrasound data), and consumer information (Kim, 1999). In assistive technology service delivery, telerehabilitation is used for preassessment screening, postassessment training in device use, and the provision of follow-up services. Transmission of telerehabilitation data may be through computer interfaces over the Internet, through telephone lines, or by satellite. For home use there are small units that resemble fax machines (Kim, 1999). These portable units allow follow-up in a consumer's home. Scheck (1998) describes several examples of the use of telerehabilitation for assistive technology service delivery, one of which is for training in augmentative and alternative communication (AAC) (see Chapter 11). In this application the speech-language pathologist uses a small "document camera" (typically used for projecting images onto a screen or photographing them for transmission) to visualize the symbol display on the AAC device. Another camera focuses on the consumer, and a microphone picks up the synthesized speech produced by his AAC device. The speech-language pathologist can provide both instruction and evaluation from his or her office while the consumer remains at home.

Burns et al (1998) describe four case studies that illustrate the application of telerehabilitation to support the use of assistive technologies in the home. The four cases are (1) seating evaluation (see Chapter 6), (2) setup of a computer access system (see Chapter 7), (3) home accessibility evaluation (see Chapter 4), and (4) training in the use of an augmentative communication system (see Chapter 11).

As Burns et al point out, telerehabilitation can overcome some of the difficulties faced by individuals who live at a distance from centers that provide assistive technology services. Low-cost video telephone technology was used in these studies. This technology, which has some limitations for studies involving full motion, was chosen because it depends only on standard telephone lines for implementation. For cases in which a family did not have a phone, cellular telephone transmission was used. Each of the cases described by Burns et al was initiated by the delivery of the telerehabilitation technology to the client's home (often by mail). The family was then instructed in the use of the equipment (by telephone from the rehabilitation center), and the consultation was conducted remotely. The results that they obtained, although preliminary, are encouraging, and they provide useful information regarding the pros and cons of distance consultation through the use of telerehabilitation technology.

The *internal operations* of a service delivery program are another characterization. These include the structure of the organization (from large corporation to small, privately owned company), the number and type of professionals employed to provide the services, and whether the consumer must come to the center for services or a van or mobile unit goes to see them.

The final descriptor of service delivery programs is how the services are funded. Some assistive technology service delivery programs are funded under the general overhead of a larger organization, such as programs based within a rehabilitation hospital. Some programs are supported by grant funding, whereas others rely on a fee for service charged to third-party payers. Sources of third-party funding and mechanisms for obtaining funding for individual consumer services and equipment are discussed in detail in Chapter 5.

Basic Research

The major goal of basic research is the generation of new knowledge. Research hypotheses are posed that address fundamental questions regarding physical or biological phenomena. There are basic research questions that underlie the successful application of assistive technologies. For example, basic neuroscience studies that help to describe movement patterns in persons with disabilities provide the fundamental basis on which new control interfaces can be designed (see Chapter 7).

The single most distinguishing feature of basic research in assistive technologies is that the outcomes are not known beforehand, although hypotheses are proposed. Basic research into the effect of disability on functional performance has implications to the design of assistive technology. Throughout this text basic research studies that underlie the successful development and application of assistive technologies are described.

Applied Research

The distinction between basic and applied research is not precise, and there is some overlap. However, in the area of assistive technology application the distinction between these two types of research is clearer than in the general case. There are many types of applied research studies in assistive technology. They can be grouped as follows: (1) testing of assistive devices under various operating conditions to answer a performance question; (2) development of new assistive devices on the basis of clinical need, basic research findings, or both; (3) research on the use of assistive technologies by persons with disabilities; and (4) research studies designed to develop new assessment or training approaches or materials.

An example of the testing of devices is the use of performance standards to test wheelchairs or other devices (e.g., Cooper, Boninger, and Rentschler, 1999). In some cases, such as wheelchairs, there are accepted standards against which devices are tested (see Chapter 12). In other cases, such as augmentative communication systems (Chapter 11), there is no generally accepted standard, but a device or series of devices can be evaluated against operational characteristics developed specifically for the research study (Dahlquist et al, 1981). Another example of an applied or clinical research study related to assistive technology use is the study of the effects of adaptive seating on eating and drinking of disabled children (Hulme et al, 1987). The purpose of this study, and of studies like it, was to determine whether positioning had any effect on the oral-motor functions of children with multiple handicaps. The results also advance the state of the art in adaptive seating systems (see Chapter 6) by providing insight into what these systems must do to facilitate positioning for functional activities.

The development of new devices may occur in a university or other research laboratory setting or in industry. In either case the objective is to design and build at least one copy of a device that will perform a specific function. In general, engineers (electrical or electronic, mechanical, or industrial) create the design and technicians carry out fabrication of the devices. The initial new device that is produced is referred to as a **prototype.** Consumers are involved in the design process and in trial testing the prototype.

Applied research studies that focus on the use of assistive technologies are abundant. Often these studies involve assistive technologies that rely on user strategies for success. For example, augmentative communication systems used for conversation use many different types of symbol systems. An applied research study might have a goal of comparing the effectiveness of these different symbol systems in facilitating conversation (see, for example, Burroughs et al, 1990). Another example is the use of computer adaptations that replace the keyboard with devices that recognize spoken words, known as automatic speech recognition (ASR). There are several different ways of accomplishing this same function, and applied research studies are carried out to compare them (Snell and Atkinson, 1987). A related example is the study of the effects of ASR on the vocal system (Kambeyana, Singer, and Cronk, 1997). Because ASR systems require abnormal speech patterns for recognition, there is concern that vocal fold damage may result from their use. Studies to determine the actual effects of prolonged usage of ASR systems contribute to both our knowledge of ASR use and to basic speech science.

Finally, some applied research has been carried out to improve the process of assessment, recommendation, and implementation for assistive technologies. Because the assistive technology field is so diverse, individuals from a variety of disciplines may conduct these studies. For example, Lee and Thomas (1990) conducted extensive research on the assessment of individuals for control interfaces suitable for accessing computers and other assistive devices. Their research resulted in an assessment protocol, a set of data collection forms, and a series of case studies usable by others. In another study, Cook and Coleman (1987) developed an assessment protocol for augmentative communication that included a hierarchy for relating the skills and needs of a person with a disability to the characteristics of devices. The research carried out to develop this hierarchy involved assessment and analysis of results from 40 children with disabilities. In both these studies the emphasis was on better application of assistive technologies as a result of improvements in the assessment process.

Product Development

Product development involves the engineering and industrial design that must be applied to a prototype device to convert it to a version that can be fabricated in small quantities and tested with potential users. Testing of this "production prototype" is commonly referred to as **alpha testing** and is normally conducted in-house by manufacturers. Once the device appears to be functioning properly, several (as few as five or as many as 100) additional replicas are fabricated. There are several goals to be achieved by this procedure. First, by making more than one copy of the same device, the manufacturer can determine what potential problems may develop during the manufacturing phase (see the next section). Second, several individuals simultaneously can engage in more extensive evaluation of this set of prototypes. This phase of evaluation is often referred to as **beta testing.** Often manufacturers of assistive devices carry out beta testing with clinicians, consumers, and others who can give the preproduction prototypes a thorough evaluation. This accomplishes several things: (1) identification of as many potential product failures as possible, (2) evaluation of product documentation (e.g., user's manual) to ensure that it is clear and useful, and (3) evaluation of the product with a variety of consumers with disabilities to identify the target population as accurately as possible.

The latter is important because new products may be developed because one individual with a disability has an unmet need, and it is not known how widely applicable the device will be. This situation is relatively unique to assistive technologies and is one of the reasons that new product development is slower in this industry than in others, such as consumer electronics.

Manufacturing

Manufacturing is the process by which a working prototype can be converted into a device that is then mass produced. Although, in the case of assistive technologies, "mass production" may mean production runs of only a few hundred units or less, this process is still quite different from producing a few beta-test prototype devices that function correctly. It is at this stage that production techniques become important. There are many fabrication techniques that are suitable for use only when many copies of an item are made. Several of these are based on the fabrication of a mold from which parts are formed. This technique can be used for polymer (plastic), metal, and ceramic materials. The cost of making the mold can often be very high ($50,000 to $200,000 or more) if the part is complex. However, once the mold is made, the individual copies of the item are quite inexpensive (from a few cents to a few dollars). This process is not feasible unless there are large numbers of parts manufactured; the cost of the mold is then amortized over the total number of parts produced. In assistive technologies this process is most often used for low-tech products such as reachers and eating utensils. Certain parts of some high-tech devices, such as wheelchair casters or the cases for augmentative communication devices, are also molded. Because the mold is a one-time cost, the size of the production run determines the cost of each part. The more pieces that are produced, the lower the cost per item. Because the cost of the molds is often very high, changes in design can also be expensive and may not be made until the original cost of the first model is recovered.

When manufacturing parts from molds, the major cost is in the production equipment; labor costs are relatively low. Other types of manufacturing are much more labor intensive. At one extreme are fabrication methods that rely exclusively on hand assembly. For example, most augmentative communication devices are fabricated one at a time by hand. There are no economies of scale in this type of process. Each device requires a certain amount of time to assemble, and the only savings in manufacturing cost are derived from the increased skill and speed of the individual worker doing the assembly. Thus production labor costs are a significant part of the cost of a manufactured item.

Both parts (materials) costs and labor costs are components of any manufacturing process. Savings in materials costs can be made by producing more units, even if they are hand assembled, because many suppliers give volume discounts for a larger order of the same part. In some assistive technologies, production runs are substantially below a level that generates a discount; for others they are much higher.

At the other extreme from hand assembly is a totally automated production process in which all fabrication and assembly are performed by dedicated machines. This ideal situation does not really exist because some human intervention in the process is necessary for all manufacturing. However, many commercial products are produced by use of a great deal of automated manufacturing. Because the automated production machines do not require a salary, the cost per item is reduced as more copies are made, that is, as the production runs get larger. The production runs necessary for true production automation are approximately 100,000 and higher, which rarely occurs in the production of assistive technology devices.

The assistive technology market is broad. The range of disabilities and the effects of those disabilities are extremely large, which result in a diversity of needs that can be served by assistive devices. Unfortunately, the number of people who have exactly the same need, and for whom the same device will meet the need, is small. This leads to small volumes of production and increased costs per device. It also has the effect of making a device seem more expensive because it is less complex but costs the same as a consumer device that is more flexible.

Many of the commercial general-use devices that are used as assistive technologies are produced by these automated manufacturing techniques. For example, personal computers often have production runs of 100,000 or greater. Thus the cost per unit for a system of this type is lower than for a device specifically designed and built for use by persons with disabilities.

Several conclusions can be drawn from this discussion. The volume in which devices are produced is directly related to their cost. This idea is reflected in two ways in assistive technologies. First, there is the direct relationship between cost and volume of production, which is why certain low-tech devices such as mouth sticks may cost in the hundreds of dollars and a high-tech electronic calculator costs less than $20. Second, the difference between devices produced in large volumes and those produced in smaller volumes is sometimes reflected in overall sophistication and capability rather than directly in price. For example, a personal computer that is capable of performing a wide variety of tasks and that uses sophisticated and complex components is often comparable in price to a much less sophisticated but more specialized assistive device. Thus more function for the price is often gained when a device is produced in larger quantities.

Distribution of Hard Technologies

Manufacturing a device is not worthwhile if consumers and service providers are not aware of its existence. Therefore marketing is an important part of the assistive technology distribution process. In contrast to consumer products, assistive technologies must be marketed and distributed to a highly specialized audience of providers (therapists, engineers, vocational rehabilitation counselors) and consumers. Marketing of assistive technologies involves significant costs, which must be recovered from the selling price of the device.

Distribution of manufactured assistive technologies can occur in several different ways. The major distribution options are (1) mail order, (2) direct sales by company representatives, and (3) distribution through a dealer or supplier. The choice of one or more of these is highly dependent on the type of product. For wheelchairs, seating and positioning systems, aids to daily living, and home care products, most distribution is through **assistive technology suppliers.** Most of these suppliers do not handle communication, environmental control, or computer access technologies.

For many low-tech devices, computer software, and some computer hardware, distribution is by mail order or via the Internet. This system is an advantage in areas where there are no suppliers providing the needed equipment. It is most effective for products for which there is no fitting or need for a prepurchase trial by the consumer. In some cases an evaluation center has devices to try, which can eliminate some limitations. Mail-order or Internet distribution can have significant costs for preparation and distribution of catalogs, for Web-based materials and brochures, and for processing orders. Another limitation to this approach is that maintenance and repair is harder to obtain for high-tech devices, such as computer systems, purchased this way.

Relatively few assistive technology products are distributed through direct company-employed representatives. Some exceptions are augmentative communication systems and aids for persons with visual impairments. Some of these have direct sales staffs, whereas others use dealers who carry several related products. In either case, this distribution network is not adequate to cover all geographical areas equally, and mail-order or Internet sales typically supplement the direct representative network. Electronic products such as augmentative communication systems, environmental control units, and feeders are often outside the range of capabilities of the standard rehabilitation equipment supplier. This situation has led to the development of more direct sales in these product areas.

Information and Referral

The ability to readily obtain current information on assistive technology services and products is essential for both service provider and consumers. The Internet has a large amount of information available in many areas, including assistive technologies. This is the good news; the bad news is that much of this information is not validated by an independent source, so both the quality and accuracy of the information accessed must be carefully evaluated. The Resources section found at the end of this book contains a list of Web sites that is intended to provide some initial information; it is not meant to be all inclusive.

ABLEDATA is the largest and most well known general source of information on products for individuals with disabilities. It contains more than 32,000 listings of devices (of which 21,000 are currently available). The ABLEDATA database also contains information on noncommercial prototypes; customized, one-of-a-kind products; and do-it-yourself designs. The scope of ABLEDATA listings is broad, encompassing sensory and motor aids, low- and high-tech devices, and applications from home care to employment. The ABLEDATA database classifies each assistive technology product by its intended function or any special features it possesses. The products are classified into the 19 areas shown in Table 1-4. Clicking on any of these topics provides a link to the major categories within that topic and then a link to specific product types in each category. Key word or phrase searching is also available. It is possible to search the ABLEDATA Web site in one of four ways: (1) by keyword or phrase, (2) by brand name of an assistive device, (3) by name of manufacturer or distributor, and (4) by Boolean search (specifying multiple features to be included in the search). If Internet access is not available, an ABLEDATA search can be requested from their information specialists by phone, fax, or mail.

ABLEDATA also publishes Informed Consumer Guides that include information on product selection and purchase of a particular type of device. References to product write-ups, standards, or comparative studies on that product class, linkages to other resources and reference materials, and reports on specific products submitted by consumers are also included. Fact sheets and Informed Consumer Guides can be viewed and downloaded from the ABLEDATA Web site. The Assistive Technology Directory lists companies with products included in the database.

Written publications such as conference proceedings, periodicals, directories, and catalogs are another way to find information on assistive technology services and products. Most manufacturers have catalogs, and it is easy to be placed on their mailing lists so that you receive updated information. In addition to their catalogs, manufacturers may also publish regular newsletters of product updates and applications, and many also have their own Web sites that are updated frequently and provide instant information regarding their products. In some cases it is possible to purchase the product directly through the company Web sites. Many of the centers that provide services in assistive technology publish newsletters and maintain Web sites as well.

Electronic listservs are formed by individuals with common interests. Each user accesses the information from his or her own e-mail system, and all messages are available to all members of the list. There are many listservs that address various areas of assistive technology applications. Some are maintained by professional associations (e.g., RESNA, American Occupational Therapy Association, American

Speech-Language Hearing Association, American Physical Therapy Association), whereas others are established and maintained by rehabilitation centers or universities. There are also user- or consumer-oriented listservs, which address either specific issues (e.g., one particular disability) or general issues. These listservs are often useful places to gain information regarding specific assistive technology questions. Four of the most useful U.S.-based conferences (all annual) are the International Conference on Technology and Disability (California State University at Northridge) Conference (held in March in Los Angeles, *www.csun.edu/cod/conf/index.html*), Closing the Gap (held in October in Minneapolis, *www.closingthegap.com*), Assistive Technology Industry Association (January, Orlando, Florida, *www.atia.org*), and RESNA (June, various locations, *www.resna.org*). International conferences include the Australian Rehabilitation and Assistive Technology Association (even years) (*http://www.e-bility.com/arata/sitemap.php*), the Association for the Advancement of Assistive Technology in Europe (odd years) (*http://www.aaate.net/*), and the Japanese conference on the advancement of Assistive and Rehabilitative Technology (odd years) sponsored by the Rehabilitation Engineering society of Japan (*http://www.resja.gr.jp/eng/*). There are also specialty conferences in specific areas of assistive technology such as the International Association for Augmentative and Alternative communication (even years) (*http://www.isaac-online.org/*) and the International Seating Symposium (annual) (*http://www.iss.pitt.edu/*).

Education

As previously stated, the growth of the assistive technology industry has meant an increased availability of devices and services for individuals with disabilities. However, it is necessary that competent professionals be involved in the delivery of these devices and services. It is also necessary that these professionals come from a variety of clinical and technical backgrounds. Many individuals practicing in the area of assistive technologies received their information on the job or through in-service training such as conferences or workshops. Formal training courses or programs as part of undergraduate or graduate educational programs have developed over the past 15 to 20 years.

For professionals currently in practice, *in-service* educational activities in assistive technologies that supplement the individual's professional training and experience are available. Typically this type of educational activity is very focused and of short duration. In-service programs have been the major type of formal educational activity for professionals applying these technologies. The variety of in-service opportunities in assistive technology applications is extremely large, and it is growing yearly. Some workshops are offered by industry, and they focus on a specific product or product line. Other workshops or seminars are offered by rehabilitation centers or universities. These workshops may include one area of application (e.g., seating and positioning or augmentative communication), or they may be broader. Often workshops are offered in conjunction with major conferences of professional associations, which can be a convenient way for conference participants to obtain in-service education in a cost-effective manner.

A major source of in-service education is conferences that focus on assistive technologies. These conferences provide a wealth of opportunities for education (see Enders and Hall, 1990). Many are regional, which makes them more financially accessible than the national meetings. Another source of continuing education is professional journals. Some professions have journals that occasionally publish

---

TABLE 1-4   **ABLEDATA Topics and Categories**

Topics	Major Categories
Aids for Daily Living (products to aid in activities of daily living)	Bathing, Carrying, Child Care, Clothing, Dispenser Aids, Dressing, Drinking, Feeding, Grooming/Hygiene, Handle Padding, Health Care, Holding, Reaching, Smoking, Toileting, Transfer
Blind and Low Vision (products for people with visual disabilities)	Computers, Educational Aids, Health Care, Information Storage, Kitchen Aids, Labeling, Magnification, Office Equipment, Orientation and Mobility, Reading, Recreation, Sensors, Telephones, Time, Tools, Travel, Typing, Writing (Braille)
Communication (products to help people with disabilities related to speech, writing, and other methods of communication)	Alternative and Augmentative Communication, Headwands, Mouthsticks, Signal Systems, Telephones, Typing, Writing
Computers (products to allow people with disabilities to use desktop and laptop computers and other kinds of information technology)	Software, Hardware, Computer Accessories
Controls (products that provide people with disabilities with the ability to start, stop, or adjust electric or electronic devices)	Environmental Controls, Control Switches
Deaf And Hard of Hearing (products for people with hearing disabilities)	Amplification, Driving, Hearing Aids, Recreational Electronics, Signal Switches, Speech Training, Telephones, Time
Deaf Blind (products for people who are both deaf and blind)	[no categories listed]
Education (products to provide people with disabilities with access to educational materials and instruction in school and in other learning environments)	Classroom, Instructional Materials
Environmental Adaptations (products that make the built environment more accessible)	Indoors, Outdoors, Vertical Lift, Houses, Specialties, Lighting, Signs
Home Management (products that assist in cooking, cleaning, and other household activities and adapted furniture and appliances)	Food Preparation, Housekeeping, Furniture
Orthotics (braces and other products to support or supplement joints or limbs)	Head and Neck, Lower Extremity, Torso, Upper Extremity
Prosthetics (products for amputees)	Lower Extremity, Upper Extremity
Recreation (products to assist people with disabilities with leisure and athletic activities)	Crafts, Electronics, Gardening, Music, Photography, Sewing, Sports, Toys
Safety and Security (products to protect health and home)	Alarm and Security Systems, Child Proof Devices, Electric Cords, Lights, Locks
Seating (products that assist people to sit comfortably and safely)	Seating Systems, Cushions, Therapeutic Seats
Therapeutic Aids (products that assist in treatment for health problems and therapy and training for certain disabilities)	Ambulation Training, Biofeedback, Evaluation, Exercise, Fine and Gross Motor Skills, Perceptual Motor, Positioning, Pressure/Massage Modality Equipment, Respiratory Aids, Rolls, Sensory Integration, Stimulators, Therapy Furnishings, Thermal/Water Modality Equipment, Traction
Transportation (products to enable people with disabilities to drive or ride in cars, vans, trucks and buses)	Mass Transit Vehicles and Facilities, Vehicles, Vehicle Accessories
Walking (products to aid people with disabilities who are able to walk or stand with assistance)	Canes, Crutches, Standing, Walkers
Wheeled Mobility (products and accessories that enable people with mobility disabilities to move freely indoors and outdoors)	Wheelchairs (Manual, Sport, and Powered), Wheelchair Alternatives (Scooters), Wheelchair Accessories, Carts, Transporters, Stretchers
Workplace (products to aid people with disabilities at work)	Agricultural Equipment, Office Equipment, Tools, Vocational Assessment, Vocational Training, Work Stations

articles on assistive technology; other journals are solely dedicated to assistive technology (see Resources). With the growth of the Internet, there is an increasing number of assistive technology courses and educational programs offered at a distance (including on-line and teleconference formats). These often involve multiple institutions (both rehabilitation centers and universities) and international linkages.

Preservice educational activities are part of professional preparation at the undergraduate or graduate level for practice in specific disciplines such as occupational therapy, physical therapy, recreation therapy, rehabilitation engineering, special education, speech-language pathology, and vocational rehabilitation counseling. In recent years the number of programs that offer instruction in assistive technology topics has increased, particularly in occupational therapy, rehabilitation engineering, and speech-language pathology (focusing on augmentative and alternative communication) programs. The scope of assistive technology instruction in preservice educational programs varies widely. There may be an assistive technology specialization within a rehabilitation discipline (e.g., OT, PT, or SLP), required or elective courses or subjects in assistive technology, assistive technology material included within a broader course, or, at the graduate level, assistive technology projects or theses. The most common programs are those that include some assistive technology material in other courses; the least common are those specializing solely in assistive technology. With the increasing role of technology in the lives of individuals with disabilities, it is crucial that newly trained professionals entering their respective fields have some level of formal training in assistive technology applications.

In rehabilitation engineering, the entry-level degree for professional practice is the master's degree. There are few universities that offer degrees in rehabilitation engineering at this level. More often, it is a subspecialization within another engineering discipline (e.g., biomedical engineering). In some cases a certificate of completion is presented to the student in addition to the master's degree in his or her field of specialization.

Rowley, Mitchell, and Weber (1997) described their experience over 6 years with one model master's level program in rehabilitation engineering. This program's curriculum has four areas of emphasis for student acquisition of knowledge and skills: (1) disability and technology, (2) major rehabilitation systems, (3) applied skills, and (4) life-long learning.

The major influence of preservice educational programs is that more individuals than ever before are entering practice in their professional field with knowledge of assistive technologies and their application. This development will have a major positive influence on the effectiveness of these technologies, the development of new and innovative devices, and the impact that these systems have on the lives of persons with disabilities.

■ PROFESSIONAL PRACTICE IN ASSISTIVE TECHNOLOGY

This section describes the person who provides assistive technology and the issues surrounding his or her professional practice. Three broad issues are discussed in this section: (1) ethics of practice, (2) quality assurance, and (3) liability. Each of these has implications both for the individual practitioner and for organizations involved in the assistive technology industry. We begin with a description of the person providing assistive technology services and devices.

Providers of Assistive Technology Services

The **assistive technology practitioner** (ATP) typically has a professional background in one of several areas, including engineering, occupational therapy, physical therapy, recreation therapy, special education, speech pathology, or vocational rehabilitation counseling. Each professional has a contribution to make to the industry based on his or her unique background. Therefore ATPs should be well grounded in their disciplines. It is equally important for each ATP to have knowledge and skills in assistive technology and familiarity with the scope of the assistive technology industry. RESNA has developed an assistive technology certification program to address this issue; it is discussed further in a later section.

Any of these professionals may be involved in any of the components of the assistive technology industry. For example, occupational or physical therapists with expertise in the area of seating may be found providing direct consumer services, consulting with manufacturers on the use and function of wheelchairs and seating systems, educating others on the prescription of seating systems, or working in research on the effect of certain body positions on functional activities. Likewise, speech pathologists may be involved in augmentative communication as a member of an evaluation team, may function as a representative for a manufacturer's particular products, or may conduct research on interactions among users of communication devices. These are just some examples of the ways in which ATPs can be involved. A similar variety of roles in the assistive technology industry are available to ATPs from other disciplines.

Having described the ATP's position in the industry as a whole, let us now look at his or her role in direct service delivery. ATPs are involved in the needs assessment, evaluation, implementation, training, and follow-up of assistive technology services in various functional areas. Examples of these areas are augmentative communication, seating and mobility, orthotics and prosthetics, sensory aids, computer access, robotics, and driving.

Because of the number of factors and the complexity involved in the delivery of assistive technology systems to the consumer, a team approach is desirable. This team may consist of as few as two professionals working together. Each individual team member brings knowledge and skills from his or her area of expertise that can be applied to the assistive technology service delivery process. Although it is tempting to view each functional service area (e.g., augmentative communication, seating, mobility) as being in the domain of one or two specific disciplines, service delivery is most effective when a **transdisciplinary team approach** is used.

In a transdisciplinary team approach, there is crossing over of professional boundaries and sharing of roles and functions. All individual team members must be well grounded in their profession but also feel comfortable enough to extend their role beyond that profession (Pronsanti, 1991). This blurring of roles can be seen, for example, during an augmentative communication assessment performed by a team consisting of a speech pathologist, an occupational therapist, and a rehabilitation engineer. Traditional roles may dictate that the occupational therapist perform an assessment of the consumer's ability to reach and point, the speech pathologist evaluate language skills, and the rehabilitation engineer design the mounting of the device. In contrast, with a transdisciplinary team, all three disciplines contribute to identification of a good control site for the individual or to mounting the device in the most appropriate location. A team discussion may also form the basis for the type of vocabulary to include in the augmentative communication device. As a result of this team collaboration, a more thorough assessment of the individual's needs and skills is likely to occur.

Although some practitioners may feel threatened that the transdisciplinary approach takes away part of their professional identity, Kangas (quoted by Mastrangelo, 1992) points out that her experience has been that this approach improves the assessment process and actually strengthens each person's professional identity through the giving and confirmation of information. This approach also encourages support, creativity, and honesty among the disciplines (Mastrangelo, 1992).

Ethics and Standards of Practice

Ethics is defined as "the study of standards of conduct and moral judgment...and the system or code of morals of a particular...profession" (McKechnie, 1983, p. 627). When applied to a field of professional endeavor such as assistive technology delivery or a profession such as occupational therapy or rehabilitation engineering, the ethical conduct of practitioners is embodied both in a code (or canons) of ethics and in standards of practice. Each ATP must comply with the code of ethics for his or her discipline (e.g., rehabilitation engineering, occupational or physical therapy, speech-language pathology, or vocational rehabilitation counseling). The code of ethics for a discipline is typically developed by the professional association serving it. As discussed, ATPs

have responsibilities in assistive technology service delivery that are not specified by their individual discipline's code of ethics. For this reason, it is important to have a code of ethics that addresses the specific issues related to the application of assistive technologies. Standards of practice differ from codes of ethics in that they describe more specifically what is and is not considered to be good practice in a given discipline.

Code of Ethics for Assistive Technologies: The RESNA Code of Ethics.   RESNA is an interdisciplinary professional association whose activities focus on assistive technologies. Its members come from many disciplines and a variety of settings, and their activities involve the full scope of assistive technology applications. In 1991 the RESNA Board of Directors adopted the code of ethics shown in Figure 1-3. This code is similar to those of other disciplines involved in rehabilitation and is based on several of them. However, it includes issues related to the provision of technology. It is presented as a reminder of the obligations that a practitioner in the assistive technology industry has to his or her consumers, others who work with and care for them, the general public, and the profession as a whole.

Standards of Practice.   Because each assistive technology practitioner belongs to his or her own discipline, it is important that the standards of practice pertaining to that specialty be adhered to. These standards are often the basis for professional certification programs. RESNA has developed the standards of practice shown in Box 1-5 for assistive technology practitioners and suppliers.

Quality Assurance

Quality assurance is a broad area of fundamental importance to the safe and effective application of assistive technologies. It involves two basic considerations: (1) the quality of the services rendered and (2) the quality of the devices supplied (Enders and Hall, 1990). Quality assurance is closely tied to reimbursement, and as the number of devices and practitioners increases, third-party payers are requiring some indication that the services and devices are necessary, safe, and effective. A comprehensive quality assurance program addresses these issues. The quality of services can be measured and evaluated by certification (of individual practitioners) and accreditation (of facilities and programs). The efficacy of devices is measured by adherence to device performance standards and good manufacturing practices. Ultimately, the quality of assistive technology services and devices is determined by measurement of outcomes resulting from both the provision of the services and devices and the use of the technologies to facilitate functional improvement and quality of life for the individual consumer.

RESNA Code Of Ethics

RESNA is an interdisciplinary association for the advancement of rehabilitation and assistive technology. It adheres to and promotes the highest standards of ethical conduct. Its members:

- Hold paramount the welfare of persons served professionally.
- Practice only in their area(s) of competence and maintain high standards.
- Maintain the confidentiality of privileged information.
- Engage in no conduct that constitutes a conflict of interest or that adversely reflects on the profession.
- Seek deserved and reasonable remuneration for services.
- Inform and educate the public on rehabilitation/assistive technology and its application.
- Issue public statements in an objective and truthful manner.
- Comply with the laws and policies that guide the profession.

Figure 1-3   RESNA code of ethics. (Modified from RESNA Ethics Committee: *RESNA code of ethics,* Arlington, VA, 1991, RESNA.)

Overview. Patterson (1989) presented the following overview of quality assurance from the perspective of The Joint Commission (TJC). The consumer, practitioner, and purchaser (of services or devices) each have a unique view of what constitutes quality. The consumer views it from his or her own point of view and, in the case of assistive technologies, judges the quality on how daily activity is improved in the specific areas of application. The practitioner generates measures of performance and then attempts to judge the quality of the services and devices against these measures. The practitioner evaluates both the technologies and the consumer because motivation, amount of effort spent on training, and so on can affect success of any device or service. The purchaser of services or devices asks the most basic of questions: are the services and devices cost-effective? This question also implies the existence of a measurable outcome, and often purchasers require the practitioner to develop such measures before funding is approved.

Patterson cites several reasons why quality assurance programs are necessary. The most important is to ensure that practice is effective and appropriate to the consumer's needs. A good quality assurance program improves practices and outcomes and consumer satisfaction. In addition, quality assurance programs are necessary to ensure accountability to the public and conformance with codes of ethics.

Quality assurance programs are implemented through both internal and external factors. Organizations that provide assistive technology services and equipment must have a philosophical commitment to quality assurance that is reflected in their mission statements, and there must be internal monitoring and evaluation. External monitoring is also important to ensure objectivity in meeting quality assurance goals. External monitoring can be accomplished through standards required by organizations that accredit the facility (such as TJC); certification of individual practitioners; standards developed by third-party reimbursement organizations; and local, state, or federal legal requirements.

Standards for Service Providers. *Professional certification* is a voluntary process in which a professional organization measures and reports the degree of competence of an individual practitioner (Warren, 1991). To establish a certification program, there must be an agreed on body of knowledge unique to the practitioners in the area to be certified. Once the body of knowledge is adequately described, a set of professional competencies must be established and a method for evaluating an individual's knowledge in these competence areas (usually a written examination) must be developed and implemented. As Warren points out, the examination process must be developed in such a way as to reflect how a person performs on the job, and it must reflect knowledge

BOX 1-5 RESNA Standards of Practice for Assistive Technology Practitioners and Suppliers

These Standards of Practice set forth fundamental concepts and rules considered essential to promote the highest ethical standards among individuals who evaluate, assess the need for, recommend, or provide assistive technology. In the discharge of their professional obligations assistive technology practitioners and suppliers shall observe the following principles and rules:

1. Individuals shall keep paramount the welfare of those served professionally.
2. Individuals shall engage in only those services that are within the scope of their competence, considering the level of education, experience and training, and shall recognize the limitations imposed by the extent of their personal skills and knowledge in any professional area.
3. In making determinations as to what areas of practice are within their competency, assistive technology practitioners and suppliers shall observe all applicable licensure laws, consider the qualifications for certification or other credentials offered by recognized authorities in the primary professions which comprise the field of assistive technology, and abide by all relevant standards of practice and ethical principles, including RESNA's Code of Ethics.
4. Individuals shall truthfully, fully and accurately represent their credentials, competency, education, training and experience in both the field of assistive technology and the primary profession in which they are members. To the extent practical, individuals shall disclose their primary profession in all forms of communication, including advertising, which refers to their credential in assistive technology.
5. Individuals shall, at a minimum, inform consumers or their advocates of any employment affiliations, financial or professional interests that may be perceived to bias recommendations, and in some cases, decline to provide services or supplies where the conflict of interest is such that it may fairly be concluded that such affiliation or interest is likely to impair professional judgments.
6. Individuals shall use every resource reasonably available to ensure that the identified needs of consumers are met, including referral to other practitioners or sources which may provide the needed service or supply within the scope of their competence.
7. Individuals shall cooperate with members of other professions, where appropriate, in delivering services to consumers, and shall actively participate in the team process when the consumer's needs require such an approach.
8. Individuals shall offer an appropriate range of assistive technology services that include assessment, evaluation, recommendations, training, adjustments at delivery, and follow-up and modifications after delivery.
9. Individuals shall verify consumer's needs by using direct assessment or evaluation procedures with the consumer.
10. Individuals shall assure that the consumer fully participates, and is fully informed about all reasonable options available, regardless of finances, in the development of recommendations for intervention strategies.
11. Individuals shall consider future and emerging needs when developing intervention strategies and fully inform the consumer of those needs.
12. Individuals shall avoid providing and implementing technology [that exposes] the consumer to unreasonable risk, and shall advise the consumer as fully as possible of all known risks. Where adjustments, instruction for use, or necessary modifications are likely to be required to avoid or minimize such risks, individuals shall make sure that such information or service is provided.
13. Individuals shall fully inform consumers or their advocates about all relevant aspects, including the financial implications, of all final recommendations for the provision of technology, and shall not guarantee the results of any service or technology. Individuals may, however, make reasonable statements about prognosis.
14. Individuals shall maintain adequate records of the technology evaluation, assessment, recommendations, services, or products provided and preserve confidentiality of those records, unless required by law, or unless the protection of the welfare of the person or the community requires otherwise.
15. Individuals shall endeavor, through ongoing professional development, including continuing education, to remain current on all aspects of assistive technology relevant to their practice including accessibility, funding, legal or public issues, recommended practices and emerging technologies.
16. Individuals shall endeavor to institute procedures, on an on-going basis, to evaluate, promote and enhance the quality of service delivered to all consumers.
17. Individuals shall be truthful and accurate in all public statements concerning assistive technology, assistive technology practitioners and suppliers, services, and products dispensed.
18. Individuals shall not invidiously discriminate in the provision of services or supplies on the basis of disability, race, national origin, religion, creed, gender, age, or sexual orientation.
19. Individuals shall not charge for services not rendered, nor misrepresent in any fashion services delivered or products dispensed for reimbursement or any other purpose.
20. Individuals shall not engage in fraud, dishonesty or misrepresentation of any kind, or any form of conduct that adversely reflects on the field of assistive technology, or the individual's fitness to serve consumers professionally.
21. Individuals whose professional services are adversely affected by substance abuse or other health-related conditions shall seek professional advice, and where appropriate, withdraw from the affected area of practice.

From RESNA, 1700 N. Moore Street, Suite 1540, Arlington, VA 22209-1903; phone: (703) 524-6686 (www.resna.org).

actually required for satisfactory job performance. Within the assistive technology field, the challenge of establishing a valid and useful certification program is complicated by the great diversity of disciplines involved. RESNA has developed a certification program in assistive technologies that addresses the special requirements of this field and that builds on other disciplines' certification and licensure, such as registered occupational therapist, registered physical therapist, professional engineer, or certificate of clinical competence–speech pathology. RESNA offers a voluntary credentialing program; on successful passage of an examination, one of two types of credentials is currently awarded. The *assistive technology practitioner certificate* is intended for service providers primarily involved in analysis of a consumer's needs and training in the use of a particular device. The *assistive technology supplier certificate* is intended for service providers involved in the sale and service of commercially available devices. The assistive technology certification focuses on the skills and knowledge required to deliver assistive technologies, assuming that the individual has already established disciplinary competence by certification or licensure. The certification process is further described on the RESNA Web site *(www.resna.org)*.

The National Association of Medical Equipment Suppliers (NAMES), an association of suppliers of rehabilitation and home health care equipment, has established a national registry for rehabilitation technology suppliers. The NAMES National Registry of Rehabilitation Technology Suppliers (NRRTS, *www.nrrts.org*) has a goal of providing a mechanism for consumers, clinicians, and third-party payers to identify qualified suppliers to ensure provision of high-quality rehabilitation technology and related services to people with physical disabilities. NRRTS defines a rehabilitation technology supplier as one who provides enabling technology in the areas of wheeled mobility, seating and alternative positioning, ambulation assistance, environmental control, and activities of daily living. To become a certified rehabilitation supplier, an individual must first join NRRTS. NRRTS membership confirms that a rehabilitation technology supplier has demonstrated work experience, received recommendations from professional associates, adheres to a stringent code of ethics, and commits to participate in continuing education to remain an NRRTS member. NRRTS awards the Certified Rehabilitation Technology Supplier certificate to a NRRTS member in good standing who has successfully completed the RESNA assistive technology supplier credentialing examination.

Although certification programs address the qualifications of individual practitioners, *accreditation* addresses the quality of services provided by facilities. The Rehabilitation Accreditation Commission (CARF) (4891 E. Grant Rd., Tucson, AZ 85712, (520) 325-1044, *www.carf.org*) accredits organizations in the rehabilitation field. This accreditation is based on the results of the organization's service delivery program, which includes hospitals, home care, mental health, long-term care, and ambulatory care. CARF views its activities as a quality improvement mechanism based on an external, impartial peer observation of current service practice. An organization's practices are measured against internationally developed and accepted quality indicators that focus on consumer-driven results, stakeholder satisfaction, and quality improvement. A CARF quality audit for accreditation serves as a framework for quality improvement, with a focus on individual consumers' outcomes and satisfaction. CARF accreditation is widely viewed as a mark of quality achievement. CARF accredits more than 20,000 service programs in the United States and Canada, and this accreditation is accepted or required for rehabilitation organizations in more than 40 states.

CARF includes standards for assistive technologies in both the employment and community services categories of their accreditation program (CARF, 1999). Standards for assistive technology services are included in the "principal standards," which apply to all types of accredited services and in specific types of community and employment services. Principal CARF standards require that each person served must have access to assistive technologies to meet his or her identified needs. If an organization cannot provide the assistive technologies required, referrals must be made to providers who can meet the needs of the persons who are served by the organization. In addition, each person's exit report must contain a description of the assistive technology services provided. CARF also has specific standards for employment assistive technology services and community assistive technology services. These services focus on achievement of employment, community access, inclusion, and independence goals. Assistive technology services may include selection, acquisition, or use of assistive technologies; information, referral, or observation of assistive technology; and exploration of alternative assistive technology strategies. CARF standards also emphasize that the accredited organization should clearly tell people what it can and cannot do to help them regarding access to assistive technologies. In addition, the organization's services should be focused on helping people get and keep a job or on community access, inclusion, and interdependence, as appropriate. Appropriate staff knowledge, training, and experience are also evaluated.

Standards for Devices.   There are several types of standards that can be developed for assistive devices. The manufacture and production of assistive technologies and other medically related equipment are regulated by federal legislation in the United States (PL 94-295). These regulations include specification of good manufacturing practices and classify devices on the basis of the risk of their use.

The Food and Drug Administration (FDA) classifies medical devices in these categories. Class I devices (e.g., wheelchair accessories) are minimal risk. Class II devices require performance standards to be met (e.g., powered wheelchairs, standup wheelchairs, and special grade wheelchairs and motorized three-wheel vehicles). Class III devices require premarket approval (e.g., a stair-climbing wheelchair) (21 C.F.R. 890.3890). The Canadian system for medical devices is almost identical, with the same risk-based classification system, Class I through Class IV.

Two types of submissions may be made to the FDA for medical devices. The premarket approval is the process that the FDA uses to evaluate the safety and efficacy of new products that pose a significant risk to the patient. A 510(k) notification is submitted for a change to an existing device that is already on the market or for a new device that is "substantially equivalent" to a preamendment device. Further information may be obtained from the FDA Web site (*www.fda.gov/cdrh*).

Most assistive technologies are judged to be minimal risk (Class I or Class II), which reduces the restrictions on their development and testing and on their approval for sale by prescription. However, in addition to paperwork and delays, there are costs associated with obtaining approval for a device at any level of risk, and these costs must be recovered from the sale of the product.

Third-party reimbursement may be refused for a device that is not FDA compliant. Repeated violations can result in fines and even jail for manufacturers who continue to market products after being informed that they needed to undergo FDA review; imported devices are often barred at the border by U.S. Customs officials if they are not cleared. Assistive technology providers and suppliers may also be at risk, from a legal perspective, if they use products that are not approved.

Devices can also be rated by development of compatibility and performance standards. *Compatibility standards* are developed to ensure that devices from different manufacturers can be used together. In assistive technologies, compatibility standards exist for control interfaces, computer-emulating interfaces, powered wheelchair controllers, and other devices. For example, control interfaces have connectors on the end of their cables that allow them to be plugged into electronic assistive technologies. For a control interface from one manufacturer to be used with a device from another manufacturer, they must both adhere to a compatibility standard that specifies the type of connector, which pins have which functions, and so on. These standards are voluntary, but it is in the best interest of a manufacturer to adhere to them to maximize the use of its products.

Performance standards are also voluntary. These standards specify how a device should perform and provide a set of tests to be used for comparing similar products from different manufacturers (Enders and Hall, 1990). For example, wheelchair performance standards specify durability, maneuverability, dynamic stability, and energy consumption (Axelson and Phillips, 1989). In some cases, such as wheelchairs, the standards become formalized and adopted by the American National Standards Institute or the International Standards Organization. Approval by one or more of these bodies indicates that the standards have received a careful and thorough review, that they embody reasonable expectations of performance, and that they address issues of safety and efficacy. There are also less formal performance standards, which may be developed by an industry or an agency. The Veterans Administration develops standards for their purchase of medical and assistive devices. Because they purchase large quantities of devices, manufacturers adhere to their standards and these purchase specifications serve as informal performance standards.

Whether standards are informal or formal, compatibility or performance, they have an influence on the success of assistive technology use only to the degree that they are voluntarily adopted by industry. The motivation for this adoption is both economic (e.g., increased sales) and altruistic (e.g., concern for safety and functional improvement). Assistive technology practitioners need to work with industry to ensure that standards are meaningful. They also need to insist that products they recommend have met applicable standards. These activities help to ensure that meaningful product standards are developed and used.

Outcomes of Assistive Technology Delivery.

Assistive technologies create unique challenges in quality assurance. For many therapies, a service is provided in a clinical rehabilitation setting and the success of the outcome is based on measures such as functional improvement, reduced hospitalization, or ability to work at average productivity. It is not possible to apply these measures directly to assistive technology services and devices because the goals of the service are different. In assistive technology service delivery, the selection of a device is based on what a person is able to do now, not what he or she will be able to do on completing a program of therapy. A device that is expected to meet the needs of the person is then recommended, and the individual consumer decides whether to use it. The device is used not in a well-controlled clinical environment, but in the larger context of employment, school, and community. To evaluate the effectiveness of this entire process, the focus should not be on the service or device individually, but on the entire assistive technology system, which includes the user, the technology, the activities being carried out, and the context (environment) in which the system is being used. The determination of the "success" of the service delivery process is based on measurement of outcomes related to the success the consumer achieves using the assistive technology system. *Outcome measures* are objective criteria, usually developed during the assessment and recommendation process, that can be used to judge the effectiveness of both devices and services during the training and follow-up phases of the service delivery process. In Chapter 2 a framework for assistive technologies that provides the basis for outcome measures is developed. In Chapter 4 the development and application of outcome measures for assistive technology services and devices are discussed.

■ SUMMARY

The definitions, history, legislation, industry, and professional issues presented in this chapter provide the foundation for our discussion of assistive technologies and their application. In the remainder of this text, a set of principles, some of which are general and some of which apply to a specific need, are presented. In addition, the practices that underlie successful application are described in detail. Many specific assistive devices are also characterized in succeeding chapters.

Study Questions

1. How are assistive technologies included within the WHO ICF?
2. What is meant by a "low-tech" and a "high-tech" assistive device? Give an example of each.
3. Distinguish between hard and soft technologies.
4. Give three examples of assistive technology appliances and three examples of assistive technology tools.
5. What is the difference between minimal and maximal technology? Give an example of each.
6. Refer to Figure 1-1. Why are standard commercially available products less expensive than special commercially available products? Why are the latter less expensive than modified or custom-designed devices? Give examples of all four classes.
7. Why do we distinguish assistive technologies from rehabilitative and educational technologies? Can one device play a role in both areas?
8. Distinguish between specific purpose and general purpose technologies.
9. What has been the influence of federal legislation on the availability of assistive technology devices and services?
10. List at least four ways in which U.S. federal legislation has affected the practice of assistive technology service delivery.
11. Compare the situation today regarding assistive technologies with that in 1972.
12. What is at the focal point of the industry of assistive technology? What are the other industry components?
13. Pick any one piece of legislation shown in Table 1-2 and describe its influence on the development and application of assistive technologies.
14. Why should the consumer be considered a "codeveloper"?
15. Assistive technology practitioners may have a background in a variety of disciplines. List some typical disciplines.
16. Define the characteristics of direct consumer service settings in assistive technology.
17. Describe how you would carry out an ABLEDATA search if (1) you know the manufacturer, (2) you know the name of the device, and (3) you only know the general name of a device.
18. Describe the benefits of a transdisciplinary team.
19. Why is it necessary to have codes of ethics?
20. How does a code of ethics differ from standards of practice?
21. What are the major elements of a quality assurance program?
22. Describe how certification and accreditation differ. What is the purpose of each?
23. What are the major features of the CARF standards in assistive technology?
24. What is the difference between a performance standard and a compatibility standard?
25. What are the two kinds of liability with which assistive technology practitioners must be concerned?

References

Assistive Technology Act of 1998, as amended, PL 108-364, §3, 118 stat 1707 (2004).

Axelson P, Phillips L: Wheelchair standards: pushing for a new era, *Homecare Magazine* pp 142-147, October 1989.

Bailey RW: *Human performance engineering*, ed 3, Upper Saddle River, NJ, 1996, Prentice Hall.

Burns RB et al: Using telerehabilitation to support assistive technology, *Assist Technol* 10:126-183, 1998.

Burroughs JA et al: A comparative study of language delayed preschool children's ability to recall symbols from two symbol systems, *Augment Altern Comm* 6:202-206, 1990.

CARF: *1999 Employment and community services standards manual*, Tucson, 1999, CARF.

Cook AM, Coleman CL: Selecting augmentative communication systems by matching client skills and needs to system characteristics, *Semin Speech Lang* 8:153-167, 1987.

Cooper RA, Boninger ML, Rentschler A: Evaluation of selected manual wheelchairs using ANSI/RESNA standards, *Arch Phys Med Rehabil* 80:462-467, 1999.

Corthell D: *Rehabilitation technologies 13th Institute on Rehabilitation Issues*, Stout, WI, 1986, Research and Training Center, University of Wisconsin-Stout.

Dahlquist DL et al: Characterization and evaluation of augmentative communication systems, *Proc 4th Annu Conf Rehab Engr*, pp 185-187, June 1981.

Desch LW: High technology for handicapped children: a pediatrician's viewpoint, *Pediatrics* 77:71-87, 1986.

Edyburn D, Higgins K, Boone R, editors: *Handbook of special education technology research and practice*, Whitefish Bay, WI, 2005, Knowledge by Design, Inc.

Enders A, Hall M: *Assistive technology sourcebook*, Washington, DC, 1990, RESNA Press.

Graves WH: NIDRR plans for the future, *Assist Technol* 5:3-6, 1993.

Goodman S: Fast facts on individualized education programs, *AT Q RESNA* 2:5-6, 1990.

Guralnik DB, editor: *Coles concise English dictionary*, Toronto, 1979, Coles Publishing.

Hulme JB et al: Effects of adaptive seating services on the eating and drinking of children with multiple handicaps, *Am J Occup Ther* 41:81-89, 1987.

Kambeyana D, Singer L, Cronk S: Potential problems associated with the use of speech recognition products, *Assist Technol* 9:95-101, 1997.

Kim H: The long view: selling providers on telerehab, *Team Rehabil Rep* 1015-19, 1999.

Lee KS, Thomas DJ: *Control of computer-based technology for people with disabilities*, Toronto, 1990, University of Toronto Press.

Mastrangelo R: Transdisciplinary treatment: crossing a bridge to better care. In *Advance for Occupational Therapists*, October 12, 1992.

McKechnie JL: *Webster's new twentieth century dictionary of the English language*, New York, 1983, Simon and Schuster.

Murphy EF, Cook AM, Harvey RF: Neuromuscular prosthetics and orthotics. In Cook AM, Webster JG, editors: *Therapeutic medical devices: application and design*, Englewood Cliffs, NJ, 1982, Prentice Hall.

North Carolina State University Center for Universal Design: *Principles of universal design*, Raleigh, NC, 2001, North Carolina State University Center for Universal Design.

Odor P: Hard and soft technology for education and communication for disabled people, *Proc Int Comp Conf*, Perth, Australia, 1984

Patterson C: *Overview of accreditation and certification*. Presented at the RESNA Annual Conference Quality Assurance Forum, Washington, DC, June 1989.

Pronsanti MP: Treating across role barriers. In *Advance for Occupational Therapists* March 1991.

RESNA: Technical assistance project, *TAP Bull*, January 1999.

Rowley BA, Mitchell DF, Weber C: Educating the rehabilitation engineer as a service provider, *Assist Technol* 9:62-69, 1997.

Scheck A: Going the distance: developments in communications technology bring telemedicine to rehab, *Team Rehabil Rep* 9:30-40, 1998.

Scherer M, Glueckauf R: Assessing the benefits of assistive technology for activities and participation, *Rehab Psych* 50:132-141, 2005.

Smith RO: Models of service delivery in rehabilitation technology. In *Rehabilitation technology service delivery: a practical guide*, Washington, DC, 1987, RESNA.

Smith RO: Technological approaches to performance enhancement. In Christiansen C, Baum C, editors: *Occupational therapy: overcoming human performance deficits*, Thorofare, NJ, 1991, Slack.

Snell E, Atkinson C: Comparison of three PC-XT based voice recognition systems, *Proc 10th Annu Conf Rehab Engr*, pp 717-719, June 1987.

Vanderheiden GC: Service delivery mechanisms in rehabilitation technology, *Am J Occup Ther* 41:703-710, 1987.

Warren CG: Quality assurance: credentialing providers of assistive technology services, *RESNA News* 3:8, 1991.

World Health Organization: *International classification of impairments, disabilities and handicaps*, Geneva, 1980, WHO.

World Health Organization: *International classification of functioning disability and health–ICF*, Geneva, 2001, WHO.

CHAPTER 2

Framework for Assistive Technologies

Learning Objectives

On completing this chapter, you will be able to do the following:

1. Define human behavior and contrast it with human performance
2. Describe the components of an assistive technology system
3. Describe and discuss the Human Activity Assistive Technology model
4. List the major performance areas in which assistive technology systems are applied
5. Discuss the contexts in which assistive technologies are used
6. Delineate the major considerations in designing an assistive technology system

Key Terms

Activity
Assistive Technology System
Contexts
Extrinsic Enablers

Function Allocation
Human Activity Assistive Technology
  Model
Life Roles

Occupation
Occupational Competence
Performance Areas
Tasks

In Chapter 1 an assistive technology *device* was defined as "an item, piece of equipment, or product system...that is used to increase, maintain, or improve functional capabilities of individuals with disabilities" (Public Law 100-407). In this chapter this base is expanded by defining an **assistive technology system** as consisting of an assistive technology device, a human operator who has a disability, and an environment in which the functional activity is to be carried out. In this chapter this concept of a system is formalized and the groundwork is laid for applying it to specific applications in later chapters.

■ HUMAN PERFORMANCE AND ASSISTIVE TECHNOLOGIES

At the most fundamental level, assistive technology systems represent someone (person with a disability) doing something (an activity) somewhere (within a context). A major goal of the assistive technology practitioner (ATP) is to recommend an assistive device that meets an individual disabled person's specific needs, is consistent with his or her skills, and accomplishes unique functions within the contexts of that person's daily life. This assistive technology system selection process emphasizes use of available function (human component) to accomplish what is desired (activity) in a given context (place, environment, people). We are not concerned as much with remediation of a disability as we are with enabling functional results and helping the individual to achieve what he or she wants to accomplish. Functional results require maximizing the skills of the person with a disability, which places human performance at the center of our system. The primary outputs of the assistive technology system are communication, mobility, manipulation, and cognition. In this chapter we discuss means of achieving these outputs in a general sense. More specific applications that may facilitate performance in these areas will be discussed in subsequent chapters.

Let's start with a case study of an individual who uses an assistive device for communication.

This case study provides a brief illustration of a situation of an individual with a disability who uses assistive technology to communicate. It hints at factors that influence whether a device will be useful in a given context and how individuals within the environment can affect the use of a device. It raises several issues involving the person using the device, the device itself, and the context in which it is used. It also points to the need for an effective evaluation that will enable selection of the most appropriate device and suggests that the interaction between the person, the device, and the contexts will influence the performance of a desired activity.

CASE STUDY

MARION

Marion is a teenaged girl who has spastic cerebral palsy that affects all four limbs. Because of these motor impairments, she is unable to speak or write. She is also unable to control her facial expressions. When her motor behavior is observed, it appears that her arm movements are random. During conversation, her facial expressions do not appear to mirror her feelings and it is difficult to interpret what she is feeling from either her arm movements or her facial expressions. Marion uses a language board (an assistive device) that allows her to communicate by pointing to letters and spelling out words. It is clear from our interaction with her that she is capable of using this device to carry out an intelligent conversation. Output using the communication board is slow. Marion is also able to use a voice output communication aid (VOCA) that generates speech electronically, thus increasing her rate of communication.

Marion communicates with others in many different contexts, including with friends and peers at school and in social situations, family at home, teachers at school, and other, less familiar individuals in a variety of contexts. When she communicates with friends in a social situation, the communication board may be the most effective device. Here, both the communication partners and the context are familiar so it is not necessary to spell out individual words. Friends can anticipate what Marion wants to say, thus increasing the rate of her communication. In less familiar situations, or with unfamiliar adults, the VOCA may be the most effective communication aid because the communication partners cannot be depended on to anticipate what Marion intends to say.

Foundation for a Human Activity Assistive Technology Model

Before a model that guides the selection and evaluation of assistive technology is described, two generic models will be presented that provide a foundation for one specific to assistive technology. These models are the International Classification of Functioning, Disability, and Health (ICF) (World Health Organization [WHO], 2001) and the Canadian Model of Occupational Performance (CMOP) (Canadian Association of Occupational Therapists [CAOT], 2002). Both these models include elements of the person, an activity, and the environment to understand a specific construct (health domains and health-related domains in the first instance and occupational performance in the second).

The ICF was described in more detail in Chapter 1. The ICF was derived from the International Classification of Disability and Handicap (WHO, 1980), with the addition of environmental factors and use of more inclusive language being two main distinctions between the two versions. It "provides a description of situations with regard to human functioning and its restrictions and serves as a framework to organize this information" (WHO, 2001, p. 7). Two components comprise factors of health and health-related states: body structures and functions and activities and participation. The framework includes two contextual factors: environmental and personal factors.

The term "body functions" refers to the functions of various systems in the body such as vision, sensation, and movement. Body structures include the anatomical structures that support the body functions (e.g., nerves, organs, and bones). Activity and participation are difficult to separate, so the ICF includes them together in its classification scheme. Activity refers to the performance of a task or action by a person, whereas participation involves performance of the activity within an individual's life roles or situation (WHO, 2001). The environmental context includes elements related to the physical, social, attitudinal, and institutional components. Finally, the personal factors include aspects such as age, sex, and lived experiences that have the potential to affect activity and participation (WHO, 2001).

Another model that is useful for understanding the relationship between the person, the activity, and the environment is the Canadian Model of Occupational Performance (CMOP) (CAOT, 2002). It conceptualizes the relationship between these three elements and their combined influence on occupational performance, which is defined as the choice, organization, and satisfactory completion of daily activities (CAOT, 2002). Components of the person factor include physical, affective (emotional), and cognitive elements. **Occupation** is composed of self-care, productivity, and leisure, whereas the environment consists of physical, social, cultural, and institutional elements. The dynamic interaction of these elements influences an individual's performance in chosen or required occupations (CAOT, 2002).

Both these models are similar in that they include elements of the person and his or her activities and environment. Assistive technology is specifically mentioned in the ICF as an aspect of the environment, specifically, products and technology for personal use in daily living, for personal indoor and outdoor mobility and transportation, communication, education, employment, and culture, recreation, and sport (WHO, 2001). It is not specifically mentioned in CMOP. These models are useful in understanding assistive technology because they identify factors that affect participation in daily activities across the life span. However, they are limited because the role and considerations of assistive technology are not specified. A model is now presented that explicitly includes assistive technology as a component of the completion of daily activities.

This model is intended to be used as a framework for the selection, implementation, and evaluation of assistive technology systems.

Human Activity Assistive Technology Model

The **human activity assistive technology (HAAT) model** is proposed as a framework for understanding the place of assistive technology in the lives of persons with disabilities, guiding both clinical applications and research investigations. The model has four components—the human, the activity, the assistive technology, and the context in which these three integrated factors exist. The human component includes physical, cognitive, and emotional elements; activity includes self-care, productivity, and leisure; assistive technology includes intrinsic and extrinsic enablers; and the context includes physical, social, cultural, and institutional contexts. Each of the components shown in Figure 2-1 plays a unique part in the total system. Consideration of each of these elements and their interaction is necessary for design, selection, implementation, and evaluation of appropriate assistive technologies and for research into various aspects of assistive technology development and use. The characterization of the model with the elements of human, activity, and assistive technology forming a collective that is nested within a physical, social, cultural, and environmental context is intended to show the dynamic interaction between the initial three factors and the pervasive influence on them, both individually and collectively of the various contexts. The interaction among the components of the HAAT model can be illustrated through application to our case study of Marion.

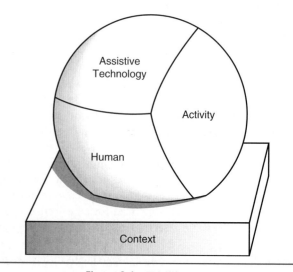

Figure 2-1   HAAT model.

MARION

One activity in which Marion needs and wants to engage is communication. She communicates in a variety of different settings, including school, home, and social situations with friends, others with whom she is familiar, and strangers. Without the use of a communication aid, Marion's speech is not readily understood by many of her communication partners. She is limited in her ability to engage in conversation, relay her needs, and express her opinions and ideas.

The communication board (the assistive technology) enables her communication by providing a means of conveying her ideas other than by spoken or written language. The communication board is particularly useful in certain contexts in which she communicates with partners with whom she is familiar and who are familiar with her use of the board. In these situations, communication can be a very quick and satisfactory process. However, the communication board is less useful with unfamiliar partners who are not familiar with its use or who may not have the patience to wait as Marion accesses the symbols on the board. Shortcuts that Marion has devised on the board will not be useful with unfamiliar partners. A voice output communication aid provides more effective communication in this latter situation because the output is clear and audible and Marion can preprogram phrases and text for quick retrieval. There are settings in which the VOCA would not be appropriate, though, such as a very noisy environment, or one in which its use would disturb others, such as a movie theater.

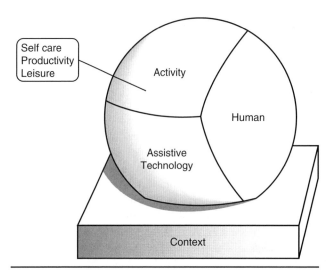

Figure 2-2 HAAT model with elements of activity component identified.

This brief example illustrates how the users' abilities are enhanced or augmented by the assistive technology to complete a desired activity. It also demonstrates that an assistive technology solution that works in one context is not as effective in another. The illustration shows that aspects of the person, the desired activity, the assistive technology, and the environment in which the technology will be used must be considered to ensure a satisfactory means to engage in daily living. What works for one person, in a particular setting for a particular activity may not be successful for another person in different circumstances. Indeed, a solution that works in one context may not transfer to another context for the same person.

■ THE ACTIVITY

The **activity** is the fundamental element of the HAAT model shown in Figures 2-1 and 2-2 and defines the overall goal of the assistive technology system. The activity is the process of doing something, and it represents the functional result of human performance. Activities are carried out as part of our daily living, are necessary to human existence, can be learned, and are governed by the society and culture in which we live (CAOT, 2002).

The profession of occupational therapy is based on the use of occupation, or activity, in the daily lives of individuals. Both the American Occupational Therapy Association (AOTA) and CAOT define these terms in the same way:

> [A]ctivities...of everyday life, named, organized, and given value and meaning by individuals and a culture. Occupation is everything people do to occupy themselves, including looking after themselves...enjoying life...and contributing to the social, and economic fabric of their communities. (AOTA, 2002; CAOT, 2002)

Activities are categorized within three basic **performance areas**: activities of daily living, work and productive activities, and play and leisure activities (CAOT, 2002). Activities of daily living include dressing, hygiene, grooming, bathing, eating, personal device care, communication, health maintenance, socialization, taking medications, sexual expression, responding to an emergency, and mobility. Included in work/productive activities are home management activities, educational activities, vocational activities, and care of others. The play and leisure area includes activities related to self-expression, enjoyment, or relaxation. Although these lists suggest that certain activities form specific categories, in reality the meaning an individual gives to an occupation determines in which performance area it is placed (CAOT, 2002; Miller Polgar and Landry, 2004). For example, gardening may be a productive activity for one person and a leisure activity for another.

Further, the meaning of an activity may vary depending on the role the individual assumes at the time the activity is performed. Christiansen and Baum (1997) define roles as "positions in society having expected responsibilities and privileges" (p. 54).

A person can have multiple roles simultaneously, and roles change throughout the person's life span. Examples of roles we hold during our lifetime include student, parent, son or daughter, sibling, employee, friend, and homemaker. Performance of an activity may differ depending on the nature of the role in which it is performed. For example, a parent reading to her child reads in a different way than when the reading is completed as part of the role of worker or student. Activities can be broken down into smaller **tasks**. The skills and abilities intrinsic to the human allow the individual to complete a series of tasks to produce the functional outcome of the activity. These skills may require any combination of physical abilities, cognitive abilities, or emotional aids for their successful completion. When an individual lacks the capacity to complete a task, the manner in which that task is completed, including the use of assistive technologies, must be changed. Understanding the activity is part of the assistive technology selection process as it requires identifying the tasks, skills, and abilities required for successful completion, the meaning the individual gives to the activity, and the different roles in which the individual uses the activity. Returning to the case study of Marion, communication is identified as the activity in which she needs to participate. She has the cognitive skills to complete the activity but not the physical ones. Further, the contexts in which she must communicate, including with different communication partners, affect her performance of this activity. Careful analysis of the activity of communication for Marion is required to identify the communication device that is most useful to her.

▤ THE HUMAN

The model in Figure 2-1 represents someone doing something someplace. Who is doing it? The individual with a disability is "operating" the system. Figure 2-3 highlights the human component of the HAAT model. Two theoretical approaches are useful when considering the human operator and his or her ability to use assistive technology: the conceptualization of the person from the CMOP (CAOT, 2002) and occupational competence (Matheson and Bohr, 1997). The CMOP conceptualizes human abilities as composed of three elements: physical, cognitive, and affective (CAOT, 2002). Physical abilities include strength, coordination, range of motion, balance, and other physical properties. Cognitive components include attention, judgment, problem solving, concentration, and alertness, whereas affect

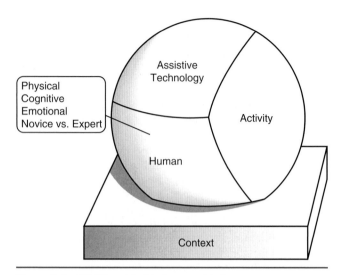

Figure 2-3 HAAT model with elements of the human component identified.

includes emotional elements. It is important to understand a person's abilities in each of these areas as they relate to the use of the desired technology. An appropriate match is needed between the person's abilities and the requirements of the technology to ensure effective use (Scherer, 1998). Where a mismatch occurs, devices will be misused or abandoned because they do not meet the user's needs.

In the HAAT model, the motor outputs of communication, mobility, and manipulation are required to accomplish the goals defined by activities. These three areas require that the human operator possess motor output skills and sensory function to perform these activities. These are akin to the physical domain of CMOP. For example, visual or auditory input is typically required for communication. If these skills are impaired, assistive technology systems can provide assistance by requiring different skills. For example, when a hearing aid compensates for reduced hearing thresholds or a Braille output system avoids visual reading, the assistive technology provides replacement or augmentation of a sensory system. Finally, central processing is required for the successful completion of activities. Components of central processing include perception, motor control, and cognition, similar to the CMOP cognitive domain. If the human's capabilities are limited, then assistive technology systems can often provide assistance in this area as well. For example, procedures for device operation may be simplified for an individual who has difficulty in sequencing tasks, or recall aids may be incorporated to assist someone who has memory deficits. Psychological function (referred to as affect in CMOP) influences performance of activities through motivation, self-efficacy, and perception of the value of the activity, as examples. These human performance components of the HAAT model are examined in detail in Chapter 3.

Occupational competence gives a dynamic context to the understanding of human abilities and how a person changes and adapts his or her engagement in activity in response to environmental demands and his or her own abilities. Although CMOP is useful to conceptualize human behavior at a given point in time, occupational competence helps understand behavior across the life span. Five constructs are important to the notion of occupational competence (Matheson and Bohr, 1997). Capacity refers to the potential skill, ability, or knowledge that an individual can apply to a given activity. Capacity changes with development, aging, or with trauma or illness. Effectance is the extent to which individuals reach or use their capacity in a given task. When a person is motivated to perform well in an activity, effectance approaches capacity. Affordances are those environmental elements that can facilitate performance of a task, providing the individual perceives them as a facilitator. Self-efficacy is a well-known concept described by Bandura (1977) that refers to an individual's belief that he or she can be successful in a particular situation. Finally, competence is the self-perception of satisfactory performance compared with some defined standard.

Collectively, these constructs contribute to occupational competence that is the ability to meet the demands that are required for successful engagement in various **life roles** (Matheson and Bohr, 1997). Thus, expectations by and of the individual, relative to performance of an activity, change as the person grows and acquires new skills, or conversely, as the person ages or experiences illness or trauma and loses skills. This notion of occupational competence illustrates the dynamic elements of physical and cognitive capacities and how they are influenced by the individual's attitudinal and motivational characteristics to meet the demands of various life roles.

Skills and Abilities

It is possible to distinguish between a person's skill and his or her ability. An *ability* is a basic trait of a person, what a person brings to a new task, whereas a *skill* is a level of proficiency, which is comparable to effectance described by Matheson and Bohr (1997). In assistive technology applications, this distinction is important. It is usually possible to obtain an assessment of a person's abilities, but it is difficult to predict the level of skill that he or she will develop using the technology. Ability can also mean transferring a skill from a related area and applying it to a new task. For example, a person with a disability might develop skill in the use of a joystick as a computer interface and then transfer this motor skill to the use of a power wheelchair. In this type of situation, the acquired skill in the first task becomes an ability that can be used in the second task.

Although it is possible for most humans to *perform* more than one task at a time, it is generally necessary to concentrate on one task to *learn* it. For example, a beginning user of an augmentive communication system may need to concentrate initially on the development of motor skills necessary to make selections with a keyboard. Eventually, he or she will have mastered this motor task sufficiently that he or she can perform it reliably while also concentrating on the language content of his or her message.

In Chapter 1 soft technologies were defined as "the human areas of decision making, strategies, training, and concept formation." In particular, strategies are part of the human skills required for the success of an assistive technology system. As Enders (1999) has pointed out, people who have disabilities use strategies to complete tasks. These can often either replace assistive technologies completely or compensate for deficiencies in the technology. For example, Marion uses strategies to enhance her augmentative communication system functionality. She may wave instead of typing "hi," or she may use prestored words to increase her speed at times and spell at other times to increase the participation of her communication partner. As in other aspects of the assistive technology system, the strategies used are highly dependent on all the other aspects of the assistive technology system. The context determines which strategies are important and useful, the characteristics of the technology affect which strategies are important to success, and the activity dictates the choice of strategies. Enders has proposed that strategies make up one side of a three-pronged approach to assistive technology applications that she calls "a human accomplishment support system." This framework is consistent with the HAAT model. The other two aspects of the framework are personal assistants and assistive technology devices.

Novice Versus Expert User

Another consideration related to the person, in the selection or evaluation of assistive technology, is whether that person is a novice or expert user of the specific technology. The term *novice* describes a user of an assistive technology system who has little or no experience with that particular system or the task for which it is used. As the user practices and gains more experience, he or she may become an *expert* user (i.e., demonstrating a high degree of skill in the use of the system). What differentiates an expert from a novice? The novice is more likely to use the system in prescribed ways, relying on soft technologies to use it effectively. The novice is less likely to generalize use of the system from one task to another and must use more conscious effort to control it. An expert takes more risks with the equipment in terms of stretching the way it is used and trying new activities with the system. For example, a skilled manual wheelchair user will take the chair up or down an escalator rather than use an elevator. A skilled communication aid operator will develop strategies to increase the rate of communication.

Understanding the differences between a novice and expert user has important implications for teaching people how to use a system and the development of strategies (soft technologies). An expert user exerts less conscious effort in the operation of the system—because he or she does not need to do so.

Analysis of the strategies of an expert user and translation of these into teaching programs can be an effective means of assisting a novice to become an expert user of a system.

■ THE CONTEXTS

Over the past several decades the models used to describe disability and the disablement process have changed dramatically (Pope and Brandt, 1997). In the 1950s the focus was on the "problem" of an inability to participate in work, play, education, and daily activities of living by the disabled person; this problem was "in the person"; that is, it was strictly the result of the impairment. More recently, there has been an increasing awareness that the difficulties experienced by individuals with disabilities result as much from environmental factors as from the impairment itself. Initially the focus was on the physical or built environment, with much effort to make curb cuts, install elevators, and so on. As individuals with disabilities began to participate more fully in society, it became evident that the social and attitudinal barriers were just as great as the physical ones. A "minority group model" of disability emerged in which the attention was shifted away from the impairment to the social, political, and environmental disadvantages forced on people who have disabilities (Brooks, 1998). Bickenbach et al (1999) conceptualized disability in a different way. In their view, disability was a universal experience, if a person lives long enough. Contrary to the minority group model, which advocated for special status for individuals with disability, the universalism concept advocated for broader social justice and policies that were more inclusive of persons with disabilities; actions that will benefit a broader segment of society. With these new perspectives, problems of societal participation were no longer attributed to the impairment of the person with a disability. Rather, lack of participation in society was viewed as resulting from limitations in the social and physical environments. The emphasis on participation in the ICF is indicative of the move away from a "problem in the person" concept to a "problem in the environment" model. In the HAAT model we have captured these external influences in the *context*.

As shown in Figure 2-4, the context includes four major considerations. These are (1) physical context, including natural and built surroundings and physical parameters, (2) social context (with peers, with strangers), (3) cultural context, and (4) the institutional context, including formal legal, legislative, and sociocultural institutions such as religious institutions. The **contexts** in which the human carries out the activity can be determining factors in whether the person successfully uses an assistive technology system. The supports and barriers in these environments are important considerations in the selection and evaluation of these systems.

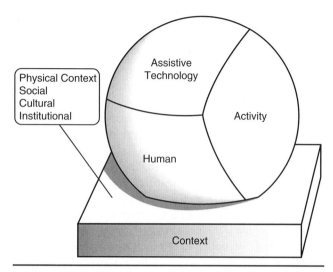

Figure 2-4   HAAT model with elements of the context identified.

One further distinction is important in the consideration of context: the level of environment. Three levels of environments have been described in the literature: microenvironment, mesoenvironment, and macroenvironment (Fougeyrollas and Gray, 1998; Law, 1991). The microenvironment refers to the closest, most intimate environments in which a person functions such as the home, school, or work setting. Here the person and his or her abilities are known, roles are defined, and rules and expectations are understood. The mesoenvironment describes those settings in which a person functions less frequently and includes various community facilities such as community centers, shopping malls, and churches. The macroenvironment refers to the broader social and cultural contexts that impose a legislative and moral behavioral framework on the person (Law, 1991). Each of these environments influences the use of assistive technology systems. It is important to understand how each aids or hinders the use of technology.

Physical Context

Perhaps the easiest environmental component to understand is the physical context. This context involves the physical attributes of the environment that enable, hinder, or affect performance of daily activities, either with or without assistive technology. It is important to identify the physical attributes of the environments in which the individual intends to use an assistive device to determine whether the device is compatible with those environments. In some cases, a device will work in one environment but not in another. Voice recognition software is an example of a device that does not readily transfer from one environment to another. In the relative quiet of an individual's home, voice recognition software may be an excellent alternative to direct input of computer keystrokes. However, it may not work in an office environment where noise interferes with the software and its use may interfere with the work of colleagues in close proximity to the individual.

A distinction that is important to understanding the physical environment is between the natural and the built surroundings. The natural surroundings include non-man-made elements such as parks. Conversely, built surroundings include those structures or elements that are man made such as buildings and sidewalks. It is critical to know whether the individual intends to use an assistive device in both built and natural surroundings because it will affect the technology selection and performance. A wheelchair with tires that facilitate travel over uneven and loose surfaces should be recommended for a person who intends to use a chair both indoors and outdoors on unpaved areas. One with smooth tires will not be useful for outdoor travel.

Assessment of the physical environment for selection or evaluation of assistive technology begins with the activities the person wants or needs to do and in which environments those activities will be performed. Within buildings, a person needs to enter and exit the building, access various locations, possibly move between levels, and perform a variety of daily activities. Further, a person needs to move from one environment to another (e.g., home to place of employment). Some of the physical aspects of the environment that should be considered include width of hallways or doorways, distances between locations the person must navigate, surface (e.g., carpet, transitions, floor surface), height and weight of devices and objects (e.g., door) the person must manipulate, and sensory cues (visual or auditory) required to successfully complete daily activities. Physical safety is an important consideration when the environment is assessed.

Three commonly measured parameters of the physical environment—heat (related to temperature), sound, and light—most directly affect the performance of assistive technologies. Many materials are sensitive to temperature and are affected by excessive heat or cold. For example, the properties of foams and gels used in seat cushions can change under conditions of very high or very low temperatures. Liquid crystal displays are affected by temperature and by ambient (existing) light.

Ambient light in classrooms or work environments can affect the use of assistive technologies. Some displays emit light and are better in conditions of reduced ambient light, whereas others reflect light and are better used in bright light. For example, lighting that is appropriate for normal classroom work may be too bright for the use of some displays, such as computer screens, because of glare.

Ambient sound (including noise) can have a major effect on the intelligibility of voice synthesizers or voice recognition systems. Sounds generated by such devices as printers, power wheelchairs, voice output communication aids, and auditory feedback from computer programs can be disruptive in a classroom. Church and Glennen (1992) discuss ways of controlling sound and lighting to avoid interference in the classroom while still facilitating the functional gains provided by the assistive technology.

Social Context

For assistive technology use, the social aspects of the context can be the most important. The social context refers to those individuals who interact with the individual using assistive technology, either directly or indirectly. Their acceptance or rejection of the assistive technology or their understanding of the purpose and need for the assistive technology is a critical component of whether the individual will be successful with technology use. As Fougeyrollas (1997) points out, social influence on individuals is related to what is considered normal or expected. Individuals who have disabilities may be stigmatized because of their disability. A frequent comment by persons with disabilities is that it is often the social environment, the attitude of others, that creates more of a handicap than the physical barriers in the environment. The use of assistive technologies can contribute to this stigmatization and lead to further isolation. For these reasons, it is important to understand the social aspects of the environments in which the individual will use the technology. If others in the environment do not support the use of the technology, the individual faces greater challenges to successful use of the device.

Relationships with others in the environment affect the use of technology. Those close to the individual, such as family, friends, teachers, or coworkers, have a better understanding of the person's capacities so use of technology is often eased. With unfamiliar people, technology use may be more complex because expectations differ as well as the understanding of how the technology works. For these reasons, it is important to determine who provides assistance to individuals using assistive technology in various environments, in particular, in key environments such as home, school, and workplace. Technology use, and consequently function, is eased when assistance is received from consistent individuals, such as family or personal care attendants, because these individuals understand the user's needs and the function of the assistive technology. When assistance is provided by several attendants, the result may be inefficient and incorrect use of the assistive technology because each successive attendant must learn the user's preferred method of completing activities and how the assistive technology is integrated into daily activities. In such situations, the user or the caregiver should be able to provide instruction to attendants.

Let's return to Marion and examine how her use of communication devices differs with various communication partners.

Communication systems are not the only type of assistive technology affected by social context. Brooks (1990) asked 595 disabled scientists and engineers to evaluate the assistive devices they used. She found that users applied devices in a variety of social settings, but use varied depending on the specific setting. For example, intimate, essential devices, such as those for personal hygiene, are not as frequently used as are those devices that assist in employment. Brooks interpreted this result as a reflection of the complex ties between the human (especially self-esteem), the technology, the activity, and the social setting. It is not possible, nor is it desirable, for us to separate the contexts (social and physical) from the other components of the assistive technology system.

A final point to consider relative to the social context is that the degree to which different types of assistive technologies contribute to stigma differs. Stigma is defined as a mark of shame. Certain devices, such as hearing aids and power wheelchairs, seem to convey greater disability than others, such as spectacles or manual wheelchairs. Consequently, persons with disabilities may choose not to use particular assistive technology within a social environment because of the stigma it conveys. If others within an environment perceive an individual as generally incapacitated because of

the presence of a specific disability, the individual may reject the use of an assistive device that brings additional attention to that disability. Consider an office worker, Ted, who has the capacity to use a manual wheelchair but who might choose to use a power chair because of the energy savings it affords. The behavior of certain colleagues in the office suggests that they perceive Ted to be less competent in performing his job tasks then he actually is. Ted's reaction may be to minimize the appearance of his disability through use of a manual wheelchair, although this choice might result in negative consequences such as excessive energy expenditure and fatigue in the short term and shoulder injury in the long term.

Cultural Context

The effectiveness of assistive technology systems is closely related to and influenced by the *cultural context*. Krefting and Krefting (1991) define culture on the basis of three concepts: (1) "culture is a system of learned patterns of behavior," (2) it is "shared by members of the group rather than being the property of an individual," and (3) it includes effective mechanisms for interacting with others and with the environment (p. 102). The first of two of these are closely related to our definition of activity or occupation. The third concept, interaction with the external world both socially and physically, illustrates the relationship of culture to the social and physical aspects of assistive technology context. Thus these three elements of culture clearly couple it with the HAAT model and emphasize the importance of cultural considerations in the design and implementation of assistive technology systems.

Krefting and Krefting (1991) point out that we all view the world through a "cultural screen" (p. 105) that is the product of our experiences, family relationships, heritage, and many other factors. This cultural screen differs for each of us, and it biases the way we interact with others and the ways in which we perceive various activities, tasks, and life roles. For example, in some cultures leisure is recognized as a desirable and socially acceptable pursuit. However, in other cultures pursuit of leisure time is thought to indicate laziness and lack of productivity. If the ATP and the consumer have differing cultural screens, they may have difficulty establishing and achieving mutual goals. For example, if the ATP views leisure as a desirable and satisfying occupation, he or she may recommend assistive technology systems that enable leisure activities, which could include modified computer or video games or an adapted wheelchair for tennis or other sports. However, if the consumer is from a culture in which leisure is viewed as being nonproductive, he or she may reject these assistive technology systems as frivolous.

There are many cultural factors that must be considered when assistive technology systems are applied. Box 2-1 lists factors that affect how assistive technology systems are

CASE STUDY

MARION

Marion may use her communication systems with her friends (familiar peers) or with her teacher (familiar nonpeer) or with a salesperson at the shopping mall (stranger). In each case her choice of vocabulary, her use of slang, and the ease with which she communicates is different. In Marion's case, she may have some stored slang words or phrases that are typically used by her friends. She may also have some more formal stored phrases that she can use in class or in a store. Additionally, because Marion and her communication partner know each other well, her friend anticipates her words, what she is spelling, which increases Marion's rate of communication and her effectiveness. A stranger who is unfamiliar with Marion's system would not anticipate her words, and the overall rate of communication would be slower. The social context directly affects total system performance. The effectiveness of her communication system is measured by the degree to which it accommodates these varied needs. Effective assistive technology systems are flexible and accommodating.

perceived and used by consumers from different cultures (Krefting and Krefting, 1991). These factors must be kept in mind by the ATP throughout the assistive technology delivery process. For example, consider three of these: importance of appearance, independence and its importance, and family roles. Wheelchair manufacturers now fabricate their products in a variety of colors, which allows choice and avoids the "institutional chrome" appearance for those who care about such things.

Another example involves Frank, a man with amyotrophic lateral sclerosis (ALS) (Murphy and Cook, 1985). Before his disability, Frank was dominant as head of his family. He was fiercely independent, and he valued his role as provider. As he lost the ability to speak because of the ALS, he used a small typewriter-like device to interact with his family. It allowed him to retain his head-of-household role, and he used his communication device to make investment decisions, plan legal affairs, and make shopping lists. His family provided the legwork to carry out his directions. As the ALS progressed, his motor control deteriorated until he could only raise his eyebrows. A new communication device, which used this limited movement, was obtained for him, but he was uninterested in using it. After repeated unsuccessful attempts to provide support for the use of this new device, those working with Frank began to realize that his role in the family had changed. Because of his dependence on aids and the difficulty in communicating with the new device, he lost all interest in his family role. His wife became the family leader, and she began to make decisions that had always been reserved for him. These changes in the family, a difficult concept for Frank because of his cultural perception of family roles, led to his

withdrawal and the failure of the assistive technologies to meet his needs.

Institutional Context

The institutional context refers to larger organizations within a society that are responsible for policies, decision-making processes, and procedures. CMOP includes economic, legal, and political components, such as government-funded services, legislation, and political regulations and policies (CAOT, 2002). The ICF section that categorizes similar aspects is labeled services, systems, and policies (WHO, 2001). Services are "benefits, structured programs and operations in various sectors of society" that meet the needs of individuals (WHO, 2001, p. 192). Systems refer to the administrative and organizational layer, at all levels of government or other authorities, that plan, implement, and monitor services. Policies are rules, regulations, conventions, and standards that regulate systems, and again, exist at all levels of government or other organizations (WHO, 2001, p. 192).

The institutional context has major implications for the acquisition and use of assistive technology. Funding is probably the most influential element in this context. Funding policies and regulations establish who is eligible to receive assistance for the purchase of devices, which devices are supported in funding schemes and who (i.e., which professional group) serves as the funding gatekeepers. Government programs also provide regulation and support for environmental modifications that enable the inclusion of persons with disabilities. Funding of assistive technology devices and services is discussed in more detail in Chapter 5.

Legislation in many countries establishes laws, policies, and regulations that enable persons with disabilities to engage in activities in various contexts with both their local community and more broadly. These laws specifically comment on environmental access issues, modifications required in employment and educational and other community settings, and the responsibility of the employer or educational system in providing accommodations for eligible individuals, including the provision of assistive technology. Examples of such legislation include the Americans with Disabilities Act (1990), Ontarians with Disabilities Act (2005), and the Individuals with Disabilities Education Act (IDEA) (1997). The implications of legislation are discussed further in Chapter 1.

A final implication of the institutional environment on assistive technology is legislation and standards that govern product design, function, and safety standards. For a product to be marketed and, in particular, for it to be included as a device for which funding assistance is provided, the developers or manufacturers must ensure that testing and other measures have been undertaken to ensure that the product meets certain technical standards. Standards for individual types of assistive technologies are discussed in later chapters.

■ EXTRINSIC ENABLERS: THE ASSISTIVE TECHNOLOGIES

The final component shown in Figure 2-1 is the assistive technology. A detailed characterization of this component is presented in Chapter 1 (see Box 1-1). Assistive technologies are also described as **extrinsic enablers** because they provide the basis by which human performance is improved in the presence of disability. The components shown in Figure 2-5, *B*, represent the flow of information and forces among the assistive technologies and the other components of the HAAT model. Interaction with the human is through the *human/technology interface* component of the assistive technology. This component represents the boundary between the human and the assistive technology. This interaction is two way; that is, information and forces may be directed from the human to the technology or vice versa. For the technology to contribute to functional performance, it must provide an output, which is accomplished by the *activity output* component. The human-technology interface and activity output are linked by the *processor*, which translates information and forces received from the human into signals that are used to control the activity output. Finally, some assistive technologies (e.g., sensory aids) must also be capable of detecting external environmental data. The *environmental interface* accomplishes this function. Once the external data are detected, the *processor* interprets and formats them so they can be provided to the user through the human-technology interface. Not all assistive technologies have all the components of Figure 2-5, *A*. However, all of them have at least one of the components, and most have two or three.

Different sets of the components shown in Figure 2-5, *A*, are required to meet the needs of different consumers. These components function together to facilitate the completion of tasks that underlie specific activities. Because the use of assistive technologies has the effect of adapting the skills required for the task to match those of the human, these technologies enable the human operator. The specific characteristics of the assistive technology components are determined by the person's needs and skills together with the goals determined by the activities to be performed. This process is described in Chapter 4 as part of the needs assessment procedures.

Human-Technology Interface

All the interactions between the human user of the technology and the device occur through the human-technology interface. As we have said, these interactions can occur in either direction (e.g., from human to technology or from technology to human), and they include both forces and information. Sometimes separate components are used to provide input to the device and output from the device. For example, a computer keyboard is used for typing and a video monitor provides feedback to the typist. Sometimes bidirectional interaction occurs in one component. For example, the computer keyboard provides tactile, auditory, and visual feedback to the typist.

Positioning devices, or *postural support systems*, are one type of human-technology interface. Any person must be stable and in a position that allows interaction with his or her environment to complete functional tasks. Some individuals with

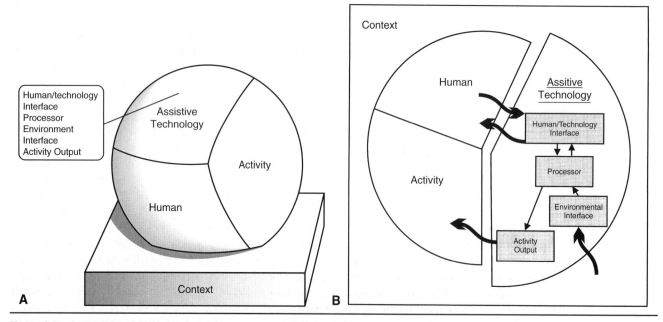

Figure 2-5   A, HAAT model with assistive technology elements identified. **B,** The assistive technology component of the HAAT model includes both the specific purpose and general purpose technologies.

disabilities have insufficient postural control to support the efficient and effective movements needed for this interaction. Provision of some form of seating or positioning system can influence their postural control. As discussed in Chapter 6, the human exerts forces on the postural support system, and the postural support system exerts forces on the human. This two-way interaction also involves the human sensory system. For example, if paralysis causes absence of sensation, the human may not detect the forces exerted by the human-technology interface (e.g., a seat cushion). If the pressures exerted on the human user by the human-technology interface are too high or are unrelieved for too long, they can lead to tissue damage. Likewise, if the human user reduces the forces that the body exerts on the device's human-technology interface (e.g., through performance of weight shifts), the total pressure at the human-technology interface is reduced, which decreases the possibility of tissue damage.

Another commonly used human-technology interface is called the *control interface,* the boundary between the user and an electronic or mechanical assistive technology device that allows the individual to operate, or control, the device. For electronic assistive technology systems, control interfaces include joysticks for power wheelchairs, keyboards for computers and communication devices, and single switches used to control household devices such as lights or radios. In addition to the motor output to the control interface exerted by the human user, sensory feedback is provided to the user during operation. This bidirectional interaction is essential to effective performance (see Chapter 7). The ways in which persons with disabilities are assessed for control interfaces, how they are selected, how they are used, and how training can be accomplished are also described in Chapters 4 and 7.

Displays that provide information to the human user are another type of *human-technology interface.* Displays are used in a wide range of technology, from power wheelchairs to computers to augmentative communication devices to environmental control systems to sensory aids. Examples include the lighted display of remaining battery energy on a power wheelchair and the lights used in a scanning display for augmentative communication. The major types of displays are visual, auditory (including synthesized speech), and tactile (e.g., Braille). Visual and tactile output modes are discussed further in Chapter 8. Speech output is discussed in Chapter 8.

Processor

Many assistive technology devices require control and processing of data to accomplish the desired functional task. The processor, often a computer, performs these actions. Many assistive devices (e.g., power wheelchairs, environmental control units) contain computers as integral components. These greatly increase flexibility and adaptability in performing functional tasks and also allow systems to be tailored to individual needs much more readily. Stand-alone personal computers also play an important role in increasing access to education, work, financial management, and recreation for persons with disabilities. The role of computers in assistive technology systems is discussed in Chapters 7 and 8. The processor in an assistive technology device may also be a simple mechanical component that links the control interface to the activity output. A common manipulation device is a mechanical reacher, which is used to obtain objects from shelves that are too high. The user controls the reacher through a hand grasp, which is coupled with a mechanical linkage that closes a gripper to reach and carry the object. In this case the mechanical linkage is the processor.

Activity Outputs

The *activity outputs* include communicating; moving from place to place; manipulating objects for self-care, work, school, or recreation; and performing cognitive activities. Each of these activities can be either replaced by a functional equivalent (e.g., a computer word processor for someone who cannot use a pencil and paper) or augmented (e.g., a holder that allows someone with limited grip to manipulate the pencil). Assistive technology systems may provide one or more activity outputs that facilitate performance. These outputs include communication, manipulation, mobility, and cognition. The activity output for communicating is transmission of information, usually provided through voice synthesis, visual display, or printed copy. Devices for manipulation are either special purpose (e.g., a modified spoon, brush, or shoe horn) or general purpose (e.g., environmental control units or robotic systems). Wheelchairs, modified driving aids for vehicles, and similar devices provide mobility outputs. Memory aids, computer sensors within the home, and computer software such as word recognition provide cognitive outputs.

Environmental Interface

The final component of the assistive technology, the environmental interface, provides the link between the device and the external world, represented by the context. This interface supports sensory performance: seeing, hearing, and feeling. For augmentation or replacement of vision, the environmental sensor is a camera capable of imaging the information to be input to the human. Two broad classes of performance are typically aided: reading and orientation and mobility for persons with visual impairments. Systems for aiding hearing often use a microphone as an environmental interface. Finally, systems designed to assist with tactile input (feeling) use transducers to detect external pressures or forces. The environmental interface is linked to the human-technology interface by a processor, often a computer.

Soft Technologies as Extrinsic Enablers

The extrinsic enablers described for general and specific purposes are hard technologies. Soft technologies can serve as extrinsic enablers, in addition to their role as strategies that were included as part of the human component of the HAAT model. For example, performance aids, written instructions, and training are all extrinsic enablers. Performance aids are often conceptual (e.g., a method of remembering vocabulary in a communication system by using pictures that can have multiple meanings). Marion, our augmentative communication system user, benefits from the use of soft technologies. With the electronic communication system, Marion must use codes to represent words or phrases. If she has many codes or difficulty remembering the codes, a list of the codes can be displayed on the device. This is referred to as a *performance* aid.

Training is often required to make a system useful. Not only the user but also the caregivers and family must be included in this training process. When adequate training in the use of an assistive device is provided to both the user and caregivers, that device is more likely to be used properly, with less likelihood of abandonment (Chen et al, 2000). Finally, written instructions and other documentation can make the difference between success and failure in the use of an assistive device. The quality of these materials varies widely. Performance aids, training, and development of written documentation are discussed in Chapter 4.

Assistive Technology Devices for Specific Applications

Specific application devices for mobility, communication, or manipulation have a *human-technology interface,* a *processor,* and an *activity output.* For example, for a manual wheelchair system, the human-technology interface includes positioning components and the push rims used for turning the wheels. The processor consists of the mechanical linkages between the push rims and wheels, and the activity output is mobility. For augmentative communication, the human-technology interface has two parts: a control interface and a user display. The processor is typically a computer with a software program that relates the control interface to stored vocabulary and controls the outputs. The output is synthetic speech, print, or visual display. An environmental aid to daily living for television, lights, telephone dialing, and other appliance control typically has a keypad or single switch and display as the human-technology interface. The processor is an electronic circuit, possibly a computer. The output is a signal or signals used to control the appliance and replace direct physical manipulation of its controls (e.g., television channel change or volume control).

Sensory aids have an *environmental interface,* a *processor,* and a *human-technology interface.* For example, a hearing aid uses a microphone as an environmental sensor, an amplifier as a processor, and a speaker (often called a receiver) as a human-technology interface. A reading machine for persons with severe visual impairments uses a camera as an environmental sensor, a computer as a processor, and a speech synthesizer as the human-technology interface.

■ APPLICATION OF THE HUMAN ACTIVITY ASSISTIVE TECHNOLOGY MODEL: DESIGNING ASSISTIVE TECHNOLOGY SYSTEMS FOR SUCCESSFUL OUTCOMES

To meet the needs of an individual, an *assistive technology system* must be designed, although this idea does not refer to the research and design process that results in the development of a new product. Rather it means the ultimate recommendation of assistive technology and how it will be used by a certain person within relevant contexts. An assistive technology system is designed through the process of assessing a consumer's needs, goals, and skills; using these to determine the necessary characteristics that an assistive technology system must have; conceiving of and planning the system for that individual; delivering the device and training in its use; and following up to evaluate success. In this section the assistive technology system is defined and then a process for designing such systems is described.

Assistive Technology System

In the previous sections each of the four components of the assistive technology human performance model was discussed. The assistive technology system is defined to be the four components shown in Figure 2-1. Needs arise from all aspects of a person's life, and the assistive technology system goals are defined by the chosen activities (see Figure 2-2). The tasks required by the activity, together with the contexts of use (see Figure 2-4) and the human operator's skills, determine the characteristics of the assistive technologies. The tasks must be matched to the human operator's abilities and skills to be completed successfully. This match is facilitated through the assistive technologies that replace or augment the human operator's function that would be precluded by his disability. The choice of the assistive technology characteristics (see Figure 2-5) and the matching of them to the skills and needs of the consumer complete the design process and the specification of the assistive technology system.

Define Key Activities

The first step in the process of designing the assistive technology system is the identification of an activity or activities that are meaningful to the consumer (Figure 2-6). These are activities that the consumer either needs or wants to do. The categories of self-care, productivity, and leisure,

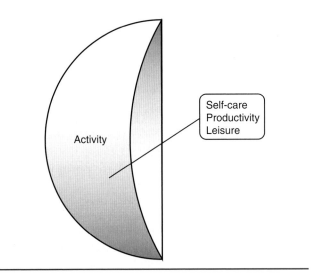

Figure 2-6 The first step in designing the assistive technology system is to define the key activities.

described earlier, are useful to help organize the evaluation and ensure that relevant activities are identified. The Canadian Occupational Performance Measure (Law et al, 1998) is a useful tool to assist with this identification. It involves the client and the ATP in a process that identifies important activities in self-care, productivity, and leisure areas and is useful to initiate a discussion of how and where these activities occur.

There are a number of questions that help define the activity. Who will perform the activity? Is it important for the client to perform the activity independently or will he or she accept assistance from others or technology? When the client will accept assistance from others, it is important to determine whether this assistance can be provided by family, friends, or a personal care attendant. If the activity is a sensitive one, such as toileting, the consumer may be very particular about the person from whom he or she will accept this assistance.

It is important to determine the meaning of the activity to the consumer and what adaptations they will accept to that activity. Klinger and Spaulding (1998) identified several different ways in which an activity could be adapted, including changing how it is completed, who does it, when and how frequently it is completed, stopping the activity, and substituting one activity for another. The consumer's acceptance of adaptation of an activity will depend on the meaning that engagement in that activity has for them. For example, a consumer who performed an activity at a highly skilled level, such as a competitive sport, may not find satisfaction with involvement in the same activity if his or her performance no longer meets previous standards. The meaning given to the activity will be a predictor of whether the consumer will accept technology as an alternate means to its completion (Spencer, 1998).

An additional factor that helps to define the activity relates to time. How frequently does the consumer engage in

that activity and will a change be accepted in that activity? One that is completed regularly and frequently is of higher priority than something that is only done infrequently. It is also useful to ask how long it takes the person to complete the task and whether the person is willing to invest that amount of time in it.

A thorough occupational or activity analysis is important for identification of the task demands. These demands are considered to be physical, cognitive, or affective skills, knowledge, or behaviors that are required for successful completion of the activity. Although they are attributes of the human, they are independent of the attributes of any specific individual. Rather, the analysis describes the skills, behaviors, and so forth required to successfully complete the activity and its subtasks. Several schemes for conducting an occupational or activity analysis are found in the literature (e.g., Blesedell Crepeau, 2003; Watson, 1997).

Consider the Perspective of the User

Once the activities have been defined, with input from the user, the focus of the system design process shifts to the human (Figure 2-7). The activity and the human are linked and it is artificial to separate the activity from the person. In this section the focus is on the attributes, perceptions, and preferences of the specific individual who will use the assistive technology. A thorough assessment should be completed of the user's physical and cognitive abilities and his or her affective state. Elements of the physical, cognitive, and affective domains and assessment specific to each of the types of assistive technologies are discussed in subsequent chapters.

Individual choice is important to determine at this stage. The consumer participates in the choice of activities in which to engage and the choice of how to adapt a specific activity. The assistive technology practitioner contributes

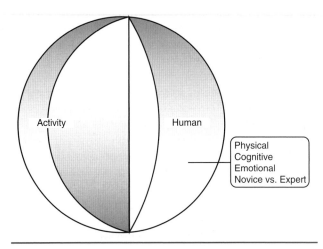

Figure 2-7 Once the activities are defined, the skills and perspective of the human user should be investigated.

expertise that assists the consumer in the choice of assistive technologies but must recognize the consumer's right to exercise that choice. How much input the ATP must have depends on many things such as whether the consumer is a novice or expert assistive technology user and the capacity of the consumer and the caregivers to understand the implications of the use of the assistive technologies for the consumer.

Choice is also seen in how a consumer completes an activity. Denison (2003) theorized that assistive technology users choose between performing a task themselves, using technology, or seeking assistance from others. For any given activity, the person may choose a combination of these three components. Let's return to the case of Marion presented at the beginning of this chapter. In some situations, she chooses to use a voice output communication aid for oral communication. When she uses this device, she performs some of the task herself (physically accessing the device), she may rely on another person to set up the device for her, and she relies on the device for oral output. In this situation, she primarily chooses to use her own abilities and the device to complete the task of communication.

What are some of the factors that influence a person's choice to complete an activity himself or herself, receive assistance from another or use technology, or, as in the example above, some combination of the three? These factors are unique to the individual user and are outside the person's actual physical and cognitive abilities. The individual may choose to complete an activity, or part of it, when the individual perceives himself or herself to have the ability to do so (i.e., self-efficacy [Bandura, 1977]). Conversely, when the person does not believe that he or she has the ability to perform a task, the person is more likely to avoid doing it altogether or rely on someone else even when he or she actually has the ability.

People make choices in their activities partially on the basis of the amount of energy they are willing to expend on the activity. For example, a person with a spinal cord injury resulting in quadriplegia who works outside the home may choose to have a personal care attendant assist with bathing and dressing in the morning when these activities would require a significant time and energy investment to be completed independently. So, even when a person is physically capable of completing a task on his or her own, it might not be worth the energy consumption if it leaves the person tired and unable to engage in activities that carry a higher personal importance. To some extent, people make choices on the basis of short- and long-term benefits and risks. The person with a spinal cord injury might be physically capable of propelling a manual wheelchair independently. However, evidence is confirming that long-term manual wheelchair use results in repetitive injuries to the shoulder (Curtis et al, 1994) that affects not only wheelchair propulsion but other important activities such as transfers. Thus, although physically capable of propelling a manual wheelchair, the client might choose to use a power chair to conserve the integrity

of the joints and energy consumption, both for the short-term gains of engaging in meaningful activities and long-term benefits of retaining physical abilities.

Features of the device itself will determine whether or how the individual chooses to use it to complete an activity. A device that is reliable (i.e., performs the task for which it is intended in a consistent manner) and one that is simple and intuitive to use is more likely to be used than one that is not (Pape, Kim, and Weiner, 2002). If use of a device conveys a stigma, then it is less likely that the person will choose to use it. Esthetics, portability, maintenance, and affordability are other device features that have been shown to influence whether a person will choose to use a device.

Elements of the social environment also affect a person's choice of how to complete an activity. Assistance is more likely to be received from another person when that person is knowledgeable of and effective with the assistance provided. In the example of Marion, her decision to use a communication board versus a VOCA was made, in part, on the basis of her specific communication partner. The communication board requires more assistance from another person (as the person must interpret the symbols or understand her abbreviations) so it was only used with more familiar partners. The VOCA, which requires less effort on the part of the communication partner, was used with less familiar partners.

Others in the environment can influence the choices an individual makes regarding task completion. For some the notion of "use it or lose it" results in the individual expending more of his or her own effort on a task. A common example is the use of a power versus a manual wheelchair. A person who chooses power over manual mobility may be seen as lazy by others, including family or therapists, even when the power chair enables more independence in other functional areas. Others may only focus on a single activity, in this case wheelchair propulsion, rather than seeing the larger picture, which may be for example, the energy expenditure of a university student propelling himself or herself across campus. In this case, the person may be so tired from propelling the chair that he or she has difficulty concentrating on academic tasks.

Finally, the choice may be dependent on what the environment will support. If a person is not available to provide assistance in a certain environment, then alternate means of completing a task must be sought. Similarly, as has been discussed previously, different environments support the use of technology in different ways. A power wheelchair may be an excellent mobility choice when moving about the community but be less effective for mobility within the confines of a home. Voice recognition software may be a very effective means of entering information at home or in a private office where ambient noise and proximity of others are limited.

Together the personal attitudes of the user, the effectiveness of the technology in supporting the activity, and the ability of the environment to support the activity all influence the choice that the individual makes when determining how to complete an activity. The assistive technology provider's role is to ask the questions and serve as a resource for the individual to assist with this decision-making process.

Consider the Environment

There are a number of important questions to answer regarding the environment when the assistive technology system is being designed. We discussed the effect that the environment has on the user's choice of how to complete the activity. Some additional questions include the following: Where will the assistive technology be used? Does the consumer expect to use it in a single environment (e.g., the home or workplace) or does the consumer need to use, and thus transport it, to different locations, in which case portability and flexibility are important? If the technology is to be used across many different environments, the effect of the environment on its use must be considered. For example, extremes of temperature will affect the performance of the materials used to construct seating systems. In northern climates, extreme cold has the potential to alter the material properties, therefore influencing the ability of the device to distribute pressure. Similarly, extremes of temperature will have a detrimental influence on any device with electronic components. Available light and sounds within the environment will also influence device performance.

The effect of the environment on the performance of the activity is another consideration. What are the differences in how an activity is or can be performed across all pertinent environments? Environments that incorporate universal design principles (see Chapter 1) facilitate performance of activities by individuals with a variety of abilities. Institutional policies and procedures can be barriers or enablers to performance of an activity and may even determine whether an individual has access to necessary technology.

When a device must be used in a variety of environments, the complexity of its setup is an important consideration. A device that is very complex to set up may not be used across various environments because the setup is too time consuming and the potential for error is great. Even when device setup is simple, such as replacing a seat cushion in a wheelchair, there is a potential for misuse if the individual replacing it is not familiar with its use. Most assistive technology providers have seen wheelchair cushions placed backward in the wheelchair, obviously compromising their performance.

Funding is another reason why it is important to determine where the device will be used. Under some funding schemes, a person is only eligible to receive a device if it is used in a specific environment such as the home. In such a situation, the ATP must determine that the device and the environment in which it is to be used are compatible. Issues such as physical access and social support for use of the device are important considerations here.

At this point, definition of the activities in which the person wants to participate, an assessment of the abilities of the user along with his or her personal choice in how to complete an activity, and the influence of the environment on the use of assistive technology have been discussed. Now, selection of the assistive technology will be discussed.

Selecting the Assistive Technology

Figure 2-8 shows the interaction of the activity, the human, and the assistive technology nested within the context. Two issues will be discussed relative to selecting the assistive technology. The first is a hierarchy of assistive technology described by Trefler and Hobson (1997) (Box 2-2). The second is the notion of function allocation (Bailey, 1996) that comes from human factors engineering.

The device abandonment literature suggests that assistive technology that is simple to use is less likely to be abandoned than that which is more complex. Trefler and Hobson (1997) describe a hierarchy that moves from simple, relatively easy-to-obtain devices to those that are more complex and more difficult to obtain. Their premise is that the ATP should recommend a device that is as simple as possible yet still meets the client's needs. As you can see from Box 2-2, these devices range from those that are commercially available for general consumption to those that are custom made for a single individual. Although it is tempting sometimes to recommend or purchase a device that promises to perform a wide variety of functions, unless the user needs or wants all the functions, a simpler device is usually the better option. Think about all the various functions that are available

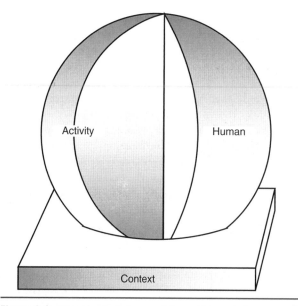

Figure 2-8   Consider the influence of the context on the human user's performance of desired activities.

BOX 2-2   A Hierarchy for Assistive Technology Selection

Adapt the activity or task.
Select a device that is commercially available for persons without disabilities.
Select commercially available rehabilitation products.
Combine commercially available rehabilitation products in innovative ways.
Modify existing commercially available rehabilitation products.
Design and create a new device for a specific individual.

Modified from Symms J, Ross D: Presented at Pacific Regional RESNA Conference, Long Beach, CA, 1991.

on current cell phones and person digital assistants. Most people do not use all these functions, even when they add to the cost. The same holds true for assistive device selection.

Allocation of Functions

In any human/device system some functions can be allocated to the human, some to the device, and some to the Personal Assistant Services (PAS). Bailey (1996) defines several approaches to **function allocation** that are used in general human factors design. Several of these are applicable to the design of assistive technology systems and are useful for both the user and ATP when determining how and what type of assistive technology will be beneficial to the individual. The simplest approach is *comparison allocation*. Here each task to be carried out is assigned completely to the human or to the device. The user's skills define the task that can be assigned to him or her; the characteristics of the technology determine which capabilities are assigned to it. For example, a standard telephone is designed with the assumption that the user can hold the handset, press the buttons to dial, hear the other person, and speak into the telephone. These are all functions assigned to the user. However, if the user cannot perform any of these tasks, the assistive technology must provide an alternative set of tasks. For example, assume that a particular consumer is able to carry out all the functions except holding the handset and dialing. A speaker phone, which avoids the need to hold the handset, together with a mouth stick for dialing, could be used. These constitute the assistive technology component of this system. Often comparison allocation is used when characteristics of technology are matched to a consumer's skills.

A second allocation approach is *leftover allocation*, in which as many functions as possible are assigned to the human and the device carries out the remainder. In assistive technology system design, this approach is often followed to give the consumer as much natural control over his activities

as possible but to provide assistance when needed. For example, some manual wheelchairs are equipped with power assist wheels that amplify the user's propulsion strokes. Thus a person who has limited strength and endurance can propel the wheelchair manually but the power assist wheels augment their abilities.

A third approach is *economic allocation*, in which the basic consideration is whether it is cheaper to select, train, and pay a personal assistant to do the activity or to design an assistive technology system for this purpose. Often the economic analysis initially favors the personal assistant because the purchase cost of the technology is relatively high. However, if the technology cost is amortized over its useful life, the technological approach may be significantly less expensive because the personal assistant cost (salary) rises over time.

The final approach that we use when designing an assistive technology system is *flexible allocation*. In this approach the consumer can vary his or her degree of participation in the activity on the basis of skills and needs. Whenever possible, we use this approach in assistive technology systems, and we couple the use of the AT system with PAS. The human and technology components are not fixed in scope; they change on the basis of specific activities and tasks to be carried out. Initially the novice operator may rely more heavily on intuitive skills to perform the desired tasks. As knowledge of the device operation increases and strategies are developed, the tasks carried out by the human operator change and system operation becomes more efficient. The role of PAS may also change over time.

As an example, consider the case of Pat.

Flexible allocation also allows for the system to change to account for decreasing human function, as in the case of degenerative disease. For example, an individual with muscular dystrophy generally regresses from walking to using a manual wheelchair and then to a powered wheelchair as the disease progresses. This loss of function often requires two new systems, a manual and a powered wheelchair. However, there are add-on powered units that can be attached to a manual wheelchair. The use of an add-on unit makes the basic manual wheelchair more flexible and allows the transfer of functions from the human (upper body strength to propel a manual wheelchair) to the device (an electric motor to power the wheelchair). Similar considerations apply to individuals whose abilities, and resulting performance, fluctuate throughout the day or from day to day because of changing neuromuscular capabilities (e.g., muscle tone, strength, attention) or fatigue. Often this fluctuation in abilities is great, and the system must compensate for these changes. If the system is able to reallocate functions flexibly, the consumer will be able to accomplish tasks with greater device assistance when he or she is tired and will be able to exert more control and independence when well rested.

Some extrinsic enablers are more flexible than others, and they allow continual alteration in the allocation between the

Pat sustained a high-level spinal cord injury that resulted in quadriplegia. He has good control of his head, but he has no functional use of his arms or legs. He uses an electronic pointing device attached to a headband to substitute for using his fingers to type on the computer keyboard. This device must be placed on his head, and a personal assistant must set up the computer. Because of his underlying abilities, Pat will always need to rely on PAS to place the device on his head. Pat will also rely on PAS as a backup if his electronic pointing system becomes inoperative. The particular device that Pat is using is equipped with a word prediction feature, which presents a choice of words based on the keys he enters. Pat's assistant may also help with some system functions as Pat is learning to use the system. As Pat gains more skill in using the system, this assistance will not be necessary. Initially Pat will use just the letter-by-letter input mode because he is familiar with that method from previous use of a keyboard. However, as he begins to learn what words are likely to be predicted when he types certain sequences of keys, he'll start using the word completion feature to speed up his selections. The advanced features of his system—in this case, word prediction—are not used until the basic features have become familiar. As Pat learns to use the advanced features, he will need to make fewer entries because the device has taken over a larger portion of the total system functions. As Pat becomes more and more skilled, he will be able to allocate more functions to the system and reserve his own energy for thinking and decision making.

human and technology. For example, computer-based devices can be altered by software to perform many functions with the same control interface. On the other hand, some extrinsic enablers, including some seating and postural support systems, are less flexible, and they must be redesigned or adjusted if the human component changes significantly (e.g., when a child goes through a growth phase).

■ SUMMARY

In the previous sections each of the four components of the assistive technology human performance model has been discussed. The assistive technology system was defined to be the four components shown in Figure 2-1. Needs arise from all aspects of a person's life, and the assistive technology system goals are defined by the chosen activities (see Figure 2-2). The tasks required by the activity, together with the contexts of use (see Figure 2-4) and the human operator's skills, determine the characteristics of the assistive technologies. Tasks must be matched to the human operator's abilities and skills to successfully complete desired activities. Facilitation of this match is accomplished through the assistive technologies, which enable the consumer to complete tasks that would be precluded by his disability. The choice of the assistive technology characteristics and the matching of them to the skills and needs of the consumer, and the influence of the context complete the design process and the specification of the assistive technology system. Figure 2-1 illustrates this integrated assistive technology system.

The following chapters will expand on aspects of human performance, evaluation of the assistive technology system and then describe specific types of assistive technology in greater detail.

Study Questions

1. Describe the three elements common to the ICF, CMOP, and HAAT models. How does the HAAT model differ from the other two? What is the purpose of the HAAT model?

2. What are the three basic performance areas defined in the HAAT model? Give an example of each.

3. Describe the relationship between tasks and activities. How is this knowledge applied to assistive technology selection?

4. Describe the five components of occupational competence and discuss how they affect the use of assistive technology.

5. What is meant by the terms *novice* and *expert*, and how do they affect assistive technology application?

6. Distinguish between *ability* and *skill*.

7. Describe the role that strategies play in the use of assistive technology systems. How can strategies compensate for the absence or inadequacy of an assistive technology?

8. Describe the four major parts of the context and how each can affect overall assistive technology system performance.

9. What are the three physical parameters of the physical context of the HAAT model? How do they affect the performance of assistive technology?

10. How do cultural considerations affect the application of assistive technology systems?

11. Explain the shift in thinking regarding societal participation by persons who have disabilities; that is, where is the "problem" with this participation thought to lie? What implications does this have for assistive technology applications?

12. What is meant by the term *institutional environment* in relation to considerations of the context of assistive technology application?
13. What are the four components of the assistive technology portion of the HAAT model?
14. Why do we refer to assistive technologies as *extrinsic enablers*?
15. Describe three factors that affect users' decision of whether to use assistive technology to assist with daily activities.
16. Describe the process of designing an assistive technology system.

17. Define the term *stigma*. How does it affect assistive technology selection and use?
18. What is the influence of the environment on assistive technology selection and use?
19. What is meant by the term *function allocation*, and how is it applied to assistive technology systems?
20. What are the major approaches to function allocation? What are the strengths and weaknesses of each approach when used in assistive technology system design?

References

American Occupational Therapy Association: Occupational therapy practice framework: domain and process, *Am J Occup Ther* 56:609-639, 2002.

Americans with Disabilities Act of 1990, 42 U.S.C. §§ 12101 et seq.

Bailey RW: *Human performance engineering,* ed 3, Upper Saddle River, NJ, 1996, Prentice Hall.

Bandura A: *Social learning theory,* Englewood Cliffs, NJ, 1977, Prentice-Hall.

Bickenbach J et al: Models of disablement, universalism and the international classification of impairments, disabilities and handicaps, *Soc Sci Med* 48:1173-1187, 1999.

Blesedell Crepeau E: Analyzing occupation and activity: a way of thinking about occupational performance. In Blesedell Crepeau E, Cohn ES, Boyt Schell BA, editors: *Willard and Spackman's occupational therapy,* ed 10, pp. 189-198, Philadelphia, 2003, Lippincott, Williams & Wilkins.

Brooks NA: Models for understanding rehabilitation and assistive technology. In Gray DB, Quatrano LA, Lieberman ML, editors: *Designing and using assistive technology: the human perspective,* pp. 3-11, Baltimore, 1998, Paul H Brookes Publishing.

Brooks NA: User's perceptions of assistive devices. In Smith RV, Leslie JH, editors: *Rehabilitation engineering,* Boca Raton, FL, 1990, CRC Press.

Canadian Association of Occupational Therapists: *Enabling occupation: an occupational therapy perspective,* ed 2, Ottawa, 2002, CAOT Publications/ACE.

Chen T et al: Caregiver involvement in the use of assistive devices by frail older persons, *Occup Ther J Res* 20:179-200, 2000.

Christiansen C, Baum C: Person-environment occupational performance: A conceptual model for practice. In Christiansen C, Baum C, editors: *Occupational therapy: enabling function and well being,* ed 2, Thorofare, NJ, 1997, Slack.

Church G, Glennen S: *The handbook of assistive technology,* San Diego, CA, 1992, Singular Publishing Group.

Curtis KA et al: Shoulder pain in wheelchair users with tetraplegia and paraplegia, *Arch Phys Med Rehabil* 80:453-457, 1999.

Denison I: Technology: How much is enough? *Proceedings of the Canadian Seating and Mobility Conference,* Toronto, 2003.

Enders A: *Technology for the next millennium: building a framework for collaboration.* Presented at the 1999 conference of the Association for the Advancement of Assistive Technology in Europe (AAATE), Dusseldorf, Germany, November 1999.

Fougeyrollas P: The influence of the social environment on the social participation of people with disabilities. In Christiansen C, Baum C, editors: *Occupational therapy: enabling function and well being,* ed 2, pp. 378-391, Thorofare, NJ, 1997, Slack.

Fougeyrollas P, Gray DB: Classification systems, environmental factors and social change. In Gray DB, Quatrano LA, Lieberman ML, editors: *Designing and using assistive technology: The human perspective,* pp. 13-28, Baltimore, 1998, Paul H Brookes Publishing.

Individuals with Disabilities Education Act Amendments of 1997, U.S.C.A. § 600, et seq.

Klinger L, Spaulding S: Chronic pain in the elderly: silence is golden, *Phys Occ Ther in Geriat* 15:1–17, 1998.

Krefting LH, Krefting DV: Cultural influences on performance. In Christiansen C, Baum C, editors: *Occupational therapy,* Thorofare, NJ, 1991, Slack.

Law M: 1991 Muriel Driver Memorial Lecture. The environment: a focus for occupational therapy, *Can J Occup Ther* 58:171-180, 1992.

Law M et al: *Canadian Occupational Performance Measure,* ed. 3, Toronto, 1998, CAOT/ACE Publications.

Matheson LN, Bohr PC: Occupational competence across the life span. In Christiansen C, Baum C, editors: *Occupational therapy: enabling function and well-being,* ed 2, pp. 428-457, Thorofare, NJ, 1997, Slack.

Miller Polgar J, Landry J: Occupations as a means for individual and group participation in life. In Christiansen C,

Townsend E, editors: *Introduction to occupation*, pp. 197-220, Upper Saddle River, NJ, 2004, Prentice Hall.

Murphy JW, Cook AM: Limitations of augmentative communication systems in progressive neurological diseases, *Proceedings of the 8th Annual Conference on Rehabilitation Technology*, pp 120-122, Washington, DC, June 1985, RESNA.

Ontarians with Disabilities Act, Bill 118, Chapter 11 of Statutes of Ontario, Legislative Assembly of Ontario, 2005.

Pape TL, Kim J, Weiner B: the shaping of individual meanings assigned to assistive technology: a review of personal factors, *Disabil Rehabil* 24:5-20, 2002.

Pope A, Brandt E, editors: *Enabling America: Assessing the role of rehabilitation science and engineering*, Washington, DC, 1997, National Academy Press.

Scherer M: The impact of assistive technology on the lives of persons with disabilities. In Gray DB, Quatrano LA, Lieberman ML, editors: *Designing and using assistive technology: the human perspective*, pp. 99-115, Baltimore, 1998, Paul H Brookes Publishing.

Spencer J: Tools or baggage? Alternative meanings of assistive technology. In Gray DB, Quatrano LA, Lieberman ML, editors: *Designing and using assistive technology: the human perspective*, Baltimore, 1998, Paul H Brookes Publishing, pp. 89-98.

Trefler E, Hobson D: Assistive technology. In Christiansen C., Baum C, editors: *Occupational therapy: enabling function and well-being*, pp. 482-506, Thorofare, NJ, 1997, Slack.

Watson DE: *Task analysis: An occupational performance approach*, Bethesda, MD, 1997, American Occupational Therapy Association.

World Health Organization: *International classification of impairments, disabilities, and handicaps: a manual for classification relating to the consequences of diseases*, Albany, NY, 1980, World Health Organization Publication Center.

World Health Organization: *International classification of functioning, disability and health (ICF)*, Geneva, 2001, World Health Organization.

CHAPTER 3

Disabled Human User of Assistive Technologies

Learning Objectives

On completing this chapter, you will be able to do the following:

1. Place the human user of assistive technologies in the proper context relative to the activities and contexts of human performance
2. Describe and apply an information processing model of the disabled human operator of assistive technologies
3. Use basic human factors and neuroscience concepts to describe the interaction between persons with disabilities and assistive devices
4. Describe how disabilities, learning (including experience), age, and changing conditions affect the human performance model and the interaction among the human, the activity, and the context
5. Apply basic principles of human performance to specific application areas (activities) and contexts

Key Terms

Abandonment	Morphology	Range
Apraxia	Motivation	Recall
Central Processing	Motor Control	Recognition
Cognition	Muscle Tone	Reluctant Users
Development	Optimal Use	Resolution
Effectors	Paralysis	Semantics
Engram	Perception	Sensors
Growth	Phonology	Spasticity
Intrinsic Enablers	Pragmatics	Syntax
Learning	Primitive Reflexes	Visual Accommodation
Memory	Psychosocial Function	

In the previous chapter the assistive technology system and the interrelationships among its component parts are described. In this chapter the focus is on the human user of assistive technologies. It is assumed that the reader has a general knowledge of normal human physiology and of disabilities, and therefore the emphasis is on those characteristics of disability that influence the use of assistive technologies. The Disability Statistics Center at the University of California, San Francisco, has provided the following statistics based on the National Health Interview Survey, a continuing national household survey consisting of 49,401 household interviews with 128,412 people in 1992 *(www.dsc.ucsf.edu)*. Data collected include information regarding basic personal assistance needs (i.e., whether people need help with activities of daily living such as bathing, eating, dressing, or getting around inside) and routine personal assistance needs (i.e., whether people need help with instrumental activities of daily living such as household chores, doing necessary business, shopping, or getting around for other purposes) as a result of chronic health conditions.

-   Approximately 15% (37.7 million) of the United States' population have a limitation that affects a major life activity such as working or going to school. These individuals report 1.6 conditions per person on average, for a total of 61 million limiting conditions.
-   More than 19 million individuals ages 18 to 69 have physical or mental conditions that keep them from working, attending school, or maintaining a household. Women report a higher number of activity-limiting conditions than do men.
-   Minorities, the elderly, and those in lower socioeconomic populations have a greater incidence of disabilities and need greater assistance in both activities of daily living (52% more than 65 years old) and instrumental activities of daily living (58% more than age 65 years).
-   A newborn infant can be expected to have 13 years of limited activity out of a 75-year life expectancy.
-   National disability-related costs are more than $170 billion annually.

These statistics indicate that activity-limiting disabilities are widespread, unevenly distributed across the general population, and expensive. Assistive technologies, if appropriately applied, can help to overcome the activity limitations imposed by disabilities. This requires a thorough understanding of human abilities and skills, especially in the presence of a disability.

In designing assistive technology systems, it is important to build on the skills of the user and provide assistive devices that augment or replace functional limitations. Because the goal is to increase functional independence for individuals with disabilities, it is important to focus on remaining function, rather than on lost function. In this chapter a description of the human user of assistive technologies is developed.

INFORMATION PROCESSING MODEL OF THE ASSISTIVE TECHNOLOGY SYSTEM USER

Human factors engineers and psychologists have developed the model shown in Figure 3-1 to describe the human component of a human-machine interaction (Bailey, 1989). This model is useful for describing the human operator of an assistive technology system. The individual blocks shown in Figure 3-1 delineate functional rather than structural components, and they are used to help identify the important considerations in human-machine interaction. Bailey (1989) lists three things that a system designer must know about the user: (1) what can be done (skills), (2) what cannot be done (limitations), and (3) what will be done (motivation). Motivation is directly related to the person's goals and needs and how well the assistive technology system meets them.

Skills and limitations in the three component areas shown in Figure 3-1 are considered when designing assistive technology systems. Taken together, these components constitute the **intrinsic enablers** for the human. Input from **sensors** is necessary for obtaining data from the environment, and limitations can arise in both the sensitivity (minimum detectable levels of light, sound, or pressure) and range (allowable variation in size, amplitude, or magnitude of the sensory input). When assistive technology system use is being considered, the visual, auditory, tactile, proprioceptive, kinesthetic, and vestibular sensory systems all play important roles. Sensory data produced by each of these systems are important for the successful use of assistive technologies. Some assistive technologies specifically address sensory loss.

For example, reading and mobility systems for the visually impaired and hearing aids for individuals with auditory impairment are designed to compensate for these specific losses (see Chapters 8 and 9). However, sensory function affects virtually all areas of assistive technology application, and it is important to consider sensory function as an integral part of the overall human capabilities required for the successful operation of an assistive technology system.

The term **effectors** will be used to describe the neural, muscular, and skeletal elements of the human body that provide movement or motor output. The result of the movement of the effectors is motor output. These elements work together to allow movement under the control of central processing and in response to sensory input. Limitations can arise from impairments in any element or combinations of them. Effectors provide the motor outputs that can be used for the control of assistive technology systems. Often, assistive technology systems are controlled by hand movements. For example, powered wheelchairs typically use joystick control activated by hand movements, and computers and augmentative communication systems use hand and finger movements for keyboard use. However, other anatomical sites may be used for control, and the components of postural control and reflexes also contribute to the generation of motor output.

Interposed between the sensors and effectors are the **central processing** functions of perception, cognition, neuromuscular control (including motor planning), and psychological factors. **Perception** is the interpretation and assignment of meaning to data received from the sensors, and it involves an interaction between information derived from sensed data and information stored in memory based on previous sensory experiences (Bailey, 1989). As Dunn (1991) points out, sensory and perceptual function provides the mechanisms by which an individual interacts with the environment. It is the combination and interpretation of data from all the sensory systems that provide a meaningful picture of the environment and our interaction with it.

The term **cognition** refers to attention, memory, problem solving, decision making, learning, language, and other

Figure 3-1   An information processing model of the human operator of assistive technologies. Each block represents a group of functions related to the use of technology. Taken together, these components constitute the intrinsic enablers for the human.

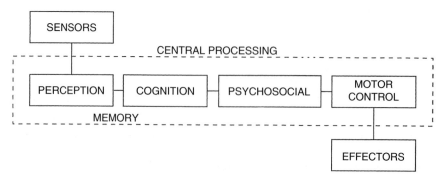

related tasks. As pointed out by Duchek (1991), virtually all aspects of performance are based on cognitive function, including performance that uses assistive technology systems and human performance in general. For example, the use of a powered wheelchair requires several types of cognitive function. The human operator must visually scan the environment, process the sensory data, make decisions as to the direction of movement desired, and activate the corresponding effector to cause the motion of the wheelchair in the desired direction. Once in motion, the user must attend to the environment to avoid obstacles and hazards and make instantaneous decisions regarding speed and direction. The user may also be required to engage in problem solving to negotiate a tight space or recover from an error. Cognitive processes involved in this example include attention, decision making, problem solving, language (e.g., spatial concepts such as left, right, forward, back), and memory. Without these capabilities, it would be difficult to control a powered wheelchair effectively.

It is also sometimes difficult to separate cognitive performance from sensory or motor performance. For example, an individual using an electric feeding device (see Chapter 14) requires sensory input to locate food on a plate, decision making to select the desired food item to be eaten, sufficient motor skills to activate a control interface that directs the spoon to the plate to pick up food and move it to the mouth, and monitoring of the path of the spoon as it travels. Because this is a complex set of tasks, it is difficult to determine whether failure to complete them successfully is caused by a sensory or a perceptual problem (e.g., difficulty in separating the food from the background of the plate), a cognitive problem (e.g., forgetting what the sequence of tasks is or inability to attend long enough to complete the task), or a motor limitation (e.g., inability to activate the control interface or inability to physically remove the food from the spoon because of lack of oral-motor control).

Motor control is the result of the integration of sensory, perceptual, and cognitive components into a motor pattern that is executed by the effectors. This process involves many degrees of feedback and feed-forward control, and there are many current theories relating to the precise mechanisms involved (see Burgess, 1989, for example). The term *motor control* refers to the central processing components of effector regulation. These components may be in the brain or spinal cord, and smooth, precise movements are possible only through integration of information from the sensors, other central nervous system (CNS) components (e.g., perception, decision making), and feedback from the effectors.

Motor planning is used to describe the process by which purposeful movements are executed to accomplish a purposeful task (Warren, 1991). This is a central processing activity that requires the highest level of motor control. For example, the tasks of writing, eating, using a hand tool, and typing all require motor planning for successful completion. *Motor learning* occurs as a task is practiced over and over, and many tasks become automatic with practice (i.e., we are not aware of the individual steps in the task). The learner must concentrate on each step to learn the task. However, although the task may become automatic or subconscious, motor planning is still involved; an individual with CNS damage may lose this ability. Thus motor output involves sensory data collection (from internal and external sensors), interpretation and integration of these data (perception), conscious planning of a movement (not always necessary), development of a movement pattern that is responsive to the plan and consistent with the sensory data (motor control), and execution of the movement (effectors). Motor control is discussed in detail later in this chapter.

Psychosocial function consists of identity, self-protection, and motivation. These factors are related to the acceptance of a disability, the approach a person takes to the assistive technology, and how effective the technology can be for the person. Concepts from self-identity and self-protection are used to describe how a person with a disability might interact with assistive technologies and how successful he is likely to be in using them. Motivation greatly influences how much an individual works to develop skill in using an assistive technology and the degree to which he or she is successful in that use.

Limitations in function can occur in any of these areas as a result of trauma, disease, or a congenital condition. A major goal of assessment for the purpose of designing assistive technology systems is to identify the disabled person's skills in the areas of sensory function, central processing, and motor output and control.

■ SENSORY FUNCTION AS RELATED TO ASSISTIVE TECHNOLOGY USE

In this section the major sensory systems that are involved in assistive technology system use are described. The emphasis is on human sensory performance and how it affects use of assistive technologies to compensate for sensory limitations. These compensatory technologies are discussed in succeeding chapters.

Visual Function

Visual function is important (but not essential) for the effective use of assistive technology systems, especially regarding access systems. For example, in using augmentative communication systems, individual items must be found in arrays of vocabulary elements, scanning cursors must be tracked, and visual feedback is often used to signify successful message generation. Likewise, to use a powered wheelchair, visual scanning of the environment must be present, and there must be adequate acuity and visual field to guide the chair around obstacles effectively, safely, and efficiently. For individuals who have visual impairments, reading print material or computer displays can be difficult or impossible, and assistive technologies can be of help.

When an individual's primary disability is visual, it is obvious that the assistive technology must accommodate needs in this area. Often other modalities must be used, typically auditory or tactile senses; general purpose visual substitution systems for mobility and reading are discussed in Chapter 8. However, as Cress et al (1981) point out, the incidence of visual impairment in individuals with severe physical disabilities may be as high as 75% to 90%. Often these visual difficulties are not identified or treated. Because assistive technology application is so dependent on the use of visual input, visual function must be carefully evaluated (see Chapter 4), and it is necessary to specify and design systems to account for special visual requirements. Several types of measurements are typically used to assess visual capability. These include visual acuity (target size), visual range or field size, visual tracking (following a target), and visual scanning (finding a specific visual target in a field of several targets). Each of these is important in the use of assistive technology systems; how they are measured is described in Chapter 4.

Visual Acuity.　The term *visual acuity* is used to refer to all those aspects of the visual system that are related to focusing an image on the retina and extracting sensory data from that image. Three factors are important in this process: (1) size of the object, (2) contrast between the object and the background, and (3) spacing between the object and surrounding background objects. One way to measure the size of an object is to determine the visual angle formed by that object when it is viewed at a known distance. Figure 3-2 illustrates the concept of visual angle. Visual angles of common objects include 13 minutes of arc for pica-typed letters,

2 minutes for a quarter held at arm's length, and 1 second for a quarter at 3 miles (Bailey, 1989). The minimal visual angle threshold for the eye is approximately 1 second of arc; however, the recommended visual angle for ease of viewing in normal light is 15 minutes of arc (21 minutes in reduced light) (Bailey, 1989).

Visual angle describes only the size of an object that is detectable. Contrast between the object and the background is equally important, and the visual threshold of interest is brightness. The minimal detectable brightness for normal human vision is a single candle seen at 30 miles on a dark, clear night (Bailey, 1989). This distance translates into measurable units of 10^{-6} millilamberts. For comparison, a tungsten filament light bulb emits 1 million millilamberts, and white paper has a brightness of 10 millilamberts in good reading light. The absolute value of the emission or reflection of light from an object is not as important as the degree to which the object differs from the background. The visual system functions best when contrast is high (Dunn, 1991). Busy visual fields have too many competing objects for the visual system to extract important visual data. In later chapters the implications of these aspects to assistive technology system assessment and design are discussed.

The eye is sensitive to colors in the visual spectrum (from violet to red), but it is not equally sensitive to all colors in this range. Also, different areas on the retina are sensitive to different colors (Bailey, 1989). If the eye is fixed and not allowed to rotate, the limits of color vision are 60 degrees to each side of the midline. Within this range, the response of the retina to colors is not equal for all wavelengths (colors). Figure 3-3 illustrates that blue objects are visible over the entire 60-degree range, whereas yellow, red, and green objects are recognizable only at points closer to the fixed (center) point of vision, which has implications for the design of systems for individuals who rely on peripheral vision or who have difficulty moving their eyes to track objects.

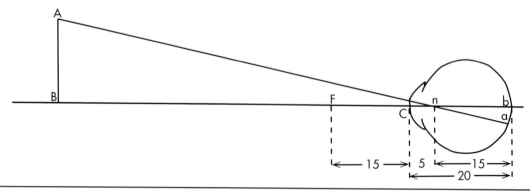

Figure 3-2　The visual angle is the angle just in front of the cornea, *C,* formed by object *AB*. (From Ruch TC,

Patton HD: *Physiology and biophysics,* ed 19, Philadelphia, 1966, WB Saunders.)

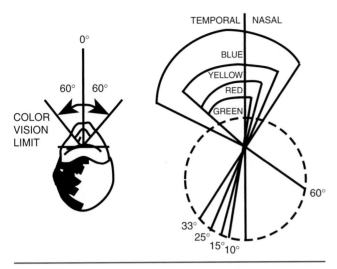

Figure 3-3   Color response of the eye differs with visual angle. (Modified from Woodson W, Conover D: *Human engineering guide for equipment designers,* Berkeley, 1964, University of California Press.)

If green or red is used, the person's ability to see the object may be limited; visibility can be increased by using blue or yellow. Contrast can also be created by using different colors for foreground and background.

Visual Field.   With the head and eyes fixed on a central point, the normal range of peripheral vision in the right eye is 70 degrees to the left and 104 degrees to the right (Bailey, 1989). If the eyes are allowed to rotate but the head remains fixed, the range is 166 degrees to each side of the central point.

This typical visual field may be altered in several ways by disease or injury to the eyes, visual pathways, or brain. The most common types of visual field deficits are shown in Figure 3-4. Visual loss may occur in one or more of the quadrants of the left or right field. Dunn (1991) discusses the major causes of these losses. These types of losses are common in persons with disabilities such as cerebral palsy, traumatic brain injury, and diseases affecting the eyes and visual system. When assistive technology systems are specified and designed, the size and nature of the individual's visual field must be taken into account.

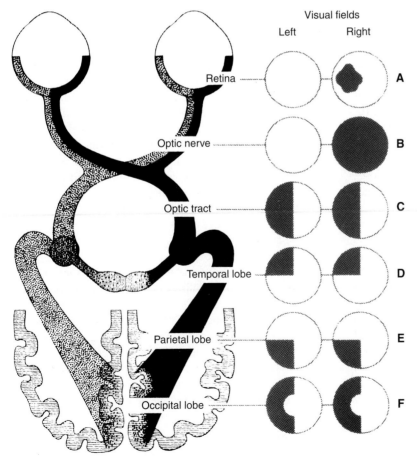

Figure 3-4   Types of visual field deficits. **A,** Retinal lesion: blind spot in the affected eye. **B,** Optic nerve lesion: partial or complete blindness in that eye. **C,** Optic tract or lateral geniculate lesion: blindness in the opposite half of both visual fields. **D,** Temporal lobe lesion: blindness in the upper quadrants of both visual fields on the side opposite the lesion. **E,** Parietal lobe lesion: contralateral blindness in the corresponding lower quadrants of both eyes. **F,** Occipital lobe lesion: contralateral blindness in the corresponding half of each visual field, but with macular sparing. (From Umphred DA: *Neurological rehabilitation,* ed 2, St Louis, 1990, Mosby, p 721. Courtesy Smith Kline & French Laboratories, Philadelphia.)

Visual Tracking and Scanning. Visual tracking is the ability to follow a moving object. This skill is necessary for many assistive technology tasks. Visual scanning differs from visual tracking in that the object does not move; instead the eyes are moved to different parts of a scene to find a specific object or location within the scene. Oculomotor function is required for normal vision and for assistive technology applications in which the eyes are used as an effector (see the section on motor control in this chapter). Conjunctive eye movements are those in which the eyes move together (e.g., saccades, vestibulo-ocular reflexes, optokinetic reflexes, and smooth-slow pursuit). In disjunctive eye movements the eyes do not track together as in vergence during refocusing. These motor behaviors all need appropriate alignment of the eye muscles in addition to the intact motor system, and this is often not the case in persons with disabilities.

Eye movements are typically classified into two sets of systems: those that stabilize the retinal image and those that transfer gaze to a new target. The optokinetic and vestibulo-ocular reflexes are in the first category. All head movements serve as adequate stimuli for these reflexes; that is, the head movement serves as the input that generates the reflex. These reflexes may be impaired for many individuals with disabilities who have difficulty maintaining a stable head or trunk position. Smooth pursuit eye movements also serve to stabilize the retinal image. Transfer of gaze is accomplished by saccades, vergence, and head movements.

Visual Accommodation.   In the normal eye at rest, distant objects are focused on the retina. As the object is brought closer, the image falls in front of the retina unless the curvature of the lens is changed. The process by which the ciliary muscles change the curvature of the lens and hence the focal point of the eye is called **visual accommodation.** Accommodation is quantified by determining the change in the power of the lens of the eye as objects are brought closer. The power is calculated as the reciprocal of the focal distance of the eye, and it is measured in diopters (D). The closest point at which an object can still be focused is called the near point. For a person less than 20 years of age with normal visual accommodation, the near point is approximately 10 cm and the accommodation is approximately 12 D. As individuals age, their accommodative ability decreases. For example, at age 50 years the near point is at approximately 30 cm and the accommodation is reduced to less than 2 D; this situation leads to the prescription of reading glasses. Many types of disabilities affect accommodation; limitations in accommodation are referred to as *accommodative insufficiency,* which can be a significant factor when assistive technologies are used. For example, if a person is using a keyboard device with a visual display, the separation of these two system components may require constant accommodation as visual gaze is directed at the keyboard and then at the display and back

to the keyboard. Appropriate placement of the keyboard and visual display can reduce the amount of accommodation that is required and can result in significantly improved overall system performance.

Common Visual Deficits.   Visual limitations are common in many types of disabilities. Two studies in this section illustrate how these limitations can affect the design of assistive technology systems. One example is of a congenital disability (cerebral palsy) and one example is of an adventitious disability (traumatic brain injury).

Duckman (1979) studied ocular function in a population of 25 children with cerebral palsy. He found that 92% of the children had ocular motor dysfunction of some type: 40% had significant refractive errors, 56% had strabismus, 100% had accommodative insufficiency, 100% had poor directional concepts, and 78% had visual perception dysfunction. These results parallel other reports in the literature, and they indicate that the visual system is far from normal in this population. Duckman states that the poor directional concepts were so severe that "most children did not even have a concept of direction on their own bodies" (p. 1015).

The high degree of accommodative insufficiency was not expected by Duckman, and he stated that "these children almost demonstrated 'paralyses' of accommodation" (p. 1015). Most of the children were unable to make shifts of as little as 0.25 D in their accommodative systems. This finding has direct bearing on tasks that require frequent redirection of gaze, such as looking at a keyboard to find the desired character and then looking at a display or screen to monitor the selections. It also helps explain the success of systems in which eye gaze is used in one plane only (e.g., vertical) rather than requiring movement horizontally and vertically (Goosens and Crain, 1987).

These considerations dictate that great care must be exercised when persons with disabilities are asked to perform visual tasks. For example, communication systems using eye gaze as a method of indicating choices typically rely on printed targets (e.g., "yes" or "no") to which the eyes must be directed (Goosens and Crain, 1987). Given the slow movements, tracking asymmetries, and difficulties with accommodation, it is not surprising that the use of these approaches is difficult for severely disabled persons and that development of these skills can take many hours of practice (see Light, Beesley, and Collier, 1988, for example).

Tychsen and Lisberger (1986) have shown that flaws in the visuomotor systems underlie deficits in the processing of visual motion. They note that the misalignment of the eye muscles (strabismus) in early life results in a permanent misalignment of the horizontal axes for both eyes, even after surgical correction of the muscle defect. Further, their tests demonstrate (1) a nasal-temporal asymmetry in the rate of smooth pursuit eye movement, given a horizontally moving target and (2) a vertical asymmetry in smooth pursuit, given a vertically moving target. Psychophysical judgments by their subjects revealed that targets were seen to move more rapidly in one direction than in the other when the targets were traveling at the same speed.

Padula (1988) describes a similar situation for individuals with traumatic brain injuries. He describes a posttrauma vision syndrome with characteristics of exotropia, exophoria, accommodative dysfunction, convergence insufficiency, low blink rate (related to attention level), spatial disorientation, and balance and posture difficulties. Individuals with this syndrome typically have diplopia (double vision), movement of objects located in the periphery, visual memory problems, poor tracking ability, and poor concentration and attention. Padula also describes remarkable improvement in functional ability when prism lens glasses are used by these individuals. These characteristics and symptoms are similar to those described by Duckman (1979) for cerebral palsy.

Auditory Function

Several types of auditory function are important for the use of assistive technology systems. *Auditory thresholds* include both the *amplitude* and *frequency* of audible sounds. The amplitude of sound is measured in decibels (dB). This unit is the logarithm of the ratio of the sound pressure being heard to the smallest sound pressure detectable by the ear (20 micropascals). This minimal threshold is equivalent to the ticking of a watch under quiet conditions at 20 feet away. Because of the logarithmic calculation of decibels, a doubling of the sound pressure level in decibels is a tenfold increase in the amplitude of the sound. Figure 3-5 shows sound pressure levels for a variety of typical sounds (Bailey, 1989).

The concept of sound pressure level and the values shown in Figure 3-5 are particularly important in consideration of the context for assistive technology use. One example of the application of these principles is Carolyn's use of an augmentative communication device that has voice synthesis output.

Impairment of auditory function has two major effects: loss of input information and inability to monitor speech output. The latter can result in significant difficulties in oral communication. There are several assistive technology approaches to providing oral communication assistance to persons who have an auditory impairment. One approach is to provide feedback, either visually or tactilely, that represents the person's speech patterns and relates them to typical speech. A second approach is to provide alternatives to oral communication, such as visual displays that are read by the listener. These and other approaches are discussed in Chapter 9.

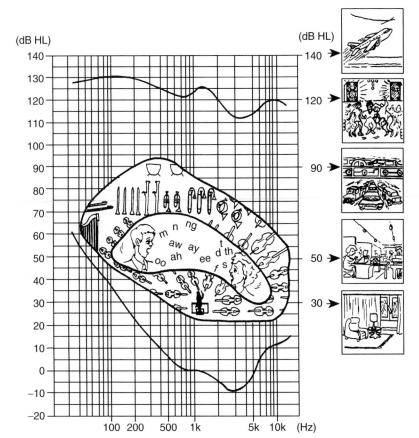

Figure 3-5   The sensitivity of the human ear to frequency is shown on the plot. This curve is normalized to 0 dB at 1000 Hz. The reference pressure is 0.0002 dynes/cm². Along each side and in the center of the plot are shown frequencies and intensities of common sounds and speech. (From Ballantyne D: *Handbook of audiological techniques*, London, 1990, Butterworth-Heinemann.)

Carolyn frequently goes shopping at a large mall (70-dB background noise) and goes out to dinner often. For dinner, her choice of restaurant may be a noisy fast food place (70 to 80 dB) or a quiet, elegant restaurant (50 to 60 dB). Because normal conversational levels are approximately 60 dB (see Figure 3-5), the quiet restaurant is more amenable to this activity. With these data, different voice output communication devices can be evaluated to see whether they will meet Carolyn's needs. For example, assume that the specification for system one is a maximum of 50 dB and for system two it is 75 dB; the greater output of system two generally results in a heavier and larger device because the speaker and the batteries must both be larger to allow greater volume output. If some other things are known about Carolyn, such as whether she is able to walk or uses a wheelchair and how stable she is when walking, the extra size and weight can be traded off against the greater output amplitude capability.

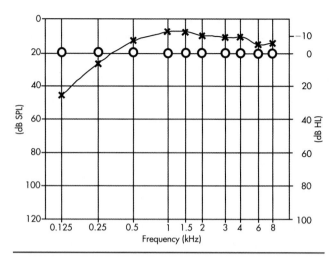

Figure 3-6   Typical audiogram test results for pure-tone testing. *SPL,* Sound pressure level. (From Ballantyne D: *Handbook of audiological techniques,* London, 1990, Butterworth-Heinemann.)

Auditory Thresholds.   The typical range of frequencies that can be heard by the human ear is 20 to 20,000 hertz (Hz) (Bailey, 1989). The ear does not respond equally to all frequencies in this range, however, and Figure 3-5 shows the response curve of a normal ear. The vertical axis of Figure 3-5 is the sound pressure measured in decibels. The horizontal axis shows the frequencies of sound applied. The curve in this figure is the minimal threshold for detecting the sound for each frequency. The tone presented at 1000 Hz requires an intensity of 6.5 dB to sound as loud as a tone presented at 250 Hz with an intensity of 24.5 dB. This curve illustrates why alarms and other audible indicators usually have a frequency near 1000 Hz.

There are several types of tests that audiologists use in assessing hearing. Pure tone audiometry presents pure (one-frequency) tones to each ear and determines the threshold of hearing for that person. The intensity of the tone is raised in 5-dB increments until it is heard; then it is lowered in 5-dB increments until it is no longer heard. The threshold is the intensity at which the person indicates that he or she hears the tone 50% of the time. A typical audiogram is shown in Figure 3-6. On the curve shown in Figure 3-6, all values are displayed as hearing loss, and the "normal" level is shown as 0-dB loss. The curve of Figure 3-5 is incorporated into the plot of Figure 3-6. Thus for 125 Hz, a tone of 90.5 dB was heard 50% of the time in the right ear (45.5-dB threshold from Figure 3-5 added to 45-dB loss from Figure 3-6). At 1000 Hz the threshold presented was 36.5 dB. This test

gives the audiologist information regarding the range of frequencies over which the person can hear.

Although the frequencies presented in the pure tone test are in the range of speech (125 to 8000 Hz), this test alone does not indicate the person's ability to understand speech. To evaluate this function, the audiologist uses a speech recognition threshold test. In this evaluation, speech is presented, either live or recorded, at varying intensity levels, and the person's ability to understand it is determined. The person is asked to repeat either words or sentences presented at these varying intensities.

Hearing Loss.   On the basis of these and other tests, the audiologist determines both the degree of hearing loss and the type of loss. Four types of hearing loss are typically defined (Mann, 1974). These are (1) conductive loss associated with pathological defects of the middle ear, (2) sensorineural loss associated with defects in the cochlea or auditory nerve, (3) centrally induced damage to the auditory cortex of the brain, and (4) functional deafness resulting from perceptual deficits rather than physiological conditions. Auditory impairment is considered slight if the loss is between 20 and 30 dB, mild if from 30 to 45 dB, moderate if from 60 to 75 dB, profound if from 75 to 90 db, and extreme if from 90 to 110 dB (Stach, 1998). Selection of hearing aids for these types and magnitudes of loss is discussed in Chapter 9.

Somatosensory Function

Somatosensory function plays an essential role in the design and selection of assistive technology systems. One view of the role of the somatosensory system is to provide information regarding "where the body ends and where the world begins" (Dunn, 1991, p. 239). As the major interface for many assistive devices, the somatosensory system plays a critical role in determining the effectiveness of assistive technology interventions. The close relationship between the motor and sensory systems is also evident in the decreased control capability exhibited in the presence of somatosensory impairment. For example, persons who have Hansen's disease (leprosy) lose peripheral sensation, which results in a loss of feedback to the motor system, and fine motor abilities are significantly compromised. Poor fine motor abilities can result in significantly compromised capabilities relative to the control of assistive technologies. Somatosensory input is received from receptors in the periphery and includes pressure, hot-cold, tactile, and kinesthetic responses.

When sensation is lost, as in spinal cord injury, somatosensory input is absent and tissue damage can result from externally applied pressures such as those generated in sitting. The inability to perceive pressure or discomfort is especially important in the design of seating systems and cushions (see Chapter 6).

Control of Posture and Position

The adequate control of posture and position in space are fundamental to successful use of assistive technologies. Movement of the limbs or head requires adjustment by the internal sensory and motor control systems to maintain a functional posture. Accommodation to external forces such as gravity or movement also requires constant adjustment. This control of posture and body position in space is an integrative function of the visual, vestibular, proprioceptive, and kinesthetic senses and the motor components of the trunk, pelvis, and extremities. As discussed in Chapter 6, a fundamental requirement for the effective use of assistive technologies is that the user be positioned appropriately.

The vestibular system provides information regarding how the body interacts with the environment (Dunn, 1991). This information is integrated with other sensory data to affect control of body position and to accommodate changes brought about by movement or changing environmental data. The sensory data provided by the vestibular system are used to relate internal sensory and motor maps to the external world. Humans constantly change their position in space to achieve greater functional control (e.g., compensating for upper extremity movement or changes in balance when picking up an object) or greater comfort or to move from place to place. When sensory or motor impairments are present, assistive technologies can be used to help compensate for postural deficits.

Likewise, the design of assistive technology systems must take into account any postural deficits present.

When changes in body position occur because of internal forces (e.g., reaching for a keyboard) or external factors (e.g., increasing the load on the arm by lifting an object), a sophisticated control system provides the necessary compensatory mechanical, neural, and sensory changes (Lee, 1989). This control system features both feedback (sensory data affects motor output) and feedforward (internal commands alter the motor system, with sensory changes following) components. Seating and positioning systems can be designed for individuals who lack the motor or sensory system function adequate for postural control to help stabilize the person and facilitate functional tasks (see Chapter 6). However, many of these systems are static, providing only one fixed position for the individual. As Kangas (1991) points out, static positioning is inconsistent with normal posture, which is dynamic and varies widely with different functional tasks. Kangas also defines a functional position, which allows movement but also stabilizes the individual to facilitate function (see Chapter 6).

As discussed earlier, Padula (1988) describes the use of prism glasses, which allow the individual to place visual and vestibular data in the proper relationship to each other. In some cases assistive technologies can be used to alter sensory perception and affect motor performance. In one case an individual had continual neck flexion and only lifted his head for short periods. When he was fitted with prism lenses, he immediately lifted his head and brought it in line with his torso. Similarly, individuals who demonstrate a consistent left- or right-leaning posture have been brought to midline by the use of horizontally oriented prism lens. In motor-disabled children and adults with disabilities such as traumatic brain injury, these lenses have resulted in postural corrections independent of any additional technological intervention such as seating systems.

The visual-vestibular coupling also can be exploited in other ways. Vestibular and visual function is closely related. The degree of this coupling is directly connected to the degree of self-produced locomotion (Campos and Bertenthal, 1987). Self-produced locomotion allows much greater correlation of visual and vestibular feedback, which has obvious implications for dependent versus independent mobility using assistive technologies. Sensory input provided by the vestibular system (in concert with visual and proprioceptive data) is significantly different when an individual is in control of his or her own movement than when a passive "passenger." A common example of this phenomenon is the observation that the driver of a car on a winding road rarely gets carsick, whereas passengers often do. Likewise, a person with a disability who is pushed in a wheelchair receives different vestibular input than when he or she is propelling the chair.

A recurring theme in this chapter is that prior experiences of the human user of assistive technology systems play a major role in both the specification and design of the system and in its success. A classic study done with newborn kittens illustrates this point for the postural control system (Held and Hein, 1963). Kittens and their mothers were reared in total darkness from birth to the initiation of visual exposure at 8 to 12 weeks of age. A special carousel was used to provide equivalent movement experiences for each kitten. Two littermates were used in each set of experiments. One kitten was allowed to move on its own; the other was moved passively by the motion of the first kitten. Only the kittens that had active movement showed fear of heights, whereas the passively moved kittens did not. These results indicate that development involving movement depends in large measure on the degree to which that movement is self-generated. An example of an assistive technology application in which these concepts are important is dependent mobility (e.g., the person is pushed by an attendant) compared with independent powered mobility.

The importance of postural and position control has other implications for the application of assistive technologies. Given that self-generated movement provides different information than passive movement, it is not surprising that children who are given access to a powered mobility system often initially spend a great deal of time turning in circles. If there is an attempt to "correct" this behavior, the child may be deprived of important vestibular, visual, and kinesthetic development. If, however, the child is allowed to experiment with the powered wheelchair and obtain the new sensory experiences associated with self-propelled locomotion, there will be greater success in getting the child to be accurate and safe with the wheelchair (Kangas, 1991).

■ PERCEPTUAL FUNCTION AS RELATED TO ASSISTIVE TECHNOLOGY USE

Perception adds meaning to sensory data. Human interpretation of sensory events is based on both physiological function and prior sensory and perceptual experiences. Assistive technologies can affect perceptual experience in many ways, some positive and some negative. Because the use of these technologies is often a new experience, a novice user who has a disability is likely to have significantly different perceptions of events and device interactions than do either more experienced users or nondisabled assistive technology practitioners (ATPs). In this section the implications of perceptual function to assistive technology use are explored.

All sensory systems have both physical and perceptual thresholds. The term *threshold* is used to describe the minimal level of input that results in an output from a sensory system. For example, the auditory system can be described in terms of the amplitude and frequency of the input information. These are physical parameters that describe the thresholds associated with sensory function. Auditory perceptual thresholds are described as loudness (related to amplitude) and pitch (related to frequency). The perceived loudness and pitch differ from individual to individual and are typical of perceptual thresholds that are often referred to as *psychophysical parameters*. Sensitivity to sound varies from person to person, and an acceptable sound for one person (e.g., a teenager listening to a rock band) may be perceived as uncomfortably loud by another person (e.g., a parent listening to the same rock music).

A major perceptual task is separating information about one portion of an image from the rest of the image, for example, picking one person out of a crowd or identifying one object in a picture when there are many objects present. This type of task is referred to as *figure-ground* discrimination because the desired object (figure) is extracted from the background (ground). Good figure-ground skill is important for many assistive technology-related activities, such as selecting one symbol out of an array of symbols on a communication device. Many disabilities interfere with the ability to make figure-ground discriminations.

Auditory localization refers to the ability to identify the spatial origin of a sound; it is based on a comparison of sound from the two ears. Separation of one source of sound from others in a noisy environment is also important for successful task completion and for the effective use of assistive technology devices in varying contexts. For example, a user of a powered wheelchair must be able to identify the location (e.g., street noise, a person approaching, a voice calling to her) of a sound if she is to respond to it. This ability is also what allows us to focus on one speaker at a party in which many conversations are going on simultaneously. Dunn (1991) uses the term *auditory figure-ground discrimination* to describe this capability.

Making discriminations of physical parameters is a perceptual task. Estimates of length, distance, and time are examples of such discriminations. Time estimates are an important part of assistive technology use, especially when single-switch scanning is used. Accurate estimates of time require active participation in the task (Bailey, 1989). An active person generally overestimates time (i.e., thinks time has passed faster), and a passive person underestimates time (i.e., thinks it has passed slower). This occurrence is a formal recognition of the old saying "time flies when you're having fun." It also underscores the importance of making the human user of assistive technologies an active participant in the training process. For example, computer-based games are often used to develop switch skills. In this approach, the disabled child is required to activate a switch to obtain interesting graphic or auditory results. Using this approach, the child may activate the switch many times in a session to obtain new results, and a training session of 30 minutes may pass very quickly. Conversely, if the switch is connected to less interesting results, such as a single light or tone, and the child is asked to practice hitting it, the training session time may drag for both the child and the teacher.

One of the major accomplishments of early childhood development is independent mobility, and early perceptual development is directly related to the acquisition of this skill. In children with motor disabilities, independent mobility is often dependent on the use of assistive technologies. Campos and Bertenthal (1987) studied the relationship between independent locomotion and perceptual development. They point out the importance of considering both growth and learning as important aspects of development. Campos and Bertenthal used an experimental paradigm that measured fear of heights (as determined by heart rate increases) in children who had developed locomotion and in those who were prelocomotor. They found that height wariness was greater in children who were independently mobile than in those who were not. They also found that the height wariness of prelocomotor infants (less than 12 months old) who had used walkers was higher than that of those who had not. In a related experiment, they studied a motorically disabled infant who had a cast and brace preventing independent mobility. When the cast and brace were removed, they found that the infant's wariness of heights increased. These and other studies demonstrate the relationship between motor experience and perceptual development and the role of assistive technologies in each. Kermoian (1998) describes evidence relating early mobility to cognitive development in young children as they actively engage in their environment. Typically developing children use creeping, crawling, and walking to obtain environmental interaction beyond their arm's reach. This interaction fosters cognitive and language development. Children who have mobility limitations can achieve similar benefits from the early use of assistive technologies for mobility (see Chapter 12).

Assistive technologies can also provide erroneous sensory data—that is, data that are not consistent with other environmental information available to the person. A classic example of this phenomenon is the use of prism glasses that reverse the image on the eye, creating a mirror image of the environment (Bailey, 1989). When these glasses are first put on, the world is reversed and the person becomes disoriented. However, as the glasses are worn for longer periods, the sensory perception is brought into conformance with the sensory data and the person begins to function as if the visual image was not reversed. When the glasses are removed, the person is initially disoriented, and a period of adjustment is required to bring sensory perception into line with the new, "normal" data.

Bailey (1989) describes another study in which subjects who wore prism glasses that displaced the visual image several inches to the left or right were asked to reach for a target. Once again, they adjusted the sensory perception to match the data, and they were able to access the targets accurately after a few minutes of practice. The most interesting result of this experiment, however, came when the glasses were removed. The subjects consistently missed the targets in the opposite direction from the original displacement provided by the glasses. Analysis of these results revealed that it was *kinesthetic* perception rather than *visual* perception that was altered, and the effect persisted for a much longer time than the original visual disorientation had. It was also determined that if one hand was observed doing a task during the wearing of the glasses and the other was not, only the hand that was observed with altered visual input was affected.

These experiments have profound implications for the application of assistive technologies. Because individuals with disabilities often have significantly different sensory experiences and sensory maps of the world than do ablebodied persons, it is difficult to predict the perceptual experience that an assistive technology system will provide to the person. Perceptual differences may result from the sensory input, as in the prism glasses experiment. For example, a person with an altered visual field may not receive visual data that provide a complete picture of the environment. If that person acts on the limited sensory data, he or she may make errors in using an assistive device. Because these errors will be reflected in motor performance, it is difficult to identify them as perceptual rather than motor. An individual who has a motor disability may have difficulty keeping the head aligned with the horizon (i.e., have a tilt of the head to the left or right), which affects sensory input. If the individual then attempts to use a computer input system that requires horizontal and vertical movement (relative to the horizon) to move a cursor on the screen, he or she may have difficulty because the sensory data provided regarding the external world are not consistent with the way in which the cursor moves on the screen. To improve performance, the sensory (visual and kinesthetic) data must be brought into conformance with the perceptual information. This conformance can be accomplished in several ways, such as orienting the screen to the same angle as the head or providing learning time that allows the person to adapt the perception of the computer task to the task of head movement.

◼ COGNITIVE FUNCTION AND DEVELOPMENT AS RELATED TO ASSISTIVE TECHNOLOGY USE

Cognitive performance plays an important role in the use of assistive technologies. In this section those aspects of cognitive performance that most often affect the design and implementation of assistive technology systems are described. There are several problems associated with adequately assessing the cognitive abilities necessary for the control of assistive technology systems. The most important of these is that the assistive technology often provides a function for which the person has no experience base. In the use of a powered wheelchair, the disabled human operator may have never been responsible for his or her own mobility and may not have experience in making the required decisions. A second difficulty is that there are many cases of effective technology use that would not have been expected given the measurable cognitive function of the user.

CASE STUDY

RICHARD

Richard, a young boy seen in our facility, was described as autistic and unable to spell. He was provided with an augmentative communication system that allowed him to use pictorial icons or spelling for choosing vocabulary (see Chapter 11). He was quite successful using this system for communicative interaction, but he was restricted to those stored utterances for which he had an iconic representation. One evening his family was deciding what game to play, and Richard was very interested in one particular game. He did not have an iconic representation of this game, so he typed in "I want to play [name of game]." His family was amazed because this incident was the first indication that Richard was capable of spelling. Needless to say, he got his choice of game that night, and his school program was expanded to include spelling.

Cognitive Development

To specify and design assistive technology systems for children, it is important to understand some fundamental concepts of cognitive development and to relate these to the use of assistive technologies by children. With the passage of federal legislation relating to early intervention and special education, services are being provided to very young (birth to 3 years) children (see Chapter 1). Many children in this age group have special needs that can be aided by assistive technologies. Although many of the principles discussed can be applied directly to this population, there are unique characteristics that must also be considered. These characteristics are discussed in this section.

Changes that occur in a child arise from both environmental influences (experience) and biological maturation (Santrock, 1997). **Growth** can be defined as change arising from physical development of the CNS. The term **learning** is used to refer to changes that occur because of contact with some environmental influence. **Development** is a function of both growth and learning. A careful consideration of development, both current status and developmental change, is crucial to the successful application of assistive technology systems.

Although there are many theories of cognitive development, the work of Jean Piaget (see Brainerd, 1978, for example) is particularly useful because of its emphasis on object manipulation in the early years and the consideration of alternative methods of problem solving as the child grows into an adult. The major stages of development proposed by Piaget are shown in Table 3-1. Although there is some controversy regarding the details of Piaget's theory, the four basic stages shown in Table 3-1 provide a useful framework for us to consider in applying assistive technologies to solve problems of children with disabilities. One of the major factors illustrated in Table 3-1 is the change in problem-solving approaches and abilities as a child develops. The very young child does not approach problems in the same way as the adult, which must be considered in the design of assistive technology systems.

One of the major controversies regarding Piaget's theory is the age at which symbolic representation emerges. This skill, necessary for cognitive functions such as problem solving, was believed by Piaget to begin with the preoperational stage (stage II in Table 3-1). However, recent work has shown that infants as young as 6 months old develop symbolic representation (Mandler, 1990). These skills are acquired by observation and by direct manipulation of objects. For example, 9-month-old infants have been shown to be capable of imitating

TABLE 3-1	Piaget's Stages of Human Development		
Stage	Age Range (y)	Title	Characteristics
I	Birth to 2	Sensorimotor	Child organizes physical action schemes for dealing with the immediate world
II	2-7	Preoperational	Child begins to use symbols and internal images; problem solving is unsystematic and illogical
III	7-11	Concrete operations	Child develops the operations to think logically but only with reference to concrete objects and activities
IV	11 to adult	Formal operations	Develops capacity to think systematically and to abstractly solve problems

actions that they have observed but not practiced. Infants are also able to remember, after a short delay, where objects have been placed. These and other similar results indicate that very young children (less than 9 months old) are capable of forming symbolic representations of objects and manipulating these representations to carry out tasks.

Goldenberg (1979) applies the idea of observational learning to the case of children whose motor abilities are severely limited and who have limited capability for further motor development. He proposes two hypothetical situations: (1) a child whose only motor response is eye movement and (2) a child whose only response is raising an eyebrow. The first child may engage the environment through movements of the eyes that cause an image to move on the retina. This motor action may or may not lead to interaction, depending on whether someone in the child's environment interprets the eye movements as meaningful and uses them as a basis for communication. In the second case, the child's action does not manipulate the environment for the child, but again its interpretation by another person may allow interaction with the environment. In each of these cases the provision of an assistive device that is sensitive to the motor actions of the child may enable development. However, in each case the importance of observational learning prevents us from saying that development is not occurring.

From the point of view of assistive technology systems, the early manipulation of objects and the use of tools are of particular importance. Table 3-2 summarizes some of the early skills in these areas. It is clear from Table 3-2 that at a very early age the normally developing child can and does interact with objects and can use an object as a tool to achieve a desired result; thus it is not surprising that assistive technologies have been used successfully with very young children. Brinker and Lewis (1982a) used the concept of co-occurrences, the provision of a contingent result when the child carries out a purposeful action, to foster the development of interaction skills in infants and very young children. They used a microcomputer to arrange events so that they could be consistently controlled by an infant's behaviors; therefore, the infant was led to believe that the world was controllable (Brinker and Lewis, 1982b). The infant used switch activation to control graphics, toys, and tape recordings of songs or voices. Data on the number of switch activations and observable behaviors (e.g., facial expressions, reaching for a toy) of the infant showed that children as young as 3 months old would develop purposeful movements to cause the contingent result. Given the skills shown in Table 3-2, these results are not surprising.

The direct manipulation of objects by robotic systems controlled by the child is an attractive contingent result in a computer-controlled and switch-activated system for very young children. Cook, Liu, and Hoseit (1990) developed a system that allowed a very young child to interact with a

TABLE 3-2 Early Object Manipulation and Tool Use in Typically Developing Children During the Sensorimotor Period of Development (Birth to 2 Years)

Developmental Age (mo)	Actions
5	Reinitiates familiar game during pause
6	Finds object hidden behind or under screen
6	Imitates novel body movement
6-8	Transfers object hand-to-hand
7	Leans forward to look for a dropped object
8-10	Anticipates circular trajectory of an object
8	Drops one object to reach for another
8-9	Moves to obtain object out of reach
8-10	Pulls support to obtain object without demonstration
9	Uses one object as a container for another
12	Pulls string to obtain object without demonstration
12-14	Retrieves object by pouring if container is too small for hand
12-15	Holds mechanical toy that another person has started
13-15	Uses string to obtain object against gravity
15	Moves around barrier to obtain object
15-18	Uses tool as extension of body to obtain object
15-18	Finds object where last seen or usually kept
15-19	Opens box to obtain object without demonstration or seeing object placed in box
18-20	Imitates two action combinations
19-20	Anticipates result of actions and adjusts behavior accordingly to situations and problems
21	Attempts to activate mechanical toy without demonstration
22	Anticipates means/end and result of applied means

small robotic arm by a single-switch activation. They investigated whether both nondisabled and disabled children would use the robotic arm as a tool. Cook et al used a continuous playback mode in which a movement was played back sequentially as long as the switch was depressed, and the arm stopped when the switch was released. Typical tasks used were bringing a cracker within reach of the child and tipping a cup to reveal its contents. If a child was attempting to retrieve an object with the robotic arm, it was concluded that he was using it as a tool if the switch was pressed to bring the object closer (in the continuous mode) and then reached for the object, and if still out of reach the switch was pressed again. Repeated use of this sequence of actions indicated the use of the robotic arm as a tool to retrieve the object. Fifty percent of the disabled children (all those with a standardized cognitive age level score of 7 to 9 months or greater) and 100% of the nondisabled children did interact with the arm and use it as a tool to obtain objects out of reach. Gross and fine motor skill levels were less related to success in using the robotic arm than were the levels in cognitive and language areas. This study illustrates the careful application of assistive technology to match the developmental level.

As children grow and develop, they are able to deal with objects and schemes of action more symbolically. These emerging skills affect the way in which assistive technology systems are specified and designed for children who are between 2 and 6 years of age (in the second stage shown in Table 3-1). For example, augmentative communication systems that require the use of symbols can be designed and the vocabulary included can be expanded over that of the stage I child. More complicated operational features such as two- and three-sequence tasks can also be included. As concepts of time begin to develop, sequential selection of objects, such as that required in scanning, can be used. For the preoperational child, it is also important for us to consider other characteristics (Brainerd, 1978). For example, children in this age range typically exhibit centration, focusing on only one aspect of an object. Often this is a surface feature such as color or flashing lights; thus assistive technology systems must be designed carefully so that the most striking features are also the most important to their use. Children in this stage also exhibit animism, attributing life and consciousness to inanimate objects. This characteristic can be exploited by making devices fun to use and giving them names. A final example is the failure of children in this stage to separate play and reality; they apply the same ground rules to each situation. If this characteristic is taken into consideration, a communication device can be used, for example, to create strange sounds (e.g., a belch), and we will not insist on always saying things properly. This approach can help the child develop skills in an interesting way and then apply them to other situations, such as moving to a given destination. Examples of characteristics of the preoperational child and their implications for assistive technology use are shown in Table 3-3.

Assistive technologies can play a role in cognitive development for children in this stage as well. Verburg (1987) studied 10 children aged 2 to 5 years who were provided with a miniature powered vehicle. The changes in scores on a developmental profile over the course of learning to use the powered vehicle were used to determine the effect of the device on cognitive development. Changes in scores were calculated in months, and those that exceeded the number of months of the training period were taken to indicate cognitive growth. For example, if a study lasted 3 months and the child's difference in beginning and ending scores was 5 months, it was decided that development had occurred as a result of the experiment. Five categories of development were used: physical, self-help, social, academic, and communication. The major effects of the use of the vehicle were in the social

TABLE 3-3	Characteristics of the Preoperational Child That Influence Assistive Technology Use
Characteristic	Assistive Technology Implications
Symbolic representation	Augmentative communication, use of language concepts in control of devices
Sequencing	Multiple symbol communication, multistep control of systems
Centration	Child may focus on color, size, or shape rather than function of assistive device
Animism	Give assistive devices a personality with names, etc.
Play equals reality	Make use of play routines to accomplish functional goals

and academic categories, with 7 of the 10 children showing gains greater than the length of the study. Communication (three children), self-help (two children), and physical (one child) showed smaller gains. This study illustrates the importance of assistive technologies in enabling learning and associated development. An added benefit of Verburg's study was that parental protectiveness decreased as the children became more independently mobile.

The older child (stage III in Table 3-1) has significantly more ways of using assistive technologies (Brainerd, 1978), and this can be captured in the specification and design process. For example, decentration is now common, and "optional" features that are secondary but useful can be included without the concern that they will distract the child from successful use of the device. For instance, a powered wheelchair controller with a high- and a low-speed feature will be more understandable by a child in stage III than by the child in stage II. A major advance for children in this stage is the ability to apply logical operations to concrete (real and observable) problems. The emergence of these skills has a direct influence on the design of augmentative communication systems to be used for writing in school. Features of word processors that allow editing of text can be included, and the child can be expected to learn to use features such as printing and saving text. It is important, however, that the design of training materials for the use of assistive technology systems be based on concrete, real situations rather than more abstract concepts. Operational principles should also be concrete. This caveat does not mean that they must be "simple" but that they rely on a logical problem-solving approach that focuses on real properties of objects and situations. Among the skills of children in this stage are the ability to carry out complex tasks consisting of several steps and recognizing that the processes are reversible, categorizing objects, combining classes of objects and extracting their common properties, recognizing that problems may be solved in more than one way, and reasoning deductively. Success in specifying and designing assistive technology systems for children in this stage of development is directly related to how carefully these and other characteristics of this age group are considered.

The adolescent (stage IV) is in transition between deductive, concrete problem solving and the inductive, systematic reasoning characteristic of adults. A key change in this stage is that problem solving and reasoning are systematic rather than random as in previous stages. The design of assistive technology systems for individuals in the early part of this age range (11 to 15 years) must include consideration of the transition from concrete to formal operations because most individuals alternate between these two during this period. The problem solving and decision making required for the use of systems can be more inductive, but allowance for basic operation that is concrete must be made.

In summary, the specification and design of assistive technology systems for children are not just a matter of simplifying the features of adult systems. Instead there are specific characteristics of children in various age groups that must be taken into account to ensure the effectiveness of systems selected for them. By taking into account the nature of childhood and its unique "lifestyle," assistive technologies can be made fun as well as useful. This design feature increases the likelihood that they will be effective. Finally, not only is the human component different in the case of children but there are activities and contexts that are unique to childhood. By incorporating the unique features of these other two components of the total system, its efficacy can be further improved.

Developmental Disabilities and Cognitive Deficits

When developmental delay or cognitive impairment caused by trauma (e.g., traumatic brain injury) is being considered, it is tempting to relate an individual's functional capability to the stages of development, such as those presented in Table 3-1. From the point of view of assistive technology use, this strategy is undesirable for several reasons. First, the individual who has a disability has a significantly different nervous system than the nondisabled person for whom the developmental sequences have been established. The developmental delay or cognitive impairment is the result of other factors, and these must be taken into account when evaluating the level of cognitive functioning. Second, it is often true that an individual with cognitive impairment exhibits significant skill in one area but has severe deficits in others. Development in the presence of an abnormal nervous system is best considered as divergent from the path considered to be typical. This is in contrast to the view that development is proceeding along the same "typical" path but is delayed. Assistive technology application is most effective when individual skills are determined through assessment

(see Chapter 4) and the system characteristics emerge from this assessment.

Individuals with congenital or adventitious cognitive impairments may have difficulties with attention, memory, problem solving, language, and other areas. When assistive technology systems are designed for these individuals, it is important to give careful attention to the cognitive demands that use of the device places on the person and to include learning and operational aids within the total system. It is generally not the goal to make things *simpler* for someone with a cognitive deficit but to make them *different*. For example, individuals who have a learning disability may benefit from alternative modes of information presentation. Often auditory information is more easily assimilated than visual information. Examples of approaches for individuals with memory loss and problem-solving limitations are described next.

Memory

Memory is important for effective use of assistive technologies. When assistive technology systems are specified and designed, the role of human memory in successful use must be considered. Human memory is often considered to have three components: (1) sensory memory, (2) short-term memory, and (3) long-term memory (Bailey, 1989). Each type of memory plays a role in the use of assistive technologies. Sensory memory describes the storage of sensory data for a very brief time after the removal of the stimulus. For our purposes, the most important types of sensory memory are visual and auditory. The afterimage that traces the path of a moving sparkler in the dark is an example of sensory memory. Visual sensory memory, typically in the form of an image, lasts for about 250 millisecond (one fourth of a second) (Bailey, 1989). Some assistive devices make use of this type of memory in their design. One example is the Pathfinder (Prentke Romich Co., Wooster, Ohio) augmentative communication system. In this device a set of 128 lights is arranged in a matrix 16 lights wide by 8 lights high. A detector is placed on the user's head, and when it is aimed at one of the lights, the Pathfinder detects it and the choice labeled by that light is activated. The device turns on the lights one at a time from the upper left corner to the lower right corner, row by row. However, although only one light is turned on at a time, the user actually sees all the lights as being dimly lit. This effect results in part from sensory memory, and without it this input method would not be feasible. Auditory sensory memory is often in the form of an echo of the original input data that lasts for up to 5 seconds (Bailey, 1989).

Short-term memory is sometimes referred to as working memory (Bailey, 1989). Its duration is generally up to about 20 to 30 seconds, and it is used for temporary storage of information necessary to complete a task. This form of memory allows us to carry out many tasks associated with assistive technologies. In assistive technologies, short-term memory is used for seldom-used device operational sequences that are looked up in a manual when needed (e.g., how to replace batteries in a hearing aid) or for remembering a piece of information briefly (e.g., a telephone number to be dialed). Because the capacity of short-term memory is approximately seven items, it is important to restrict the amount of information required to be stored in short-term memory. Individuals have difficulty remembering more than seven items if they do not have the opportunity to rehearse and transfer the information to long-term memory. Information stored in short-term memory arises from both external and internal sources. For example, reading this sentence requires using stored information regarding letters and their combination into words, together with visual input from the page. Information in short-term memory is generally believed to be stored in an encoded form. The code may be a form that makes use of longer-term stored information or one that is more easily recalled than the original form of the information. There is evidence that some visual information, such as words, is actually stored in auditory form, by memory of their sounds rather than what they look like. This evidence has implications for individuals who are unable to use oral language or who have not heard oral language because of a congenital hearing impairment, and this must be taken into account when assistive technology systems are designed for them.

When designing systems, several steps can be taken to help the human operator maximize use of short-term memory. One strategy involves grouping information into short sequences and use of patterns that are related to stored information. For example, an assistive device for writing may have several functions, such as entering text, storing text, and printing. If the system is designed so that each of these tasks follows a similar, consistent sequence of actions, then the use of the system will be more easily learned. Bailey (1989) also discusses the use of rehearsal and patterns in codes as aids to users of systems. Rehearsal is the repeating of a new piece of information (e.g., a phone number) to ensure that it is not forgotten. Another strategy groups number or letter sequences into short (three- or four-character) groups and includes similar patterns in the groups. Examples of useful patterns for numbers are groups that end in the same number; for letters the groups may spell short words or be remembered as acronyms.

Long-term memory stores information that has lasting value. Although short-term memory consists of "throwaway" information that is used only once, long-term memory is important for things used often. Examples of the use of long-term memory in assistive technologies include recalling codes used for storage of information, remembering how to turn on a device and use its features, and remembering where to go and how to get there with a powered wheelchair. Long-term memory differs from the other two types primarily in the duration of the stored information. This type of memory is permanent although we forget it. There is evidence indicating that loss of information from long-term memory is a problem of access rather than actual loss of stored information (Bailey, 1989). Designers of assistive technology systems need to be aware of several memory processes related to remembering and forgetting: (1) encoding, (2) storage, and (3) retrieval. Each of these plays a major role in the design and use of assistive technology systems.

Encoding is the way in which information to be stored is organized, and it is important in retrieval of the stored information. System designers can help with this process by relating steps, tasks, or information to be remembered to the person's experience. Because each person has unique, and sometimes limited, experiences, careful attention must be paid to assessing the best ways to encode information for easy retrieval. For example, with speed dialing, in which one digit is used as a code for a stored phone number, it may be easier if phone numbers for certain people are recalled by letters instead of by the digit. Mom's number could be stored under *M*, sister Tammy under *T*, work under *W*, and so on. This method of encoding helps with recall because there is a relationship between the stored number and the code.

There are many theories regarding how and why we forget. From a systems design point of view, these are important, especially in relation to training individuals to use assistive technologies. One of the most important factors affecting forgetting is what the person does between the time the information is learned and the time that it is used (Bailey, 1989). The term *interference* is used to describe the process of forgetting. Bailey discusses two types of interference: proactive and retroactive. Proactive interference occurs when information acquired before the learning of new material interferes with the use of the new material in performance. This type of interference often occurs in assistive technology system use. For example, Tom has learned to use one type of mechanical feeder, which requires that a switch be pushed to the right to rotate the plate and to the left to raise the spoon to mouth level. The spoon action is automatic once the switch has been activated. A new feeder is introduced that gives Tom more control because the second switch must be continuously pressed to scoop the food and raise the spoon, and it can be stopped at any point and restarted. This process can make eating more efficient because, if the spoon misses the food, it is not necessary to go through an entire cycle before trying again to get food. Tom has *proactive interference* if he persists in pushing the second switch only once because this was a previously learned strategy rather than maintaining switch activation until the food reaches mouth level. Even if Tom is able to adapt to the new strategy, he may revert to the old strategy if he is tired or stressed.

Retroactive interference occurs when a person learns to do task A, then learns task B, and finally is asked to perform task A. He or she may forget how to do task A because of concentrating on task B. This situation can occur when a person is trained to use an assistive technology system that has multiple functions or tasks. This type of problem can be avoided by allowing enough practice and use time for task A before task B is introduced. For example, a person with a visual impairment is being trained to use a screen reader. This is a device that provides speech output instead of visual output. The person has learned how to scan through the text by using the arrow keys on the keyboard (task A). Now he is trained to save a file and retrieve it (task B). When he goes back to task A, he may have forgotten how to do it or forgotten details of this task. This is called retroactive interference.

It is important to distinguish between **recall** and **recognition**. The task of recalling information relies exclusively on the person's abilities, with no assistance from the system. Recognition requires the person to identify the proper or desired item from a list presented by the device. This difference is evident in two types of computer user displays, which are discussed in Chapter 7. In one type of interface, called the command line interface, the computer screen merely displays a "prompt" and the user must type in the information desired, such as the name of a file to be retrieved or a program to be run. The second type of user interface is called a graphical user interface (GUI). In this approach the user is presented with a series of icons on the screen and a selection is made by moving a pointer to the desired icon and pressing a button. This list then produces a list of items from which the user can choose by pointing at the desired item and pressing a button. The command line interface approach depends on recall, and the GUI makes use of recognition. Because recognition is easier than recall, it should be included in assistive technology system design whenever possible.

Human memory includes information from all the senses. For example, somatosensory long-term memory plays a role in many aspects of assistive technology application. The feel of a switch or joystick is remembered, and a new, improved control may not be as effective because it is unfamiliar. Tactile memory is also important in seating and positioning systems. Often persons who have had one seating system for a long time are not comfortable in a new seating system although it is more functional. The tactile memory of the old system is present, and the new system must be introduced gradually to ensure acceptance.

When an individual has memory deficits, it is necessary for us to alter the way in which we design assistive technology systems. Batt and Lounsbury (1990) present a case study in which they describe the development of computer use by an individual who had memory deficits as a result of a cerebral vascular accident. He and his wife were both concerned that he had no activities other than watching television, and they wished to make use of his personal computer

for writing and correspondence. This activity was limited because he could not remember any verbal commands, and his cognitive deficits prevented him from using the owner's manual supplied with his computer. The word processing program that he wanted to use featured a menu approach with eight options, which perplexed the user because of his impaired memory. A simple color-coded flow chart was designed to break the complex list of options down into a manageable form (Figure 3-7). This chart allowed the user to progress through his choices without having to remember the previous selections or having more than one option for the next choice. By using the flow chart and a training program, the user was able to learn to write letters and his own memoirs. Writing his memoirs helped him deal emotionally with his disability, and it led to an increase in his self-esteem and a perception on his part that his memory and cognitive processing had improved.

Language

A language is any system of arbitrary symbols that are organized according to a set of rules agreed to by the speaker and the listener (Miller, 1981). This set of symbols may be the familiar alphabetical written language (referred to as *traditional orthography*) or it may be a set of pictographic symbols conveying meaning (such as hieroglyphics or other special symbols) or a set of hand movements (sign language) or gestures. Speech is the oral expression of language.

Language consists of five basic elements: (1) phonology, (2) morphology, (3) syntax, (4) semantics, and (5) pragmatics. **Phonology** describes the sounds used in any particular language and the rules for their organization. The smallest group of language sounds that can be considered unique is called a *phoneme*. To produce English speech with an electronic speech synthesizer requires approximately 60 phonemes (Fons and Gargagliano, 1981). However, different synthesizers or analysis methods may use a larger or smaller number. Phonemes and letters do not have a one-to-one relationship because phonemes represent spoken language and letters portray written language. There are, however, computer programs that convert written text to spoken language (Allen, 1981). Because there is no one-to-one correspondence between phonemes and letters, all these programs require both a set of rules and a large number of exceptions to convert from text (letters) to speech output. (Voice synthesis is discussed in Chapter 11.) Words often have fewer phonemes than they do letters. For example, the word "night" has three phonemes: (1) *n*, (2) *igh*, and (3) *t*. We refer to the generation of language by the selection of phonemes as the *segmental* characteristic of spoken language. Some electronic speech synthesizers use allophones (combinations of phonemes) rather than phonemes. In this case it may take up to 130 allophones to generate an unlimited vocabulary in English (Smith and Crook, 1981). Prosodic or suprasegmental

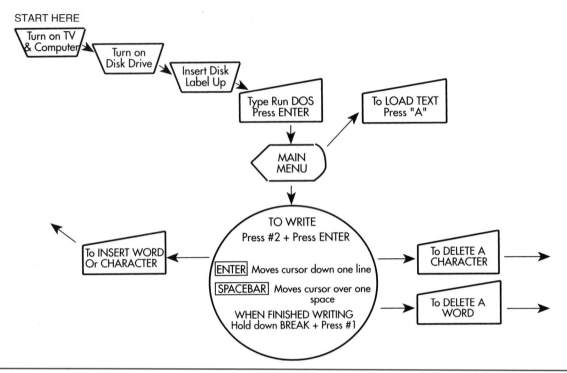

Figure 3-7 A flowchart used to assist a person with memory deficits to use a word processing program. (From Batt RC, Lounsbury PA: Teaching the patient with cognitive deficits to use a computer, *Am J Occup Ther* 44:366, 1990.)

features such as pitch, duration, and amplitude give richness and add meaning to spoken language (Miller, 1981). These features convert a statement into a question by raising the pitch at the end of a sentence or increasing the amplitude and duration of a word to stress it in a sentence.

Morphology describes the rules for organizing the smallest meaningful units of language, which are called morphemes. *Free morphemes* are complete words that may stand alone (e.g., *run*); *bound morphemes* must be coupled to another morpheme (e.g., *-ing*) to form a complete word. *Words* are articulated sounds or series of sounds that are used alone as units of language; they symbolize, communicate, and have meaning. **Syntax** refers to the rules for organizing words into meaningful utterances. Taken together, morphology and syntax constitute grammar, which is the set of rules for speaking and writing a language. Various grammatical rules are used by linguists to describe language usage (Miller, 1981) and by designers of augmentative communication systems to enhance communicative ability.

Semantics describes the relationship between words and their meaning. This is the "definition" of a word. The *lexicon* of a language is a list of all the words in that language. Semantics describes the meaning of the words. There are approximately 100 concepts that have a word in every language (Miller, 1981). The relationships between a word and its meaning can be complex. For example, the word *gold* may mean the color, the metal, or the concept of wealth

(e.g., "good as gold"). This flexibility is what makes natural languages (as opposed to computer languages, music, etc.) powerful. These languages allow us to talk about anything, even without precise definitions.

Pragmatics is the relationship between language and language users. By understanding the rules of pragmatics, a user of a language is able to observe social conventions. No matter how many words a person knows, the words are not functional unless the person knows when and how to use them to convey ideas. This use of language is fundamental to effective communication, but the rules are not intuitive, which is especially important when a person obtains an augmentative communication system for the first time. He or she may not understand how effective language is used, and extensive training may be required just to develop adequate strategies of use.

Both semantics and pragmatics are important in applying assistive technology systems. Barnes (1991) uses the term "motoric language" to describe the language necessary to drive a powered wheelchair. She describes two categories of vocabulary that apply to wheelchair use: relational and substantive. *Relational vocabulary* refers to concepts such as *in, on, between, under,* or *over; substantive vocabulary* refers to the appropriate use of nouns, verbs, and adjectives. Interestingly, Barnes and her colleagues have found that a good substantive vocabulary is more predictive of success in powered mobility than is a good relational vocabulary.

Because mobility involves the use of spatial concepts, relational concepts would be expected to be more important. However, the relational concepts are generally more complex and difficult to understand, so they may develop later.

Language Development

The development of language begins very early in a child's life. At 1 or 2 months of age an infant can distinguish between speech and nonspeech sounds, and there is an inherent predisposition to be interested in communication (Miller, 1981). It is generally believed that skill in language use is developed primarily through practice. Children who are unable to speak because of a disability still develop language. First words are typically tied to gestures such as the direction of eye gaze. The direction of gaze leads to arm or other limb movement in the direction of the object, and this leads to vocalizing (e.g., whining) until the object is given to him and he can manipulate the object. The linguistic functions of requesting and asserting that are performed at this early age by gestures are those later performed by oral language. Table 3-4 lists several important stages in the development of early language (Chapman, 1981; Santrock, 1997).

Infants show an interest in sounds and respond to voices between 3 and 6 months of age. Babbling (producing sounds such as "goo-goo" and "ga-ga") follows during the next 3 to 6 months. Babbling is thought to be a result of biological maturation and not hearing, care giver interaction, or reinforcement (Santrock, 1997). The purpose of this early communication is to attract the attention of parents and others. An infant's receptive vocabulary, or the ability to understand words, begins to develop in the second half of the first year and increases dramatically in the second year.

The first vocalizations begin to appear at 10 to 15 months. Typically, communicative competence (e.g., requesting, asserting, protesting) develops before linguistic competence (e.g., the use of symbolic representations such as words). Vocalizations during the first year are generally more in a play than a communication context, and the child develops a greater variety of sounds than are needed in adult speech.

During the second year, vocalizations and communication begin to merge as the child learns to control the vocalizations sufficiently to communicate ideas and to manipulate his or her world. Not surprisingly, the first words uttered by most children fall into one of two categories: (1) names for concrete objects, usually those that have been manipulated and (2) words for social interactions, such as *move, up,* and *bye.* At 16 to 18 months, vocalizations have several communicative intents, as listed in Table 3-5 (Chapman, 1981). By 2 years of age the child has begun to develop imaginative uses of language and to explore its manipulative potential. For children who have difficulty speaking, the design of augmentative communication systems must take into account these very early language skills. By providing means of achieving language skills that are alternatives to speech, assistive technologies can have a major impact on both functional competence and long-term development. For example, early communication systems should give the child the opportunity to carry out as many of the communicative intents shown in Table 3-5 as possible, even if the child is unable to speak.

As the child continues to develop, the conversational use of language increases and the categories of use are expanded. Box 3-1 lists two of several categorizations of speech acts (Chapman, 1981). These primitive speech acts and conversational uses of language are typically learned by the young child through practice. For the child who has difficulty with speech or motor control, the ability to perform these acts becomes a joint venture between the human and the augmentative communication device. In Chapter 11 we discuss the use of augmentative communication systems.

Problem Solving and Decision Making

Problem solving is an important aspect of the use of assistive technologies. Bailey (1989) defines problem solving as "the combination of existing ideas to form a new combination of ideas" (p. 119). This definition emphasizes the importance of prior experience in developing a solution to a new problem. A problem is a situation for which the person has no ready

TABLE 3-4	Early Development of Language
Approximate Age (mo)	Language Use
8-10	Communicative intent by gestures
3-6	Babbling sounds (e.g., "goo-goo," "ga-ga")
9-15	Utterances expressing communicative intent
16-22	Utterances with discourse function (see Table 3-5)
24+	Utterances with symbolic function (symbolic play, evoking absent objects or events, etc.)

TABLE 3-5	Early Communicative Intents With Discourse Functions
Intent	Example
Instrumental	"I want"
Regulatory	"Do as I tell you"
Interactional	"Me and you"
Personal	"Here I come!"
Heuristic	"Tell me why"
Imaginative	"Let's pretend"
Informative	"I've got something to tell you"

response (Bailey, 1989). Decision making, on the other hand, is choosing between already defined alternatives. Assistive technology systems may require the use of problem solving, decision making, or both. Problem solving is the discovery of a correct solution in a new situation; decision making is the weighing of alternative responses in terms of desirability and the selecting of one alternative. When a novice is learning to use an assistive device, he or she uses problem-solving strategies. However, when an expert uses a system in daily life, he or she applies decision making more frequently than problem solving. Our recommendation and design of assistive technology systems must take into account the skills of the potential user in these two areas. Well-conceived and well-executed training programs can facilitate the development of both problem-solving and decision-making skills in the user. The emphasis of both problem solving and decision making on past events implies a dependence on memory skills.

Bailey (1989) discusses several steps in problem solving that can be aided by computers, and we can apply these to assistive technology system specification and design. These are (1) problem recognition, (2) problem definition, (3) goal definition, (4) strategy selection, (5) alternative generation, (6) alternative evaluation, and (7) alternative selection and execution. To alert the user to the fact that there is a problem (problem recognition), the system must provide information regarding only relevant changes. Assistive devices can facilitate problem recognition in several ways. The most common is through warnings that are displayed to the user. For example, some computer-based powered wheelchair controllers (see Chapter 12) have a visual output that displays a flashing light when there is something wrong (Figure 3-8). This display alerts the user to the existence of a problem. The visual display also shows a code indicating the type of error (e.g., joystick disconnected, battery low). This is the problem definition stage because the device has told the user what the problem is. Strategy selection is based on the first two steps—the recognition of a problem and the definition of the nature of the problem. In this example, a troubleshooting chart in which the error code is listed together with possible causes and solutions may aid strategy selection. This problem-solving aid can then be combined with the user's experience with similar problems to develop a strategy for solving the problem. The problem-solving strategy generally

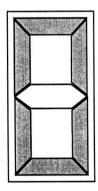
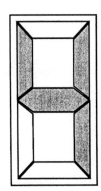

Troubleshooting Chart		
Code	Probable Cause	Correction
01	No power to motor	Check cable Check fuse
02	Weak battery	Recharge
03	Left motor cable disconnected	Reconnect cable
04	Joystick disconnected	Reconnect cable
•		
•		
•		

Figure 3-8   A display and troubleshooting chart used in diagnosing a malfunction in a powered wheelchair. The display is part of the wheelchair controller, and the chart is included in the user's manual.

yields a set of alternatives (alternative generation) from which the most likely cause can be chosen (alternative evaluation). Finally, an alternative is chosen (e.g., disconnected joystick) and the error is corrected. This final stage is alternative selection and execution. If the alternative provides a solution to the problem, then all is well. If not, then additional alternatives must be evaluated and executed until the problem is solved. The problem-solving aids provided by the technology, in this case a warning display and code and a troubleshooting chart, help to convert a difficult problem into a series of decision-making steps. Whenever possible, we should include aids for problem solving in our design of assistive technology systems.

It is possible to compensate for poor problem solving on the part of the user by incorporating some "intelligence" into the device. For example, in the design of an augmentative communication system for a person with aphasia, the combination of pictures or other symbols and categorization can help avoid the dependence on recalling a specific word. A "food" picture can be selected, which leads to the presentation of different types of food (e.g., fruits, meats) or eating situations (e.g., breakfast, lunch). Once a secondary category is selected, the choice can be more specific (e.g., pear, apple, banana). This approach converts a problem-solving or memory task (recalling the correct word or phrase) to a decision-making process (choosing one of several alternatives). By carefully designing the system to accommodate the possible number of choices and steps in a sequence of activities, the system can provide significant improvement in communicative performance.

■ PSYCHOSOCIAL FUNCTION AS RELATED TO ASSISTIVE TECHNOLOGY USE

How the human interacts with assistive technology involves more than the physical and cognitive components. Psychosocial factors have a significant influence on assistive technology use as well. Psychosocial function is composed of both intrinsic and extrinsic factors. The intrinsic psychosocial characteristics of an individual are hard to separate from the influences of the person's social environment. In the human activity assistive technology model, these intrinsic psychosocial factors are discussed in relation to the human, and the person's social environment is seen as a part of the context (see Chapter 2).

In an attempt to understand the psychosocial factors that influence human performance, Depoy and Kolodner (1991) organize the information into three major areas: self-definition or identity, self-protection or maintenance, and motivation for action. These areas can also be applied to assistive technology and can help us understand how psychosocial factors influence human performance related to assistive technology use.

Identity and Self-Protection

In terms of identity the main question that is asked is "Who am I?" The answer to this question involves notions such as self-concept, locus of control, well-being, emotion, environment, and performance (Depoy and Kolodner, 1991). Of primary importance to the successful use of assistive technology is a clear self-concept on the part of the person with a disability. Robertson (1998) defines self-concept as "our definition of the goals, values, and beliefs that give direction and meaning to life" and states further that "knowing who we are unifies our actions, pulls the various parts of ourselves into a cohesive whole" (p. 452). The individual with a well-developed self-concept has clearly defined goals and expectations for the assistive technology system and is more likely to be successful in using the technology.

An individual's self-concept is closely linked to physical attributes. Any changes in physical skills and features as a result of illness or disability can have a profound effect on how an individual feels about himself or herself. Individuals who acquire a disability go through various emotional stages of loss before accepting the disability. Different authors have identified these stages as shock, anxiety, denial, depression, internalized anger, externalized hostility, acknowledgment, and adjustment (Livneh and Antonak, 1990, 1991). The sequence in which these stages are experienced and the duration of each stage vary depending on the individual (Livneh and Antonak, 1991). For example, a woman who sustains a stroke later in life will go through the stages in the process of adjusting to her disability. Her ultimate acceptance of the disability requires a balance between acknowledging her loss and appreciating her remaining abilities to participate in activities of daily life (Sabari, 1998). If she is in the stage of depression when it is time to select an assistive technology device, she may not be capable of exercising good judgment (Scherer, 1998). Furthermore, assistive technology that is recommended before acceptance of the disability may be seen as a reminder of the independence that she has lost and consequently may be avoided or abandoned altogether. On the other hand, a person who has grown up with a disability, such as cerebral palsy, does not experience this same type of process. As Scherer (1993) points out, the person who is born with cerebral palsy is more likely to have adjusted to the disability. This individual is inclined to view assistive technology as opening up new opportunities.

A second critical psychosocial factor is self-protection. The fundamental purpose of the self is "to regulate behavior, to maintain mental health, and [to] maximize each person's productive contributions in valued roles in society" (Robertson, 1998, p. 452). To achieve stability and protect himself or herself from internal and external psychological harm, the individual uses mechanisms of self-protection, such as defense mechanisms and adaptive strategies (Depoy and Kolodner, 1991).

Protecting oneself can factor into assistive technology use as well, particularly if a person does not feel comfortable using the device. For example, there are individuals with spinal cord injuries who may have lived more in their body than in their mind before their injury (Scherer, 1993). As a result, these individuals may have had limited exposure to computer technology and now are being asked to use it for functional activities. If a person is uncomfortable using an assistive technology device, dependency on it can be anxiety producing. To protect himself or herself and reduce the anxiety, this person may avoid or abandon the device.

Motivation

Bailey (1989) defines **motivation** as "any influence that gives rise to performance" (p. 154). In the context of assistive technology systems, motivation may result from the human, the activity, the context, or the assistive technology components of the system. Lack of motivation by the consumer to use the device or perform the task is one of the principal reasons an assistive technology device is abandoned (Scherer and Galvin, 1996). We can define both internal motivating factors and external factors. Internal factors include desire to succeed, and external factors include praise and task-related effects such as feedback generated by the task. Feedback that results from the performance of a task can serve three purposes: (1) provision of knowledge regarding performance, (2) motivation to continue, which is the current state and does not equal the ultimate goal, and (3) reinforcement. A *reinforcer* is a stimulus whose occurrence tends to strengthen the response through a close temporal relationship.

Assistive technologies can provide motivation in many ways. It is often useful to couple social interaction with the occurrence of a desired result.

Because motivation is so important to the effective use of assistive technologies, the goals of the potential user must be carefully defined and devices chosen that meet these goals in a manner that is meaningful and motivating to the person. Depoy and Kolodner (1991) provide an overview of the major psychological theories relating to motivation. They define six factors that determine motivation for action: (1) elicitors of behavior, (2) symbols, (3) beliefs and perceptions, (4) cultural norms and expectations, (5) intrinsic motivation, and (6) history of experience (p. 313). Although the major schools of psychological thought view each of these factors somewhat differently, the factors can be used as a basis for discussing motivation as it applies to assistive technologies.

As we have discussed, elicitors of behavior can be either *intrinsic* (e.g., the desire to please) or *extrinsic* (e.g., synthetic speech feedback), and they are the forces that cause or trigger behavior. In assistive technology systems, external elicitors

CASE STUDY

MARY LOU

Mary Lou was particularly passive, and her use of a switch to activate graphics, toys, and sounds was inconsistent and slow (in some cases minutes). Mary Lou was especially fond of her father, and this relationship was used to motivate her motor performance. A computer and voice synthesizer were used to allow her to generate a spoken phrase by activating a switch. The phrase used was "Come here, Dad." Her father was asked to leave the room, and Mary Lou used her switch to activate the stored phrase and request that her father return to the room. She found this task to be highly motivating, and her response times were rapid. The social reward facilitated by the technology provided the necessary motivation for her to activate a switch, a difficult motor act for her. In this case all three of the purposes of feedback were accomplished, and each played an important role in her success. First, the provision of external feedback provided Mary Lou with the knowledge that she could summon her father. Second, she was motivated to act by the social reward of interacting with her father. Finally, the spoken phrase activated by her switch provided reinforcement for the accomplishment of the motor act, and she was motivated to repeat the action to repeat the social reward.

of behavior may include those resulting from social outcomes (the context) or successful completion of an activity. Examples of social results include conversational interaction, achieving a goal (e.g., moving a wheelchair to a given location), and reinforcement (e.g., getting a high grade). These social effects result because the individual completes an activity such as conversational communication, mobility, or studying for an examination.

From a psychological point of view, *symbols* are abstract representations of reality. Many actions in daily tasks are symbolic, and they are carried out to conform to expectations. For example, a major goal of communication is social politeness, in which the content of the communication is less important than the conformance to social norms (Light, 1988). For a person whose goal is social politeness to be motivated to use an augmentative communication system, the device must be capable of providing rapid and simple output that facilitates social interaction. This goal differs from the use of a system for making requests, in which the user's motivation is to receive a specific result. As Depoy and Kolodner (1991) point out, the degree to which the symbols are shared between the user of the assistive technology system and his or her communication partner has a major impact on the effectiveness of an interaction.

Beliefs have a strong effect on motivation. In relation to assistive technologies, a system must be designed so that is consistent with the person's belief system for the person to be motivated to use it. Among the most highly valued beliefs is acceptance by others. Assistive technology systems can either facilitate or impede acceptance. A simple example is the choice of color in a wheelchair for a child. If the child is allowed to have a wheelchair whose frame is in his favorite color, he may be more accepted by his peers than if the wheelchair is the standard "hospital chrome." A more significant problem in acceptance was (and still is to a large extent) presented by the limited availability of female synthetic voices used in augmentative communication systems. Women have often acquired but not used communication systems with male voices, which is at least partially related to the social acceptance of the total assistive technology system when a disparity exists between the person's characteristics and the quality and gender of her voice.

As emphasized throughout this chapter, *experience* plays a major role in the successful use of assistive technologies. The ways in which these experiences are perceived can also have a large impact on motivation. Our perceptions give us an understanding of events and also provide the basis by which we ascribe meaning to them. These perceptions can be motivating in several ways. Negative experiences can lead to avoidance of events, tasks, or actions. For example, a child who is introduced to a powered wheelchair without adequate preparation and training may have difficulty using the system and may be frightened by errant movements or collisions. This experience can dissuade the child from attempting to use the system. Alternatively, a child who has a positive experience in his or her first attempt at powered mobility will be highly motivated to repeat the actions.

The final factor underlying motivation is adherence to *cultural norms and expectations.* Assistive technology systems must foster such adherence if they are to be motivating and useful. Depoy and Kolodner (1991) describe cultural norms and expectations as "shared, common environmental elements that underpin behavior" (p. 317). Many individuals who have disabilities live in segregated group homes and spend the majority of their time in "special" educational or adult programs. This culture differs significantly from the world in which the majority of us live, and these two cultures may have widely different norms and expectations. One of the major goals of assistive technology application is to normalize the performance of an individual with a disability to facilitate greater independence and broader exposure to the world at large. To approach this goal, the influence of cultural norms and expectations on motivation for performance when using the assistive device must be carefully considered. In some cultures—Asian,

for example—if an elderly person becomes disabled as a result of a stroke, the person's continued independence is not viewed as being important. The extended family now perceives their role as taking care of that person. In this situation, outside intervention, including that provided by assistive technology, may not be seen as necessary. As another example, consider devices intended for self-feeding (see Chapter 14). These devices are imperfect, and a severely disabled person who uses one may achieve independence at a cost of neatness. It may be more "acceptable," in a public place such as a restaurant, for the disabled person to be fed by a human attendant, resulting in less mess. The person may choose to sacrifice independence, as obtained using the mechanical feeder, to achieve cultural acceptance. Alternatively, in a group home setting, an individual may choose independence (the use of the mechanical feeder) over neatness because his or her peers are more accepting than strangers in the restaurant. Another person may be less influenced by cultural acceptance and choose to use the mechanical feeder in both locations. Because no assistive device will be used effectively if the person is not motivated, these factors are important.

In her book *Living in the State of Stuck: How Technology Impacts the Lives of People with Disabilities,* Scherer (1993) presents the milieu personality technology model, which describes personality characteristics as one aspect influencing an individual's use of assistive technology. The three factors described earlier (identity, self-protection, and motivation) are all incorporated into these personality characteristics. **Optimal use** of the technology occurs when the individual is proud to use the device, motivated, cooperative, and optimistic; has good coping skills; and has the skills to use the device. It is predicted that those individuals who are unmotivated, intimidated by technology, embarrassed to use the device, or impatient or impulsive, or who have low self-esteem, unrealistic expectations, or limitations in the skills needed may become partial or **reluctant users.** Nonuse of the assistive technology occurs when the individual either avoids it altogether or abandons it after initial use. Characteristics of the person who avoids using a device may include someone who does not have the skills to use the device and someone who is depressed, unmotivated, embarrassed to use the device, uncooperative, withdrawn, or intimidated by technology. The personality characteristics related to the **abandonment** of a device can be attributed to an individual who is depressed, angry, embarrassed to use the device, withdrawn, or resistant; who has low self-esteem or poor socialization and coping skills; or who lacks the skills and or training to use the device. Being aware of the psychological factors that affect assistive technology use can facilitate the matching process for the ATP and optimize use of assistive technology systems.

Assistive Technology Use Over the Life Span

The person's developmental stage at the time that assistive technology is being considered influences the decision-making process and use of the device. Child development and its implications for assistive technology use were discussed earlier in this chapter. In this section, factors that change over the life span and their implications for assistive technology use are considered.

King (1999) characterizes how learners across the life span approach technology. Children from birth to 3 to 4 years of age are eager to explore and play. They will be motivated to engage in assistive technology by this need to explore. It is for this reason that very young children who are being introduced to powered mobility should be encouraged to explore with the mobility device rather than being asked to follow instructions for a particular protocol (Janeschild, 1997). Children of this age may have some fear of sounds or movement, but they have little or no fear of failure and embarrassment (King, 1999). At this age, they will use any and all parts of their bodies to interact with devices. As children age and their motor skills become more refined, so does their ability to control a device. The fingers and hands are then more likely used as control sites.

From childhood to the early teenage years, children remain eager to explore and are interested in trying out control interfaces (King, 1999). As children approach adolescence, they become more motivated by the desire to be competent than by the need to explore (Early, 1993). Consequently, persons at this age will practice over and over even when they fail. They are not embarrassed about making mistakes or worried about the time involved in developing their skills. Their desire to learn how to interact with technology drives them to seek and accept instruction from adults and older or more skilled children.

The next age span described by King (1999) is the young adult to middle-aged adult, which encompasses roughly age 20 years to age 65 to 70 years. Individuals in this phase of the life cycle are typically engaged in job pursuits and are motivated by the need to achieve (Early, 1993). The young adults in this group (age 20 to 30 years) have grown up with technology and in general are not intimidated by it. They remain eager to explore technologies and are fairly confident in their approach. The middle-aged adults in this group (age 50 to 70 years) did not grow up with computer or video games. However, through their work they have most likely been exposed to some type of technology, and in most cases keeping their job depends on their ability to use technology. Those middle-aged adults who use technology are comfortable with it and not intimidated to use it. However, those who are not familiar with technology are uncomfortable using it and can find it threatening. These individuals prefer to learn about the technology and practice it in private, without being observed or supervised while gaining the needed skills.

Older adults (age 65 to 70 years and older) have similar characteristics as the group just described (King, 1999). They may have had little exposure to new technologies and tend to use devices and tools that they are familiar with. When it comes to using a new tool or device, they may be extremely fearful. Part of this fear is related to the belief that they may do something to the technology that will damage it or result in costly repairs. Given one-on-one training, encouragement, and practice, these individuals have the potential to become highly skilled in the use of new technologies. As these individuals age, however, they are likely to have sensory, motor, and cognitive deficits that affect the learning and use of technology. Older adults are motivated by a need to explore the past, review life accomplishments, and investigate current capabilities through leisure activities (Kielhofner, 1980). Someone who is otherwise fearful of using a computer may be motivated to overcome that fear if given the task of writing his life story or using it for genealogy research.

To maximize the use of assistive technology, the ATP must take into consideration the learning characteristics of each stage in the human life span and be able to select technologies and interventions that match the individual's age group.

■ MOTOR CONTROL AS RELATED TO ASSISTIVE TECHNOLOGY USE

As stated above, *motor control* refers to all the central processing functions that lead to planned, coordinated motor outputs. Many aspects of motor control are important in the use of assistive technologies. To perform a control task, the human operator must be able to locate a target, plan a movement to that target, and produce a desired action once the target is reached. This process involves both sensory and motor components. Sensation is involved in both the scanning of the environment to locate the target and in the regulation of the movement through sensory feedback during the task. For example, one of the tasks involved in writing is to pick up a pencil. The pencil is the target, and the steps in picking it up follow the sequence described above. These motor actions to targets are called *aimed* movements.

As a movement is repeated many times, *motor learning* takes place, and both the speed and accuracy of the movement improves. Another effect of motor learning is changes that occur in the variability of the path of movement or trajectory. Initially the path used to move to the target varies widely from trial to trial. As the movement is learned, the trajectory becomes much more uniform and consistent from trial to trial. This motor learning is made possible by the formation of **engrams,** which are preprogrammed patterns of centrally represented muscular activity (Pedretti, 1996). Engrams develop when there are many repetitions of a specific movement or activity. With repeated, consistent movements, the conscious effort of the person is reduced and the movements become more automatic.

For the sensory and motor components of these movements to be integrated, there must be maps of both the person's own internal neuromuscular system and the external worlds. These maps also consist of engrams, and they are constructed as the person encounters the environment through experience.

This section considers the role of motor control in the use of assistive technology systems and the effects abnormalities may have. The emphasis is on those aspects of motor control that are most important for the successful application of assistive technology systems.

Aimed Movements to Targets

Control of assistive devices is achieved through aimed movements carried out by the user. This control requires the successful completion of a number of sensorimotor tasks. A set of targets *(selection set)* must be visually or auditorily scanned, the desired element chosen, and the element selected, activated, or manipulated through a motor act. This process applies equally to the use of devices in which several choices are to be made (e.g., a wheelchair joystick with four directions or a television remote control with a group of buttons, in which the targets are physical locations) and to objects to be manipulated (e.g., fork, washcloth). It also applies to systems in which the targets are on a screen (graphic) or spoken (auditory) and are presented one at a time for the user to select. The movement to and activation or manipulation of targets may be through any of the effectors discussed in the next section.

Speed and Accuracy of Movements.   Human factors engineers often use speed and accuracy to measure motor performance in moving to targets (Bailey, 1989). In general, these two parameters are inversely related: as speed increases, accuracy decreases. The level of experience the person has also affects this relationship between speed and accuracy. For a novice, the inverse relationship generally holds. However, for experienced users of systems, increasing speed does not necessarily result in decreased accuracy. For example, Klemmer and Lockhead (1962) found that the fastest (and most experienced) keypunch operators were twice as fast as the slowest (and least experienced) operators. Surprisingly, the fastest operators were also ten times as accurate as their slower colleagues. Thus, it cannot be assumed that because a task is completed faster it is necessarily less accurate.

Fitts (1954) found that the time to move to a target decreases for closer or larger targets and increases for more distant or smaller targets. This relationship, called Fitts's Law, "appears to hold under a wide variety of circumstances involving different types of aimed movements, body parts,

manipulanda [types of controls], target arrangements, and physical environments" (Meyer, Smith, and Wright, 1982, p. 451). Jagacinski and Monk (1985) found that Fitts's Law was a good predictor of the speed-accuracy tradeoff for control of two-dimensional cursor movements on a video screen. This relationship held for both a helmet-mounted control and a hand-controlled joystick.

Using Fitts's Law, Radwin, Vanderheiden, and Lin (1990) evaluated both mouse movement and a head-mounted pointer for computer entry. They found that mouse input was faster and generally required less movement than the head pointer for able-bodied subjects. For disabled subjects they found that the speed and accuracy of head control were both dramatically affected by proper trunk stability provided through a seating system. Figure 3-9 is a plot of movement time (the distance from the origin radially outward) versus the direction of cursor movement on a computer screen. Both the dotted and solid lines are for the same subject, who had cerebral palsy. The solid curve represents the speed of head movements when the subject had inadequate thoracic support; the dotted curve shows that movement times were much faster and more symmetrical

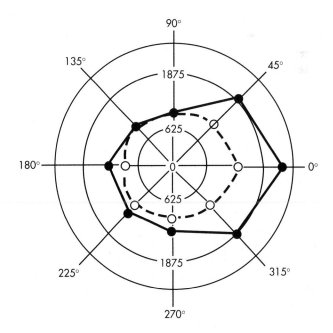

MOVEMENT TIME (ms) vs. DIRECTION (degrees)

Figure 3-9 A plot of movement time, from the origin radially outward, versus the direction of cursor movement, shown in degrees, for a head pointer controlled cursor on a computer screen (From Radwin RG et al: A method for evaluating head-controlled computer input devices using Fitts' Law, *Human Factors* 32, 1990. Copyright 1990 by The Human Factors and Ergonomics Society.)

from left to right when adequate support was provided for the subject. This type of study underscores the importance of providing a stable position as a base of support for control tasks.

Reaction Time. Although the inverse speed-versus-accuracy relationship holds for movement time to a target, it does not generally apply to reaction times. Reaction time can be broken down into contributions from the major information processing stages, as shown in Table 3-6 (Bailey, 1989). From this table, we can see that the majority of the reaction time is taken up by "cognitive processing," with much smaller contributions from sensors, neural conduction, and effectors (muscles). Central processing is largely perception and motor control in our stage processing model (see Figure 3-1). The ranges shown in Table 3-6 indicate differences on the basis of the type of sensory input. For example, reaction to an auditory stimulus is faster than that to a visual or tactile stimulus. Fastest reaction times occur when multiple sensory stimuli are available simultaneously.

The values in Table 3-6 are for nondisabled subjects; the presence of a disability can dramatically affect the results. For example, individuals who have sustained a stroke or head injury or who have cerebral palsy often exhibit **apraxia,** a motor planning deficit in which the peripheral components necessary to execute the motion are generally intact (Trombly and Scott, 1977). In these cases, reaction time can be significantly increased, and it is often difficult to separate central causes (e.g., apraxia) from peripheral (e.g., sensory or effector) factors. The use of assistive devices that depend on reaction time must take these factors into account. For example, some individuals with motor disabilities find it easier to release a switch than to activate it when asked to choose from sequentially presented choices. Alternatively, a step approach in which the user hits the switch repeatedly to move through the choices works better for some persons because it does not depend on their reactions being rapid. This method brings the operation of the device under the control of the user to a

greater degree, and it can result in improved performance. This type of selection method also allows the user to get into a motor pattern that is more automatic. These topics are discussed further in Chapter 7.

Development of Movement Patterns Through Motor Learning

Movement trajectories provide important information regarding motor control and motor learning. Although there are a large number of potential trajectories in an aimed movement task, only a few are actually used (Georgopoulos, Kalaska, and Massey, 1981). To understand this concept, place a pencil or pen on the table. Now think about all the different paths that your arm can take as you reach for the pencil. Although all these paths or trajectories are possible, there are only a few that would ever actually be used. As the movement is practiced over and over, the variability of path trajectory decreases; that is, fewer of the possible trajectories are actually used in accomplishing the movement. Georgopoulos, Kalaska, and Massey also found that reaction times increased as the number of targets increased, but the change in reaction time was smaller than the change in the number of targets. This finding means that use of a keyboard with many targets results in slower reaction times than a single target presented by one switch, which helps to explain why, with some types of disabilities, it is easier for the individual to select from a group of targets once he is positioned near them (e.g., his hand is over the keyboard) than it is to move to the array of targets from a rest position (e.g., his hand is in his lap).

In a similar study, Flash and Hogan (1985) examined the configuration of the arm and hand in space during two-dimensional arm movements. They also found that, with practice, only a few of the many trajectories from a rest position to a target are actually used and that variability decreases with practice in nondisabled subjects. If similar relationships exist in disabled persons, then assessment and training of consumers to use devices that require aimed movements should include tasks designed to identify and emphasize trajectories for which motor performance is optimized. An individual seen at our center presents a striking example of the application of these concepts to augmentative communication system use.

Some assistive technology systems involve uncertainty in target locations, which must be considered if the technology is to be used effectively. An example is augmentative communication systems with dynamic displays in which the selection set on the touch screen changes with each selection. Each time the user makes a choice, he or she is confronted with a totally new set of choices on the display. If the choices are totally random, then motor learning relative to movement to the targets will not occur. However, if the choices are *predictable*, although they change from screen to screen, then motor patterns can develop and speed and accuracy can both improve with practice.

TABLE 3-6	Reaction Times Related to Stages of Human Processing
Delay	Typical Times (ms)
Sensory receptor	1-38
Neural transmission to CNS	2-100
Cognitive processing delays (CNS)	70-300
Neural transmission to muscle	10-30
Muscle latency and activation time	30-70
Total delay	113-528

From Bailey RW: *Human performance engineering,* Englewood Cliffs, NJ, 1989, Prentice Hall, p 43.

CASE STUDY

DOUG

At the time of assessment, Doug was a very proficient user of the HandiVoice 120 (Phonic Ear, Inc., Mill Valley, California). His overall communication rate, determined during an interview, was 26 words per minute. He used whole words and phrases (selected with a single three-digit code) approximately 65% of the time and individual phonemes 35% of the time. Because of his cerebral palsy, he had some difficulty in hitting the keys, and our initial naive assumption was that by providing the equivalent of the three-digit codes on individual keys and therefore reducing the number of keystrokes, his overall rate would increase dramatically. This solution was addressed by placing the individual phoneme and word or phrase labels on the keys of a computer, with the corresponding words or phrases of the phonemes being spoken on key activation. To our surprise, he was unable to use these labels; they were no longer meaningful to him. We then substituted the three-digit codes for the word or phoneme labels. Once again, Doug was unable to access the vocabulary with which he had demonstrated such facility when using the HandiVoice directly. At Doug's suggestion, we placed the HandiVoice next to the computer keyboard, and he looked at the keyboard, visualized the movement required, and then entered the correct word or phoneme codes to generate his message. He had, in fact, developed a set of motor patterns or engrams that he used with the HandiVoice, and he no longer made use of either the phoneme or word labels or their corresponding codes; his motor learning associated with the use of the HandiVoice had progressed to the stage of maximizing motor performance in the absence of cognitive attention to target locations. This skill had developed over long periods of practice with a carefully designed training program using the HandiVoice. This outcome, in retrospect, was predictable on the basis of the concepts of aimed movements and reduction in hand path variability with practice described by Georgopoulos, Kalaska, and Massey (1981) and Flash and Hogan (1985). It is also consistent with the common experience of not being able to recall a phone number but being able to dial it once the motor pattern is begun.

Relationship Between a Stimulus and the Resulting Movement

In the use of assistive technologies, there are many situations in which a device generates an output that requires a response by the user. This output can be thought of as a *stimulus* and the user's resulting movement as a *response*. For example, most computers now use a GUI that displays a set of small pictures (icons) depicting the action to be taken. There are icons for loading a file, running a program, erasing a file, and many others. An icon is selected by moving an on-screen pointer by using a mouse—an aimed movement to a target. The relationship between the stimulus (in this example, an icon) and the response (movement of the cursor with the mouse) is important. Fitts and Deininger (1954) used the term *stimulus-response (S-R) compatibility* to describe improvements in motor performance that resulted from a close relationship between the stimulus and the response. Fitts and Deininger used the task of a radial movement from the center of a circle to one of eight targets located around the circle to study S-R compatibility. The subject was asked to move to one of the eight locations as quickly as possible after a stimulus that represented one of the eight locations. Four stimulus sets were used in this experiment: (1) eight lights arranged in a pattern around a circle, corresponding to one of the eight target locations (spatial two-dimensional set); (2) numbers corresponding to locations around a clock face (1:30, 9:00, etc.) (symbolic two-dimensional set); (3) a horizontal string of eight lights (one-dimensional stimulus set); and (4) eight three-letter first names, each assigned to one of the eight locations (symbolic nonspatial set). Fitts and Deininger recorded reaction time and number of errors for each stimulus set to determine whether any of them led to increased performance (faster times and fewer errors). The fastest response times and fewest errors were obtained with the spatial two-dimensional stimulus set (clock face). This set was familiar to the subjects. The symbolic two-dimensional set (common three-letter names) was second best, followed by the one-dimensional and symbolic nonspatial sets. Therefore, the sets with the least similarity to the task were the slowest and least accurate.

The implication for the design and use of assistive technologies is that motor performance can be improved if the correspondence between the stimulus and required response is high. For example, in a GUI a stored file can have a picture of a file folder and the data file system can be portrayed as a filing cabinet. Because of the limited motor experiences of many disabled persons, S-R compatibility may be considerably different from that of subjects without motor impairments (e.g., manipulation of objects may have been limited and file folders may be meaningless). As motor experience increases, the number of available motor responses may increase, and this creates more options for stimuli that match desired responses.

▇ EFFECTOR FUNCTION AS RELATED TO ASSISTIVE TECHNOLOGY USE

The human operator controls the assistive technology through the various effectors, and the effectors enable manipulation of the environment in a variety of ways. The presence of disability dramatically alters the use of effectors. Several factors are important to keep in mind when effector use is considered for the purpose of controlling assistive technologies. First, there are a variety of ways of accomplishing the same task. For example, people type using fingers, toes, head wands, mouthsticks, and many other methods. This diversity in accomplishing tasks opens up many options that would not be considered if we were restricted to the common ways of doing things. Second, effector function cannot be interpreted from the point of view of a nondisabled person. We must attempt to obtain the perspective of the person with a disability; this underscores the importance of including this person in the process of service delivery.

Description of Effectors

Effectors provide the motor outputs that underlie both stabilization and control. The large muscles of the trunk and pelvis provide strength for stabilization of the body. This stabilization is required for manipulation, or control. Control effectors include hand or finger, arm, head, eye (oculomotor control), leg, foot, and respiration and phonation. These effectors are described in this section, and the processes by which an individual person's capabilities in the use of these effectors are assessed are discussed in Chapter 4.

Figure 3-10 shows the body sites that can be used to control a device. These are referred to as *control sites.* Each control site is capable of performing a variety of movements. The mouth can be used in a number of ways, depending on the individual's capabilities. The flow of air can be used as a control signal. This regulation of air flow requires chest muscles and diaphragm control; to use air flow as a control signal, the individual must be able to control his or her *respiration.* Respiratory flow can be detected by sip (inhaling) or puff (exhaling) switches. Air flow that also includes sound production by the vocal folds is referred to as *phonation.* Phonation may produce sounds (including whistling) or speech. Sounds can also be detected by various control interfaces. If the individual is able to use speech, we can use *speech recognition* as a control interface. Tongue movements can also be used for control.

For many persons with severe disabilities, eye gaze techniques are the first that are used as control signals in augmentative communication systems, and this method of communicative output can be developed to a high degree of competence (Goossens and Crain, 1987; Nolan, 1987). Often the first communication after a major injury (such as a traumatic brain injury) is yes/no questions answered by eye blinks or eye movement. The eyes can also be used in the control of assistive devices by use of control interfaces that detect eye movements. For these reasons, oculomotor function is included with other effectors. Erhardt (1987) uses the following terms, which emphasize the role of the oculomotor

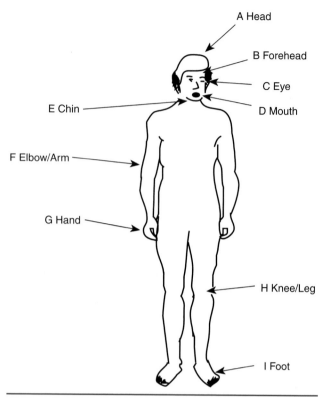

Figure 3-10 Anatomical sites commonly used for control of assistive technologies. (From Webster JW, Cook AM, Tompkins WJ, Vanderheiden GC: *Electronic devices for rehabilitation,* New York, 1985, John Wiley and Sons, p. 207.)

system as an effector: *visual approach* (localization), *visual grasp* (fixation), *visual manipulation* (ocular pursuit), and *visual release* (gaze shift). When the role of the oculomotor system is considered in these terms, its role as a control site is clear. For example, identification, selection, and indication of vocabulary elements in augmentative communication systems involve all these oculomotor tasks. For eye movements to be used to access an assistive device, the eye movement must be detected and it must be used as a signal for communication or control. Often eye movements are observed by another person, and the control or communication is carried out by that person (see Goossens and Crain, 1987, for example). However, there are also electronic systems that can measure eye position and use it as a control signal. Control interfaces for all these effectors are described in Chapter 7.

The head can be used as a control site in a number of ways. Movements of the head include tilting side to side, vertical movement, horizontal rotation, and linear forward and backward movement. Very few functional movements are purely horizontal or vertical or purely rotational with no tilt; most movements of the head are combinations of these components. Upper extremity sites include the movements of the shoulder, elbow, forearm, and hand and finger. Shoulder movements include elevation, flexion, extension, abduction (away from the body), and adduction (toward the body). The movements of the elbow are flexion and extension. The movements of the forearm consist of pronation (turning the palm down) and supination (turning the palm up). The wrist can flex or extend or move from side to side (radial deviation or ulnar deviation). The fingers can individually flex and extend or, together, perform a grasp and release movement. The thumb can flex and extend, abduct and adduct, and oppose each of the fingers. Control movements used in the lower extremities include raising and lowering of the leg at the hip (e.g., hip flexion and extension), knee flexion and extension or knee abduction and adduction, foot plantar flexion (toes point down) or dorsiflexion (toes point up), and foot inversion or eversion (side to side).

When the interaction between a person with a disability and an assistive device involves relatively fine control, the hand and fingers are the preferred control site because they are typically used for manipulative tasks. Even if hand control is limited, it may still be possible to enhance the existing function by using assistive technologies, which makes it possible to use hand movements for control. If the hand is not controllable, then the use of the head as an interface site is preferred. With pointers of various types as control enhancers (e.g., a head pointer), it is possible to obtain relatively precise control with the head. Oculomotor control is most often used for indicating choices in augmentative communication when no other control site is available for pointing. Eye-controlled switches can be used for gross control by using the eyes. Voice allows for relatively fine control with many possible control signals. Simple air flow with no speech is generally more gross and restricted to a few signals. For some individuals, fine control of the foot is possible. For fine manipulative tasks, the foot is less desirable than the hand or head because visual monitoring can be difficult and the foot is generally not as finely controlled as the hand. The use of the arm or leg is less desirable for precise tasks because these represent naturally gross movements controlled by large muscle groups. For this reason, they are the least desirable for manipulative functions.

Although generally an individual's "best" available control site is used, in some cases more than one control site must be identified. This situation most often occurs when one person uses several types of assistive technologies. For example, head control may be used for augmentative communication and foot control for a powered wheelchair. In other cases, such as with some neuromuscular disabilities (e.g., amyotrophic lateral sclerosis), multiple sites need to be identified because of progressive paralysis. The course of this progression can vary from months to years. The variation in ability to use effectors over the course of the disease makes it necessary to find flexible control interfaces that can be used with multiple control sites or to find separate control interfaces for several sites initially (see Chapters 4 and 7).

Factors Underlying the Use of Effectors

Two primary factors underlying the use of effectors are automatic movements and muscle tone. The former consists of primitive reflexes, righting reactions, and equilibrium reactions (Hopkins and Smith, 1993).

Primitive reflexes are characterized by immediate and automatic movement performed at a subconscious level (Hopkins and Smith, 1993). They are usually initiated by sensory stimulation. Present at birth or shortly thereafter, these reflexes are inhibited or (more often) integrated into volitional movements to control posture and perform basic movement patterns as the infant develops. Neurological damage before or at birth may affect the degree to which the infant is able to integrate or inhibit these reflex patterns, resulting in delayed motor development and impaired motor control (Fiorentino, 1978). Neurological damage later in life can also reduce the individual's ability to inhibit some of these primitive reflexes, resulting in impaired postural control and movement patterns.

Hopkins and Smith (1993) tabulate 17 primitive reflexes, including their initiation, stimulus, response, and adaptation in later life. The primitive reflexes that most commonly influence effector use are the asymmetrical tonic neck reflex and the tonic labyrinthine reflex (Trefler, 1984). The asymmetrical tonic neck reflex occurs when the head is turned to one side, the arm on that side is extended, and the opposite arm is flexed. This reflex makes it difficult for the person to hold his trunk and head in midline, prevents use of both hands together, and contributes to scoliosis (Trefler, 1984). The tonic labyrinthine reflex is displayed by increased extensor tone in the supine position and increased flexor tone in the prone position. When sitting, the result is increased extensor tone in the lower limbs, trunk, and neck, causing the person to slide forward in the chair (Davies, 1985).

Righting reactions and equilibrium reactions respond to more global stimuli, and they persist throughout life (Hopkins and Smith, 1993). *Righting reactions* support the vertical position of the head, alignment of the head and trunk, and alignment of the trunk and pelvis. These reactions are essential for the effective control of assistive technologies. Hopkins and Smith also list nine righting reactions. One reaction that can interfere with assistive technology use is the *positive supporting reaction*, which is elicited by pressure on the toe pads or ball of the foot. The pressure from the footrest of a wheelchair, for example, can elicit this reaction. Increased extensor tone of the lower extremities follows simultaneously with contraction of the flexor muscles. The result is strong extension of the legs, which affects upright posture.

Equilibrium reactions provide balance when the center of gravity is disturbed, such as by leaning to one side. As the nervous system matures, equilibrium reactions serve to regain balance. These reactions include the counterrotation of the head and trunk away from the direction of a displacement of gravity (e.g., by leaning) and the use of the extremities to gain balance by abduction. Hopkins and Smith (1993) describe 12 equilibrium reactions.

Muscle tone is defined as the resistance to stretch provided by neural activity, viscoelastic properties of muscle and joints, and sensory feedback to the CNS (Brooks, 1986). Normal muscle tone is high enough so that the individual can resist gravity and low enough to allow for movement (Bobath, 1978). Tone varies with age, level of activity, stress, and other factors. Muscle tone in infants is generally decreased, or *hypotonic,* and infants begin to develop more normal tone as the nervous system develops. As people age, the amount of tone generally decreases for many reasons, including changes in muscle fibers, sensory receptors, and CNS function (Farber, 1991).

Disabilities can also lead to changes in muscle tone. Depending on the level of damage to the nervous system, impaired muscle tone can include flaccidity, spasticity, and rigidity. A reduction in normal muscle tone is referred to as *flaccidity* or *hypotonicity.* When muscle tone is increased, it is referred to as *hypertonicity* or **spasticity.** Several types of disorders can result in spasticity. Increased muscle tone is often accompanied by exaggerated reflexes and imbalances between the antagonistic muscle pairs controlling joints. With *rigidity* there is an increase of muscle tone in both the antagonist and agonist muscles at the same time, resulting in resistance to passive range of motion throughout the range and in any direction (Undzis, Zoltan, and Pedretti, 1996). It is possible for a person to exhibit a mixture of types of muscle tone and for the tone to fluctuate throughout the course of a day. This fluctuation has a direct consequence on effector use and therefore on the control of assistive technologies.

Trauma to or disease of the CNS that results in abnormal muscle tone, the presence of primitive reflexes, or abnormal righting or equilibrium reactions affect the individual's ability to maintain a stable upright posture and perform smooth, coordinated movements. When an individual does not have the ability to stabilize the body, assistive technologies can be used externally to obtain balance and functional positioning (discussed in Chapter 6). Lack of coordinated volitional movements may dictate the use of specialized controls that are enlarged or positioned in locations of maximal control (see Chapter 7).

Characterization of Effector Movements

The movements of effectors can be characterized in several ways, as listed in Table 3-7. By defining the resolution, range, strength, and flexibility for an anatomical site, we can relate these to the skills required for the use of control interfaces.

Resolution.   **Resolution** is used to define the degree of fine control, and it describes the smallest separation between

TABLE 3-7	**Effector Characteristics**			
Effector	Resolution	Range	Strength	Versatility
Fingers	High	Small	Low	Very high
Hand	Moderate	Moderate	Moderate	Moderate
Arm	Low	Large	Large	Low
Head	Moderate	Moderate	Moderate	High
Leg	Low	Moderate	High	Low
Foot	Moderate	Large	High	Low
Eyes	High	Small	NA	Moderate

NA, Not applicable.

two objects that the effector can reliably control. For example, the spacing of individual keys on a keyboard requires relatively fine motor control and an effector with good resolution. Alternatively, a 6-inch diameter single switch used to turn on a toy requires much lower resolution on the part of the effector. All the components of effector use that we have described contribute to the generation of high-resolution fine movements.

Range.   The maximal extent of movement possible is **range.** Some tasks require large range and others require small range. For example, the use of push rims on a manual wheelchair requires a relatively large range of movement, whereas the use of a computer mouse requires a relatively small range. The combination of resolution and range allows us to define the workspace of the effectors. These are both affected by disease or injury. For example, *contractures,* a shortening of the muscles and tendons that limits joint range of motion, may occur as a result of increased tone.

Strength.   Another measure of effector performance is *strength* of movement. Designers of assistive technology systems must take into account the strength of the effector that is being considered for control of the system. In general, the upper extremities function best when precision and control are required, and the lower extremities are best suited for power and strength. Control of assistive technology systems may require that a minimal level of strength, as reflected by the force required to activate a control interface, be available. Even if the necessary resolution and range are available, there may be insufficient strength to activate the control.

In some disabilities, strength is significantly reduced (or absent). For example, **paralysis** resulting from a spinal cord injury prevents the use of certain effectors, depending on the level of the injury (Table 3-8). In this case the major goal is to find an effector that is not paralyzed; head or chin control may be required, rather than a control interface activated by hand function. Partial paralysis or *paresis* is a muscle weakness that makes it difficult to move but does not prevent movement as paralysis does. In this case the assistive

TABLE 3-8   **Motions and Functions Available at Different Levels of Spinal Cord Injury**

Level of Injury	Active Motion Available*	Possible Functions
C3	Neck motion	Unable to perform personal care
	Chin control	Directs others in transfers, personal care
		Uses mouth or chin control for assistive technologies, ventilator on wheelchair
C4	Neck motion	Same as C3 except:
	Shrugs shoulder	No ventilator
		Shoulder switch available
C5	Some shoulder motions	Assistance for bathing/dressing, bladder/bowel care, transfer
	Flex elbow, no extension	Uses mobile arm support for feeding, hygiene, grooming, writing, telephone (must be set up by attendant)
		Uses chin or mouth control for assistive technologies
		Can propel manual wheelchair short distances with hand rim projections
C6	Wrist extension	Independent transfer, dressing, personal hygiene
	Forearm pronation	Manual wheelchair possible with adapted rims, hand splints for writing, feeding, hygiene, grooming, telephone, typing
	Full shoulder motions	
C7	Wrist, elbow, shoulder motions; no finger grasp	Independent sitting
		Drive with adapted controls; uses hand splints for manipulation
C8	No intrinsic hand muscles; limited sensation in the fingers	Limited hand grasp with splints
T1	Paralysis of intrinsic hand muscles; limited flexibility of hand	Weak unaided grasp
T2-T12	Full use of upper extremities; increasing lower extremity function at lower levels; increasing trunk control at lower levels	Manual wheelchair; may use reachers; trunk supports required for higher levels

Modified from Adler C: Spinal cord injury. In Pendleton HM, Schultz-Krohn W, editors: *Pedretti's occupational therapy: practice skills for physical dysfunction,* ed 6, St Louis, 2006, Mosby.
*At each lower level, all the functions of higher levels are available plus those listed for the given level.

technology control interfaces must be modified to accommodate for reduced effector capabilities. For example, an adapted door handle could be used to require less force to be applied to turn the doorknob. In diseases such as muscular dystrophy, fine control is often available but muscle weakness results in very low levels of strength, which may lead to restricted movement over large distances, but fine movements such as those required for a contracted keyboard or a short-throw joystick may be possible.

It is also possible that strength is too great for adequate control. This situation often occurs when the foot is used for fine control such as typing on a keyboard. However, excessive strength is not restricted to the lower extremities. Spastic movements are poorly controlled, and they often lead to force in excess of that required for control. Because many control interfaces, such as joysticks, are designed for normal upper extremity levels of force, the excessive forces generated by spastic movements can result in damage to the assistive technology system, as well as to poor performance.

Endurance.   ATPs are also interested in the ability of an individual to sustain a force. In contrast to strength, which is an indicator of the maximal force that can be exerted by an effector, *endurance* refers to the ability to sustain a force

and to repeat the application of a force over time. In other neuromuscular disabilities, such as myasthenia gravis, the problem is one of *fatigue,* and initial strength may be within a normal range. However, as the individual repeats a movement, there is a continual decrease in performance until total fatigue occurs. Aspects of the assistive technology system design can minimize the effect of fatigue in several ways. First, the interface between the human and the device can be designed to minimize the amount of fatigue by requiring low energy expenditure. The device can also be designed so that it is flexible and reduces the amount of effort as the person tires. An example of the first approach is a joystick for a wheelchair, which requires very little travel and small force. An example of adaptation to fatigue is a variable scanning rate so that when the user is fresh, the scanning is rapid (and selections can be made quickly), but when the person tires, the scan rate slows down to accommodate. The slowdown could be automatically triggered by erroneous entries or manually selected by the user or an attendant. These approaches may be necessary to allow continued functional performance in the presence of fatigue. The careful consideration of the strength and endurance available to move an effector is crucial to the successful application of assistive technology systems.

Versatility. Some effectors are capable of being used for a variety of tasks and in a variety of different ways for the same task. This characteristic is called *versatility*. For example, both the hand (fingers) and foot (toes) can be used to press a key or switch. However, the hand can also be used to grasp a handle (e.g., a joystick). Thus the hand is more versatile than the foot. The higher the versatility, the more options provided for the use of the effector to control an assistive device, which is directly reflected in our choice of control interfaces (see Chapter 7) and in the overall design of the human-technology interface.

■ SUMMARY

The emphasis of this chapter has been on the human operator of assistive technologies. The use of the basic information processing model shown in Figure 3-1 allows us to describe the many components that underlie human performance. This model is also used in succeeding chapters as we discuss specific assistive technology systems. The next chapter explores the assessment of these areas of performance for the purpose of matching assistive technologies to the skills and needs of persons with disabilities.

Study Questions

1. Distinguish between sensation and perception.
2. Assume that you determine the total reaction time for an upper-arm reaching task. Referring to Table 3-6, how would you expect the various components of this total to change (i.e., increase or decrease) given the following conditions: (a) muscular dystrophy, (b) spinal cord injury at the T2 level, (c) traumatic brain injury, (d) cerebral palsy, (e) Hansen's disease (loss of peripheral sensation)?
3. What is the difference between visual tracking and visual scanning? How do the oculomotor mechanisms that underlie them differ?
4. What is visual accommodation, and how can it affect assistive technology use?
5. What are the three major characteristics that can be changed to increase visual input?
6. If you knew that a person with whom you were working had a severe peripheral visual loss, what color of stimulus would you use to try to maximize visibility (refer to Figure 3-3)?
7. If a person is reported as having a 40-dB hearing loss at 2000 Hz, what was the actual intensity of sound applied to the ear (refer to Figure 3-6)?
8. How is the degree of self-produced locomotion related to integration of visual and vestibular sensory function? Relate this to dependent and independent wheeled mobility.
9. Explain why prism glasses experiments produce the results they do, including the effects on kinesthetic perception.
10. Assume that you are trying to develop a word processing program for use as an augmentative writing system. How would your design differ for a preoperational, concrete operational, and formal operations person? Focus on the user interface (screen commands, loading files, etc.) to the system and special features that you would or would not include. Also include the method you would use to introduce the program to each group.
11. Is motor capability necessary for the development of cognitive skills? If yes, how much capability is required? Explain and justify your answer.
12. What are the major notions involved in self-concept?
13. How is self-concept related to the physical abilities and attributes of the assistive technology user?
14. List and describe the stages of loss typically experienced by a person who has sustained an injury or disease that results in permanent disability.
15. How is the concept of self-protection related to the acquisition and use of assistive technologies?
16. How can difficulties in self-concept or self-protection lead to abandonment of assistive technologies?
17. What are the six factors that affect motivation? How can each of these be incorporated into an assistive technology system? Give an example for each factor.
18. What are the three types of memory distinguished on the basis of time?
19. What is the difference between recognition and recall? How does each apply to assistive technology device use?
20. What are the five basic elements of language? Distinguish between speech and language.
21. What is the difference between problem solving and decision making?
22. Design a flow chart similar to Figure 3-7 for a program of your choice. Assume that the user has short-term memory deficits that make it difficult to follow a sequence of steps.
23. Explain the meaning of the solid and dashed curves in Figure 3-9. What type of curves would you expect if the individual lacked good trunk support to each side?
24. What are the implications of a decrease in motor path variability on assistive technology use?
25. Distinguish between range and resolution for an effector system.
26. How does the age at which an individual is introduced to assistive technology influence acceptance and successful use of assistive technologies?
27. How does the age at which an individual is introduced to assistive technologies relate to the possibility of abandonment of those technologies?

References

Allen J: Linguistic-based algorithms offer practical text-to-speech systems, *Speech Technol* 1:12-16, 1981.

Bailey RW: *Human performance engineering*, ed 2, Englewood Cliffs, NJ, 1989, Prentice Hall.

Barnes KH: Training young children for powered mobility beyond the standard joystick, *Devl Disabil Spec Interest Sect Newsl Am Occup Ther Assoc* 14:1-2, 1991.

Batt RC, Lounsbury PA: Teaching the patient with cognitive deficits to use a computer, *Am J Occup Ther* 44:364-367, 1990.

Bobath B: *Adult hemiplegia: evaluation and treatment*, ed 2, London, 1978, William Heinemann Medical Books.

Brainerd CJ: *Piaget's theory of cognitive development*, Englewood Cliffs, NJ, 1978, Prentice Hall.

Brinker RP, Lewis M: Discovering the competent infant: a process approach to assessment and intervention, *Top Early Child Ed* 2:1-16, 1982a.

Brinker RP, Lewis M: Making the world work with microcomputers: A learning prosthesis for handicapped infants, *Except Child* 49:163-170, 1982b.

Brooks VB: *The neural basis of motor control*, New York, 1986, Oxford University Press.

Burgess MK: Motor control and the role of occupational therapy: past, present and future, *Am J Occup Ther* 43:345-348, 1989.

Campos JJ, Bertenthal BI: Locomotion and psychological development in infancy. In Jaffe KM, editor: *Childhood powered mobility: developmental, technical, and clinical perspectives*, Washington, DC, 1987, RESNA Press.

Chapman RS: Exploring children's communicative intents. In Miller JF, editor: *Assessing language production in children*, Baltimore, 1981, University Park Press.

Cook AM, Liu KM, Hoseit P: Robotic arm use by very young children, *Assist Technol* 2:41-57, 1990.

Cress PJ et al: Vision screening for persons with severe handicaps, *TASH J* 6:41-49, 1981.

Davies PM: *Steps to follow: a guide to the treatment of adult hemiplegia*, New York, 1985, Springer-Verlag.

Depoy E, Kolodner EL: Psychological performance factors. In Christiansen C, Baum C, editors: *Occupational therapy*, Thorofare, NJ, 1991, Slack.

Duckek J: Cognitive dimensions of performance. In Christiansen C, Baum C, editors: *Occupational therapy*, Thorofare, NJ, 1991, Slack.

Duckman R: Incidence of visual anomalies in a population of cerebral palsied children, *J Am Optom Assoc* 50:607-614, 1979.

Dunn W: Sensory dimensions in performance. In Christiansen C, Baum C, editors: *Occupational therapy*, Thorofare, NJ, 1991, Slack.

Early MB: *Mental health concepts and techniques for the occupational therapy assistant*, ed 2, Raven Press, New York, 1993.

Erhardt RP: Sequential levels in the visual motor development of a child with cerebral palsy, *Am J Occup Ther* 41:43-49, 1987.

Farber SD: Neuromotor dimensions of performance. In Christiansen C, Baum C, editors: *Occupational therapy*, Thorofare, NJ, 1991, Slack.

Fiorentino MR: *Normal and abnormal development: the influence of primitive reflexes on motor development*. Springfield, IL, 1978, Charles C Thomas.

Fitts PM: The information capacity of the human motor system in controlling the amplitude of movement, *J Exp Psychol* 47:381-391, 1954.

Fitts PM, Deininger RL: S-R compatibility: correspondence among paired elements within stimulus and response codes, *J Exp Psychol* 48:483-492, 1954.

Flash T, Hogan N: The coordination of arm movements: an experimentally confirmed mathematical model, *J Neurosci* 5:1688-1703, 1985.

Fons K, Gargagliano TA: Articulate automata: an overview of voice synthesis Gelfan, *Byte* 6:164-187, 1981.

Georgopoulos AP, Kalaska JF, Massey JT: Spatial trajectories and reaction times of aimed movements: effects of practice, uncertainty, and change in target location, *J Neurophysiol* 46:725-743, 1981.

Goldenberg EP: *Special technology for special children*, Baltimore, 1979, University Park Press.

Goosens CA, Crain SS: Overview of non-electronic eye-gaze communication, *Augment Altern Commun* 3:77-89, 1987.

Held R, Hein A: Movement-produced stimulation in the development of visually-guided behavior, *J Comp Physiol Psychol* 81:394-398, 1963.

Hopkins HL, Smith HD, editors: *Willard and Spackman's occupational therapy*, ed 8, Philadelphia, 1993, JB Lippincott.

Jagacinski RJ, Monk DL: Fitts' law in two dimensions with hand and head movements, *J Mot Behav* 17:77-95, 1985.

Janeschild M: Early power mobility: evaluation and training guidelines. In Furumasu J, editor: *Pediatric powered mobility: developmental perspectives, technical issues, clinical approaches*, Arlington, VA, 1997, RESNA Press.

Kangas KM: Seating, positioning and physical access, *Dev Disabil Spec Interest Sect Newsl Am Occup Ther Assoc* 14:4, 1991.

Kermoian R: Locomotor experience facilitates psychological functioning. In Gray DB, Quantrano LA, Lieberman ML, editors: *Designing and using assistive technology*, Baltimore, 1998, Paul H Brookes Publishing.

Kielhofner G: A model of human occupation, 2: Ontogenesis from the perspective of temporal adaptation, *Am J Occup Ther* 34:657-663, 1980.

King TW: *Assistive technology: essential human factors*, Needham Heights, Mass, 1999, Allyn & Bacon.

Klemmer ET, Lockhead GR: Productivity errors in two keying tasks: A field study, *J Appl Psychol* 46:401-408, 1962.

Lee WA: A control system framework for understanding normal and abnormal posture, *Am J Occup Ther* 43:291-301, 1989.

Light J: Interaction involving individuals using augmentative and alternative communication systems: state of the art and future directions, *Augment Altern Commun* 4:66-82, 1988.

Light J, Beesley M, Collier B: Transition through multiple augmentative and alternative communication systems: a three-year case study of a head injured adolescent, *Augment Altern Commun* 4:2-14, 1988.

Livneh H, Antonak R: Reactions to disability: an empirical investigation of their nature and structure, *J Appl Rehabil Counsel* 21:12-21, 1990.

Livneh H, Antonak R: Temporal structure of adaptation to disability, *Rehabil Counsel Bull* 34:298-319, 1991.

Mandler JM: A new perspective on cognitive development in infancy, *Am Sci* 78:236-243, 1990.

Mann RW: Technology and human rehabilitation: prostheses for sensory rehabilitation and sensory substitution. In Brown JHU, Dickson JF, editors: *Advances in biomedical engineering*, New York, 1974, Academic Press.

Meyer DE, Smith KJ, Wright CE: Models for the speed and accuracy of aimed movements, *Psychol Rev* 89:449-482, 1982.

Miller GA: *Language and speech*, San Francisco, 1981, Freeman.

Nolan C: *Under the eye of the clock*, New York, 1987, St. Martin's Press.

Padula WV: *A behavioral vision approach for persons with physical disabilities*, Santa Ana, CA, 1988, Optometric Extension Program Foundation.

Pedretti LW: *Occupational therapy: practice skills for physical dysfunction*, ed 4, St Louis, 1996, Mosby.

Radwin RG, Vanderheiden GC, Lin ML: A method for evaluating head-controlled computer input devices using Fitts' law, *Hum Factors* 32:423-431, 1990.

Robertson SC: Treatments for psychosocial components: intervention for mental health. In Neistadt ME, Crepeau EB, editors: *Willard and Spackman's occupational therapy*, ed 9, Philadelphia, 1998, Lippincott-Raven.

Sabari JS: Occupational therapy after stroke: are we providing the right services at the right time? *Am J Occup Ther* 52:299-302, 1998.

Santrock JW: *Life-span development*, Madison, WI, 1997, Brown and Benchmark.

Scherer MJ: *Living in the state of stuck: how technology impacts the lives of people with disabilities*, Cambridge, Mass, 1993, Brookline Books.

Scherer MJ: The impact of assistive technology on the lives of people with disabilities. In Gray DB, Quatrano LA, Lieberman ML, editors: *Designing and using assistive technology: the human perspective*, Baltimore, 1998, Paul H Brookes Publishing.

Scherer MJ, Galvin JC: An outcomes perspective of quality pathways to the most appropriate technology. In Galvin JC, Scherer MJ, editors: *Evaluating, selecting and using appropriate assistive technology*, Gaithersburg, MD, 1996, Aspen Publishers.

Stach BA: *Clinical audiology*, San Diego, 1998, Singular Publishing Group.

Smith W, Crook SB: Phonemes, allophones, and LPC team to synthesize speech, *Electron Des* 25:121-127, 1981.

Trefler E: *Seating for children with cerebral palsy*, Memphis, 1984, University of Tennessee Press.

Trombly CA, Scott AD: *Occupational therapy for physical dysfunction*, Baltimore, 1977, Williams & Wilkins.

Tychsen L, Lisberger SG: Maldevelopment of visual motion processing in humans who had strabismus with onset in infancy, *J Neurosci* 6:2495-2508, 1986.

Undzis MF, Zoltan B, Pedretti LW: Evaluation of motor control. In Pedretti LW, editor: *Occupational therapy: practice skills for physical dysfunction*, St Louis, 1996, Mosby.

Verburg G: Predictors of successful powered mobility control. In Jaffe KM, editor: *Childhood powered mobility: developmental, technical and clinical perspectives*, Washington, DC, 1987, RESNA Press.

Warren M: Strategies for sensory and neuromotor remediation. In Christiansen C, Baum C, editors: *Occupational therapy*, Thorofare, NJ, 1991, Slack.

PART 2

Service Delivery in Assistive Technologies

CHAPTER 4

Delivering Assistive Technology Services to the Consumer

Conclusions

SUMMARY

APPENDIX 4-1A: SAMPLE OF A WRITTEN QUESTIONNAIRE

APPENDIX 4-1B: ASSESSMENT FORMS

Learning Objectives

On completing this chapter, you will be able to do the following:

1. Describe principles related to assessment and intervention in assistive technology service delivery
2. Describe the methods used to gather and analyze information during assistive technology assessment and intervention
3. Understand the relationship between the consumer's life roles and performance areas and his or her needs for assistive technology
4. Identify and describe each of the steps in assistive technology service delivery
5. Discuss the matching of device characteristics to consumer needs and skills
6. Understand the need for training and how to develop effective programs
7. Define outcomes as related to assistive technology
8. Understand why outcomes in assistive technology need to be measured
9. Discuss the principles of outcome measurement and their relationship to service delivery and system effectiveness
10. Understand how measurement of outcomes in related disciplines can contribute to knowledge and development of assistive technology outcome measurements
11. Understand the unique outcomes measurement needs of the field of assistive technology
12. Describe the primary outcome measurement tools developed for outcome assessment in assistive technology service delivery programs

---

Key Terms

Assessment
Client-Centered Practice
Criteria for Service
Criterion-Referenced Measurement
Device Characteristics
Expert Systems
Functional Performance Measures
Follow-Along

Follow-Up
Health-Related Quality of Life
Implementation Phase
Needs Identification
Norm-Referenced Measurements
Operational Competence
Outcome Measures
Performance Aid

Qualitative Measurement
Quality-of-Life Measures
Quantitative Measurement
Referral and Intake
Strategic Competence
Technology Abandonment
User Satisfaction
User Satisfaction Measures

Service delivery is the provision of hard and soft assistive technologies to the consumer. Chapter 1 delineated the components of the assistive technology industry, which has at its core the consumer and service delivery programs. This chapter describes the process by which the consumer obtains assistive technology devices and services. Chapter 2 described a model that is used as the basis for assistive technology assessment and intervention (human activity assistive technology [HAAT] model) and discussed the principles of assistive technology system design. This chapter builds on the HAAT model by delineating systematic methods of assessment and intervention that help the assistive technology provider (ATP) define the components of the model and integrate them into an effective assistive technology system for each individual consumer. The intrinsic enablers of the human and his or her relationship to the use of assistive technologies, as discussed in Chapter 3, provide the foundation for the discussion of evaluation of consumer skills in this chapter.

To effectively provide these services to the consumer, the ATP should be knowledgeable in the following areas:

1. The principles related to assessment and intervention and methods of gathering and interpreting information
2. The service delivery practices used to determine the consumer's needs, evaluate his or her skills, recommend a system, and implement the system

3. The measurement of outcomes of the assistive technology system that indicate whether the identified goals have been achieved

4. The identification and attainment of funding for services and equipment

In this chapter and in Chapter 5 general principles and practices related to each of these areas are presented.

PRINCIPLES OF ASSISTIVE TECHNOLOGY ASSESSMENT AND INTERVENTION

The assistive technology intervention begins with an **assessment** of the consumer. Through this assessment, information about the consumer is gathered and analyzed so that appropriate assistive technologies (hard and soft) can be recommended and a plan for intervention developed. Information is gathered regarding the skills and abilities of the individual, what activities he or she would like to perform, and the contexts in which these activities will be performed. The assessment also yields information regarding the consumer's ability to use assistive technologies. On the basis of the assessment results, a plan for intervention is developed. This plan includes implementation of the system, follow-up, and follow-along. Basic principles that underlie assessment and intervention in assistive technology service delivery are listed in Box 4-1.

Assistive Technology Assessment and Intervention Should Consider All Components of the HAAT Model: Human, Activity, Assistive Technology, and Context

Often assistive technology assessment focuses on the assistive technology only, which can lead to later rejection or abandonment of the technology. One way to reduce the probability of abandonment or misuse is to consider systematically all four parts of the HAAT model. Needs and goals are often defined by a careful consideration of the activities to be performed by the individual. However, it is rare that the activity will be performed in only one context, so it is important to identify the influence of the physical, sociocultural, and institutional elements in the contexts in which the activities will be performed (see Chapter 2). Thus the careful evaluation of the activities to be performed and the contextual factors under which that performance will occur are key to success. Once the goals have been identified, an assessment of the skills and abilities of the human operator (the consumer) must be identified. Only after consideration of these three components (activity, context, and human) can a clear picture emerge of the assistive technology requirements and characteristics. The assessment process must also include an assessment of the degree to which these characteristics match the consumer's needs. Chances of success in implementation of an assistive technology system are enhanced by attention to all four parts of the HAAT model during the service delivery process.

Assistive Technology Intervention Is Enabling

The *primary* purpose of assistive technology intervention is not remediation or rehabilitation of an impairment but provision of hard and soft technologies that *enable* an individual with a disability to be functional in activities of daily living. This principle places the focus on functional outcomes. Through the application of the HAAT model we can develop goals for the assistive technology intervention, and these goals ultimately are used to measure the functional outcomes of the intervention. Approaching intervention from this perspective requires that the ATP determine the individual's strengths and capitalize on them instead of focusing on deficits or impairments. For example, in functional activity of typing, in a rehabilitation approach the goal would be to improve hand and finger control sufficiently to allow for typing, with the intervention focusing on exercises and activities for the fingers and hands. From an assistive technology perspective, however, the objective becomes enabling the person to perform the functional activity of typing regardless of how it is done. The impairment in the hands and fingers that causes the disability is not necessarily addressed. The disability of being unable to type is what is addressed in the assistive technology approach. Through the use of assistive technology, alternative approaches to using the fingers for typing are considered, such as using a mouthstick, head pointer, or a speech recognition system instead of the hands.

This focus on function does not mean an individual's potential for improvement is ignored. The *parallel interventions model* (Angelo and Smith, 1989; Smith, 1991) demonstrates

BOX 4-1	Principles of Assessment and Intervention in Assistive Technology

- Assistive technology assessment and intervention should consider all components of the HAAT model: the human, the activity, the assistive technology and the context.
- The purpose of assistive technology intervention is not to rehabilitate an individual or remediate impairment but to provide assistive technologies that *enable* an individual to perform functional activities.
- Assistive technology assessment is continuous and deliberate.
- Assistive technology assessment and intervention require collaboration.
- Assistive technology assessment and intervention require an understanding of how to gather and interpret data.

how technology can be used to promote the dual objectives of enabling function and improving an individual's skill level. In one track, assistive technologies are provided that are based on the consumer's current skills and needs and that maximize function. Simultaneously, a second track provides intervention that focuses on improving skill level to minimize the reliance on technology. Some individuals who have a severe physical disability may never have had the opportunity to develop their motor skills, and training to develop these skills can take months or years (Cook, 1991). A common example is an individual whose evaluation shows that he or she is able to use the head to activate a single switch to make simple choices on a computer. With training and a period of experience in using this switch, head control may improve to the point where the individual can use a light beam positioned on the head to make direct choices with a dedicated communication device. The latter means of control would more quickly provide access to choices on a device and would be much less demanding cognitively.

Assistive Technology Assessment Is Continuous and Deliberate

Although assessment is typically considered a discrete event in the direct service delivery process, it is actually a continuous process. Assistive technology assessment entails a series of activities linked together and undertaken over time. The activities that occur and the decisions that are made during the intervention are deliberate rather than haphazard. Information is gathered and decisions are made from the moment of the initial intake referral through follow-along.

The ATP re-evaluates progress toward the goals of the intervention plan and makes necessary revisions. For example, during training, observation may reveal that the consumer can access the control interface more effectively if it is positioned at an angle instead of flat. As decisions are implemented, their influence is continuously assessed and revisions are made to the intervention. The ideas of **client-centered practice** (Canadian Association of Occupational Therapists, 2002) highlight the importance of involving the client at all stages of assessment, from the initial framing of the activities in which the client wishes to engage to the recommendation of an assistive technology system. The client refers to the individual and others in the environment such as family and caregivers (Canadian Association of Occupational Therapists, 2002). Assessment continues not only while the consumer is actively involved in the service delivery process but also potentially throughout the consumer's life. Because many individuals have life-long disabilities, they will be in need of assistive technology throughout their lives. It is important not only to recommend assistive technology that enables the individual today but also to predict the technology that will be necessary to enable the individual in the future. The components of the HAAT model change over

each individual's lifetime. Changes may occur in the individual's skills and abilities, life roles, and goals; the capabilities of technology; and the context in which the assistive technologies are used. By using the HAAT model as a framework, the ATP can predict some of these changes and plan for the consumer's future technology needs.

Assistive Technology Assessment and Intervention Require Collaboration and a Consumer-Centered Approach

Given the nature of assistive technology and its influence on the consumer's activities of daily living, it is essential that the assessment and intervention be a collaborative process. McNaughton (1993) defines a collaborator as "one who works with another toward a common goal" (p. 8). Furthermore, she states that collaboration requires that (1) all participants be equal partners, (2) a problem-solving attitude be shared by all participants, (3) there be mutual respect for each other's knowledge and the contributions each person can make as opposed to the titles he or she holds, and (4) each participant have available the information necessary to carry out his or her role (McNaughton, 1993).

Frequently, assistive technology services are provided through consultation, in which the ATP is called into a situation on a limited basis to specifically address the assistive technology needs of the consumer. There may be several people already involved with the consumer, including family members, teachers, vocational counselors, employers, therapists, and representatives from the funding source. The assistive technology assessment and intervention is more successful when these significant others are identified and involved at the beginning of the process.

There is a delicate balance between the opinion and "expertise" of the ATP (based on technical knowledge and experience with a variety of people) and the opinion and "expertise" of the consumer and family relating to the specific needs and goals of the person. The role of the ATP is to educate the consumer of the choices available so that the consumer can make decisions related to the assistive technology in an informed manner. The challenge for the ATP is to do this without unduly influencing the client's choice. The value of this approach is that the consumer and the ATP inform each other throughout the process and develop a shared responsibility for the outcome. This approach has been referred to as the "educational model" of intervention (as opposed to the "expert" and "consumer-driven" models, which take one extreme position or the other). Lysack and Kaufert (1999) describe this process and its benefits.

The ATP should initiate the collaborative process by identifying significant others as a part of the intake referral phase. For example, Jerry, who has a developmental disability, lives in a small group home. During the intake, the ATP discovers there are several key people who need to be involved in the assistive technology intervention for Jerry: staff at his home, staff at the day program he attends, an occupational therapist who consults with his residential program, his caseworker at the department of developmental services, and his parents, who live out of town. Each of these individuals is invited to participate in the initial assessment and decision-making process. Different participants will be working with the consumer to accomplish different goals. Communication among the collaborators regarding their respective goals for the consumer is critical. It is important to identify the ways in which the goals of the assistive technology intervention can be accomplished without interfering with other goals. Sometimes compromises need to be reached. For example, two professionals working with the consumer may be focusing on different goals, and compromises may need to be made by all parties in working toward these interdependent goals. One therapist may be working with a child on improving the strength in his or her neck muscles to improve head control, whereas the ATP's goal may be to support and position the head in an upright position to prevent deformity and allow optimal position for functional activities. The success of the assistive technology system depends on coordination and teamwork among all the individuals involved with the consumer.

Beukleman and Mirenda (1998) discuss the importance of building consensus among the user, family members, and other team members. Negative consequences, such as a lack of vital information for intervention, lack of "ownership" of the intervention resulting in poor follow-through with the recommendations, and distrust of the service provider, may result if the process of consensus building is not begun during the initial assessment. Initiating this process early helps to avoid problems in the future with regard to the acceptance and use of a device.

Assistive Technology Assessment and Intervention Require an Understanding of How to Gather and Interpret Data

It is both possible and desirable to measure human performance, and much of what is described in this chapter is directed toward that end. In assistive technology service delivery we need to be careful that we know what we are measuring. In some cases, as in determining the effectiveness of our service delivery process and outcomes, we want to measure the performance of the entire assistive technology system. Because this system has been defined to be the four components of the HAAT model (human, activity, context, and assistive technology), measurements and outcomes that apply to the entire system must be developed. In other cases (e.g., during an initial assessment) *human performance* rather than system performance needs to be measured. Measuring human performance can be

general or task specific (Sprigle and Abdelhamied, 1998). An individual's *general abilities* are measured when separate components of the sensory, perceptual, physical, and cognitive systems, such as range of motion, sensation, strength, tone, or memory, are evaluated. Task-specific measurement involves the evaluation of the individual's *functional skills.* The ability of the person to complete a functional task, such as entering text into a computer document, requires a level of skill that combines physical, sensory, and cognitive abilities. In this case clear objectives must be established for each task, a clinical standard to be applied must be developed, and then measures that evaluate the performance must be developed.

In this section we focus on the principles associated with measurement in assistive technology service delivery. These include the purposes, types, standards, and methods of measurement.

Quantitative and Qualitative Measurement. Information gathered by the ATP throughout the assistive technology intervention can be by either **quantitative measurement** or **qualitative measurement.** The philosophies of qualitative measures and quantitative measures are quite different. Quantitative measures assign a number to an attribute, trait, or characteristic (Nunnally and Bernstein, 1994). The assumption of quantitative measures is that the construct of interest can be measured in some meaningful way. For example, a test can be constructed that measures the joint range of motion (the construct) that an individual has available to control a computer access device. Joint range is expressed as degrees of motion and a common understanding exists regarding what is meant when a specific joint range of motion is described. Here the construct can be assigned a number that is meaningful to individuals using and interpreting the test. Alternatively, a test can be constructed that intends to measure boredom. It is possible to develop a scale and have individuals rate their boredom on a four-point scale (for example). But what does a score of 4 mean on such a scale? We can assign a number on a scale but it is difficult to interpret the meaning of that number.

Qualitative assessments assume that each individual has a different experience and that it is important to provide the opportunity to capture that experience. There is no attempt to measure a particular construct. Rather, the purpose is to describe and understand the user's experience with the technology. Qualitative assessments may include observation, either directly or by videotape or interview with the client and others. Qualitative assessments often capture those experiences that cannot be directly quantified or for which quantification holds little meaning. They provide the client with the opportunity to identify issues, experiences, or goals that may not be previously identified on a quantitative measure.

Both qualitative and quantitative assessment formats are important in the AT assessment process and for evaluation of the outcomes of AT use. Quantitative measures allow comparison of experiences of a large number of individuals and a well-constructed instrument is essential in building evidence to support the efficacy of AT use. Qualitative methods provide a rich description of the experiences of AT use, which may not be readily apparent from the use of quantitative instruments alone. Together these methods can provide strong support for AT use, both on an individual and collective basis.

Norm-Referenced and Criterion-Referenced Measurements. Two commonly used standards are available for measuring performance (for both the human and the total system): norm referenced and criterion referenced. In **norm-referenced measurements** the performance of the individual or system is ranked according to a sample of scores others have achieved on the task. Norm-referenced measures usually produce a percentile rank, a standardized score, or a grade equivalent that indicates where the individual stands relative to others in the representative sample (Witt and Cavell, 1986). When selecting a norm-referenced test for use, it is important to review how the norms were developed. Norms need to be relevant to the population for which the instrument is being used. They need to be recent and representative (Wiersma and Jurs, 1990). In other words, the characteristics of the sample used to develop the norms must be similar to those of the client group for which

the assessment is being used. The items that form the instrument need to be relevant to the client group. For example, assessing visual-perceptual skills by using blocks is not relevant for most adults. Similarly, use of outdated questions or materials will not give an accurate picture of the client's abilities. For example, testing keyboarding skills on a typewriter will give some information on keyboarding skills but does not cover the full range of skills required to use a computer (Miller Polgar, 2003). An alternative way to assess human or system performance is to rate the performance according to a specified criterion or level of mastery, which is referred to as **criterion-referenced measurement,** and the person's own skill level in using the system is used as the standard. As an example of this approach, Jagacinski and Monk (1985) evaluated joystick and head pointer use by young adult nondisabled subjects. They found that skill in using these devices is acquired with some difficulty over many trials. The criterion used was whether the individual's performance (time to move to target) did not change by more than 3% over a period of 4 consecutive days (Figure 4-1). In Figure 4-1, the horizontal axis represents the elapsed practice time and the vertical axis represents how quickly the person has been able to use the joystick or head pointer to move to a target. The horizontal dotted line is the final level of performance and serves as the criterion of performance. Using this criterion, they found that joystick use required 6 to 18 days and head pointer use required 7 to 29 days of practice to reach the criterion level of performance.

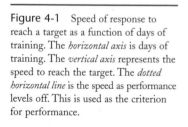

Figure 4-1   Speed of response to reach a target as a function of days of training. The *horizontal axis* is days of training. The *vertical axis* represents the speed to reach the target. The *dotted horizontal line* is the speed as performance levels off. This is used as the criterion for performance.

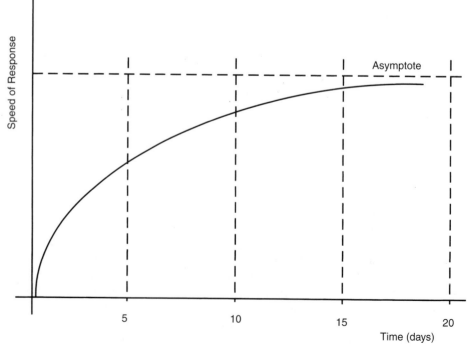

When the criterion-referenced approach to measurement is used, two desirable goals are accomplished. First, the assessment of progress is based on the person's unique set of skills and there is no attempt to relate this performance to a normalized standard. In this example, the two alternative ways of accomplishing the same task (joystick and head pointer) are compared to determine which method is likely to result in a higher skill level. The second goal is accomplished by using the person's own performance as a standard for measuring progress. Goal attainment scaling (King et al, 1999) is one standardized process of developing criteria that are specific to the client and task that are then applied to evaluate outcomes.

Methods for Gathering and Interpreting Information.
There are several methods used to gather and interpret quantitative and qualitative information about the consumer: (1) collection of the initial database, (2) interview procedures, (3) clinical assessment, and (4) formal assessment procedures (Dunn, 1991). Often, more than one method is used to gather information about the same aspect of a consumer's skills, the context, the activity, or the use of assistive technology. For example, information on an individual's hand function can be collected through each of these methods. The use of multiple sources of information is illustrated by Sam, a 22-year-old man with quadriplegia secondary to a complete C6 lesion of the spinal cord, who is being evaluated for his ability to access a computer.

Information collected for the *initial database* may include the reason for referral, medical diagnosis, and educational and vocational background information. This information is collected during the referral and intake phase of the service delivery process; its purpose is to provide preliminary data for planning the assessment. Sam's medical diagnosis is complete quadriplegia at the C6 level. If we refer to a text describing the effects of spinal cord injury at the C6 level on arm function (see Table 3-8), we expect Sam to have scapular movements, shoulder flexion, elbow flexion, and wrist extension but to lack finger flexion and extension. Most medical histories do not provide information on the consumer's assets and functional abilities. In some cases we may unintentionally limit the consumer's potential if we fail to look beyond the expectations we have acquired on the basis of the medical diagnosis. As Christiansen (1991) points out, a medical diagnosis may provide guidelines for the assessment and expectations regarding the nature of the consumer's impairments, but it is inadequate for planning intervention.

The *interview*, another way to collect information, can occur at different points in the service delivery process. Typically, an initial interview takes place during the needs identification phase as a means of gathering information regarding the consumer and his or her needs. It is important that the consumer, family members, rehabilitation or education professionals, and other care providers be interviewed. In Sam's case, during the initial interview his goals and his particular needs related to using a computer are determined. The tasks with which he has difficulty performing are identified. Finding out whether Sam currently uses any adaptive equipment, or has in the past, to complete functional tasks also provides valuable information about his hand function. For example, Sam is able to sign his name by using an adapted splint to assist with grasping the pen, but it is difficult for him to write and he tires quickly. This difficulty has led him to pursue the use of a computer to facilitate taking notes at school and completing homework assignments. Another stage in which the interview is important is follow-up. At this stage, interviewing the consumer or caregivers provides valuable information on whether the device is being used and how. It is important that the ATP develop the ability to conduct interviews so that useful information is gathered.

Formal assessment procedures are administered in a prescribed way and have set methods of scoring and interpretation. Therefore, they can be duplicated and analyzed. Through formal assessment procedures, Sam's arm and hand abilities can be quantified. For example, Sam's muscle strength in his upper extremities can be evaluated by performing a manual muscle test (Daniels and Worthingham, 1986). Formal assessments should use standardized tests whenever possible. The ATP who uses such tests should evaluate the instrument development and psychometric properties to determine whether they are applicable to the client population and that the interpretation of the scores will be meaningful. Frameworks exist that guide a clinician's critique of an evaluation (e.g., Miller Polgar and Barlow, 2002). These frameworks identify aspects of test construction, psychometrics, and clinical utility that are important considerations of an instrument's usefulness in a given situation. *Clinical assessment techniques* involve skilled observation of the consumer and are used throughout the assessment and intervention process. The ATP may structure these techniques so that a series of steps is followed to determine specific skills or they may be intentionally left unstructured to see what takes place. Observation can be done during a simulated task in a clinic setting or in a context familiar to the consumer (e.g., classroom or workplace). Through skilled observation during the structured task of a series of typing tests, it may be observed that Sam's typing speed and accuracy improve when he stabilizes himself with his left forearm and types with his right hand. Observation complements information obtained from standardized tests.

All these considerations lead to one very important conclusion: In the application of assistive technology systems, success is largely the result of the combined efforts of knowledgeable and competent clinicians who, in collaboration with informed consumers and caregivers, make decisions on the basis of both specific knowledge and experience. The complexity of the total system, including the diversity of the individual and of disabilities, technologies, and contexts of use, dictates that, when an assistive technology device is designed, best practice is often a matter of using clinical reasoning combined with results of established assessments.

■ OVERVIEW OF SERVICE DELIVERY IN ASSISTIVE TECHNOLOGY

Regardless of the type of service delivery model (see Chapter 1), there is a basic process by which delivery of services to the consumer occurs. Figure 4-2 illustrates the steps involved in this intervention process. The first step is **referral and intake.** At this point, the consumer, or someone close to him or her, has identified a need for which assistive technology intervention may be indicated and contacts an ATP to make a referral. The service provider gathers basic information and determines whether there is a match between the type of services he or she provides and the identified needs of the consumer. Funding for the services to be provided is also identified and secured at this stage. Once the criteria for intake have been met, the *evaluation phase* begins. A more detailed specification of the consumer's assistive technology needs is the first step in this phase, which is referred to as *needs identification.* After a thorough identification of the consumer's needs, the consumer's sensory, physical, and cognitive skills are evaluated. Technologies that match the needs and skills of the consumer are identified, and a trial evaluation of these technologies takes place. The evaluation results are summarized and *recommendations* for technologies are made on the basis of consensus among those involved. These findings are summarized in a written *report,* which is used to justify funding for the purchase of the assistive technology system.

When funding is secured, the consumer proceeds with the intervention in the **implementation phase.** At this phase, the equipment that has been recommended is ordered, modified, and fabricated as necessary, set up, and delivered to the consumer. Initial training on the basic operation of the device and continuing training of strategies for using the device also take place during this phase.

Once the device has been delivered and training has been completed, whether the system as a whole is functioning effectively must be determined. This step normally occurs during the follow-up phase, in which it is determined whether the consumer is satisfied with the system and whether the goals that have been identified are being met. The follow-up phase actually closes the loop by putting in place a mechanism by which regular contact is made with the consumer to see whether further assistive technology services are indicated. When further AT services are required,

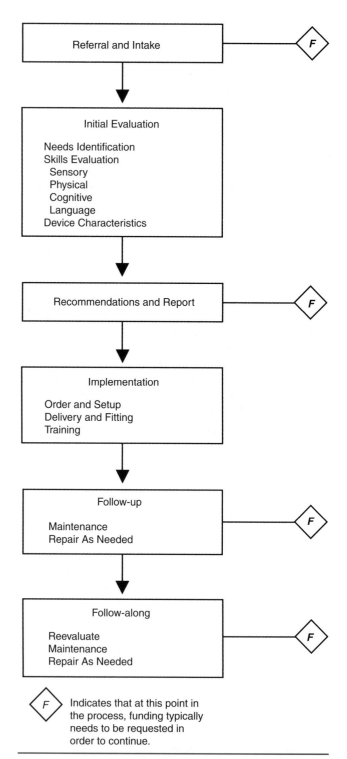

Figure 4-2   Steps in the service delivery process.

the referral, intake, and implementation phases are repeated. Building this final phase into the service delivery process ensures that the consumer's needs are considered throughout the life span. A more in-depth look at each of these steps follows.

Referral and Intake

The purpose of the referral and intake phase is to (1) gather preliminary information on the consumer, (2) determine whether there is a match between the needs of the consumer and the services that can be provided by the ATP, and (3) tentatively identify services to be provided (Gaster, 1992).

The consumer, or the person making the referral on the consumer's behalf, recognizes a need for assistive technology services or devices, which triggers the referral to the ATP. These identified needs are called **criteria for service,** and they define the objectives for the intervention. A third party involved in the referral, such as a state vocational rehabilitation agency, will have a set of policies and procedures that governs who is eligible to seek assistive technology intervention and what devices and services they cover. Langton and Hughes (1992) describe a framework called "tech points" for inclusion of assistive technology in the vocational rehabilitation case management process. They identify key points during the consumer's vocational rehabilitation at which technology should be considered. This approach is valuable because it includes a mechanism through which the vocational case manager can monitor whether a criterion for assistive technology services exists for individuals in his or her caseload. Depending on the policies of the ATP, referrals are accepted from a variety of sources. These sources include the consumer, a family member or care provider, a rehabilitation or educational professional, or a physician. At this time, information regarding the consumer's background and perceived assistive technology needs is gathered for the initial database. This information includes personal data (e.g., age, place of residence), medical diagnosis and health information, and educational or vocational background. Information related to the individual's medical diagnosis and health information that may guide the assessment includes whether the condition is expected to remain stable, improve, or decline. The appropriateness of the referral is viewed from the perspective of both the ATP and the referral or funding source. When exchanging information about the consumer's needs and the services provided by the ATP, each party can determine whether there is a match. One outcome is that the needs of the consumer do not match the services provided by the ATP. For the consumer's benefit, this mismatch should be acknowledged and the consumer referred to another source that can more appropriately address his or her needs. The assistive technology provider should have, within the organization's mission statement, a policy that establishes what services are provided and who is eligible to receive services. For example, some assistive technology service providers specialize in certain disabilities (e.g., visual impairment), and others focus on specific technologies (e.g., seating technologies). Professional codes of ethics and standards of practice (see Chapter 1) require that ATPs practice within their specialization and not try to provide services outside of this realm.

The other outcome is that there is a match between the needs of the consumer and the services provided by the ATP. In this case, funding is sought and plans are made to move forward with the initial evaluation, starting with a thorough identification of the consumer's needs. From the information provided, the ATP also determines the level of service that would be most beneficial to the consumer. There are a number of scenarios. First is the individual who has never used or been evaluated for assistive technologies, which could be an individual who is newly disabled or someone with a long-standing disability. An individual with a long-standing disability who may not have previously been a candidate for assistive technology services may now be able to access assistive devices because of recent advances in technologies. In this situation an in-depth assessment is warranted. Referrals may also be received from consumers who have used technology for some time and would like to evaluate current commercially available technologies. If this person's functional status has remained stable, it may not be necessary to conduct a complete evaluation. In some cases the assistive technology is not working or has been abandoned by the consumer and he is seeking a referral to see if modifications to the system can aid in making it more functional. Sometimes the consumer may only require further training or re-evaluation of how he or she is using the current system to see whether training in new strategies would be beneficial. Similarly, there may be a new care provider who needs training or technical assistance.

Initial Evaluation

Through a systematic evaluation, the ATP gathers information and facilitates decisions related to eventual device use. Because of the cost of the assistive technology to the consumer (or third-party funding source), it is essential that the ATP be able to assist the consumer in making informed decisions in the selection of a device. Current knowledge of the available technology and use of a systematic process facilitate the ATP's ability to make such decisions. This section focuses on the type of information gathered and the procedures used during the evaluation. Examples of assessment forms that capture most of the data discussed here are included in Appendices 4-1A and 4-1B.

Needs Identification

Through the **needs identification** process, the individual's needs and goals, which provide the basis for the assistive technology intervention, are determined. Identifying the needs of the consumer is the most critical component of the service delivery process and it is completed at the onset of evaluation. The information collected during needs identification is the cornerstone for measuring the effectiveness of the final outcome. Therefore, it is important to take this step seriously and ensure that there is a consensus among those involved as to the nature and scope of the problem to be addressed by the assistive technology intervention and the goals identified to target these problem areas.

Information gathered during needs identification is also used by the ATP to justify purchase of services and equipment. Third-party payers who fund services and equipment want to know what the problem or need is and how the equipment is going to address the need. Finally, the needs identification process results in the development of a plan for completing the remainder of the evaluation, which includes composition of the evaluation team, determination of needed evaluation tools and devices, and identification of further information required (either through evaluation of the consumer or by request from outside sources).

Figure 4-3 provides a model for gathering and analyzing information regarding the person's life roles, performance areas, related activities, and tasks. The consumer's life role at the time influences his or her needs and goals. Is the individual a child or an adult? What are his or her life roles? Life roles include student, parent, employee, volunteer, and so on. It is important to note that, as the individual's life roles change over time, so may the technology that is needed.

Changing life roles, and therefore technology needs, is one of the reasons that consumers may return after a time to be re-evaluated.

In relation to the consumer's life roles, there are performance areas (self-care, work, school, play, leisure) in which activities are accomplished. Identifying these performance areas helps the ATP to define the activities for which the consumer needs assistance. For example, play (performance area) is very important for a young child (life role), and a child with a disability may be precluded from manipulating toys (activity). Identifying the context in which the consumer will perform these activities is also critical. In Figure 4-3 we show needs identification for a student who is attending college. A major activity for this student is reading the material assigned from the textbook. The major part of this activity will take place at home for him, but he will also need to do some reading at school.

A task analysis of the skills required to complete the activity is conducted. The consumer and others identify to the best of their ability which tasks the consumer can likely perform himself or herself and which tasks may need to be assisted with technology. This information may be unknown in some cases, and the evaluation can determine which tasks the individual needs assistance with. In our example the activity of reading is broken down further into small tasks.

Life Roles/ Performance Areas	Activities	Difficult Tasks to Perform	Contexts	Prior Technology History
1. College student education	1. Reading class assignments in textbook	1a. Holding the book 1b. Turning the pages	1a. Home 1b. Library	1. Has used mouthstick and bookholders in the past; encountered problems positioning book and mouth becoming tired from holding mouthstick

Intervention Goals:	Directions:
1. Evaluate alternatives for holding reading material and turning pages in order to increase Joe's independence in reading.	1. Identify consumer's life roles and performance areas. 2. Identify activities consumer is interested in performing. 3. Identify the specific tasks the individual has difficulty performing. 4. Identify the contexts in which these activities are carried out. 5. Determine if consumer has used technology in the past for the activity and what the outcomes were.

Figure 4-3   Identifying consumer needs with the HAAT model.

If the student has a physical inability to hold the book and turn the pages, resulting in the need for manipulation of reading material, we identify this inability as a need in the third column. Another student who may have difficulty with the activity of reading because of a visual impairment will require different technologies to meet this need.

The consumer's prior history with technology should also be discussed as part of the needs identification. Useful information can be gathered from the consumer's previous success or failure with using assistive technology. Has he or she had experience in using technology before, and if so, what technology was used and was the experience successful? If not, why? In our example the student had attempted to turn the pages of different books with the use of a mouthstick, which turned out to be unsuccessful. It is important to identify and discuss reasons why the mouthstick did not work for the individual. Perhaps the mouthstick was cumbersome and uncomfortable to use for any extended period, or perhaps the individual could physically perform the task with the mouthstick but did not like the esthetics of it.

Beukelman and Mirenda (1998) discuss the need to identify actual or potential "opportunity barriers" and "access barriers" for the consumer. Although their model specifically targets consumers with augmentative communication needs, it also holds true for other areas of assistive technology. *Opportunity barriers* are imposed by individuals or situations that are not under the consumer's control. Generally the provision of assistive technology does not result in the elimination of these barriers. Beukelman and Mirenda (1998) identify five types of opportunity barriers: policy barriers, practice barriers, attitude barriers, knowledge barriers, and skill barriers. Policy barriers are legislative, regulative, or agency policies that govern situations in which consumers find themselves. For example, there are regulations in some school districts that restrict the use of school-purchased assistive technology to use in the school, preventing it from being taken home. Practice barriers refer to routine activities that are not dictated by policy but that constrain the use of assistive technologies. If the school's policy does not *require* that the device stay in the school, but the local teacher or principal has the practice of keeping the devices in the school, the result is the same as if it were a policy. Attitude, knowledge, and skill barriers all apply to those individuals with whom the consumer interacts and on whom the effective use of the device depends. If the consumer's job supervisor has a negative attitude regarding the use of automatic speech recognition because it is distracting to other workers, it is an attitude barrier that prevents the consumer's participation in that job. Alternatively, the supervisor may have insufficient knowledge or skill regarding automatic speech recognition to ensure that it is effectively installed and made available to the consumer. The approach taken by the ATP to overcome opportunity barriers is very different depending

on the type of barrier. It may involve training (for skills or knowledge), lobbying (for policy, attitude, or practice barriers), or a combination of the two.

Access barriers are barriers related to the abilities, attitudes, and resource limitations of the consumer or his or her support system (Beukelmen and Mirenda, 1998). During the needs assessment before an augmentative communication evaluation, for example, all the consumer's current ways of communicating can be identified. Known constraints related to user and family preferences and the attitudes of communication partners are other access barriers that should be identified. A potential barrier to accessing technology, one commonly seen during augmentative communication assessments, is resistance on the part of parents to pursue an augmentative communication device because they are worried that the use of such a device will inhibit the child's development of natural speech. As discussed later in this chapter, the ability to find funding for assistive technology systems and services may also pose a barrier. Identifying potential and actual barriers (both opportunity and access) during needs assessment will help the ATP formulate strategies for assessment and intervention.

The information for the needs assessment can be derived from an interview or through a written questionnaire completed by the consumer or his representative. In Appendix 4-1A we provide one example of a questionnaire. Instruments such as the Matching Person and Technology Assessments (Scherer, 1998) can also be used by the ATP to identify the areas of the individual's needs and his or her predisposition to use assistive technology. If the information is gathered through a written questionnaire before the ATP actually meets the consumer, it should be reviewed at the time of the first meeting with the consumer. The purpose of reviewing this material at the first meeting is to ensure that all the necessary information has been provided and to analyze the information to develop the goals. The total team should also be present at this meeting, and everyone's input regarding the needs and goals of the consumer can be discussed and a consensus reached.

Skills Evaluation: Sensory

As discussed in Chapter 3, auditory, tactile, and visual senses all play a role in the use of assistive technology. In recommending assistive technologies, the ATP needs to be aware of the consumer's sensory abilities and limitations. The ATP is not expected to diagnose sensory impairments such as hearing loss or visual impairments. Consumers who have sensory impairments have usually undergone evaluation by a specialist (e.g., audiologist, ophthalmologist, or optometrist) and are able to provide the ATP with a report that details the degree of impairment. If this testing has not occurred, the ATP should make a referral to an appropriate source before proceeding.

The ATP needs to be able to identify sensory functions that are available. If the primary disability is sensory, an alternative sensory pathway may need to be used, so the ATP needs to know what the consumer's sensory capabilities are. For example, in the case of a consumer who is blind and who needs to read, the ATP must evaluate tactile and auditory skills that can substitute for vision during reading (see Chapter 8). In other cases a consumer may have a sensory disability resulting from either a physical or a cognitive limitation. For example, if a consumer is hard of hearing, the ATP needs to know how this will affect interaction with technology. This includes everything from hearing warning beeps when a computer error is made to understanding voice synthesis on a communication device.

Evaluation of Functional Vision. The most critical visual skills needed for assistive technology use are sufficient acuity to see the symbols used in the system of choice or to identify small objects in the environment; adequate visual field to allow input of information from a display (e.g., the keyboard or the monitor) or the environment; and sufficient visual tracking ability (e.g., for reading or tracking a moving cursor). During the initial interview, known visual problems should have been identified, but a visual screening may also identify previously undetected deficits. The ATP can evaluate the effect of these deficits related to the use of technologies.

Identifying any *visual field deficits* a consumer may have is extremely important in the application of assistive technology. Visual field is commonly assessed by having the consumer look straight ahead and then indicate when he or she first sees a moving stimulus appear in the peripheral visual field. The stimulus is held approximately 18 inches away and moved in an arc toward the consumer's midline. This testing is typically done for the right and left peripheral fields and the upper and lower fields. Peripheral field vision is considered intact if the stimulus is seen when it is parallel to the person's cheek and impaired if the individual does not indicate that he or she sees the object as it approaches the center of his or her face (Dunn, 1991).

In some cases it is difficult to identify the effects of visual field limitations on assistive technology use. For example, individuals with a visual field deficit may make errors in typing because they do not see the whole keyboard. If the ATP is not careful, this performance may be interpreted as a physical limitation instead of a visual field deficit. If motor limitations were assumed, the keys may have been made larger so that the consumer could hit them more easily, an expensive and unnecessary step.

Visual tracking is the ability to follow a moving object. This skill is necessary for many assistive technology tasks, such as following a moving cursor on a screen, following the rotation of a plate with food in a feeder, or following objects in the environment while driving a wheelchair. Visual tracking is usually tested by having the consumer follow a moving object with the eyes. The object is held approximately 18 inches in front of the consumer and moved horizontally, vertically, and diagonally. The ATP notes whether the two eyes track together, whether the eye pursuits are smooth or jerky, whether there is a delay in the tracking, and whether the eyes can track without head movement.

Limitations in visual tracking ability may significantly reduce the options for specifying and designing an assistive technology system. In particular, these results have implications for the use of scanning augmentative communication systems in which the cursor moves left, right, up, and down (four-way directional scanning). It may be that an individual with a disability is able to track more easily to the right and down than to the left and up. In this case, two-way directional scanning, right and down, is preferable to using all four directions. When the cursor gets to the extreme right of the display, it automatically wraps around and begins from the left side again. Similarly, when it gets to the bottom, it wraps around to the top.

Visual scanning differs from visual tracking in that the object does not move; instead the eyes are moved to view different parts of a scene to find a desired object or location. This skill is used, for example, to locate obstacles during mobility and to scan a keyboard to find a specific key. The eye movements used in visual scanning are the same as those used in tracking. We often assess this capability by presenting arrays of pictures, symbols, words, or letters and asking the consumer to choose one item from the array. In Chapter 3 we described *visual accommodation* as the ability of the eyes to adjust to objects near and far. This component is impaired in many persons with disabilities, and it is important to be aware of possible accommodative insufficiency during the assessment process. A visual accommodation impairment may be observed by changing the visual focus between a monitor and keyboard. If the monitor and keyboard are far apart, the person may have more difficulty than if these objects are visually close. An individual's ability to see objects (visual acuity) is affected by (1) the size of the object, (2) the contrast between the object and the background, and (3) the spacing between the object and surrounding background objects. These three considerations apply to symbols as well as to objects. For testing of visual acuity, actual objects, photographs, line drawings, orthographic symbols, letters, and words are used. It is helpful to have a set of materials that includes objects of 3 to 4 inches high; large letters, pictures, and symbols 1 to 2 inches high; and letters and words down to the size of standard typewritten letters (an eighth of an inch) (Cook, 1988). Information gathered from the initial interview can guide the ATP as to the type and size of symbol to start with. The goal is to find the smallest size of symbol that can be seen well by the consumer and that results in accurate selections, which are tested by presenting two items of the selected size and symbol type at a time to the consumer. The individual is asked to identify one of the two items using the manner in which he or she usually indicates a choice (e.g., eye gaze, pointing, yes/no). Three trials of each size and symbol are completed before proceeding to the next smaller size, until the individual is no longer able to identify the item successfully. It is desirable for the consumer to be able to see a small size for a number of reasons. First, the smaller the size, the larger a given array of symbols can be. Second, this allows greater options in hardware and software, including standard keyboards and software that have been developed for the nondisabled population.

If the consumer is able to read but appears to have difficulty seeing words, the effects of various foreground-background combinations (to improve contrast) and letter spacing can be assessed by using computer displays and software designed for this purpose (see Chapter 7). For example, most word processing software allows alteration in the background and foreground (letters) colors. Special software designed for persons with visual impairments also adds size variation to these capabilities. For computer applications, these features can improve performance.

We can improve visual performance by using enlarged graphics or text and by designing control panels with dark backgrounds and light lettering or controls. Identifying switches or keys with colors more distinguishable to the individual may be helpful. Switches can be light colored and placed on a dark background to improve recognition, and language board arrays can have bold dark letters or pictures on a white background, or vice versa. Likewise, video screens and the input array need to be carefully planned so that the amount of information presented is not cluttered.

Evaluation of Visual Perception.
As discussed in Chapter 3, visual perception is the process of giving meaning to visual information. Visual perceptual skills that need to be considered during assessment include depth perception, spatial relationships, form recognition or constancy, and figure-ground discrimination. Visual perception is an important consideration when considering the client's ability to interpret information presented in a visual display or to safely navigate a mobility device in the environment. Formal testing of the consumer's visual perception may have been completed before the assistive technology assessment, and results of this evaluation can be gathered during the initial interview. It is necessary to observe the consumer during functional tasks and note any apparent perceptual problems. If there is still some concern regarding the exact nature of the problems, a formal evaluation such as the Motor Free Visual Perception Test (Colarusso and Hammill, 1972) can be used.

Evaluation of Tactile Function.
There are three particular circumstances in which attention needs to be paid to the evaluation of tactile sensation. These occur during seating and positioning assessments, when evaluating tactile input for the use of control interfaces, and when considering the use of tactile alternatives to vision or hearing.

Somatosensory input is necessary for detecting forces or pressures exerted on the surface of the skin. Individuals who lack sensation may sit for prolonged periods without shifting position, which can result in skin breakdown. The ATP needs to be aware of an individual's sensory status in these situations and be able to evaluate pressure on the sitting surface. Dunn (1991) presents a specific testing protocol for tactile response. Additionally, observation and monitoring of the skin surface is necessary. Tactile functions that are included in a somatosensory protocol include one-two point discrimination, perception of light touch versus deep pressure, perception of temperature, joint position sense, and localization of tactile stimulation. Somatosensory function is responsible for providing information regarding the location of a control interface, the movements required to activate it, and whether it is successfully activated. Lack of ability to receive appropriate sensory input (e.g., because of Hansen's disease, nerve injuries, or sensory loss from aging) can severely limit the effective use of control interfaces. The initial interview generally reveals whether somatosensory deficits are present. During functional tasks, the ATP's skilled observation can identify limitations caused by sensory deficits. Dunn's (1991) sensory testing protocol can also be applied in this situation. In the case of decreased tactile sensation, the control interface needs to provide adequate feedback so that it compensates for the loss of sensory function (see Chapter 7). When visual or auditory function is inadequate for the input of information, we often use tactile substitutes (see Chapters 8 and 9). To determine whether this alternative sensory input is viable for an individual, tactile function must be evaluated. In particular, the skin response on one or more fingers is evaluated by using two-point discrimination and similar tests. This evaluation is necessary because certain diseases (e.g., diabetes) that result in loss of vision also cause reduced tactile sensation.

Evaluation of Auditory Function.
The ATP, through the initial interview and observation during functional tasks, should be aware of any significant auditory impairments that may affect device use. In cases of suspected hearing loss, a formal evaluation by an audiologist should be requested. Basic information sought by the ATP should include whether the individual responds to auditory stimuli, is distracted by some or all sounds, recognizes specific auditory stimuli (e.g., someone calling his or her name), and responds appropriately to auditory stimuli (Dunn, 1991). For example, many augmentative communication devices emit a beep when a selection is made. For some individuals, this cueing is helpful; however, for others the beep may produce a startle reflex that interferes with the succeeding motor movement. The individual may eventually habituate to the beep, but it is

important to consider a device that has the option of disabling it.

Skills Evaluation: Physical

The overall goal of the *physical skills evaluation* is to determine the most functional position for the individual and evaluate his or her ability to access a device physically. At a very basic level, physical skills include range of motion, muscle strength, muscle tone and the presence of obligatory movements. Many protocols exist for evaluation of range of motion. Both passive and active ranges of motion are assessed. Range of motion is important in consideration of positioning needs for function and the amount of movement available to access a device or perform a task. Related to range of motion is muscle strength. Again, many protocols are available for testing muscle strength. Muscle strength is graded in a range from unable to move independently, moves with gravity eliminated, able to move against gravity, and moves against different degrees of resistance. It is important to note that the presence of a neurological disorder such as cerebral palsy, stroke, or traumatic brain injury will affect both range of motion and muscle strength. Typical protocols for testing these components are not generally useful for these populations because the position of the individual affects muscle tone and subsequently range of motion and muscle strength. For example, a child with cerebral palsy may seem to have limited flexion range of motion in the lower extremities when lying in supine. However, when turned on the side, the ability to flex the legs is much easier. In supine, the influence of the tonic labyrinthine reflex increases extensor tone. This influence is not present in side lying, making flexion much easier.

Muscle tone and the presence of obligatory movements are important considerations for individuals with neurological disorders. As described above, the position of the individual affects the available movement. Muscle tone is assessed in various functional positions, particularly prone, supine, sitting, and standing. Obligatory movements, or reflexes, are assessed to determine how they might affect function. Key reflexes or obligatory movements include the asymmetrical and symmetrical tonic neck reflexes, tonic labyrinthine, extensor thrust, bite, and grasp reflexes. The ability to right the head when moved out of a vertical alignment, either lateral or in the anterior-posterior plane is another component. Postural control is a related component that refers to the ability to maintain the trunk in a vertical alignment. When completing an assessment to determine function in various positions, it is important to handle the client and to challenge his or her balance and postural control to determine the degree of support he or she will need to work in a given position and the movement available in that position.

Sitting and standing balance are additional considerations. The ability to maintain balance in these positions is determined through observation of the ability to maintain the position independently and the response to challenges to balance in these positions. Sitting balance is described as hands free, where the individual can maintain balance and function without using hands to support himself or herself; hands dependent, where he or she needs to support himself or herself with one or both hands to maintain sitting; and propped or dependent sitting, where he or she cannot sit without external support. Sitting balance is an important component of a seating and mobility assessment (Chapters 6 and 12).

Gross and fine motor assessments generally test higher-level motor skills. Gross motor skills include balance on one foot, performing symmetrical and asymmetrical movements of the upper and lower extremities, coordinating one side of the body, lifting and carrying objects, rapidly alternating movements, and running, skipping, and hopping. Fine motor assessment includes rapidly alternating finger movements, performance of isolated finger movements, manipulation of objects of different sizes, and performance of specific fine motor tasks. The Bruinicks-Oseretsky Test of Motor Proficiency (Bruininks, 1978) and the Movement ABC (Henderson and Sugden, 1992) are two examples of comprehensive motor evaluations appropriate for children. The Gross Motor Function Test (Russell et al, 2002) is designed specifically for children with neurological impairments. Once again, if a neurological condition is present, it is important to remember that function is dependent on the client's position.

Identifying Potential Anatomical Sites for Control.
In Chapter 3 we identify the control sites that can potentially be used by the consumer to operate a device (see Figure 3-10) and describe the various movements that each control site is capable of performing.

When individuals with physical disabilities are evaluated, it helps to keep in mind the movement capabilities of each of these anatomical sites and the hierarchy in which these sites are considered. The hands and the fingers are the preferred control sites because they are naturally used during manipulation tasks and finer resolution can be achieved. If the hands are not an option for control, the head and mouth are considered next. With the use of mouthsticks, head pointers, or light beams, it is possible to achieve the fine resolution and range needed to control a device. The next option to consider is the foot. Some individuals are able to develop fine control of the foot for typing (Figure 4-4); however, problems with positioning the device so that the user can see it make this site less desirable than the hands or the head. The least desirable sites are the legs or the arms because they are controlled by larger muscle groups, so the movements of these sites are gross in nature compared with the fine movements of smaller muscles (Cook, 1988).

Simulation of functional tasks is used to evaluate the types and quality of movement an individual possesses.

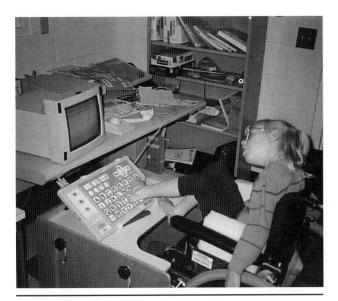

Figure 4-4   Child using her foot to control an expanded keyboard.

Functional tasks are chosen for evaluation because they are often more meaningful to the consumer than physical performance components such as strength and joint range of motion. They also provide the ATP with an opportunity to gather qualitative information regarding the consumer's movements, and results of such tasks are more likely to reflect the consumer's true abilities.

We present a model based on clinical experience to determine the best anatomical site for accessing a control interface. The hands, being the control site of choice, are the first to be assessed. Basic hand function can be observed and rated by using a "grasp module" (Figure 4-5), which includes

a total of seven functional grasp patterns. The consumer's ability to complete each grasp pattern is rated (unable, poor, fair, or good). Notations are also made regarding how the consumer completed the movement and the factors that made it successful or not. For example, did the object need to be positioned in a particular way for the consumer to grasp it? Was there a delay in initiating the movement? Did the consumer have difficulty releasing the object? Was the movement pattern isolated or synergistic in nature? Did the consumer appear to have problems with depth perception when reaching for the object?

If the consumer has the potential for hand use, it is then necessary to determine the minimal and maximal arm range within a workspace and the resolution in hitting a target. A range and resolution board, as shown in Figure 4-6, can be used to measure both of these. If possible, the consumer is asked to use the thumb or a finger to point to each corner of each numbered square. If the consumer is unable to point to the corners, he or she is asked to touch each square with the whole hand. This provides information regarding the approximate size of the workspace and the best locations for a control interface and a rough measure of accuracy of movement. Both arms are evaluated as appropriate.

If the hands are eliminated as a control site, other anatomical sites must be considered. For example, we can also measure range and resolution for the foot and head. With a range and resolution board of smaller dimensions, the same task can be used to evaluate foot range and targeting skills and the consumer's range and resolution with a mouthstick, light pointer, or head pointer. Appendix 4-1B shows a sample assessment form for documenting the information gathered during the physical skills evaluation. After completion of this component of the skills evaluation, the ATP

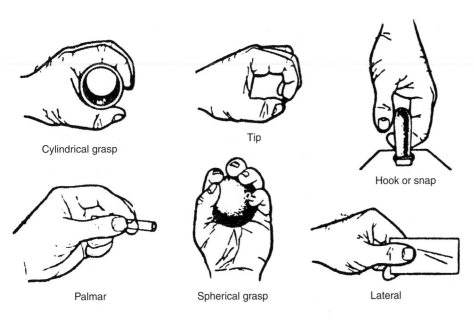

Cylindrical grasp

Tip

Hook or snap

Palmar

Spherical grasp

Lateral

Figure 4-5   Functional grasp patterns for evaluating hand use.

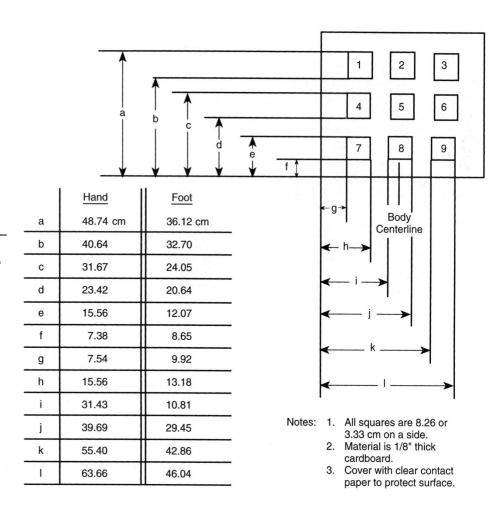

	Hand	Foot
a	48.74 cm	36.12 cm
b	40.64	32.70
c	31.67	24.05
d	23.42	20.64
e	15.56	12.07
f	7.38	8.65
g	7.54	9.92
h	15.56	13.18
i	31.43	10.81
j	39.69	29.45
k	55.40	42.86
l	63.66	46.04

Notes: 1. All squares are 8.26 or 3.33 cm on a side.
2. Material is 1/8" thick cardboard.
3. Cover with clear contact paper to protect surface.

Figure 4-6 Range and resolution board used for evaluating the ability to hit a target using a given control site.

should have a good idea of the user's physical skills and the anatomical sites that can best be used to control an interface.

Selecting Candidate Control Interfaces. Once the ATP has identified anatomical sites that the consumer can potentially use, the next step in the process is to select control interfaces that have potential to be used successfully by the consumer. In Chapter 7 we present a set of control interface characteristics that are useful in selecting interfaces that most closely match the consumer's available anatomical sites.

Comparative Testing of Candidate Control Interfaces. Once potential anatomical sites and candidate control interfaces have been chosen, next the consumer's ability to use these interfaces is measured. Comparative testing provides the ATP with data on the consumer's speed and accuracy in using particular control interfaces. These data can be used to compare different interfaces operated with a given site. If a control enhancer (e.g., mouthstick, head pointer) or modification (e.g., keyguard) is being considered, its use should also be evaluated (Chapter 7). This is one area where gathering

quantitative information on the person's ability to use the control interface is extremely valuable and can assist the ATP in making decisions regarding the selection of a control site and interface. It is also important to note the consumer's preferences during this process.

During the assessment process, speed of response is often used to compare control interfaces. *Speed of response* is a temporal (time-based) measurement that can be quantified. Because these measurements are typically made in the controlled setting of the clinic, they must be carefully applied to contexts outside the clinic. Another measure used to compare control interfaces is *accuracy of response*. This is often based on moving to the correct position, and it is therefore a spatial measurement, rather than a temporal (time-based) measure. Measurement of accuracy requires a standard of performance. This is usually the number of correct responses out of the total number of trials. Speed of response and accuracy are generally inversely proportional to each other for novice users.

When these two basic parameters are defined, methods for measuring them can be described. The selected control interface is first placed in a position where the consumer can activate it. It may be necessary to try different locations for the control interface before finding the position at which the consumer has the greatest control. The consumer's time to move from a rest position to target the control interface can be measured with a stopwatch.

Computer-assisted assessment provides several useful features. First, data collection and analysis can be automated, relieving the clinician of tedious record keeping. Performance measures for each possible control site/interface pair can be obtained. The effects of different positions for the control interface or the use of control enhancers and modifications can also be measured. Because several different control site/interface combinations can be evaluated, this data collection process can facilitate the choice of interfaces on the basis of measured results. Second, the computer can provide a variety of contingent results (including graphics, sound, and speech) when the control interface is activated. This variety of results not only makes the task more interesting, but it also can allow assessment of visual and auditory capabilities.

Skills Evaluation: Cognitive

Chapter 3 describes the major cognitive skills associated with assistive technology use. Although there are standardized test batteries that are used for cognitive assessment (Duchek, 1991), in general we do not use them for evaluating consumer's cognitive skills related to assistive technologies. Instead, clinical observation is the major strategy used for the collection of information regarding a consumer's cognitive function. Clinical observation yields information that is often not provided by standard tests. For example, by observing a consumer using a switch-activated program on the computer, the ATP can obtain an indication of the consumer's level of attention, understanding of cause and effect, degree of motivation, and ability to follow directions. Assessment of cognitive skills is important when determining whether the client will be able to learn how to use the technology and whether he or she has the capacity to use it effectively in the long term.

All three types of memory discussed in Chapter 3 (sensory, short-term, and long-term) are important for the use of assistive technologies. Memory tasks related to assistive technology can be evaluated by structured clinical observations. For example, the ATP can have the consumer memorize a group of codes and then note the consumer's ability to remember these codes during an encoding task.

Problem solving can also be measured during functional tasks. For example, when an electric feeder is used, it is necessary to rotate the plate to position the food so that the spoon can pick it up. Proper use of this technology requires a high degree of problem-solving skills. If the person lacks these skills, use of the device becomes frustrating and an alternative should be considered. The value of this type of

cognitive assessment is that it occurs during completion of a functional task, which may be predictive of assistive technology system use.

Skills Evaluation: Language

The evaluation of language skills required for the use of assistive technology devices focuses on both expressive and receptive abilities. In addition, the ability to sequence items, use symbol systems, combine language elements into complex thoughts, and use codes is important in operating various types of assistive technologies. Although the most extensive language evaluation is carried out for augmentative communication system recommendations (see Chapter 11), language skills and use are also important in using other assistive devices such as mobility systems (see Chapter 12) or systems for manipulation (see Chapter 14). Also, language and hearing are closely coupled, and assistive technologies intended for persons with hearing impairments must address language and auditory skills (see Chapter 9).

Specific areas that are evaluated include categorization, sequencing, matching, social communicative skills (e.g., degree of interaction), receptive language skills (e.g., recognition of words or symbols, understanding of simple commands), motor speech skills, and pragmatic language skills. Advanced language capabilities (e.g., syntax and semantics) are also evaluated when possible. The evaluation of these skills for augmentative communication device use is discussed in Chapter 11.

Matching Electronic Device Characteristics to the User's Needs and Skills

The assessment process to this point provides the basis by which the ATP and the rest of the assistive technology service delivery team carefully define the goals to be accomplished and determine the skills the consumer has available for assistive technology system use. It is necessary to systematically transform these goals and skills into characteristics of assistive technology devices. In this section those aspects that are specific to the characteristics of electronic devices are considered. The term **device characteristics** refers to general properties of the technology. A *feature* is a particular implementation of a characteristic. Characteristics of automobiles include, for example, engine, color, size, performance (acceleration, gas mileage), and doors. Features for these same characteristics might include four-cylinder engine, blue color, compact size, 35 miles per gallon, and two doors. Consumers have certain needs, and they match those needs to general characteristics to select specific features of interest. They also have skills that apply to the selection. For example, a consumer may not be able to use a standard manual transmission and chooses only automatic transmission cars for consideration. Life roles also play a part in the selection decision.

For instance, parents with small children may choose a minivan rather than a compact car.

In assistive technology service delivery, a similar matching process can be used to choose features that match the consumer's needs and skills. This systematic approach is superior to using trial and error with all the possible devices that *may* work and then trying to pick one. To use this approach, however, a set of characteristics to be considered must be defined. A generic set of assistive technology device characteristics is listed in Box 4-2. The categories in this box parallel those used in Figure 2-5 to describe the components of the assistive technology portion of the HAAT model. In the following chapters more specific characteristics are considered for certain areas of assistive technologies: seating systems, control interfaces, computer adaptations, augmentative communication systems, mobility devices, manipulation devices, and sensory aids.

Human/Technology Interface. The human/technology interface is the portion of the device with which the consumer directly interacts. The most general human/technology characteristics, which apply to all devices, are the physical properties. These include the force exerted by the human/technology interface on the person and the force exerted by the person on the interface, the size and weight of the interface, and its texture and hardness. A seating system may be too hard or soft to be effective, and this feature can be related to the needs of the individual consumer. All human/technology interfaces must be attached either to the person, to a wheelchair, or to a stable work surface. Consideration of this "mountablilty" characteristic can often mean the difference between success and failure of the human/technology interface. For example, if a consumer has very limited range of arm movement, a switch must be positioned within this range.

Just as the human user exerts forces on the human/technology interface, the human/technology interface provides feedback to the user. This may be as a direct consequence of the interface. For example, a seat cushion exerts a certain force, depending on its materials, design, and construction. In other cases the user feedback is a separate component, such as a flashing light indicator on a television control or a tactile display on a reading device for a person with total visual impairment. Human/technology user feedback sources can be described in terms of the characteristics of magnitude, type, and origin. These characteristics can be matched to the consumer's needs. For example, the *magnitude* of a visual display is the brightness of the light. The *types* of human/technology interface feedback are other characteristics and include visual, auditory, and tactile varieties. Each of these can be matched to the corresponding user skill. The *origin* refers to the source of the feedback, such as that provided by a seat cushion or the voice output provided from the screen reader.

The next three characteristics listed in Box 4-2 apply to human/technology interfaces used with electronic assistive devices (including power mobility). The *number of inputs* required to operate any device is a characteristic. This characteristic is referred to as the *size of the input domain* (see Chapter 7). There are many types of control interfaces available, with varying numbers of inputs and requiring different physical skills for activation. The most appropriate control interface for any given consumer is largely determined by the physical and interface assessments that are described here and in Chapter 7.

Depending on the size of the input domain related to the consumer's needs and skills, a *selection method* can be chosen. In Chapter 7 two basic selection methods are described: direct and indirect. In direct selection, all the choices are presented to the user at one time and the user has the physical ability to choose any one element directly. With indirect selection, there are intermediate steps required for the user to make a selection. If the number of input signals required (on the basis of needs) is greater than the number the consumer can control (on the basis of physical skills), then some form of indirect selection must be used. Individual devices may have both these methods or they may be restricted to only one method. Direct selection requires greater physical skill than indirect selection; however, indirect selection requires greater cognitive, visual, perceptual, and possibly auditory abilities. The consumer's skills must be taken into account when specific device features are chosen.

BOX 4-2	**Assistive Device Characteristics**

HUMAN/TECHNOLOGY INTERFACE
Physical properties
Mountability
User feedback
Number of inputs
Selection methods
Selection set

PROCESSOR
Commands
Control parameters
Data or information processing

ACTIVITY OUTPUT
Magnitude
Precision
Flexibility

ENVIRONMENTAL INTERFACE
Range
Threshold

PHYSICAL CONSTRUCTION
Mountability
Portability
Packaging

Selections are made from a *selection set* consisting of the choices available to the consumer. Features of this set include size, number of choices, format (e.g., print, tactile), and type of symbol (real objects, pictures, computer icons, line drawings, traditional orthography, or symbols used to represent an idea). The type of symbol system that is most appropriate to a given individual is determined during the language assessment. The question of symbol system type is obviously essential for augmentative communication devices, but it is also important in other applications. For example, in electronic aids to daily living (EADL), the devices to be controlled must be labeled, and often symbols are used rather than words to make the systems available to persons who have difficulty in reading. Speech labels, generated by synthetic speech, are also used in the selection set for individuals who have either visual or cognitive limitations. Along with determining the type of symbols used in the selection set, the size of the selection set is also determined. The number of choices required is often dictated by the consumer's needs and by other factors such as how many will fit on a display given the consumer's visual acuity. The choice of these features for a consumer is based on his or her skills in several areas, including sensory, cognitive, and language.

The Processor.   Recall that the processor is the element of the assistive technology device that relates the human/technology interface to the other components. Sometimes this is simply a mechanical linkage (e.g., in a reacher), and in such cases there are not many choices in characteristics. However, processors for electronic devices have several characteristics that must be carefully matched to the consumer's needs and skills. The first of these is the basic set of *commands* that are necessary to operate the device. It is important to ensure that the consumer can use these so that the system will be functional for the consumer. For example, in a powered wheelchair system the basic commands are forward, backward, left, and right. In a communication device, some basic commands include printing a document and speaking. In an EADL the commands may include lights on and off, TV channel selection, and telephone dialing. These are essential for operation. The greater the number of commands, the more flexible the system is to the user. For example, an EADL that can control the television with three functions (power, volume, and channel), turn three appliances on and off (lights, drapes, and door lock), dial a telephone (three commands), and access an emergency message machine has 10 functions. The more commands included, the more confusing the system can become. The consumer, family, care providers, and ATP need to evaluate the effect of a specific command size during the assessment.

A second characteristic of the processor is the *control parameters*. In contrast to commands, control parameters allow adjustments to be made to the system; they are nice to have but not always essential. Control parameters include

such things as variable speed for forward and reverse or indoor and outdoor speed levels in a powered wheelchair. In an augmentative communication device, control parameters adjust the voice synthesizer pitch, voice type, and rate to affect the way the speech output sounds. A control parameter also provides the ability to switch between different applications for multiple activity outputs. For example, it is possible to operate an EADL, communication device, and computer access system from a powered wheelchair controller. Individual control parameters need to be presented to the consumer for the systems being considered, and both the consumer and the ATP need to evaluate their effectiveness.

The final general processor characteristic is *data or information processing*. In this case the device is internally processing information rather than dealing with commands or control signals. One example, used in augmentative communication systems and screen readers for the blind, is the generation of spoken output from text using software programs. By listening to several speech systems, the consumer can determine the intelligibility of each and identify which one is preferred.

Another type of information processing is word prediction, in which the software program guesses at the desired word on the basis of the entries the consumer makes. This type of application can also adapt to the user by learning his or her most frequently used words. Encoding involves the use of a symbol (e.g., number, letter, mnemonic, color) to represent a vocabulary item or a command (e.g., TV ON in an EADL). The user selects the code instead of directly selecting the element, which can increase the user's rate of data entry. Encoding schemes can be cognitively difficult, and the consumer should try them during the assessment. The consumer may indicate a preference of one encoding method over another after having a chance to try several.

Information processing is also used in sensory systems to convert the input from the environmental sensor to a form that can be presented to the user. For example, a hearing aid uses a microphone to detect voices, amplifies them (data processing), and presents the amplified signal to the ear (see Chapter 9). Different hearing aids have different data processing, and the consumer can evaluate this characteristic.

Environmental Interface.   As discussed in Chapters 2, 8, and 9, the environmental interface is that portion of the assistive technology system that is used to take in information from the external world for use in a sensory substitution system. For example, when the person has a visual limitation, we use a camera, and when a person has an auditory impairment, we use a microphone. Characteristics that apply to this element include the *range* of the input signal (i.e., how big or small the signal can be and still be detected). The smallest signal that can be discerned from background noise is the *threshold.* As an example of how these characteristics can be applied, consider the two problems of reading and mobility for persons with severe visual impairments. For reading, the device needs very little range because only one letter or line of text needs to be viewed at a time. However, for mobility the environmental sensor needs to take in a variety of sizes (e.g., from a dish to a tree). For reading, the threshold is low (a letter in fine print), but for mobility the threshold can be much higher.

Activity Output.   The activity output is what the system accomplishes for the consumer (e.g., communication, mobility, manipulation). The first characteristic that describes the activity output is its *magnitude*. This includes the volume for a speech synthesis system, the force or torque generated by a powered wheelchair, and the brightness of a video screen display. *Precision* is a measure of how accurately the system performs the functions and how exactly it accomplishes its task. For example, a reacher may be able to pick up a cup but not a button. If the consumer needs to pick up the button, then this particular reacher has insufficient precision to accomplish the task. If an output can be used in different contexts or can be used to accomplish different goals for the consumer, we would say that it is *flexible*. Flexibility can be an important factor when the consumer has many tasks to perform. Careful consideration of context must also be included in choosing specific activity output features.

Physical Construction.   The final category of characteristics is physical construction. No matter how well a system works in an assessment session, it will not be effective in everyday use unless the person has access to it at all times. This is determined primarily by the *mountability* of the system. Special consideration must be given to both the mounting of the system (or placement on a desk) and the attachment of any components to a wheelchair. For example, mounting of a communication system to a wheelchair must be considered during the assessment to ensure that the chosen system is compatible with the consumer's wheelchair.

Portability is a measure of the degree to which the device can be moved from place to place. This characteristic includes a consideration of size, weight, and power source. For electronic devices, portability often requires that the device be battery operated and that it be small and lightweight enough to be carried or attached to a wheelchair. If the person is ambulatory, his or her ability to carry the device needs to be assessed. There are differences in batteries (e.g., life may be a few hours or a few days between charges) and size and weight. For mobility devices, the ability to transport the wheelchair in the trunk of a car may need to be considered. Some wheelchairs fold so that they can be transported in a car trunk, whereas others, such as powered wheelchairs, do not typically fold.

Generally consideration of the characteristics of color, shape, and overall design are done last when a recommendation for

assistive technologies is developed for a consumer. We refer to these as *packaging* characteristics. Consideration of the consumer's preferences in this area can contribute to motivation to use the system and to overall user satisfaction. However, the consumer's packaging preferences cannot always be integrated into the system (e.g., the wheelchair may not come in bright orange). All these features should be discussed with the consumer and others to ensure that the device selected will meet the consumer's needs.

Evaluating the Match Between Characteristics and the Consumer's Skills and Needs.   It is our premise that a large part of the assessment up to this point is best completed without the introduction of specific devices. The focus of the assessment remains on the functional results to be achieved by the technology instead of on the secondary features of technology, such as color, size, and design. Once the basic functional characteristics have been determined, differences in the secondary factors of size, weight, color, and overall design become important, and they may be the basis for a final decision. After the assessment phases described earlier, one or more devices that have the potential to meet the consumer's skills and needs are identified for the consumer to evaluate. There are two primary ways in which the ATP can evaluate specific technologies for use by the consumer: (1) trial using the actual device and (2) simulation of device characteristics.

Ideally the consumer will have the opportunity to try the devices being considered and evaluate their usefulness before a recommendation is made. However, because of the expense, it is not always possible for the ATP to have access to every available device, nor is it a prerequisite for conducting a skilled assessment. It is desirable that the ATP have available a set of devices that represents a broad range of characteristics. A service delivery program can carefully choose equipment to be used for evaluations, making it possible to address the major characteristics of devices during consumer assessment. Sometimes a short trial during a one-time assessment is not adequate and it is necessary to have the consumer use the device for an extended period. In some cases a local manufacturer's representative might loan a device to the ATP for a consumer trial. Other manufacturers and service delivery programs lease devices for this purpose. If these devices are available, it is helpful to demonstrate the various features to the consumer and have the consumer try them. There may be two or three devices being considered, and, if possible, each device should be tried and evaluated by the consumer. In lieu of having the actual device available, the ATP can simulate device characteristics. Simulation requires that the ATP be knowledgeable about the characteristics and features available for specific assistive technologies. For computer-based products, the assistive technology adaptations are often software based, and demonstration disks can be obtained from manufacturers or downloaded from a manufacturer's Web site. These demonstration programs illustrate the essential features of the software, but they are not fully functional and their use is time limited.

To position a control interface for simulation during assessment, universal mounting systems that can be adjusted and placed in various positions can be used. This step is important to ensure that the control interface is in a functional position for the consumer and that it remains stable during the assessment.

Effects of Errors in Assistive Technology Systems.

An important operational characteristic of assistive technology systems is the way in which they deal with errors. Two types of errors are of concern. *Random errors* are infrequent and are generally chance occurrences. An example of a random error is the consumer's inability to understand a voice synthesizer because of high amounts of ambient noise. If the noise is not present, there is no error, and even if there is noise it may not lead to an error in interpretation. It is only the random co-occurrence of the need to use the voice synthesizer, the presence of noise, and a listener who does not understand the output that creates the error. Random errors may recur, but they are not consistently present in the system. We can do very little to avoid this type of error in the assistive technology system design process.

Of greater concern are *periodic*, or regular, *errors*, which occur under predictable conditions. These errors may also be infrequent, but they are foreseeable. As an example, many letter-to-speech software programs make mistakes in pronunciation when used with voice synthesizers. The mispronunciation always occurs whenever the particular word is entered. This type of error can be dealt with in the design process. For our example of mispronunciation, exception tables are typically used so that the utterance sounds correct although the letter-to-speech rule makes an error. There are several effects of errors on assistive technology system performance, including loss of information, injury, and embarrassment. All three of these can occur in the same system, and they may be due to the human, the activity, the context, the assistive technology, or the interaction of all of these components. For example, a power wheelchair will not function if the user does not regularly charge the batteries. The user must somehow cause the action that results in the batteries maintaining a charge, and the power wheelchair system must provide accurate information about the degree to which the batteries are charged. Error-free function here relies on the successful integration of the human with the technology. Loss of information is a common effect associated with augmentative communication systems (see Chapter 11) and sensory aids (see Chapters 8 and 9). Loss of information refers to an interruption in the output of the system, whether it is auditory or visual, as in a voice output communication aid, or physical, as in the power to propel an electrically powered wheelchair. It can occur because the human operator makes

an error in motor, sensory, or cognitive performance or as a result of a device error. Although the net effect on system performance of either of these errors (human or device) may be the same, it is important to distinguish between them to correct the problem.

When the human operator makes the errors, the distinction needs to be made as to whether the cause is lack of capacity (e.g., inability to control excessive tremor resulting in erroneous selections or visual limitations in reading a display) or lack of skill (inadequate experience or practice in using the device). If the problem is the capacity of the user, then modifications must be made in the system (e.g., using a keyguard to prevent erroneous entries or an enlarged display screen to improve visibility). If the problem is one of skill, training may help reduce the number of errors.

Physical injury is a more serious effect of a system error. This type of error can occur in a mobility system (see Chapter 12) if, for example, a braking system fails or a motor fails to turn off. Consideration of this type of error leads us to the concept of "fail-safe" design. This approach attempts to anticipate the types of errors (termed *failures* when caused by the device) and to ensure that, if they do occur, the probability of injury is minimized. For example, if a power wheelchair controller fails, it should fail in the off state. If it fails in the on state, the user may be injured because the chair cannot be controlled. Similar to loss of information, the capacity or the skill of the user can cause physical injury. A final general effect of assistive technology system errors is embarrassment. This effect is somewhat unique to assistive technologies, and it is a direct result of the role that assistive technology systems play in the daily life of the user who has a disability. Because the tasks being performed cannot be accomplished without the system, its use is continuous throughout the day. Over a long period, system errors leading to embarrassment are inevitable. The embarrassment may be relatively minor, such as a manipulation system dropping a spoonful of food. In other contexts, it may be much more significant. For example, an augmentative communication device may fail and produce the wrong utterance. If the context is a presentation in an important meeting and the mistaken utterance is an obscenity, the consequences are potentially very negative. To place the importance of this type of error in perspective, recall that the device is often perceived by both the user and other people as being a part of the user. Thus, the user is held responsible for an inappropriate utterance just as if he or she had used his or her own voice to produce it.

The errors and their resulting effects may arise from any of the components of the assistive technology system or their interaction. The human error may be related to capacity or skill. The device may malfunction, in which case the error is related to the design. The context may cause an error. For example, the pressure relief properties of a wheelchair cushion may be impaired if the cushion is exposed to extremely cold environments for a prolonged time and the cushion materials freeze. An example of an error that is caused by the interaction of the components of the HAAT model relates to devices that have many functions, with complex commands required for successful activation. In part, the error is caused by the capacity of the user to learn how to operate the device. It is also caused by the design of the device that requires complex actions for successful operation. Some of the concepts related to human factors that were discussed in Chapter 2 are relevant here.

It is clear from this discussion that identification and reduction of errors can occur at several points in the assistive technology process. Initially, incorporating a design and accompanying soft technologies that are congruent with universal design principles can minimize errors. Errors can be identified and possibly corrected through use of a thorough evaluation that leads to a suitable device recommendation, coupled with a trial period. Finally, errors in the assistive technology system are identified and reduced through follow-up with individual users and after market research into the effectiveness of the system.

Decision Making.   To propose a set of candidate assistive technology devices for a consumer, it is necessary to choose characteristics of these systems that will meet the needs and be consistent with the skills possessed by the consumer. The most important principle in this process is the relationship between the tasks the assistive technology device must accomplish for a person (embodied in the consumer's goals) and the characteristics that must be contained in the device for those tasks to be accomplished. Each goal may be accomplished only if a set of essential characteristics is included in the assistive technology system. For example, the goal may be mobility, and the characteristics of the type of cushion, wheelchair type, and color all contribute to the accomplishment of this goal.

Many characteristic-goal relationships are subtler, however, and generic characteristics of devices are not always equivalent to specific features of commercially available assistive technologies. For example, a generic characteristic of all EADLs is turning lights on and off. However, different manufacturers of EADLs may accomplish this function in different ways. Developing recommendations and a plan for implementation should be based on the consideration of device characteristics that have been evaluated by the consumer.

Computer-based **expert systems** that assist in the decision-making process for assistive technologies are being developed. Depending on the expert system, collection and interpretation of data are incorporated. Expert systems use artificial intelligence to guide the ATP through the assessment and decision-making process. Expert systems attempt to mimic the skills of an ATP by using software programs that are capable of making decisions much like humans do.

In assistive technologies, several preliminary systems have been developed. Garrett et al (1990) have developed an expert system called VOCAselect for use in selecting augmentative communication systems for specific consumers. Their system is based on 17 features that are determined during the assessment process. In addition to features related to consumer performance (e.g., input method, vocabulary size), they include physical construction (e.g., portability) and information regarding available support services (e.g., acceptable price range, training availability). These factors are then related to specific features of each available communication device. The expert system matches the specific requirements of the user, on the basis of goals and needs and on assessment of skills, to appropriate devices. By including the weight of factors (e.g., characteristic A is twice as important as characteristic B) and a scale of responses (e.g., priority for speech output is nine out of 10), this type of expert system can focus on specific options even more closely. Garrett et al report that preliminary trials indicate exact agreement in device selection between the expert system and a speech-language pathologist.

Stapelton and Garrett (1995) carried out an evaluation of this system. Respondents to a survey indicated strongly (greater than 79%) that this system would be of value in making recommendations for augmentative communication systems. They also present an example of the use of this program for a specific case. Stapelton et al (1995) extended the VOCAselect concept to the selection of computer adaptations (see Chapter 7). This computer program is similar to VOCAselect, but it is built on characteristics of devices and software used to make computers accessible to individuals who cannot use a keyboard or mouse for entry or the standard screen for output. In operation this software is functionally identical to VOCAselect. Stapelton et al (1995) present an example of the use of this system.

Regardless of whether an expert system is used, the process we have described is highly effective in defining the features of a recommended system. It is important to recognize that the features that are most limiting must be considered first, followed by those that are less restrictive. For example, in an augmentative communication system, the type of symbol system is often the most limiting characteristic. If a consumer requires pictures as a symbol, many devices are eliminated immediately. In contrast, spoken output as a characteristic is not as limiting because most devices use similar speech synthesizers. For each type of assistive technology, it is important for the ATP to identify a set of general characteristics that fit within the categories of Box 4-2. These are presented in later chapters. If the characteristics are generic, then specific features can be selected in sequence to define the final assistive technology system. The major advantage of the assessment methods described here is that they are based first on a consideration of the consumer's goals and skills and second on a consideration of assistive technology system characteristics. Thus the system is matched to the consumer (within the limits of current technology) rather than the consumer being forced to adapt to the system. Without a structured approach such as the one presented here, however, it is very difficult to meet consumer's goals.

It is clear that many characteristics of devices should be considered, and the features (and their costs) will differ from one system to the next. In addition to specific features of the device, other important factors include the contexts of use, the amount of training required before the device can be used effectively, cost, availability of a family member or caregiver to support and facilitate the training and implementation of the device, and ease of use of the device.

Recommendations and Report

The recommendations summarize the information gathered during the evaluation and suggest a design for the assistive technology system. At the conclusion of the assessment, everyone involved should sit down to review it and come to a consensus regarding the final recommendation. A written report is prepared that details the assessment and recommendations for an assistive technology system. The written report synthesizes the assessment process, and it starts out by defining the needs and goals that have been addressed. A summary of the consumer's skills applicable to device use is provided, with a description of generic characteristics to be incorporated into a device. This summary is followed by specific recommendations for equipment, including descriptions, part numbers if applicable, manufacturer's name, any modifications that need to be made, and cost. Recommendations for soft technologies are also included in the written report. These may include recommendations for developing skills that are necessary before purchase of a device, training once the device has been purchased, and strategies for incorporating the technology into the individual's context. Finally, a plan for implementation of the recommendations is provided. This includes logistics such as seeking funding from the appropriate sources and who will take responsibility for implementing the recommendations.

Often the written report is aimed at various individuals, thus presenting a unique challenge for the ATP writing it. The report, first of all, needs to be geared toward the consumer, who may not be familiar with medical or technical jargon. Rehabilitation or educational professionals working with the consumer may also be receiving the report and its recommendations. These professionals typically need information on what the consumer's skills have been in using the technology and what skill areas they may need to address to facilitate the use of the device. Some of these professionals may be very knowledgeable in assistive technology, but for others this may be their first experience with it. The contact person for the funding source will also be reading the report, and his or her interest is typically in the "bottom line," or what it is going to cost. This person wants evidence that the system recommended is going to meet the consumer's needs at the lowest possible cost. In the section on funding in this chapter, we describe how to write a report to a third-party payer to justify the purchase of an assistive technology system.

▦ IMPLEMENTATION

Once the recommendations have been made and funding is obtained, the implementation phase begins. This aspect of the delivery process consists of ordering specified equipment, obtaining commercially available equipment or fabricating custom equipment, making needed modifications, assembling or setting up equipment, thoroughly checking it as a system, fitting the device to the consumer, and training the consumer and caregivers in its use.

Ordering and Setup

Many recommended interventions have components from several manufacturers, and these must be integrated into a total system. Some of these may be standard commercially available components and others may be commercial assistive technologies. These devices are ordered from the manufacturer or equipment supplier and may take up to 6 weeks to be received after ordering. The recommendation may have also included a custom device or devices that require an adaptation. Examples of custom modifications include mounting a switch to a wheelchair or table, making a cable for connecting two devices together (e.g., a communication device and an EADL), programming a device for unique vocabulary, and adapting a battery-powered toy so that it can be controlled with one switch. The design and fabrication of these system components can occur during the waiting time for the delivery of the commercially available technologies. Once all the individual devices and adaptations are available, it is necessary to assemble them into a total package. For example, a wheelchair obtained from one source and a seating system from another will need to be interfaced to each other. The complexity of this assembly process varies widely, and some systems require much more effort than others.

Delivery and Fitting

Once the equipment is obtained, modified, or adapted as necessary and integrated into a system, the system is ready to be delivered to the consumer. This may occur in a clinic setting, in a school or at a job site, or in the consumer's living setting. The choice of locations depends on the nature of the equipment, the ease of transport of the consumer, and the complexity of the system (i.e., what support services of technicians and tools are required). We refer to all system deliveries as a "fitting" because we are interfacing the human (consumer) with the rest of the system. In some cases, such as custom seating systems, the process resembles a fitting for an orthotic or prosthetic device. In other cases the fitting focuses on installation of the system, mounting the control interface and the device to a wheelchair, and interconnection of the various components. The fitting phase may also include some amount of assessment as adjustments are made to optimize the consumer's ability to use the system. An example of this is the use of head switches to control a power wheelchair. The head switches must be attached to the wheelchair and wired into the controller unit. This is done before the fitting, and during the fitting, the location of the head switches (e.g., how close they are to the consumer's head) is adjusted to maximize performance.

The complexity of many assistive technology systems may require more than one session to obtain all the proper adjustments, mountings, and fittings. The ATP must be prepared to continue making adjustments and adaptations in the system until the consumer's goals and needs are met. This phase of the delivery process often involves some reassessment, but its success is directly related to the quality of the initial assessment and recommendations, and difficulties experienced at this time can often be traced to incomplete or inaccurate assessments.

Facilitating Assistive Technology System Performance

A major concern of everyone involved in the delivery of assistive technology services is whether the device recommended is going to meet the stated goals. It *cannot* be assumed that intervention ends with the delivery of the device. Most users of technology, even those with previous technology experience, require assistance in facilitating their performance with the device. The ATP, as the designer of the system, is responsible for providing the means to facilitate human performance. The soft technology described in Chapter 1 is relevant here.

Bailey (1989) identifies three methods that facilitate human performance: written instructions, performance aids, and training. He describes the major difference among each of these facilitators as "the time that elapses between when information is presented and when the performance takes place" (Bailey, 1989, p. 325). A performance aid is used immediately and written instructions are read and also used fairly quickly, but information presented during a training session may not be used until months later. In designing performance facilitators for individual users, the ATP should keep this difference in mind. The ATP also needs to know how to provide a balance among these facilitators. For example, many manufacturers of augmentative communication devices develop an abundance of written instructions.

Even if the user were to read all this information, most of it would be forgotten. It has been found that when workers on a job site need information that can be found in similar documents, they either take a guess at the solution or ask someone else (Bailey, 1989). The same thing happens with assistive technology users. An example of this is a person who is hard of hearing and obtains a hearing aid. It may work fine for a relatively long period; then the batteries are discharged and need to be replaced. Often the user merely puts the hearing aid in a drawer because it "doesn't work anymore" instead of replacing the batteries. If the user does replace the batteries, it is generally because he asked someone else what to do or was instructed in the process when the aid was sold to him, not because he looked it up in the user's manual. Bailey admits that there are few guidelines to help the ATP determine when to use performance aids, written instructions, or training but emphasizes that "the best decisions are made when as much as possible is known about the potential users, the activity to be performed, and the context in which the performance will take place" (p. 326). As applicable, each of the following chapters has a section on specific training ideas.

Training.   Bailey (1989) defines training as "the acquisition of skills, knowledge, and attitudes that will lead to an acceptable level of human performance on a specific activity in a given context" (p. 387), which is referred to as *performance-based training*. In the field of assistive technology, prior authorization from the funding source to conduct training is usually required. For a funding source to authorize training, an estimate of the amount of time that will be needed is typically required, with the result that training becomes *time based* rather than performance based. Time-based training is completed within a specified period, regardless of whether the user achieves a level of skill. Without adequate training, there is an increased likelihood that the device will be abandoned. The training process is facilitated if the ATP starts out by developing a set of well-defined, measurable objectives for training. These objectives help focus the training sessions and serve as an indicator for termination of training. It is also important that there be one person affiliated with the consumer who takes on the role of the facilitator and learns the operation of the device and basic concepts so that he or she can assist with the use of the device as needed.

Training oriented toward establishing **operational competence** is initiated at the delivery and fitting (Pallin, 1991). This phase of training is intended to make it possible for the user of the technology, his or her care providers and family, and any other support person to begin using the assistive technology system. Examples of considerations included in training for operational competency for the consumer are (1) how to turn an electronic device on and off, (2) making adjustments in operational parameters (e.g., adjusting a scanning rate), (3) loading an initial vocabulary in an augmentative communication system, (4) explaining basic maintenance (e.g., battery charging, cleaning), (5) introducing basic functions and how they work (e.g., choosing what to say on a communication device, using an adapted telephone dialer), and (6) basic troubleshooting so that the consumer and others have some strategies to use if problems develop with the system. It is important to present information in small doses to avoid overwhelming the consumer and others, particularly for a complex system. At the initial fitting session it is only necessary to present enough information so that the consumer can begin to use the system. Subsequent training addresses the acquisition of the necessary skills for more advanced operations.

In addition to basic operational competence, it is necessary for the consumer to develop strategies that maximize the effectiveness of the system. To facilitate this, the ATP provides training for **strategic competence.** The training focuses on the *application* of the system rather than on basic operation. As this phase of training progresses, the consumer begins to develop his or her own set of strategies. For example, the person using a manual wheelchair will develop strategies for navigating curbs or inclines and the user of an augmentative and alternative communication (AAC) device will develop strategies for communicating in a noisy restaurant.

CASE STUDY

TRAINING

Marilyn is a 45-year-old woman who sustained a brain-stem stroke. Her only available control site is very slight movement of her right thumb. She will use this movement to control a computer that provides both verbal and written augmentative communication (see Chapter 9) and EADL (see Chapter 14). She resides in a skilled nursing facility where she has daily visits from family and church members. One session a week for 4 weeks will be carried out. Her training program will include the following:

Session One
Basic operational competence: Instruction in how to connect the switch to the AAC system and to mount the switch for independent access; discussion of setup of software parameters for scanning; presentation of an overview of system features; instruction in charging of batteries and the use of the swing-away mounting systems for the computer and the switches.
Basic linguistic competence: Instruction in how to use commands in the word processor to load, save, edit, print, use pictures and use different fonts; instruction in how to retrieve and use vocabulary; and selection of preliminary vocabulary.
Basic strategic competence: Discussion of when to use features to maximize effectiveness of the AAC device.
Basic social competence: Discussion of how augmented communication differs from speech.

Session Two
Intermediate operational competence: Instruction in storage and retrieval of vocabulary in the electronic AAC device.
Intermediate linguistic competence: Instruction in how to use advanced features of the word processor and how to add vocabulary to the system.

Intermediate social competence: Discussion of how to be a good communicator.

Session Three
Advanced operational competence: Instruction in how to load and use new vocabulary files and how to print. Instruction in how to use the AAC menu to select and control the EADL; demonstration of how to connect devices to remote control receivers and how to make phone calls by using the AAC device.
Intermediate strategic competence: Discussion of how to use strategies for conversations with visitors. Development of strategies for conversations with nursing staff.

Session Four
Advanced linguistic competence: Practice with word processor for writing. Instruction in how to use special features to enhance speech output.
Advanced strategic competence: Discussion of when to use different system features. Development and use of conversational repair strategies, and effective use of commenting (see Chapter 11).
Advanced social competence: Instruction in how to vary conversational vocabulary and moods for differing categories of interaction and partners, and how to select vocabulary and modes for differing social situations.

Marilyn, her husband, and the staff of the long-term care facility in which she is currently living will devote the period between the sessions to practice. Before the start of each session, information from the prior session will be reviewed to see whether Marilyn has any questions. At the fourth session Marilyn will be evaluated to see how she is doing in using the device and to determine whether she has further training needs.

Performance Aids. A document or device containing information that an individual uses to assist in the completion of an activity is called a **performance aid.** By decreasing the amount of information to be remembered, the performance aid reduces the amount of cognitive processing required to complete an activity. With a performance aid, the user does not have to rely as much on long-term memory, which results in reduced errors, increased speed for certain tasks, and a reduced amount of training required. Performance aids do not necessarily have to be written; picture symbols can also be effective for individuals who cannot read. Bailey (1989) describes five quality standards for performance aids: (1) accessibility, (2) accuracy, (3) clarity, (4) completeness and conciseness, and (5) legibility.

Performance aids are commonly used with individuals who have memory deficits as a result of damage to the brain. One type of performance aid is simple step-by-step instructions that assist the user in carrying out a sequence of tasks. For example, Tim is a young man who has sustained a head injury. He uses a computer to complete school assignments but has problems remembering the sequence of steps to get into his computer word processing program. The steps to do this have been simply written and are posted next to his computer. Because Tim also has visual acuity problems, the instructions are printed in large, bold letters. For Tim, this simple performance aid has meant the difference between success and failure in using his computer.

Another type of performance aid assists in remembering several items of information. An example of this type of aid is a printed list of codes with their meanings, which an individual may have stored in his or her augmentative communication system. Often such a list such is attached to the side of the device so the user can view it easily as needed. Sometimes codes and their meanings are built into software programs and presented on the screen each time the user selects a letter.

Written Instructions. Written instructions should be considered an integral part of the system and be available to the user at the time of the system delivery. Instructions are helpful when step-by-step directions with detailed information are required or when graphic information needs to be presented. Written instructions may be compiled and presented in the form of user manuals, handbooks, or computer software. The ATP must not assume that the instructions provided by the manufacturer are going to be adequate. Written instructions provided by the manufacturer of the system may include too little or too much information or they may be difficult to follow by the user. It is recommended that instructions from the manufacturer be reviewed and supplemented as needed. When the manufacturer's documentation is overwhelming, the ATP can review the documentation and condense it into a quick reference sheet that provides simplified and frequently used information.

Bailey (1989) provides detailed guidelines for developing the various types of written documents, including software documentation. It is important to remember to keep the audience in mind and to write the instructions for the people who will use them. For example, if the primary person facilitating the performance is the parent, the instructions may be different from those generated if the facilitator is a teacher. In the field of assistive technology, this may mean a new or revised set of instructions for each individual consumer, even for use of the same device.

■ FOLLOW-UP AND FOLLOW-ALONG

Once the system has been implemented, it is tempting to think that the intervention has been completed. This perception, however, is totally false; the delivery of the system marks the beginning of the time of use, and it therefore signals the beginning of the evaluation of system effectiveness. The term **follow-up** refers to activities that occur during the period immediately after delivery of an assistive technology system and that address the effectiveness of the device, training, and user strategies. The term **follow-along** is used to describe those activities that take place over a longer period. This phase addresses factors such as changes in needs or goals, availability of new devices, and other concerns.

A formal follow-up phase is included in the delivery process for several reasons: (1) assistive devices can seldom be used right out of the box without ever needing to be adjusted, (2) electronic devices are not 100% reliable, and a significant portion of them require repair during the first year of use, (3) training programs seldom proceed flawlessly, and questions arise during the initial period of use, and (4) perceived device failures are often the result of operator error caused by a lack of device understanding. A carefully developed follow-up program will identify these problems easily and address them quickly.

Repair and maintenance are often conducted during the follow-up phase. *Repair* refers to action taken to correct a problem in a system. *Maintenance,* on the other hand, is a systematic set of procedures that is aimed at keeping the device in working order. Examples of maintenance functions are proper battery charging, cleaning, tightening mounting hardware, and lubrication of moving mechanical parts. A regular schedule will ensure that necessary maintenance takes place. Assistive technology system failures result in a major disruption of the consumer's life. For example, a consumer depends on a power wheelchair for mobility. If it fails, he or she may have a manual wheelchair as a backup, but the consumer's independence may be significantly reduced. Repair of assistive technologies is most often carried out either through manufacturer's representatives or directly through the manufacturer. In the latter case, the device must be returned to the factory for repair, and the consumer may be without it for several days or even longer. Prompt attention to repair needs of consumers is an important part of follow-up.

As part of a formal follow-up program, contacts with the consumer (by telephone, on the job site, in the home, or in the clinic) are scheduled on a regular basis, such as at 1, 3, 6, and 12 months after delivery. These contacts occur regardless of whether there is a perceived problem, and they are in addition to other activities such as training or repair. This regularly scheduled contact is important because there may be unnoticed problems, or more often there are underused features that are discovered during the follow-up sessions. Mortola, Kohn, and LeBlanc (1992) found in a follow-up study that, because of mechanical reasons, 63% of 196 assistive devices delivered by their center were not being. In most of these cases the consumer had not informed the ATP of the device failure.

As we have defined it, follow-along has a much longer time frame than follow-up does. Although follow-up typically covers the first year of operation of an assistive technology system, follow-along is carried out over the individual's lifetime. Consumers may return for service after a period of years for several reasons. They may have found that the device is not working as they would like and is not meeting their functional goals. Another reason is to obtain information about advances in technology since they obtained the device. In other cases the consumer may have changed in significant ways. This change is often seen in children who have grown significantly and need a revision in their seating system. Change can also be the result of a degenerative condition such as amyotrophic lateral sclerosis, and in these cases the device may need to be altered to accommodate decreased physical function. In other cases the change in consumer condition is a result of the development of new skills that make it possible to consider new device features. For example, a consumer who has had a traumatic brain injury may initially receive a communication device that is based on very simple replay of sentences. As he or she recovers, the ability to spell effectively may improve and a device with this capability should be considered.

There are other reasons for follow-along. One of the most important of these is a change in the life roles and context of the consumer. For example, Martin, who has severe cerebral palsy and has used an AAC device for several years, decides to move into an apartment on his own. The success of this transition could depend heavily on the availability of assistive technologies. An EADL would allow him to control lights and appliances, answer and dial the telephone, and control the television, DVD, and other entertainment devices. This re-evaluation is dictated not by changes in his condition but by changes in his life roles and the context in which he will be using his technology.

As opposed to follow-up, follow-along is often initiated by the consumer rather than by the ATP. This is because the ATP is not aware of the changing physical, sensory, and cognitive conditions in the consumer. On the other hand, the consumer cannot possibly be aware of changes in technology. For this reason, it is important that the ATP develop a mechanism to maintain contact with consumers to inform them of changes in technology. This mechanism should empower each consumer to take personal responsibility for his or her long-term assistive technology needs. One frequently used method for doing this is a regular newsletter that is sent to consumers by the ATP.

Another reason for both follow-up and follow-along is to evaluate the effectiveness of the assistive technology system by measuring outcomes. This evaluation provides a measure of how well the system meets the original needs identified during the assessment. The next section describes the measurement of outcomes.

■ EVALUATING THE EFFECTIVENESS OF ASSISTIVE TECHNOLOGY SERVICES AND SYSTEMS

Measuring the outcomes of assistive technology services is a primary focus in the industry today and will continue to be in the forefront of assistive technology service delivery. Consumers want measures that reflect their needs for improved function and quality of life. Payers seek efficient provision of services using the fewest possible resources, and providers seek information on how to deliver efficient and effective assistive technology services. To provide evidence of the effectiveness of assistive technology services and systems, well-developed and sound outcome measures are required.

Fuhrer et al (2003) suggest that a comprehensive conceptual framework will guide the development of useful outcome measures. They describe a model that will help researchers and clinicians identify assumptions, variables, and populations when developing, considering, and implementing assistive technology outcome measures. Outcome of device use is considered to be the frequency and duration of device use.

The model considers different time frames when evaluation is important: initial procurement of the device and the introductory period leading to short- and long-term outcomes. Three aspects are considered when a device is obtained: (1) the need for the device, (2) the type of device, including its intrinsic and extrinsic properties, and (3) the services involved when obtaining the device (Fuhrer et al, 2003). A number of constructs are considered in evaluating short- and long-term outcomes, including effectiveness, efficiency, satisfaction with the device, psychological function, and subjective opinion of the contribution of the device to the client's well-being (Fuhrer et al, 2003). If the user is not satisfied with the device, it may be abandoned in either the short or the long term. The constructs related to the *International Classification of Functioning, Disability, and Health* (ICF) (World Health Organization [WHO], 2001) are mediating factors in the short and long term. This classification is described in Chapter 1.

When outcome measures for assistive technology systems are considered, the ATP needs to develop measures and standards of performance that allow a careful determination of the effectiveness of such systems. For instance, a child who is evaluated for a power wheelchair (see Chapter 12) will have a level of accuracy, speed, and reliability that can be measured. Speed of response and accuracy are both used to assess power wheelchair performance. The speed of response is important in describing how quickly a disabled consumer reacts to obstacles, and accuracy is a measure of how well the consumer can navigate a specific course. If this is used as the baseline performance, progress over time can de determined by comparing performance with this baseline. In a clinic or laboratory setting, these measures can be used to select a control interface (see Chapter 7) and to determine such things as the feasibility of safe powered mobility. However, to determine the success of the desired functional outcome (independent mobility), measures must be made in the intended context. This requirement raises several additional questions, such as what is the standard for accuracy of power wheelchair use in a shopping mall? Is it a minimal number of collisions with people and objects? If so, how many are acceptable? Is it being able to successfully negotiate a crowded store? If so, what is being measured to assess success (e.g., minimal breakage, no collisions, how fast the user gets to the door)? Obviously, measuring and assessing assistive technology system performance in the real world is not an easy task. In the remainder of this chapter the focus is primarily on the measurement of outcomes of the use of assistive technology devices and the provision of services.

Overview

The effectiveness of assistive technology systems in meeting the needs of consumers is related to many factors. Sackett (1980) identifies four types of evaluation to consider: effectiveness, efficacy, availability, and efficiency. These can each be related to different questions and to different assessment instruments. For evaluating *effectiveness* we ask the question, does it work? Effectiveness is measured in terms of the impact of the product on the consumer's life and needs. Therefore the outcome measurements that we collect must begin with and focus on the consumer and the results of the assistive technology intervention. These outcomes allow us to determine the *efficacy* of the service delivery structure and process. Efficacy is the ability to produce a desired result or effect; the question to be asked is, can it work? This aspect

is what is measured in evaluation of a service delivery structure and process. It provides useful information on how services are being delivered so that necessary revisions can be made.

The entire assistive technology industry is evaluated by the success of service delivery and assistive technology system use by the consumer. As described above, the consumer and the delivery of assistive technology services are at the core of the assistive technology industry (see Figure 1-2). Gathering information on outcomes should be included as a regular part of the service delivery process so that this information can be used as feedback to the rest of the industry. For example, a manufacturer could be determined to have good manufacturing practices and meet all industry standards; however, the most meaningful standard is the effectiveness of the equipment for consumers. Likewise, the effectiveness of the equipment is only as good as the service provider who delivers it. If, as a whole, there are problems with consumer use of assistive technology, all the industry will be affected. This aspect is related to evaluation of *availability*, which asks the question, is it reaching those who need it (Sackett, 1980)?

Finally, the question, is it worth doing? needs to be answered. This addresses the relative importance of the service being provided by comparing it with other programs that could be purchased with the same resources. This evaluation measure is referred to as *efficiency*. Third-party payers want to know that the assistive technology services and devices are worth paying for. It is the ATP's responsibility to provide this justification.

A wide range of outcome data needs to be collected, and determinations need to be made regarding what measures will be used, how many measures are needed, and how focused the measures need to be (Smith, 1996). When outcome measures are developed for assistive technology devices and services, it is important to be clear about who the stakeholders are in this process (DeRuyter, 1995). This is not as obvious a question as it first seems. If outcome measures are used to inform funding sources, are these funding sources consumers of the outcome results or stakeholders in the process? Likewise, providers may be considered either consumers or stakeholders, depending on the type of outcome measure used and the implications for its implementation. If user satisfaction is to be used as an outcome measure, is that a measure that relates to the provider, the funding source, or the user? Certainly the user of the technology is a consumer, but not all outcome measures are user centered. In the remainder of this section those measures that have been demonstrated to have reliability and validity in the measurement of outcomes at several levels are discussed.

Structure, process, and outcome measures in assistive technology delivery can be distinguished among. The *structure* of the delivery system refers to aspects such as the staffing, staff expertise, equipment on hand, budget, and range of services provided. The *process* of assistive technology delivery includes the stages of assessment and intervention described in this chapter. Process measures ascertain whether these stages have occurred and whether the procedures meet an acceptable standard. **Outcome measures** evaluate the end result of the assistive technology intervention. Figure 4-7 illustrates the interrelationships among the assistive technology system, the service delivery process, and their outcomes.

There are a number of different levels at which we can evaluate the effectiveness of both devices and services by measuring outcomes. Traditionally, at the clinical level the question being asked is, did the intervention remediate the individual's impairment? This is the impairment level of the ICF classification of the WHO (see Chapter 1). In the provision of assistive technologies, this level is seldom the major focus, but it is important because assistive technologies can lead to improvement in impairment and thus in function. The *parallel interventions model* (Angelo and Smith, 1989; Smith, 1991) described earlier in this chapter illustrates how intervention to affect the level of impairment is related to the use of assistive technologies. The next level is the functional level, when the question is, can the individual accomplish tasks that he or she could not do without the assistive technology? This is the activity level of the ICF classification of the WHO. In this case, **functional performance measures** are typically used to determine effectiveness.

When services were primarily clinical and delivered in institutional settings, measures of impairment and functional measures were the focus of outcome evaluation. However, over the past decade there has been a move toward community-based services in rehabilitation. This has been driven by rising costs of institutional care and is being addressed by shortening stays and transferring more care to the community. As described in this chapter, many services, including most of assistive technology services, are more appropriately delivered in the community where they will be used.

Community-based services are also being driven by an emerging alliance between the largely institution-based rehabilitation establishment and the largely community-based disability community. This alliance has implications for responsibility for care, including responsibility for choices of assistive technology devices and services (Lysack and Kaufert, 1999). As described in Chapter 1 and in this chapter, consumers play a larger role in decision making regarding what they receive and the evaluation of the quality of both the devices and services. The question being asked by the consumer at this level is, do the assistive technology services and devices provided meet my needs? To answer this question, **user satisfaction measures** related to assistive technology services and devices have been developed.

As discussed in Chapter 1, the classification of disability over the past 20 years has begun to focus on its social dimensions (Fougeyrollas and Gray, 1998). This social model, now incorporated into the WHO ICF classification (WHO, 2001), provides a richer and more complete view of both disability and the role of assistive technologies in the lives of people who have disabilities. It is no longer important to achieve success only in the clinic or laboratory. The real test is in daily community use of the technologies. The question being asked at this level is, what is the impact of this assistive technology device or service on quality of life? The primary outcome measures used for assessing the effectiveness of assistive technology devices and services in this broader social context are **quality-of-life measures.**

Each of these primary types of measurement of assistive technology device and service outcomes is discussed in the following sections.

Measuring Clinical and Functional Outcomes

In the past, health care and rehabilitation quality of service was measured by looking at factors such as timeliness and the completeness of the services provided (e.g., whether a discharge summary was completed for the consumer within 1 week of discharge). These are actually process measures, and they do not reflect outcomes of the assistive technology intervention. Within the past decade or so, rehabilitation service providers have begun to focus more on the functional

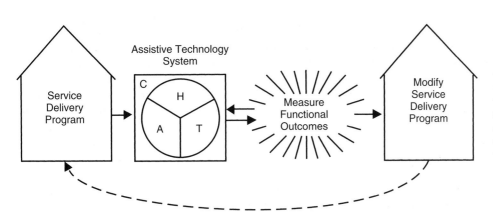

Figure 4-7 Interrelationship among the assistive technology system, the service delivery process and structure, and their outcomes. *H*, Human; *A*, activity; *C*, context; *T*, assistive technology.

outcomes achieved by the consumer as a result of intervention. Because the focus of assistive technology practitioners is on reducing disability and maximizing an individual's functional status, it is only natural that one of the factors to measure is functional outcome related to assistive device use.

There are a number of tools that have been developed and studied that measure functional outcomes of individuals who have been through the rehabilitation process. Examples of functional outcome measures include the Barthel Index (Mahoney and Barthel, 1965), the Klein-Bell ADL Scale (Klein and Bell, 1979), and the Functional Independence Measure™ (FIM) (Uniform Data System for Medical Rehabilitation, 1997).

Unfortunately, many of these traditional tools used in the field of rehabilitation do not document the efficacy of technological intervention (Christiansen, Schwartz, and Barnes, 1988; Smith, 1996). As Smith (1996) points out, many instruments are limited in their scope in three ways: (1) they tend to be developed for a particular population, such as individuals who have sustained a stroke, (2) many instruments are developed for a particular health care setting, such as long-term care or acute rehabilitation settings, and (3) they frequently focus on a specific functional area, such as hand function or self-care.

Functional Independence Measure. The FIM™ Instrument is an example of one functional outcome measure. We have chosen the FIM™ as an example because it is widely used in assessing the outcomes of rehabilitation interventions. The FIM™ is based on a medical model of assessment that places importance on cure (Smith, 1996). The FIM measures the individual's performance on 18 items under the categories of self-care, bowel and bladder management, transfers, locomotion, communication, and cognition (Uniform Data System for Medical Rehabilitation, 1997). The scoring of the FIM™ is on a seven-point scale. The individual only obtains the full seven points if he or she does not require any assistance or assistive device to perform a function. Thus the FIM™ is not directly applicable to assistive device outcome measurement because its maximal score in any category can only be obtained if the person does not use any technology. Use of technology automatically implies that the person is not totally functionally independent. This appraisal of functional independence is inconsistent with the current view that an individual is independent if he or she can manage his or her own life (Smith, 1996). Another concern regarding the FIM™ and other tools that measure function is that they do not impart information regarding the impact of assistive devices on the quality of life of the user (Jutai et al, 1996).

User Satisfaction as an Outcome Measure

Any discussion of assistive technology effectiveness must consider the recommended system and how well it meets the consumer's needs. Therefore, the measures must be consumer oriented, which means that the factors used to evaluate the effectiveness of assistive technology systems must be based on criteria that are important to the consumer. **User satisfaction** is the consumer's perception of the degree to which the assistive technology system achieves the desired goal. This is a multidimensional phenomenon that requires qualitative measures (Demers, Weiss-Lambrou, and Ska, 1996). In addition, general user satisfaction scales are global, and they do not take into account various factors that affect a person's use or nonuse of assistive technologies. In assistive technology applications, on the other hand, rating scales that address specific aspects of use are used (see Brooks, 1990, for example). For a large sample of users, these surveys can be statistically analyzed to determine the most important factors in achieving user satisfaction. These group statistics may indicate a significant lack of satisfaction, and this information can be used to make changes in the service delivery structure and process to improve user satisfaction. For any individual assistive technology system, satisfaction is one parameter to be evaluated during the follow-up and follow-along processes. One limitation with satisfaction survey instruments is that they often "top out"; that is, individuals use either the highest or lowest score, and the range of a scale is lost. For example, assume that a five-point scale is used, with levels of "very dissatisfied," "dissatisfied," "neutral," "satisfied," and "very satisfied." Most individuals will reduce this to a three-point scale, using the two ends and "neutral." This is especially true if several parameters are measured with the same scale. Also, user satisfaction scales are one dimensional, measuring only satisfaction. Multidimensional scales can be more informative (Jutai, personal communication, 2001).

Canadian Occupational Performance Measure. The Canadian Occupational Performance Measure (COPM) (Law et al, 1998) assesses the client's perception of the importance of self-identified occupational performance goals and his or her satisfaction with that performance. The measure uses an interview format to identify goals in the areas of self-care, productivity, and leisure. The client rates the importance of each of these goals and their satisfaction. The instrument can be used before and after intervention. It is quite flexible because it allows the user to adapt the instrument for a specific purpose. The user can ask the client to think specifically of self-care, productivity, and leisure activities that he or she wants or needs to do when using a particular type of assistive technology. Miller Polgar and Barlow (2002) used this instrument as an outcome of seating and mobility intervention. Its utility was somewhat limited unless the client was asked to think about goals that specifically involved the use of assistive technology. This instrument has been used with many different client populations. Once the client becomes comfortable with identifying his or her own goals, the COPM is a very useful outcome measure.

Quebec User Evaluation of Satisfaction With Assistive Technology.

Five criteria were used in the development of the Quebec User Evaluation of Satisfaction with Assistive Technology (QUEST) (Demers, Weiss-Lambrou, and Ska, 1996). The first is the recognition that user satisfaction is a multidimensional phenomenon that includes a broad range of variables, each of which can affect the user's satisfaction with assistive technology. The second criterion relates to the inclusion of three types of variables: those involving the environment (context in the HAAT model), pertinent features of the person's personality (the human), and the characteristics of the assistive technology itself. The third criterion is the recognition that the user should determine the relative importance of the satisfaction variable. This reflects the highly subjective nature of the user satisfaction measure. The fourth criterion provides for the user to express his or her opinion freely within the constraints of an interview context. Finally, the QUEST was designed to be simple to understand and easy to use by ATPs when evaluating satisfaction. The QUEST requires approximately 30 minutes to administer and is guided by a three-part form.

The first part of the instrument is the general information questionnaire. This form is designed to determine the context in which the user's satisfaction or dissatisfaction developed. It consists of 18 open-ended questions designed to include the three domains of environment (context [e.g., living arrangements, social supports, funding considerations]), user characteristics (human [e.g., sex, age, nature of disability, types of functional problems]), and assistive technology characteristics (e.g., when the device was acquired, frequency and patterns of use or nonuse, number and types of assistive technologies used).

The second part of the QUEST instrument is an assessment of satisfaction. This includes a set of 27 variables that represents the factors most likely to affect user satisfaction with assistive technologies. Each of the variables represents a specific category, but they are randomly ordered in the presentation to the user. This ensures that the user's answers are not artificially influenced by the category of the question. Three tasks are used in this part of the evaluation. In the first task, the person is asked the degree of importance that he or she attributes to each variable. Each of the variables is printed on a card. There is a board for classifying the variable from very important (a score of 3) to no importance (0). The evaluator asks the user where he or she would like each card placed and then circles the response on the form. After completing the 27 variables, the user is given an opportunity to add other satisfaction variables that he or she feels are important. This task personalizes the assessment in terms of the individual's preferences. The second task requires that the evaluator reorganize the variables according to the three

categories, and only the variables selected as being quite or very important (scores of 2 or 3) are included. For this task, a six-point scale (0 [very dissatisfied] to 5 [very satisfied]) portrayed on a semicircular dial is used. For each of the variables included from Task 1, the user is asked to indicate his or her satisfaction by moving the dial or instructing the evaluator where to place it. The evaluator then circles the result on the summary form. Finally, the user is asked to express a global satisfaction score for the device. This task, as in Task 1, personalizes the assessment to the individual user. The third and final part of the QUEST requires that the evaluator reorganize the results from Part 2 into the three global categories (environment, person, and assistive technology). Only the values for those variables rated as quite or very important in Task 1 are included. The summary sheet then serves to facilitate the interpretation and use of the data in assessing satisfaction and addressing those areas in which satisfaction is low.

Weiss-Lambrou et al (1999) used the QUEST to determine satisfaction of consumers with seating aids. They describe the application of QUEST to this situation with a group of 24 subjects who used modular seating aids (see Chapter 6). They found that the most important variable (user comfort) was also rated as the least satisfying. This study illustrates the value and importance of a consumer-driven measure of user satisfaction. Weiss-Lambrou et al describe the application of QUEST in this context in detail.

Assistive Technology Abandonment.

One of the most tangible indicators of lack of consumer satisfaction is when the consumer stops using a device although the need for which the device was obtained still exists. This situation is called **technology abandonment,** and it is useful to look at some of the factors that lead to it. Phillips and Zhao (1993) surveyed more than 200 users of assistive technologies and identified four factors that were significantly related to the abandonment of assistive technologies: (1) failure of providers to take consumers' opinions into account, (2) easy device procurement, (3) poor device performance, and (4) changes in consumers' needs or priorities.

More recent research examined personal and social factors that predict assistive technology abandonment. Pape, Kim, and Weiner (2002) conducted a review of the literature related to assistive technology abandonment to look at how the personal meaning attributed to assistive devices influences their integration into the user's daily life. They found that psychosocial and cultural variables were primary factors in determining the meaning individuals assigned to assistive technology. In particular, their expectations of how the device would function, the social costs of using the device (i.e., cost/benefit of device use), and an outlook that disability did not define the user as a person were the primary factors that contributed to whether a person integrated assistive technology into his or her life (Pape, Kim, and Weiner, 2002). Reimer-Weiss and Wacker (2000) examined factors that predicated assistive technology use in individuals with disability. They found that the relative advantage of the assistive technology in the user's life and the user's involvement in the device selection process were predictors of device use or discontinuance.

Scherer et al (2005) have developed a group of measures that help determine the match between the individual and technology. The Matching Person and Technology assessment is described shortly. A recent study examined the validity of the assumptions that guided the development of this instrument. The results of the study supported these assumptions, specifically that personal characteristics related to mood, self-esteem, self-determination and motivation, and psychosocial characteristics related to friend and family support (as examples) were significant predictors of device use (Scherer et al, 2005). Collectively, the earlier studies of Phillips and Zhao (1993) and the more recent work of Pape et al (2002), Reimer-Weiss and Wacker (2000), and Scherer et al (2005) provide evidence that characteristics of the device, the person, and their environment predict whether the client will use a device or abandon it.

Quality of Life as an Assistive Technology Outcome Measure

ATPs, assistive technology suppliers, and assistive technology manufacturers often claim that their services or devices "improve the quality of life" of the consumer. This is an appealing concept. Who wouldn't want to do this? There are, however, several difficulties with this concept when there is an attempt to actually measure it. In fact, the term *quality of life* is itself controversial and subject to misuse (Wolfensberger, 1994). Despite these limitations, it is tempting to want to measure quality of life. It is being applied with increasing frequency to outcomes measurement in medicine and rehabilitation (Oldridge, 1996). In a medical service context, quality of life is often related to life expectancy and optimal life quality during the time a person is alive. In rehabilitation the concept of quality of life takes on a bit of a different meaning because the goal is not "repair" or cure but rather maximizing function and independence for the individual. In both cases the concept of health is important. The WHO defines health as "a state of complete physical, mental and social well-being, not merely the absence of disease" (WHO, 1948). Assistive technologies can certainly contribute to both quality of life and a healthy life. Measures designed to assess the degree to which this goal is achieved have begun to emerge over the past decade, and we are in a position to evaluate the assertion that a service or device actually does improve a consumer's quality of life. Several measures of quality of life are discussed in this section.

Health-Related Quality of Life. The concept of **health-related quality of life** (HRQL) refers to the impact of health services on the overall quality of life of

individuals, and it represents the functional effect of an illness and its consequent therapy on an individual as perceived by the person receiving the therapy (Oldridge, 1996). It measures one dimension of quality of life. Others are independence, income, adequate housing, and a safe environment. The definition of HRQL is "the value assigned to duration of life as modified by impairment, functional states, perceptions and social opportunities that are influenced by disease, injury, treatment or policy" (Patrick and Erickson, 1993; quoted by Oldridge, 1996). Rehabilitation in general, and assistive technologies in particular, addresses the long-term effects of disease and injury. Therefore both rehabilitation and assistive technology affect HRQL as defined here. However, as Oldridge points out, there are many instruments that have been developed to measure HRQL. Many of these are medically oriented and unsuited to assistive technology outcomes measurement. However, the general concepts underlying HRQL do have relevance to assistive technology outcomes measurement, and there is a need to develop new instruments that are more sensitive to the impact of assistive technologies on HRQL. Oldridge (1996) describes the types of HRQL measurements, their application, and the underlying principles on which this construct is based.

Psychosocial Impact of Assistive Devices Scale. To address the need for quality of life–related measures in assessing assistive technology outcomes, Day and Jutai (1996) developed the Psychosocial Impact of Assistive Devices Scale (PIADS). The development of the PIADS was based on information obtained through focus groups on the experiences of users of assistive technology (Day and Jutai, 1996). The initial set of constructs was developed and evaluated by a set of users. The scales were modified to include both positive and negative impacts on quality of life of assistive technology users by defining a scale from −3 (maximal negative impact) to +3 (maximal positive impact). The final version of the PIADS is a 26-item self-rating scale intended to measure the impact of rehabilitative technologies and assistive devices on the quality of life of the users of these products. Three subscales are included in the PIADS. These are competence (the effects of a device on functional independence, performance, and productivity), adaptability (the enabling and liberating effects of a device), and self-esteem (the extent to which a device has affected self-confidence, self-esteem, and emotional well-being). This multidimensional aspect of the PIADS contributes to its reliability and validity as a measure of the psychosocial impact of assistive technologies on the consumer.

The PIADS has been applied to measurement of outcomes with a variety of assistive technologies. The original study focused on eyeglass and contact lens wearers (Day and Jutai, 1996). In subsequent studies it has been demonstrated that the subscales of the PIADS remain consistent over populations and types of disabilities (stroke, amyotrophic lateral sclerosis, cerebral palsy) or types of assistive technologies. For example, Jutai et al (2000) used the PIADS to evaluate the psychosocial impact of EADLs (see Chapter 14). The goal of this study was to determine the perceived benefit of EADLs to the consumer's quality of life. Two groups were included: users of EADLs and those for whom EADLs were appropriate but who had not yet received them. Users' perceptions were measured at two points 6 to 9 months apart to determine the stability of the perception of psychosocial impact. Jutai et al found that EADLs produced similar degrees of positive impact on users and positive perceptions of anticipated impact on those without EADLs. The two measures of those using EADLs indicated that the psychosocial impact was stable over the time frame used. This study demonstrated the utility of the PIADS as an instrument for quantifying the psychosocial impact of assistive technologies.

Jutai et al (1996) discuss the use of instruments such as the PIADS to evaluate the outcomes of service provision in assistive technologies. The importance of quality-of-life outcome measures, in addition to clinical, functional, and user satisfaction assessments, is demonstrated through a series of case studies related to ease of implementation, clear definition of the desired outcomes, ethical considerations, and responsibility to the user of the assistive technology.

Matching Person and Technology Model. The Matching Person and Technology (MPT) model and assessment instruments have been developed to allow consumers to prioritize their own outcomes in relation to measurable changes in the perceived quality of life as opposed to the absence of disease or sickness or functional ability (Galvin and Scherer, 1996). This instrument has much in common with the QUEST and PIADS. The developers of the QUEST used the MPT as one of the theoretical bases for their work (Demers, Weiss-Lambrou, and Ska, 1996). As in these other measures, the MPT is a multidimensional instrument that taps domains related to overall impact on quality of life. Three domains are included in the MPT (Galvin and Scherer, 1996). The *milieu* dimension assesses characteristics of the environment and psychosocial setting in which the assistive technology is to be used. The *personality* dimension focuses on the individual's personality, temperament, and preferences. Finally, the *technology* component addresses characteristics of the assistive technology itself. Like the QUEST and PIADS, the MPT is designed to be applied across a wide range of disabilities and assistive technology types. The multidimensional nature of the MPT makes it possible to separate influences of the technology, environment, and personal preferences. For example, a consumer may have characteristics (goals, skills, and abilities) typically associated with assistive technology nonuse as measured by the

milieu/environment variable but may appear to be an optimal user according to characteristics identified for personality and technology. In this case the milieu/environment influences may need to be addressed before the consumer can gain maximal benefit and satisfaction from the use of the assistive technology. Galvin and Scherer (1996) describe the MPT instrument and its application in detail. The MPT has been shown to have reliability and validity in determining the factors related to device abandonment and in assessing the impact on quality of life of assistive technology use.

Relationship of Outcome Measures to the Human Activity Assistive Technology Model

The framework used throughout this text is the HAAT model. This framework is useful in placing the various outcome measures described in an overall structure. Each HAAT element can be related to outcome measures. The *activity* defines the consumer goals to be achieved on the basis of a consideration of life roles, performance areas, and tasks. There may be several goals for one consumer because he or she has several different life roles (e.g., worker, parent, husband or wife). Goals that are defined form the basis for a consumer-driven outcome assessment. Important questions to be addressed in this domain include (1) was the goal achieved? how well was it achieved? (outcome measures) and (2) were the needs adequately addressed during the assessment to allow definition of goals? (process measure).

Constraints that are placed on the achievement of goals are defined by the HAAT context. This is directly related to the milieu of the MPT and the environment of the QUEST and the adaptability subscale of the PIADS. Outcome measures arising from the context include whether the system is able to function in the required contexts and how well. These may relate to the physical context (e.g., heat or cold, bright light, noisy environment), settings (e.g., home versus employment), or social factors. The inclusion of social factors links the process to society as a whole through cultural considerations (see Chapter 2). One aspect of culture is the funding priorities that are mandated by society's attitudes toward persons with disabilities. Society as a whole determines funding priorities. If the consumer obtains a system purchased though a particular source, he or she is obligated to comply with the mandate of that funding source. For example, vocational rehabilitation agencies fund services and devices if they are related to employment, and a consumer who receives a computer from this source is obligated to use it for employment rather than for recreation. However, if a consumer uses his or her own money to buy the services or system, he or she can use them as she sees fit. Thus the funding source is linked to the assistive technology system through the social context. The area of funding is discussed further in Chapter 5.

The human component of the HAAT model is directly related to the personality dimension of the MPT, the self-esteem and competence subscales of the PIADS, and the personality feature of the QUEST. Each of these instruments taps a slightly different perspective on the human element of the HAAT model and relates to the overall perception of consumer satisfaction and improvement in quality of life as a result of the acquisition of an assistive technology system.

The desired assistive technology characteristics, the final element of the HAAT model, are defined by the combination of consumer skills, goals, personality, and contextual constraints. The QUEST addresses these through its assistive technology characteristics criterion, the MPT through the technology dimension, and the PIADS through the adaptability subscale. These characteristics are based on the consumer tasks that must be accomplished; the personality, perceptual, and motivational characteristics; and the characteristics of the assistive technology relevant to device use or nonuse. Questions of importance that can be addressed by the various outcome instruments include (1) were the skills accurately determined? (2) were these characteristics able to accommodate for contextual constraints? (3) were the characteristics and associated tasks consistent with the consumer's skills? and (4) if the identified tasks are successfully completed, is the goal achieved?

Process and structure can also be evaluated by determining how well the needs and goals; human skills, perceptions, and motivation; and contextual constraints described by the HAAT model are identified. The assessment determines the human skills available to meet the goals. One typical process measure is how accurately these skills were determined. An example outcome measure is the degree to which these skills apply to the use of assistive technologies. For example, assume that it is determined during the assessment that a consumer can use a standard keyboard (see Chapter 7). By evaluation of his or her success in performing functional daily tasks with the keyboard, both the outcome and the process can be measured. If the consumer is physically unable to use the keyboard, then the assessment procedures must be reviewed to see whether the assessment process is sound. If the process is all right but an error in ATP judgment was made, then the structure needs to be altered by providing more staff training to increase the likelihood that correct recommendations will be made. When the effectiveness of training is being considered, a process goal, such as the degree to which the consumer has moved from novice to expert status with a given system, can be measured. Alternatively, the consumer may be able to use the keyboard physically, but the total system may not meet his or her needs, so the consumer may be dissatisfied with the overall result. This outcome will have an impact on process and structure as well, but it also may require revision in the system to make it functional.

Conclusions

The effectiveness of the assistive technology system and the efficacy of the ATP to provide services are both measured by their ability to meet the needs of the consumer. Obviously this is appropriate. However, it is easy to lose sight of this emphasis if a program is built from a perspective of "experts" providing a service for consumers rather than collaborating with the consumer, family, and others to meet a goal. The collaborative approach releases the ATP from the burden of having all the answers and accepting total responsibility. Responsibility for successful outcomes is shared with the consumer and others. This avoids the paternalistic protection of the consumer and empowers him or her to take responsibility for the outcome. Each member of the team becomes 100% responsible for success. This encourages cooperation, communication, and interaction, all factors that are essential for effective use of the system. The most effective service is operated from the point of view of establishing desired outcomes and then developing the structure and process to realize them. Too often ATPs and other professionals tend to protect their services from scrutiny rather than welcoming evaluation and its implications for improvement.

The development of appropriate process and outcome measures for assistive technology service delivery is still at an early stage. Since the mid 1990s, however, a number of new tools have been developed and validated and are now available for the ATP to use in evaluating the effectiveness of assistive technology systems. The outcome measures described in this chapter have been developed to allow determination of skills, abilities, and motivation; functional performance requirements and skill levels; consumer satisfaction with the recommended system; and overall impact on the quality of life of the consumer and significant others. Each of these measures has been developed and validated to focus on different aspects of assistive technology outcomes. As demonstrated, several of these have common characteristics. Work is under way to relate three measures, the PIADS, QUEST, and MPT, to each other and to develop a common understanding of the important variables leading to successful assistive device application and use (Jutai, 2001). Continued research and development, particularly on the psychosocial aspects of assistive technology use and nonuse, will continue to inform our assessment of outcome measures and the development of assistive technologies that are more effective in meeting the needs of consumers.

■ SUMMARY

This chapter describes the principles of assessment and intervention and the service delivery process to the consumer. The steps in the process include referral intake, needs assessment, evaluation, recommendation, implementation, follow-up, and follow-along. The current state of outcome measurement in the field of assistive technology is also discussed.

Study Questions

1. Describe the five principles for assistive technology assessment and intervention.
2. Distinguish between quantitative and qualitative assessment procedures.
3. What are the four methods of gathering assessment information?
4. What is the difference between clinical and formal assessment procedures?
5. What is the meaning of the term *criteria for service* as used in assistive technology referral?
6. List the steps involved in assistive technology service delivery and write a brief description of each one. Which of these steps is the most important? Justify your choice.
7. Describe the difference between opportunity barriers and access barriers. Give an example of each.
8. List three types of opportunity barriers and how they can be addressed during the assessment process.
9. What consumer skills do we evaluate during the assistive technology skills assessment?
10. Describe the ideal relationship between the consumer and the assistive technology practitioner in the assessment and recommendation process for assistive technologies.
11. What visual functions do we measure during the sensory assessment, and how does each of these apply to the use of assistive technologies?
12. Describe the major components of a physical evaluation.
13. What are the major areas that are assessed in the cognitive evaluation for assistive technologies? Why do you think these areas were chosen?
14. Why is a separate "device characteristics" section included in the assessment? What are the outcomes of this portion of the evaluation?
15. Who are the audiences for the written assessment report? What challenges does this present?
16. Describe the major steps in implementation of an assistive technology system.
17. What are the major types of performance facilitators? When is each type used? What is the role played by each?
18. What are the major goals of a follow-up program, and how does this differ from follow-along?
19. What is the difference between repair and maintenance?
20. What are the three major domains in which outcome measures are used in assistive technology service delivery?
21. How do the three measurement domains of Question 20 relate to an improvement in the service delivery process?
22. What are the limitations in the use of the Functional Independence Measure™ Instrument for assessing the outcome of assistive technology interventions?
23. What are the strengths of the COPM in relation to determination of consumer needs and satisfaction?
24. Describe the major features of the QUEST and how it is used to assess user satisfaction.
25. What are the most common reasons that consumers abandon technology?
26. What is the HRQL, and how is it related to assistive technology outcome measures?
27. What are the three subscales of the PIADS? Why does the inclusion of these three scales increase the usefulness and validity of the PIADS?
28. Describe the relationship of the four HAAT model components to the outcome measures described in this chapter.
29. What are the roles and responsibilities of the ATP in determining the effectiveness of assistive technology services and devices?

References

Angelo J, Smith RO: The critical role of occupational therapy in augmentative communication. In American Occupational Therapy Association, editors: *Technology review '89: Perspectives on occupational therapy practice*, Rockville, Md, 1989, American Occupational Therapy Association, pp 49-53.

Bailey RW: *Human performance engineering*, ed 2, Englewood Cliffs, NJ, 1989, Prentice Hall.

Beukelman DR, Mirenda P: *Augmentative and alternative communication, management of severe communication disorders in children and adults*, Baltimore, 1998, Paul H Brookes.

Brooks NA: User's perceptions of assistive devices. In Smith RV, Leslie JH, editors: *Rehabilitation engineering*, Boca Raton, FL, 1990, CRC Press.

Bruininks RH: *Bruininks-Oseretsky Test of Motor Proficiency*, Bloomington, MN, 1978, Pearson Assessments.

Canadian Association of Occupational Therapists: *Enabling occupation: an occupational therapy perspective*, ed 2, Ottawa, ON, 2002, CAOT Publications/ACE.

Christiansen C: Occupational therapy, intervention for life performance. In Christiansen C, Baum C, editors: *Occupational therapy*, Thorofare, NJ, 1991, Slack.

Christiansen CH, Schwartz RK, Barnes KJ: Self-care: evaluation and management. In DeLisa JA, editor: *Rehabilitation medicine principles and practice*, Philadelphia, 1988, JB Lippincott.

Colarusso RP, Hammill DD: *Motor free visual perception test manual*, Novato, CA, 1972, Academic Therapy Publications.

Cook AM: Assessing physical and sensory skills necessary for augmentative communication. In Coleman CL, editor: *ACTion augmentative communication training modules*, Sacramento, CA, 1988, Assistive Device Center.

Cook AM: Development of motor skills for switch use by person with severe disabilities, *Dev Disabil Spec Interest Sect Newsl* 14, 1991.

Daniels L, Worthingham C: *Muscle testing: techniques of manual examination*, ed 5, Philadelphia, 1986, WB Saunders.

Day H, Jutai JW: Measuring the psychosocial impact of assistive devices: the PIADS, *Can J Rehabil* 9:159-168, 1996.

Demers L, Weiss-Lambrou R, Ska B: Development of the Quebec User Evaluation of Satisfaction with Assistive Technology (QUEST), *Assist Technol* 8:3-1, 1996.

DeRuyter F: Evaluating outcomes in assistive technology: do we understand the commitment? *Assist Technol* 7:3-16, 1995.

Duchek J: Assessing cognition. In Christiansen C, Baum C, editors: *Occupational therapy overcoming human performance deficits*, Thorofare, NJ, 1991, Slack.

Dunn W: Assessing sensory performance enablers. In Christiansen C, Baum C, editors: *Occupational therapy overcoming human performance deficits*, Thorofare, NJ, 1991, Slack.

Fougeyrollas P, Gray DB: Classification systems, environmental factors and social change: the importance of technology. In Gray DB, Quatrano LA, Lieberman, ML, editors: *Designing and using assistive technology: the human perspective*, Baltimore, 1998, Brookes Publishing.

Fuhrer MJ et al: A framework for the conceptual modeling of assistive technology device outcomes, *Dis Rehabil* 25:1243-1251, 2003.

Galvin JC, Scherer MJ: *Evaluating, selecting and using appropriate assistive technology*, Gaithersburg, Md, 1996, Aspen Publications.

Garrett R et al: Development of a computer-based expert system for the selection of assistive communication devices, *Proc RESNA 13th Ann Conf*, pp 348-349, June 1990.

Gaster LS: Continuous quality improvement in assistive technology. Presented at RESNA International Conference, June 1992, Toronto.

Henderson SE, Sugden D: *Movement ABC*, London, 1992, Psychological Corporation.

Jagacinski RJ, Monk DL: Fitts' law in two dimensions with hand and head movements, *J Motor Behav* 17:77-95, 1985.

Jutai J et al: Outcomes measurement of assistive technologies: an institutional case study, *Assist Technol* 8:110-120, 1996.

Jutai J et al: Psychosocial impact of electronic aids to daily living, *Assist Technol* 12:123-131, 2000.

King GA et al: Goal attainment scaling: its use in evaluating pediatric therapy programs, *Phys Occup Ther Pediatr* 19:31-52, 1999.

Klein RM, Bell B: *The Klein-Bell ADL Scale mannual*, Seattle, 1979, University of Washington Medical School Health Sciences Resource Center.

Langton A, Hughes JK: Back to work, *Team Rehab Rep* 3:14-18, 1992.

Law M et al. *Canadian Occupational Performance Measure*, ed 3, Toronto, 1998, CAOT/ACE Publications.

Lysack C, Kaufert J: Disabled consumer leaders' perspectives on provision of community rehabilitation services, *Can J Rehabil* 12:157-166, 1999.

Mahoney RI, Barthel DW: Functional evaluation: The Barthel Index, *Maryland State Med J* 14:61-65, 1965.

McNaughton S: Connecting with consumers, *Assist Technol* 5:7-10, 1993.

Miller Polgar J: Critiquing evaluations. In Crepeau E, Cohn E, editors: *Willard and Spackman's occupational therapy*, ed 10, Philadelphia, 2003, JB Lippincott Co, pp. 299-313.

Miller Polgar J, Barlow I: Measuring the clinical utility of an assessment: the example of the Canadian Occupational Performance Measure. *17th International Seating Symposium*, Vancouver, BC, 2002.

Mortola PJ, Kohn J, LeBlanc M: Success through client follow-up, *Team Rehabil Rep* 3:49-51, 1992.

Nunnally JC, Bernstein IH: *Psychometric theory*, ed 3, Toronto, 1994, McGraw-Hill.

Oldridge NB: Outcomes measurement: health-related quality of life, *Assist Technol* 8:82-93, 1996.

Pallin M: Techniques for the successful use of augmentative communication systems. Presented at *Demystifying Technology Workshop*, Sacramento, CA, 1991, Assistive Device Center.

Pape TL, Kim J, Weiner B: The shape of individual meanings assigned to assistive technology: a review of personal factors. *Dis Rehabil* 24:5-20, 2002.

Patrick D, Erickson P: *Health status and health policy: quality of life in health care evaluation and resource allocation*, New York, 1993, Oxford University Press.

Phillips B, Zhao H: Predictors of assistive technology abandonment, *Assist Technol* 5:36-45, 1993.

Reimer-Weiss ML, Wacker RR: Factors associated with assistive technology discontinuance among individuals with disabilities. *J Rehabil* 66:44-50, 2000.

Russel DJ et al: *Gross motor function measure*, Cambridge, 2002, Cambridge University Press.

Sackett DL: Evaluation of health services. In Last JM, editor: *Mosley-Rosenau's public health and preventive medicine*, ed 11, New York, 1980, Appleton-Century-Crofts.

Scherer M: *Matching person and technology: a series of assessments for evaluating predispositions to and outcomes of technology use in rehabilitation, education, the workplace and other settings*, Webster, NY, 1998, Institute for Matching Person and Technology.

Scherer MJ et al: Predictors of assistive technology use: the importance of personal and psychosocial factors, *Dis Rehabil* 27:1321-31, 2005.

Smith RO: Technological approaches to performance enhancement. In Christiansen C, Baum C, editors: *Occupational therapy*, Thorofare, NJ, 1991, Slack.

Smith RO: Measuring the outcomes of assistive technology: challenge and innovation, *Assist Technol* 8:71-81, 1996.

Sprigle S, Abdelhamied A: The relationship between ability measures and assistive technology selection, design, and use. In Gray DB, Quatrano LA, Lieberman ML, editors: *Designing and using assistive technology: the human perspective,* Baltimore, 1998, Paul H Brookes.

Stapelton D, Garrett R: VOCAselect version 1.0: an AAC device selection tool, *Proc Aust Conf Technol People Disabil* 114-116, 1995.

Stapelton D et al: Computer access selector: a tool to assist in the selection of computer access devices, *Proc Aust Conf Technol People Disabil* pp 129-131, 1995.

Uniform Data System for Medical Rehabilitation: *Functional Independence Measure, version 5.1,* Buffalo, NY, 1997, Buffalo General Hospital, State University of New York.

Weiss-Lambrou R: Wheelchair seating aids: how satisfied are consumers? *Assist Technol* 11:43-53, 1999.

Wiersma W, Jurs SG: *Educational measurement and testing,* ed 2, Boston, 1990, Allyn and Bacon.

Witt JC, Cavell TA: Psychological assessment. In Wodrich DL, Joy JE, editors: *Multi-disciplinary assessment of children with learning disabilities and mental retardation,* Baltimore, 1986, Paul H Brookes.

World Health Organization: *Constitution of the World Health Organization: basic documents,* Geneva, 1948, WHO.

World Health Organization: *International classification of functioning, disability and health: ICIDH-2,* Geneva, 2001, WHO.

Wolfensberger, W: Lets hang up "quality of life" as a hopeless term." In Goode D, editor: *Quality of life for persons with disabilities: international perspectives and issues,* Cambridge, Mass, 1994, Brookline Books.

Sample of a Written Questionnaire

BACKGROUND INFORMATION QUESTIONNAIRE

This questionnaire will help us in providing the services that the client may need. Please answer all applicable questions and return the form as soon as possible so that an evaluation may be scheduled.

General Information

Form completed by: _____   Relationship to client: _____

Client's name: _____   Date: _____

Address: _____   Birth date: _____

City/State/Zip: _____   Phone: _____

Language(s) spoken: _____

Please mark the ethnic group that applies (optional):

☐ Asian   ☐ American Indian   ☐ African American

☐ Caucasian   ☐ Hispanic   ☐ Other

Spouse/parent/guardian: _____   Phone: _____

Address: _____   _____

City/State/Zip: _____   _____

Residence:

☐ Home: ____ Alone   ____ With Family   ____ With Attendant   ☐ Group Home

☐ Skilled Nursing Home   ☐ Rehab Facility   ☐ Extended Care Facility   ☐ Other _____

Referral Information

Referred by: _____   Relationship to client: _____

Address: _____

_____

Phone: _____

How did you learn about our services?

☐ Professional   ☐ Friend   ☐ Conference   ☐ Yellow Pages   ☐ Other _____

Reason for Referral:

☐ Communication   ☐ Computer Access   ☐ Ergonomics (Work Site)

☐ Postural Seating/Wheelchair   ☐ Environmental Control   ☐ Lease/Rent Device

☐ Pressure Management/Wheelchair ☐ Powered Mobility   ☐ Repair Device

☐ Other _____

Goals/Expectations:

Medical/Health Information

Primary Diagnosis	Other Condition		Onset Dates	Specifics/Comments
☐	☐	Amyotrophic Lateral Sclerosis	_____	_____
☐	☐	Traumatic Brain Injury	_____	_____
☐	☐	Muscular Dystrophy	_____	_____
☐	☐	Multiple Sclerosis	_____	_____
☐	☐	Spinal Cord Injury	_____	Level: _____
☐	☐	Stroke	_____	_____
☐	☐	Cerebral Palsy	_____	_____
☐	☐	Developmental Delay	_____	_____
☐	☐	Emotional/Behavioral Disability	_____	_____
☐	☐	Learning Disabiltiy	_____	_____
☐	☐	Cognitive Impairment	_____	_____
☐	☐	Hearing Impairment	_____	_____
☐	☐	Seizures	_____	_____
☐	☐	Other	_____	_____

Anticipated Course of Condition: ☐ Stable   ☐ Improving   ☐ Deteriorating   ☐ Fluctuating

General Health Condition: ☐ Excellent   ☐ Good   ☐ Fair   ☐ Poor

Medications: _____

List any joint dislocations, deformities, other orthopedic problems, and past or pending surgeries:

_____

_____

Services Currently Receiving: ☐ OT   ☐ PT   ☐ Speech Therapy   ☐ Other _____

Sensory/Perceptual Abilities

<u>Vision</u>

Visual deficits?	☐ Yes	☐ No	Comments: _____
Wear glasses or corrective lenses?	☐ Yes	☐ No	Comments: _____
Perceptual deficits?	☐ Yes	☐ No	Comments: _____
Lighting affect vision?	☐ Yes	☐ No	Comments: _____
Can fixate vision on stationary object?	☐ Yes	☐ No	Comments: _____
Can follow a moving object?	☐ Yes	☐ No	Comments: _____
Can look right/left without moving head?	☐ Yes	☐ No	Comments: _____
Preference for placement of objects?	☐ Yes	☐ No	Where in visual field? _____

<u>Hearing</u>

Known hearing loss?	☐ Yes	☐ No	If yes, include audiology results
Wears hearing aid?	☐ Yes	☐ No	Comments: _____
Reacts to sounds?	☐ Yes	☐ No	Comments: _____
Understands speech?	☐ Yes	☐ No	Comments: _____

Activities of Daily Living

☐ School: _____ Full Time _____ Part Time _____ Grade Level _____

☐ Day Program: _____ Days per Week _____

☐ Work: _____ Position _____

     Full Time _____ Part Time _____

☐ Other Program: _____

Please indicate how many hours per day are spent in the following:

	Hrs.		Hrs.		Hrs.
a regular chair/couch	____	driving/riding in a car	____	a manual wheelchair	____
powered wheelchair	____	standing unsupported	____	standing frame	____
lying in bed	____	sitting on the floor/mat	____	sitting at a desk	____
other _____	____				

Social Interaction, Learning, and Behavior

Choose one that best describes level of alertness:

    ☐ No interest in surroundings

    ☐ Little interest in surroundings

    ☐ Sometimes observant; sometimes sees humor in situations

    ☐ Very alert; observant; sees humor in situations

For children, choose one that best describes his/her social play:

    ☐ Unoccupied behavior   ☐ Play among others; little interaction

    ☐ Onlooker behavior   ☐ Interaction with other peers

    ☐ Solitary independent play

Can he/she:

Sit and concentrate on a task for appropriate amount of time?	☐ Yes	☐ No
Concentrate within a distracting environment?	☐ Yes	☐ No
Make eye contact with people and/or tasks?	☐ Yes	☐ No
Classify different objects into categories?	☐ Yes	☐ No
Carry out tasks of 2 or more steps?	☐ Yes	☐ No
Understand concept of direction? (i.e., up, down)	☐ Yes	☐ No
Know his/her actions can cause something else to happen?	☐ Yes	☐ No
Make choices when 2 objects or activities are presented?	☐ Yes	☐ No
Follow directions or commands given?	☐ Yes	☐ No

List activities/objects/people that the client finds motivating or interesting.

_____

Comments about social behavior:

Functional Abilities

Feeding: ☐ Independent   ☐ Assisted   ☐ Dependent   ☐ Tube Feed   ☐ Electric Feeder

Chewing/
Swallowing: ☐ Independent   ☐ Assisted   ☐ Dependent

Dressing: ☐ Independent   ☐ Assisted   ☐ Dependent

Transfers: ☐ Independent   ☐ Assisted   ☐ Dependent

If assisted: ☐ Two-Man Lift   ☐ Sliding Board   ☐ Stand-Pivot

Motor Skills

Does the client have motor control in the following:

Eyes   ☐ Yes   ☐ No   Mouth   ☐ Yes   ☐ No
Neck/Head   ☐ Yes   ☐ No   Trunk   ☐ Yes   ☐ No
Right Arm   ☐ Yes   ☐ No   Left Arm   ☐ Yes   ☐ No
Right Hand ☐ Yes   ☐ No   Left Hand ☐ Yes   ☐ No
Right Leg   ☐ Yes   ☐ No   Left Leg   ☐ Yes   ☐ No
Right Foot ☐ Yes   ☐ No   Left Foot ☐ Yes   ☐ No

Which part of the body is best controlled? _____

Are there any positions or supports that help control movement?   ☐ Yes   ☐ No

If yes, describe: _____

Please mark all capabilities below (and dominant side when applicable):

☐ Write with pen or pencil ☐ R ☐ L   ☐ Point with a finger   ☐ R ☐ L
☐ Type with one digit   ☐ R ☐ L   ☐ Type with more than one digit ☐ R ☐ L
☐ Grasp/release object   ☐ R ☐ L   ☐ Hold objects   ☐ R ☐ L
☐ Use both hands for a two-handed activity ☐ Type with head or mouthstick
☐ Reach capabilities: ☐ Forward   ☐ Sideways   ☐ Backward

Problems that may interfere with motor function:

☐ Incoordination/poor balance   ☐ Endurance/fatigue   ☐ Tremor
☐ Tone: ☐ Too little   ☐ Too much   ☐ Reflexes   ☐ Joint contractures

Mobility/Positioning

Check all that apply:

☐ Sits independently in regular chair   ☐ Unable to sit upright

☐ Sits in wheelchair without support   ☐ Walks independently

☐ Sits in wheelchair with support (describe below)   ☐ Walks with assistance

_____ ☐ Depends on wheelchair for mobility

☐ <u>Manual Wheelchair:</u>   (Used Where? _____)

     Brand Name/Manufacturer: _____ Date Obtained: _____

     Model: _____

     Funding Source: _____

     How Propelled: ☐ Hands   ☐ Feet   ☐ Assisted/Dependent

     Type/Description of Seating System: _____

     Accessories (e.g., Laptray): _____

     Problems with Wheelchair: _____

     _____

☐ <u>Power Wheelchair:</u>   (Used Where? _____)

     Brand Name/Manufacturer: _____ Date Obtained: _____

     Model: _____

     Funding Source: _____

     Controlled By: ☐ Joystick   ☐ Sip & Puff   ☐ Chin Switch   ☐ Switch Array

     Control Site: ☐ Hand   ☐ Head   ☐ Foot   ☐ Other _____

     Type/Description of Seating System: _____

     Accessories (e.g., Laptray): _____

     Problems with Wheelchair: _____

     _____

Is there a history of pressure sores?   ☐ No   ☐ Yes   (Current? ☐ No   ☐ Yes)

Please check all means of <u>transportation</u> that are used:

☐ Car   ☐ Family van   ☐ Day program's vehicle

☐ Van/bus for wheelchairs   ☐ Public transportation   ☐ Paratransit

Communication Skills

Select all methods used to communicate:

☐ Speech   ___ Sounds   ___ Single Words   ___ Phrases   ___ Whole Sentences

Intelligibility: ___ To All Listeners   ___ Only to Familiar Listeners

☐ Gestures   ☐ Eye Gaze   ☐ Facial Expressions

☐ Sign Language

    Type: ___ ASL   ___ SEE   ___ Other _____
    Number of signs used ___
    List 5 most commonly used signs _____

☐ Pointing   (How? with finger? foot? eye gaze? _____)

☐ Handwriting   ☐ Drawing   ☐ Typing

☐ Communication Board or Notebook: (Symbols Used: ☐ Pictures   ☐ Words   ☐ Letters)
    Number of symbols used ___ Approx. size of symbols _____

☐ Electronic Communication Device: _____

    Symbols Used: ☐ Pictures   ☐ Words   ☐ Letters   ☐ No. of Symbols ___
    How long has this device been used?: _____
    Is this successful/How successful has it been? _____

What is the client's means of indicating "YES": _____   "NO": _____

Can the client spell?   ☐ Yes   ☐ No   (Approx. grade level ___)

Is communication spontaneous?   ☐ Yes   ☐ No

To whom can the client reliably communicate the following:

	All	Friends	Family/Caregiver	No One	Method:
Attract attention	☐	☐	☐	☐	_____
Pain/discomfort	☐	☐	☐	☐	_____
Frustration/happiness	☐	☐	☐	☐	_____
Hunger/thirst	☐	☐	☐	☐	_____
Fatigue/boredom	☐	☐	☐	☐	_____
Refusal	☐	☐	☐	☐	_____
Choice of items	☐	☐	☐	☐	_____
Convey new information	☐	☐	☐	☐	_____
Discuss past/future events	☐	☐	☐	☐	_____

Can the client convey medical needs to professionals?   ☐ Yes   ☐ No

How would you like to see the client's communications skills improve? _____
_____

Assessment Forms

■ INITIAL EVALUATION FORM ASSESSMENT SECTION

I. Motor
   A. Grasps
      1. Finger, hand, and wrist movement
         a. Check the following finger/hand movement functions for both the right (R) and left (L) hands. For numbers 1, 2 (or 2a) and 3, place the object on the table and ask the person to hand it to you. If the person cannot pick the object up, then hand it to him or her. For numbers 4, 5, and 6, hold the object in a comfortable location oriented as shown and ask the person to grasp it, move it from front to back and side to side, and release it. For number 7, place the push button on the table and ask the person to press it. Place a number in the box as follows: 1, poor; 2, fair; and 3, good.

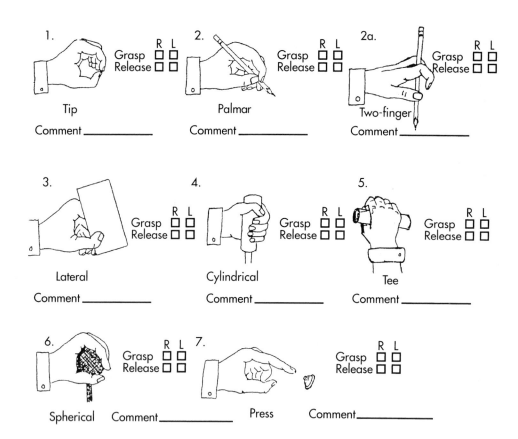

B. Range: Hand

Present hand range sheet. Locate the sheet with the client's midline centered on square 8.

The squares are numbered and each corner is lettered as shown. The targets are the corners. Use the sequence: touch the square then 1A/1B/1C/1D and repeat for all squares within the person's range. Circle locations reached. For children, it may be necessary to use the smaller (foot) range sheet.

Compare your impression of the time required to reach the square (tracking time) to the time required to move among the corners A, B, C, D (select time).

Use the distance table (see Figure 4-5) to fill in the following block.

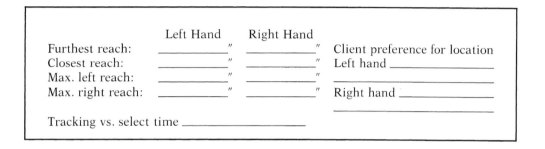

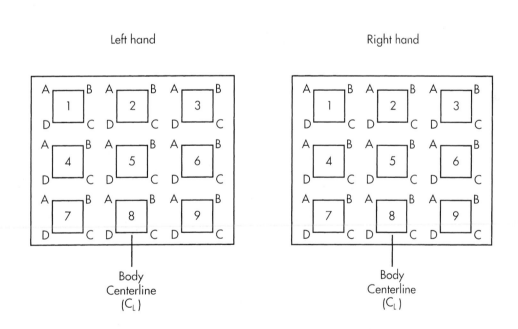

C. Body part movement and control

For each movement requested place a + (present) or – (absent) in the appropriate column. Note whether required movement can be initiated (I), controlled (C), and terminated (T).

	Left			Right			
ARM	I	C	T	I	C	T	COMMENTS
Tasks: Tester places object (cup, toy, etc.) at person's midline 10″ from his or her body and instructs. Reposition if necessary and note new position.							
Lift 6″							
Extend by reaching							
Rotate as if to pour (put object in cup to be poured)							
Rotate in the opposite direction							
Turn upright again							
Move 6″ to the left							
Move 6″ to the right							
Pull back							

If adequate arm and hand movement are available, omit the following tasks:

KNEE	I	C	T	I	C	T	COMMENTS
move knee to the left							
move knee to the right							
JAW							
open							
close							
MOUTH							
blow through a straw							
sip through a straw							
VOICE							
produce a sound							
produce a variety of words							

D. Range: Foot

Present the foot range sheet unless the interview indicates there is no foot movement possible or hand movement is adequate. If foot control appears to be feasible, then repeat the same tasks that were done with the hand. Start by locating the heel of the foot at the site labeled "X." Allow the person to move the entire foot as necessary to complete the task.

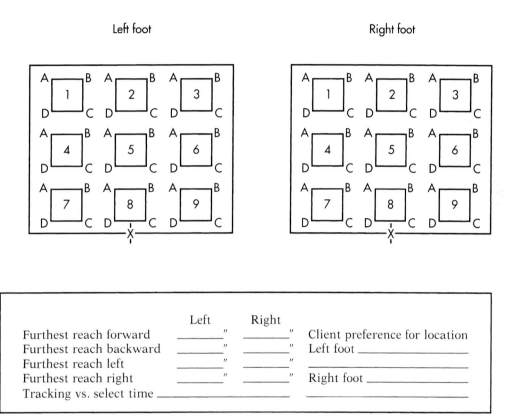

	Left	Right	
Furthest reach forward	_____"	_____"	Client preference for location
Furthest reach backward	_____"	_____"	Left foot _____
Furthest reach left	_____"	_____"	_____
Furthest reach right	_____"	_____"	Right foot _____
Tracking vs. select time _____			_____

E. Head control

Measure range of movement in the planes shown. Check the space representing the person's degree of movement to indicate if he or she has no movement, partial movement, or full range of movement.

Directions

Movement plane	left			right			
	None	Partial	Full	None	Partial	Full	Comments
Horizontal							
	Up			Down			
Vertical							
	Left			Right			
Tilt							

Is a headpointer used now? _____ If so, describe: _____

_____

If the client has used one before but doesn't now, explain why: _____

_____

Reflexive head movements noted: _____

_____

Restraints to head
movement:

_____

_____

Sketch

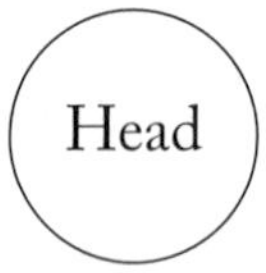

(Head)

List those
anatomical sites
appearing to be
most suitable
for interfacing

Most suitable _____
Next most suitable _____
Third most suitable _____

II. Symbol Location, Type, and Size
   A. *Symbol location task*
      1. *Peripheral*
         Instruct the person to keep head and eyes fixed straight forward. Ask the person to indicate when he or she can see your finger or pointer without moving his or her eyes. If the person cannot keep the eyes fixed, provide an object to stare at. Start with your finger or pointer approximately 12 inches from the side of his/her head (at the ear) and move it around the head toward the face. Mark the areas in which the person can see your finger.

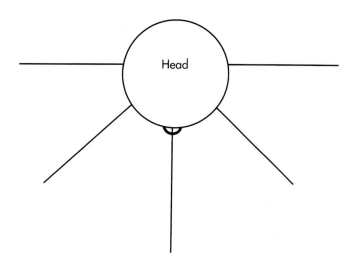

      2. Tracking
         Using your finger or pointer, have the person track horizontally at the level of the eyes. Begin at the nose and go left/right. To track vertically, begin at the nose and go up/down.

	Yes	Comments
Can the person track horizontally?	_____	_____
Can the person track vertically?	_____	_____

   B. Symbol size verification
      1. Instructions
         Select the stimuli according to the information available. If information is lacking, begin with a more "basic" symbol system (e.g., select pictures over words or letters) and begin with the largest size set. Place the stimuli approximately 18 inches from the subject's eyes. Determine the method of selection and explain it to the consumer.

Present two stimuli to the consumer and say, for example, "Please point to (look at) the comb," or "Is this a comb?" Three trials should be run. If no errors are made, the size of the stimuli should be reduced, with three trials run at each size tested. A more advanced symbol system may then be tested if appropriate. If some errors are made, a more basic symbol system should be tested and the positioning of the stimuli should be reexamined.

2. Data sheet

   Use a plus mark in the choice column to designate a correct response and use a circle to designate an error. Be sure to note a symbol system and stimulus size for all trial groups.

	Symbol System	Size	Trials + ○ Correct/Incorrect
a.	_____	_____	1. _____ 2. _____ 3. _____
b.	_____	_____	1. _____ 2. _____ 3. _____
c.	_____	_____	1. _____ 2. _____ 3. _____
d.	_____	_____	1. _____ 2. _____ 3. _____

Optimal symbol type: _____

Optimal size: _____

If you were not able to establish an optimal stimulus, explain why.

CHAPTER 5

Funding Assistive Technology Services and Systems

Chapter Outline

Learning Objectives

On completing this chapter, you will be able to do the following:

1. Identify the major categories of funding for assistive technology services and equipment
2. Describe the types of assistive technology devices and services covered by each category of funding
3. Distinguish between categories of funding as they relate to specific consumer characteristics

4. Describe the process for procuring funding
5. Describe the process by which funding decisions can be appealed

---

Key Terms

Appeals Process	Medical Necessity	Public Funding Sources
Diagnosis Codes	Medicare	Third-Party Payer
Fee for Service	Plan for Achieving Self-Sufficiency	Tricare
Managed Care	(PASS)	
Medicaid	Procedure Codes	

As discussed in Chapter 1, there is an established assistive technology industry that provides services and devices for individuals with disabilities. Evaluation, implementation, and maintenance and repair of assistive technologies can be costly, and most consumers do not have the financial resources available to purchase the necessary services and equipment. Therefore, funding by third-party sources is necessary for individuals to procure assistive technology services and equipment. Fortunately, funding for many assistive technology services and devices is widely available, and accessing that funding is generally a matter of following a straightforward process. Assisting with the acquisition of this funding is an inherent part of the assistive technology practitioner's (ATP) role as a service provider.

In most countries assistive technology services and devices are funded by numerous sources rather than by a system solely dedicated to the funding of assistive technology services and equipment. For any given individual, equipment and services may be funded solely from one source or through a combination of sources. Funding for assistive technology is usually rendered through agencies that have been primarily developed for the provision of other types of health, education, or social services programs.

In this chapter funding for assistive technologies in several countries (United States, Australia, and Canada) is described. Funding programs in these countries are representative of those in many other countries with local modifications of elements of the programs. The various funding sources can be categorized as three general types: public, private, and other.

▥ PUBLIC SOURCES OF FUNDING

U.S. Public Sources of Assistive Technology Funding

Public funding sources for assistive technology funding in the United States include federal, state, and local government agencies; several public sources of funding are listed in Box 5-1. There are more than 30 programs established by the U.S. Congress that affect U.S. residents with disabilities and more than 12 agencies on the federal level that oversee these programs

(Morris and Golinker, 1991). Typically, Congress authorizes funding through a specific piece of legislation, such as the Medicare Act, and designates a federal agency to determine the scope and criteria for the program. Other programs are examples of a principle called "cooperative federalism." For them, Congress passes a law that is broadly administered by a federal government agency but administered on a day-to-day basis by the states. These programs also will be jointly funded by the federal and state governments. Medicaid and vocational rehabilitation are examples of cooperative federalism programs. A third model extends the federal presence to local levels of government where day-to-day decision making occurs. The Individuals With Disabilities Education Act (IDEA), which sets standards for the education of children with disabilities by local schools, is an example of this type of program.

Medicare. **Medicare** is the health insurance program operated by the federal government. Coverage, benefits, and program operation for this program are described in Chapter 1. Medicare funds *durable medical equipment* (see Chapter 1 for definition). Some assistive technology equipment, such as speech-generating devices, the full range of mobility aids and accessories, hospital beds, and patient lifts, are covered under Part B as durable medical equipment.

Medicaid. **Medicaid** is a public welfare program whose coverage, benefits, and program operation are described in Chapter 1. Assistive technology services and devices are within the scope of each state's Medicaid program (Golinker and Mistrett, 1997). The federal definitions of the intent and scope of mandated and optional services should be used as a starting point to determine the basis of Medicaid funding for assistive technology. To receive federal funding for Medicaid, all states must comply with these definitions of services. Golinker and Mistrett (1997) identify 11 services among the list of mandatory and optional Medicaid services under which funding for assistive technology and services may qualify (see Box 1-3). These services are early and periodic screening, diagnostic treatment services; home health care

---

BOX 5-1   U.S. Assistive Technology Financing Options

PUBLIC PROGRAMS
Medicare
Medicaid
  Required and optional services
  Intermediate care facilities for persons who are mentally
    retarded
  Early and periodic screening, diagnosis, and treatment
  Home- and community-based waivers
  Community-supported living arrangements
Maternal and child health
  Maternal and child health block grant to states
  Children with special health care needs
  Special projects of regional and national significance
Education
  Individuals with Disabilities Education Act state grants (Part B)
  IDEA programs for infants and toddlers with disabilities and
    their families (Part H)
  State-operated programs
  Vocational education
  Head Start
Vocational rehabilitation
  State grants
  Supported employment
  Independent living Parts A, B, and C
Social Security benefits
  Title II: Social Security Disability Insurance
  Title XVI: Supplemental Security Income
  Work incentive programs
Developmental disability programs
Department of Veterans Affairs programs
Older Americans Act programs

ALTERNATIVE FINANCING
Revolving loan fund
Lending library
Discount program

Low-interest loans
Private foundations
Service clubs
Special state appropriations
State bond issues
Employee accommodations program
Equipment loan program
Corporate-sponsored loans
Charitable organizations

U.S. TAX CODE
Medical care expense deduction
Business deductions
Employee business deductions
Americans with Disabilities Act credit for small business
Credit for architectural and transportation barrier removal
Targeted jobs tax credit
Charitable contributions deduction

PRIVATE HEALTH INSURANCE
Health insurance
Workers' Compensation
Casualty insurance
Disability insurance

CIVIL RIGHTS
Americans with Disabilities Act
Rehabilitation Act, Section 504

UNIVERSAL ACCESS
Rehabilitation Act, Section 508
Decoder Circuitry Act

TELECOMMUNICATIONS
Telecommunications for the Disabled Act of 1982
Telecommunications Accessibility Enhancement Act of 1988

From the National Council on Disability: *Study on the financing of assistive technology devices and services for individuals with disabilities,* Washington, DC, 1993, The Council.

---

services, prosthetic devices; occupational therapy; physical therapy; speech-language pathology; rehabilitative services; preventive services; skilled nursing facility; and services and intermediate care facility services for persons with mental retardation, developmental disabilities, and related conditions. Because assistive technology devices and services are not listed as such in the Medicaid vocabulary, it is recommended that use of these terms be avoided when applying for funding under Medicaid (Golinker and Mistrett, 1997). Instead, the device being requested should be identified by its specific name in all documentation and any descriptive terms used should match those in the definition of one of the Medicaid services listed above.

One of the general criteria for funding of all Medicaid services is that the requested equipment or service be considered a medical necessity. Another general criterion for funding of Medicaid services is that prior approval or authorization is required for nearly all services and equipment. Before commencing any services or purchasing any equipment for a Medicaid beneficiary, the ATP needs to request approval from Medicaid for the purchase of such services or devices. In some states a certain amount of occupational and physical therapy services may be provided without prior authorization. Because the ATP may not know whether this threshold has already been reached, it is generally safer from a reimbursement standpoint to get prior approval for the services to be provided.

Children's Medical Services. Medical and related services are provided to children under the age of 21 years who have chronic disabling conditions and who meet income limitations. These services are funded by the federal government under Title V of the Social Security Act. All children are eligible for medical diagnosis and evaluation.

In some states, funding of assistive technologies is provided by Children's Medical Services.

Programs for the Developmentally Disabled. Within each state, programs for the developmentally disabled provide a range of services, including case management, advocacy, community living, and purchase of other services. Assistive technology services and equipment may be funded from these programs.

Tricare (formerly CHAMPUS). The **Tricare** program, formerly known as the Civilian Health and Medical Program of the Uniformed Services (CHAMPUS), is a federally funded program that provides medical benefits to active duty military service members and their dependents and to military retirees and their dependents. Tricare contracts with various health insurance companies to administer this program, which provides medically necessary equipment and assistive technology services.

Education. As discussed in Chapter 1, the Education for All Handicapped Children Act of 1975, the Handicapped Infant and Toddlers Act of 1986, and the 1991 reauthorization of these statutes through IDEA are vehicles through which assistive technology and related services can be provided to children with disabilities. Children from birth to 2 years of age must have an Individualized Family Service Plan (IFSP), and children 3 years to 21 years old must have a written Individual Education Plan (IEP) (see Chapter 1). Assistive technology must be considered in the development of the child's IEP. If assistive technology is identified as being necessary for a "free and appropriate public education," it must be included in the IEP and this service must be provided.

Vocational Rehabilitation. The federal government provides states with funds to administer programs that help individuals with disabilities to enter, remain in, or return to employment. An Individual Plan for Employment (IPE, formerly called an Individual Written Rehabilitation Plan) that outlines the individual's vocational objectives and services to be provided is required. Those who need assistive technology to complete training in a vocational rehabilitation program or to obtain or retain employment (competitive, supported, or sheltered) are eligible for funding of assistive technology equipment and services. Statutory amendments to this program create a strong presumption that an employment outcome always is possible, if the right services, including assistive technologies, are provided. For this reason, greater attention is expected to be directed to developing services plans and vocational outcomes for individuals with more severe disabilities. However, staff of vocational rehabilitation programs may not be aware of the benefits of assistive technology, and efforts by ATPs to provide continuing training can increase their awareness regarding assistive technology.

Plan for Achieving Self-Sufficiency. The **Plan for Achieving Self-Sufficiency (PASS)** is a program that allows individuals to put aside income for equipment or services that will assist them in achieving a vocational objective. This includes assistive technology services and devices such as augmentative communication devices and adapted computer equipment. The Social Security Administration oversees this program and must approve the PASS before it can go into effect. The Social Security Administration excludes the money earned to pay for the devices from earned income, which allows the consumer to continue to receive applicable benefits. The consumer develops a written plan that identifies needs and feasible occupational goals, with a timetable for attaining these goals.

Department of Veterans Affairs. The Department of Veterans Affairs (DVA), formerly the Veterans Administration (VA), directly provides assistive technology equipment and related services and contracts with outside programs to provide these services. Individuals who have a service-connected disability are eligible for purchase of assistive technologies by the VA.

Workers' Compensation. Expenses incurred as a result of work-related injuries are covered by Workers' Compensation benefits. Under certain conditions, equipment, home modifications, and services are covered. Workers' Compensation benefits are financed jointly by individual employers or groups of employers and state governments (Burton, 1996). A designated state agency or board develops the regulations for Workers' Compensation and private insurance companies typically administer the program.

Canadian Provincial and Territorial Sources of Assistive Technology Funding*

In Canada the delivery of health services is the responsibility of the provinces and territories. Although there are federal programs, most assistive technology funding is allocated and managed at the provincial/territorial level. Most federal programs have clauses about funding only what the provinces and territories do not fund. Table 5-1 shows the breakdown of public funding sources for assistive technologies in Canada by jurisdiction. It is clear that there are major differences in programs across the country. In general, funding

*Deb Finn of the Assistive Devices Industry Office, Industry Canada, made major contributions to the sections on Canadian funding.

TABLE 5-1	Canadian Public Funding Sources by Province or Territory			
Province/ Territory and Relevant Departments	Assistive Devices Funded	Special Conditions or Program Features	Eligibility	Web Links
Alberta: Alberta Aids To Daily Living	Back supports, bathing and toileting equipment, electrolarynx, hearing aids, orthotic braces, prosthetic devices, specialized seating devices, speech-generating communication devices, wheelchair cushions, wheelchairs (manual and power), walkers	Cost share: 25% of cost of benefits, maximum $500 per family per benefit year, clients on income supplement programs and those with low income are exempt from cost sharing	Disability lasting 6 months or more, a chronic illness or a terminal illness, Alberta resident, valid Alberta Personal Health Care Number	*http://www.seniors.gov.* *ab.ca/AADL/index.asp*
British Columbia: At Home Program Set BC Red Cross Aids to Independent Living Program (AILP)	Alternate positioning devices, bathing and toileting aids, hearing aids, lifts, mobility equipment, orthotics and bracing, specialized car seats, speech-generating devices, scooters, wheelchairs, and walkers	Programs for children under 17 years (At Home, Set BC) and low-income homes and active in their communities and participate in social activities	New or good quality recycled devices,	*www.mcf.gov.bc.ca/* *at_home/* *www.setbc.org* *http://www.redcross.ca/* *article.asp?id=011086* *&tid=078*
Manitoba: Prosthetics and orthotics, hearing aid, telecommunications	Prosthetics and orthotics, hearing aids, adapted telephones, TTY	$75 deductible	Prescription by a medical practitioner	*http://www.gov.mb.ca/* *health/mhsip/*
New Brunswick: Seniors' Rehabilitation Equipment Program Health Services Program, Training and Employment Support Services (TESS)	Canes, crutches, hearing aids, raised toilet seats, tub transfer benches, grab bars, walkers, wheelchairs, drop seats, wheelchair accessories (trays, brake extensions, and cushions), speech aids	Senior (65 years and over) residing at home, special care home, or nursing home, whose care is subsidized and who is in financial need	A health card with rehabilitation equipment as an eligible benefit, medical necessity TESS: goal is to assist persons with disabilities to obtain or resume employment	*http://www.gnb.ca/0017/* *Health%20Services/* *index-e.asp*
Newfoundland and Labrador: Special Assistance	Orthotics and equipment, walkers, lifts, hearing aids, power wheelchairs and scooters, manual wheelchairs, custom seating systems, noncustom seating components and accessories, augmentative and alternative communication	To alleviate the costs of supportive health services for clients in the community that would ordinarily be a benefit extended to persons in hospitals or nursing home	Clients who meet the financial eligibility criteria, payer of last resort	*http://www.gov.nf.ca/* *health/*
Northwest Territories: Extended Health Benefits for Seniors Extended Aid for Specified Diseases	**Seniors:** Prostheses, hearing aids, manually operated wheelchairs, walking aids, grab **Specified diseases:** Prosthetic appliances, communication aids (hearing and telephone aids, bliss board), walkers, crutches, canes, manual and electric wheelchairs, wheelchair trays, transfer boards, armrests, cushions, seating inserts, transfer bars,	Registered with the NWT Health Care Plan, permanent NWT resident, be non-Native or Metis, have a specified disease	Payer of last resort	*http://www.hlthss.gov.* *nt.ca/*

Continued

TABLE 5-1   Canadian Public Funding Sources by Province or Territory—cont'd

Province/ Territory and Relevant Departments	Assistive Devices Funded	Special Conditions or Program Features	Eligibility	Web Links
	toileting aids, patient lifters, grab bars, bars, other equipment or devices that are medically necessary (may be covered on a case-by-case basis)			
Nova Scotia: Specialized Equipment Program (SEP) Department of Health service program available and administered through the Canadian Red Cross	Wheelchairs (specialized/custom) plus accessories, scooters, specialized transfer aids (e.g., transfer boards), walkers, resident-specific lifts/slings	Approved residents may be required to pay a monthly income-based fee for the equipment being provided through the SEP	Regular bed resident of a Department of Health long-term care facility; requires covered equipment, has been assessed by an occupational or physical therapist	https://www.gov.ns. ca/health/ccs/ltc.htm
Nunavut	Assistive devices are usually acquired through third-party insurance	Most people in Nunavut are covered with Health Canada's Non-Insured Health Benefit (Table 5-2)	See Non-insured benefits, Health Canada in Table 5-2	
Ontario: Assistive Devices Program	**Communication devices:** Electrolarynges, communication boards, mounting systems, signaling aids, teletypewriters for the speech impaired, voice amplifiers voice output devices, voice prostheses, writing aids **Hearing aids:** Bone anchored hearing aid, cochlear implant processors, hearing aids, personal FM systems, TTY **Orthotic devices:** Custom standing frames, custom-made braces **Prosthetic devices:** Body-powered leg and arm prostheses, electric and myoelectric arm prostheses **Visual aids:** Braillers, computer hardware and specialized software, enlarging optical systems (CCTVs), magnifiers, telescopes, binoculars, optical character recognition, specialized glasses, specialized lenses/contact lenses, specialized peripherals (e.g. Braille embossers, refreshable Braille displays), spectacle-mounted low vision and field enhancement aids, standard orientation and mobility canes, audio book playback machines	Most devices must be authorized by a qualified health care professional registered with the program. Registered authorizers work in hospitals, home care agencies or private practice, 25% client copayment	Eligibility includes any Ontario resident who has a valid Ontario Health card and who has a physical disability of 6 months or longer, specific eligibility criteria which apply to each device category	http://www.health. gov.on.ca/english/ public/program/adp/ adp_mn.html

TABLE 5-1	Canadian Public Funding Sources by Province or Territory—cont'd			
Province/ Territory and Relevant Departments	Assistive Devices Funded	Special Conditions or Program Features	Eligibility	Web Links
	Wheelchairs, positioning and ambulation aids: Manual wheelchairs, power wheelchairs, electric scooters, power add-on devices for manual wheelchairs, positioning devices (cushions, back and head supports, etc.), dynamic positioning devices (power tilt and recline), forearm crutches, wheeled walkers, specialized pediatric walkers, strollers, standers			
Prince Edward Island: Department of Education Student Services Division	Assistive technologies for control of the environment, augmentative communication, accessing computer programs, vision aids, hearing aids, aspects of motor and mobility aids, seating and positioning, accessing sports equipment, learning self-help and independent living skills, participation in social interactions	An assistive technology recommendation is made collaboratively with parents, school, and department personnel, occupational therapy, speech language pathology; training and technical support for assistive technology is provided by or arranged for by the Student Services Division	Students with special educational needs	
Quebec	Walking aids, standing aids, locomotor assists and posture assists, orthotics and prosthetics, crutches, canes, walking frames and walkers, standing aids, manual and powered wheelchairs, wheelbase systems, orthomobiles and children's strollers, posture assists, hearing devices, visual devices	Assessment and device distribution services provided in special facilities, accredited by the government	Insured under the Québec Health Insurance Plan, physical deficiency, medical prescription from a specialist	http://www.ram.q. gouv.qc.ca/en/citoyens/ assurancemaladie/ serv_couv_queb/serv_ couv_queb.shtml
Saskatchewan: Saskatchewan Aids to Independent Living Program			Saskatchewan resident, valid Health Services card; referred by an authorized health care professional; not be eligible to receive the service from any other government agency such as First Nations and Inuit Health (Health Canada), Workers' Compensation Board, Saskatchewan Government Insurance or Department of Veterans' Affairs	
Yukon: Health and Social Services Education	Manually operated wheelchairs, walking aids, grab bars and support rails, commodes, artificial eyes, hearing aids Other equipment or devices that are medically necessary may be covered		The physician must apply for benefits on behalf of the patient	http://www.hss.gov. yk.ca/

is provided for children through a children's services ministry or an education ministry. For older adults, the major funding is for seniors in a social services department or, in some jurisdictions, a senior's ministry. Table 5-1 lists the covered assistive technologies. This list is not complete in all cases because some jurisdictions list devices as examples and consider each request on the basis of medical necessity. Eligibility for funding is also listed in Table 5-1. Assistive technologies are generally funded only for conditions lasting 6 months or longer. In most cases an approved health provider must make a recommendation or generate a prescription for the appropriate assistive technology. Although this is often a medical doctor, many jurisdictions also accept recommendations from occupational therapists, physical therapists, or speech-language pathologists, depending on the type of technology being recommended. Some jurisdictions recycle assistive technologies. This only applies to technology that can be cleaned, reconditioned, and upgraded (e.g., with new software in an electronic system) to meet current levels of performance. Some communication devices, wheelchairs, and selected types of aids to daily living are routinely recycled. Customized seating systems, prosthetics and orthotics, and aids to daily living used for self-care and eating are not generally recycled.

Canadian Federal Sources of Assistive Technology Funding

Federal or national Canadian programs are listed in Table 5-2. These programs may have slightly different forms in each province.

Health Canada—First Nations and Inuit Health: Uninsured Health Benefits.   The Federal Department of Health (Health Canada) provides funding to persons of Native Canadian descent for uninsured provincial or territorial items *(http://www.hc-sc.gc.ca/fnih-spni/nihb-ssna/benefit-prestation/2004-2005_rpt_e.html)*. Under the Canada Health Act, provinces and territories are responsible for delivering health care services. First Nations and Inuit people access these insured services through provincial and territorial governments. There are a number of health-related goods and services, including assistive technologies, that are not insured by provinces and territories or other private insurance plans.

TABLE 5-2   Canadian Federal Programs That Fund Assistive Technologies

Program	Assistive Devices Funded	Special Conditions or Program Features	Eligibility	Web Links
Aging and Seniors	Depends on province or territory	Benefits related to provincial/territorial programs		*http://www.phac-aspc.gc.ca/ seniors-aines/pubs/info_sheets/ assistive/index.htm#who*
Workers' Compensation Board	Devices necessary for return to work	One for each province and territory	Workplace injuries including work-related accidents or diseases that require medical treatment or time away from work	Varies by province or territory
Health Canada— First Nations and Inuit Health: Non-Insured Health Benefits	A variety of mobility devices, aids to daily living items not listed on the benefit list may be considered on a case-by-case basis with written medical justification	Device is listed by program; intended for use in a home or other ambulatory care settings; not available through any other federal, provincial territorial, or private health or social program; prescribed by health professional licensed to prescribe; provided by a recognized provider	Canadian resident and one of the following: (1) registered Native Canadian according to the Indian Act, (2) Inuk recognized by one of the Inuit Land Claim organizations, or (3) infant less than 1 year of age whose parent is an eligible recipient	*http://www.hc-sc.gc.ca/fnih-spni/nihb-ssna/index_e.html*
Veterans' Affairs	Aids to daily living, canes, walkers; foot boards, overbed tables, raised toilet seats, bath benches	Available devices may vary by province	**Group "A" clients:** Pension from Veterans' Affairs Canada **Group "B" clients:** Established eligibility for treatment of nonpensioned conditions, established health need, benefits not covered by province	*http://www.vac-acc.gc.ca/ clients/sub.cfm?source= health/fallsp/assistdev& CFID=8156146& CFTOKEN=36150877*

Health Canada's Non-Insured Health Benefits Program supports First Nations people and the Inuit in reaching an overall health status that is comparable to that of other Canadians by providing coverage for a limited range of these goods and services when individuals are not insured elsewhere. Assistive technology devices and services may be funded under this program on a case-by-case basis. A benefit will be considered for coverage when the conditions shown in Table 5-2 are met.

Veterans Independence Program. The Veterans Independence Program is administered by the DVA. As shown in Table 5-2, this program is available to all veterans who require it for their pensioned conditions, wartime pensioners who are seriously or medium disabled, pensioners with multiple health conditions, war veterans with low income, former prisoners of war, and overseas service veterans waiting for a priority access bed. The program covers the provision of wheelchairs, some activities of daily living (ADL), and other self-care equipment.

Opportunities Fund for Persons With Disabilities. The Opportunities Fund for Persons With Disabilities has a primary objective of assisting persons with disabilities to prepare for and obtain employment or self-employment and to develop the skills necessary to maintain that new employment. The program works with employers to assist them in making their work setting accessible to persons with disabilities and with individuals to prepare them for work or for starting their own businesses. The program also partners with private sector organizations to develop programs that enhance employability for persons with disabilities. Among the benefits listed are expenses related to university tuition, equipment, transportation, and living expenses while in training.

Australian State Government Funding Schemes

The funding programs that are provided through the state governments of Australia have been designed specifically to provide for people with disabilities and include assistive technology in the lists of approved items. The state programs have evolved quite independently in each Australian state or territory and therefore are not uniform. The schemes are administered through various state government departments and are funded from state/territory sources. Although all these programs have similar objectives, there is variation in the level and range of assistance that they provide to people with disabilities. These programs also vary in their level of means testing. The Australian state funding schemes and their Web links are summarized in Table 5-3. Details of Australian public sources of funding for assistive technology devices and services are shown in Table 5-4.

Text continued on p. 160

TABLE 5-3   **Australian Funding Programs by State/Territory**

State	Assistive Technology Funding Program Name	Managing Authority	Web Site
New South Wales	Program of Appliances for Disabled People	New South Wales Department of Area Health and Community Services	http://www.health.nsw.gov.au/health-public-affairs/factsheets/pdf/padp.pdf http://www.health.nsw.gov.au/policies/pd/2005/pdf/PD2005_563.pdf
Victoria	Victorian Aids and Equipment Program	Department of Human Services	http://nps718.dhs.vic.gov.au/ds/disability site.nsf/sectionfour/equipment_service_providers?opendocument
Western Australia	Community Aids and Equipment Program	Disability Services Commission	http://www.dsc.wa.gov.au/2/234/67/Community_Aids_.pm
Queensland	Medical Aids Subsidy Scheme	Queensland Health	http://www.health.qld.gov.au/mass/default.asp
South Australia	Independent Living Equipment Program	Disability Services South Australia	http://www.ilc.asn.au/ilep/
Tasmania	Community Equipment Scheme	Department of Health and Human Services	http://www.dhhs.tas.gov.au/services/view.php?id=352
Northern Territory	Territory Independence and Mobility Scheme	Department of Health and Community Services	http://www.nt.gov.au/health/docs/reference/ADS_DisabilityReviewBackgroundPaper_Feb2006.pdf
Australian Capital Territory	Australian Capital Territory Equipment Subsidy Scheme	Aged Care and Rehabilitation Service	http://health.act.gov.au/c/health?a=sp&pid=1059610195 http://www.health.act.gov.au/c/health?a=sendfile&ft=p&fid=1059627567&sid= http://www.health.act.gov.au/c/health

TABLE 5-4 State and Territory Funding Programs for Assistive Technology in Australia

	New South Wales	Victoria	Western Australia	Queensland	South Australia	Tasmania	Northern Territory	Australian Capital Territory
Program Name	Program of Appliances for Disabled People (PADP)	Victorian Aids and Equipment Program	Community Aids and Equipment Program (CAEP)	Medical Aids Subsidy Scheme (MASS)	Independent Living Equipment Program (ILEP)	Community Equipment Scheme (CES)	Territory Independence and Mobility Equipment (TIME) Scheme	Australian Capital Territory Equipment Subsidy Scheme (ACTESS)
Eligibility Assessment	Resident of New South Wales with a disability as defined by the Australian Disability Services Act	Resident of Victoria, holds Medicare card, long-term disability (medical practitioner verifies disability), require aids from the list	Permanent resident of Western Australia, clients must have a long-term disability and hold one of the following: Pensioner Concession Card, Health Care Card, Commonwealth Seniors Card, or receives a Carers Payment, live in a residential situation that is structured to encourage independent living and live in the community the majority of the time	Permanent resident of Queensland and have a permanent and stabilized condition or disability and hold one of the following cards: Centrelink Pensioner Concession Card, Veterans' Affairs Pensioner Concession Card (conditions apply), Centrelink Health Care Card, Queensland Government Seniors Card, Centrelink Confirmation of Concession Card, Entitlement Form (conditions apply)	Permanent resident of South Australia, people who have permanent disabilities, no means test but an age limit of 65 years, are living in or returning to community accommodation such as client's own home or a group home	Permanent Tasmanian resident having a long- or indefinite-term disability and living at home in the community or require equipment to enable discharge from hospital or nursing home to live at home in the community and a recipient of the following benefit card entitlements: Health Care Card, Pensioner Concession Card, Health Benefit Card, children with access to a Health Care Card are eligible	Resident of the Northern Territory, permanent or long-term duration defined as likely to last more than 12 months, living in or returning to the community (includes clients residing in individual dwellings, group homes, and residents of aged care facilities assessed as low-level care), hospital in-patients, being discharged back to the community are eligible for assistance if they meet other TIME Scheme eligibility criteria, in-patients requiring customized or specialized equipment, such as a modified wheelchair can be referred to TIME Scheme before discharge to enable equipment to be in place on discharge, require equipment on a permanent or long-term basis	Permanent resident in the Australia Capital Territory ≥6 months, permanent disability that will last at least 12 months, lives permanently in the community, meets financial criteria (currently receiving Commonwealth Centrelink payment), current Commonwealth Centrelink* Health Care Card, not eligible to receive assistance from other funding sources for disability equipment, such as DVA, EACH packages, private health insurance, third-party payers for injury/compensation

Means Testing	Eligibility categories are defined on the basis of income; entitlement and priority are defined for each category of eligibility	Victorian Aids and Equipment Program subsidizes aids and equipment for eligible people	If the client is a not a holder of one of the above cards, they can apply for consideration on the grounds of financial hardship	MASS subsidizes aids and equipment for eligible people	No means test	If not a holder of one of the above cards, can apply for consideration on the grounds of demonstrated financial need	Clients do not have to pay to register, but you may be asked to contribute toward the cost of some items and modifications	Currently require applicant to be receiving Commonwealth Centrelink payment such as pension, Carer Allowance, Carer Payment, Disability Support Pension, Age Pension
Children	Children under the age of 16 years are eligible regardless of parental/carer income	Children are eligible for subsidy	Children are eligible	Different eligibility applies for children aged less than 16 years for some aids/equipment depending on the child's age	Age 18 years downwardfunded by ILEP	Children with access to a health care card are eligible	Age under 16 years and family member is in receipt of Centrelink Carer Payment or Carers Allowance or approved as eligible on basis of financial hardship. Children who are in the care of the minister, who meet all other eligibility criteria are eligible for TIME Scheme assistance, irrespective of their foster parents' income	Children meeting eligibility criteria are eligible for 80% of subsidy ceiling for equipment if the parent(s) receive Centrelink benefit; otherwise child receives 20% of funding
Individuals Not Eligible for the Program	Hospital outpatients, clients with far advanced progressive disease, clients receiving community nursing assistance, those receiving health insurance funds, compensable clients, residents of department of community services, programs,	Residents of a Commonwealth funded residential care facility, those receiving a Community Aged Care Package, people who receive aids and equipment through other government-funded programs,	Current hospital in-patient, outpatient, or day patient, current recipients of any Commonwealth Aged Care funding including resident in a high-care facility (nursing home) or low-care facility (hostel); or Commonwealth Aged Care Packages (e.g., EACH), Flexible Care	Recipients of WorkCover, DVA card holders, residential aged care facility, recipients with a classified high need for aids and equipment or those who are one of the following: hospital inpatients, palliative care–eligible persons, ostomy	Clients able to receive equipment from another funding source, specifically: clients entitled to compensation, DVA Gold Card holder and eligible to receive equivalent item from DVA Rehabilitation Appliances Program, people who require assistive technology	Residents who are occupying a Commonwealth-funded residential aged care place. On admission to a residential aged care facility equipment previously supplied through CES should be returned (discretionary); hospital clients are ineligible while inpatients; veterans eligible for assistance from the	People who have received compensation or damages to provide equipment in respect of their disability; people who can obtain the prescribed item under another program: DVA provides eligible White and Gold Card holders with basic aids and equipment entitlements,	People resident in other than hostel-type accommodation in a Commonwealth-funded aged care facility; recipient of EACH Package; people eligible for DVA assistance with disability equipment; people in receipt of private health insurance for disability equipment,

*Centrelink delivers the social security services to the Australian public.

Continued

TABLE 5-4 State and Territory Funding Programs for Assistive Technology in Australia—cont'd

	New South Wales	Victoria	Western Australia	Queensland	South Australia	Tasmania	Northern Territory	Australian Capital Territory
	facilities for people with developmental disabilities, residents in Commonwealth hostels and nursing homes	those who are recipients of or are entitled to receive any form of compensation, people able to claim the cost of the aid through a private health insurance provider, people who have been discharged from a public hospital or extended care center, individuals needing aid or equipment specifically for use at work or in educational settings	and Community Aged Care Packages and similar programs, recipients of a compensation settlement, and those eligible for equipment through other funding programs (e.g., DVA), funding is not for vocational purposes	association persons, those with compensation claims	for discharge from hospital, people living in Commonwealth-funded Aged Care Accommodation (high- and low-level care), people who require the equipment specifically and only for work, study, or recreation	Rehabilitation Appliances Program; motor vehicle accident insurance board compensable clients; clients with spinal injury may have access to regional Spinal Accounts for assistance with aids, clients who are able to claim for aids from their private health care fund, recipients of Commonwealth EACH packages	people eligible to use other agencies that provide aids and equipment, including the Commonwealth Rehabilitation Service, private health funds provide some aids and equipment to their members, people who are high-care residents of a residential aged care facility	compensation payment for injury; people receiving Workers' Compensation for workplace injury
Funding Limits for Electric Wheelchair: Communication aid: Year 2006	Electric wheelchairs and communication aids: must be greater than $A800, $A100 Co-contribution. Over 16 YO means tested. No upper limit stated.	Electric wheelchair: $A6000 Communications aid: $A6000	Electric wheelchair: $A7700 Standard Wheelchair: $A11,000 Complex WC: $A5000 Power assist wheelchair Communication aids: $A7150 Committee will also consider aids that exceed	Electric wheelchair: $A5100 Communication aid: $A3000	Electric wheelchair: $A8500 Wheelchair only: $A11,000 Wheelchair plus complex seating communication aid: $A4000 Can apply for overrun	Electric wheelchair: $A6000 Communication aid: $A2000	Electric wheelchair: $A7000 Communication aid: $A3000	Electric wheelchair: $A6000-$A9500 Communication aid: $A6000

								Australian Capital Territory Health Web site
Information Available to the Client (see Table 5-2 for Web site)	Information brochure and policy available on New South Wales Health's Web site	the funding limits set by the program provider. Service Providers acting for CAEP remain responsible for device maintenance. The program funds are used for this purpose. Web site includes a brochure detailing application process, eligibility, and equipment available	Web site includes brochure, application form, and program guidelines	Web site provides detailed information, includes application form, eligibility, procedures, application process, and publications	Web site informs clients of the prerequisites for referral to the ILEP. Needs assessment performed before visiting ILEP. Telephone numbers to locate an assessor are provided.		See Web site or telephone: Darwin—08 8922 7224 East Arnhem—08 8987 0416 Katherine—8973 8778 Barkly—08 8962 4201 Alice Springs—8951 6734	
Application Process	Form obtained from lodgment center. Prescription required from appropriate health professional. Lodgment center staff determines test eligibility. Equipment list defines aids and equipment categories. Lodgment center processes application and orders equipment.	Applicant obtains referral from physician or health care professional (known as "referrer"). Referrer sends referral to a "specifier" requesting an assessment of the applicant's specific needs. A specifier is a CAEP-recognized health professional. Specifier will recommend the correct item of equipment	Client's health care professional refers to Victorian Aids and Equipment Program service provider. Service provider establishes whether applicant is within target population; if yes, forwards application form. It is the responsibility of client to collect all documentation required. General practitioner certifies diagnosis of disability.	Inquiries should be directed to the local MASS service center. Authorized prescribers provide justification of functional need for the requested aid or any accessories or modifications. Prescribers complete all application forms and in detail explain the applicant's functional/clinical need	Completing the ILEP application form (referral section) or by telephoning ILEP where application details will be recorded. On receipt of the referral the ILEP arranges a consultation for the client with an appropriate health professional. An application form (needs) is completed at this meeting and forwarded to ILEP.	Assessment by an appropriately qualified health professional usually from a public hospital or other government service. The health professional must complete the application to CES for funding	Prescriptions for the issue of an appliance are completed by a prescriber using the TIME scheme prescription form. Service provider must develop procedures to process and approve prescriptions for CES funding	Applicant completes application form that can be downloaded from the health ACT Web site (see Table 5-2) and provides evidence of eligibility. Physician must sign to indicate applicant has a permanent, stabilized disability. Applicant's allied health professional provides report on function and information on aids trialed and item that meets client's requirements.

Continued

TABLE 5-4   State and Territory Funding Programs for Assistive Technology in Australia—cont'd

	New South Wales	Victoria	Western Australia	Queensland	South Australia	Tasmania	Northern Territory	Australian Capital Territory
		Victorian Aids and Equipment Program do not fund the cost of the assessment of the client's needs and prescription of the aids and equipment. It is the responsibility of the client to organize and, when necessary, pay for the assessment, which forms part of the application. Application returned to service provider for consideration.	and ensure that funding approval is forthcoming from a service provider. A service provider is an organization who provides services to a specific disability type or range of types.	for the chosen aids and equipment in the home. This includes completion of the manufacturer's specification form (if applicable), including any accessories or modifications to detail the product to be supplied to the applicant. Applications should be directed to the local MASS service center.				
Prescriber for Aids and Equipment Requirements	Policy guidelines specify qualifications required for assessors in relevant equipment categories.	Specialist assessors provide assessments in the relevant categories. Applicant pays costs incurred.	Select health professions determine the requirement for aids or equipment.	There are designated MASS prescribers for each category of aid or equipment who submit an application to MASS for consideration for subsidy funding and who are responsible for application and training. MASS clinical advisers can assist prescribers.	Specialist assessors provided through case management agency.	Search facility on Web site will locate the closest health care professional who can prescribe assistive technology	Access to the scheme is based on assessment of need by an authorized prescriber. This may be a physiotherapist, occupational therapist, specialist nurse, or other recommended prescriber.	Prescribers are designated for each equipment category (occupational therapist, physiotherapist, speech pathologist, registered nurse, orthotist, etc.).

Co-payment							
An annual co-payment of $100 is required (there are some exclusions and variations to this). Co-payments or part payments can be negotiated in some circumstances, where applicants request a more costly item than would normally be funded.	If the item exceeds the subsidy cost, the service provider advises the supplier and client that a separate invoice covering the difference must be issued to the client. If a client has contributed more than 50%, they can retain ownership of the item and be responsible for the cost of maintenance and repairs, or transfer ownership and costs of repairs (excluding tires and tubes for wheelchairs) to Victorian Aids and Equipment Program.	Joint funding conditions include that equipment that is recyclable remains the property of the service provider. If the applicant has contributed greater than 50% of the device, then the applicant owns the item. Maintenance remains responsibility of service provider. If the family/applicant has made a significant contribution to the initial purchase of an item, they will not be required to contribute to the replacement or updating of basic and essential features if item is still on list.	Co-payment conditions include that MASS retains ownership of aids and equipment when MASS has contributed more than 50% toward the cost of the item. If the applicant has contributed more than 50% toward the cost of the item as a co-payment, the client can accept or reject MASS's offer for ownership. This means that the applicant may retain ownership of the item and be responsible for the cost of maintenance and repairs or can transfer ownership of the item to MASS and the costs of repairs (except large tires and tubes for manual wheel chairs) will be covered by MASS. There are certain items that MASS will only consider subsidizing if the applicant accepts ownership (e.g., voice-output communication devices).	Co-payment is unusual.	If the cost of the required item is in excess of the ceiling allowed, the client will be expected to arrange to meet the deficit. They can consider a range of options including top-up funds from Disability Services. Equipment provided by regional CES outlets remains the property of the statewide CES. When no longer required by the client, it must be returned. Repair and maintenance of equipment issued through the scheme is part of the Duty of Care of CES. Duty of Care contribute up to $50 in a 12-month period for this Duty of Care in addition to the hire/loan fee.	Where the client contributes 50% or more toward the cost of the item, then the client gains ownership. Any financial contribution (less than 50%) made by the client toward the purchase or repair of any item does not entitle the client to ownership or part ownership of that item. Equipment no longer required or suitable for the client must be returned to TIME scheme.	Client subsidy contribution is on a sliding scale of 10% at lower cost end through 2.5% at the ceiling cost and above. Client pays balance of subsidy ceiling to purchase price.

Continued

TABLE 5-4   State and Territory Funding Programs for Assistive Technology in Australia—cont'd

	New South Wales	Victoria	Western Australia	Queensland	South Australia	Tasmania	Northern Territory	Australian Capital Territory
Prioritization of Funding	Policy guidelines set priority for funding on the basis of eligibility category.	Priority ratings include No waiting category: —Clients who meet the clinical eligibility criteria of the oxygen program. —Wheelchair repairs; high urgency category: —Aids and equipment critical to the safety of client or injury prevention in daily living activities —Nonavailability will lead to a deterioration of the client's health or functioning —Nonavailability will lead to excess demands on carers in caring for person Low urgency category: —Length of waiting period —Clinical factors as indicated by prescribing therapist.	Priority ratings set to suit service providers' specific clientele (i.e., specific disability type or range of types).	Category 1: —Enabling a Queensland public hospital discharge to occur. —At risk for imminent hospitalization because of safety or medical need. —Repairs or maintenance to existing MASS aids and equipment. —Modifications or accessories to MASS aid for a MASS client who is at risk. —Replacement of a MASS aid that is unsafe for use. Category 2: —All other categories.	A score of 0 to 15 is assigned to each of the factors below to determine the priority for a client's need for a particular device: —Health and safety —Independence and function —Need for services/ institutional care —Rate of use —Area of use —Rapidly deteriorating condition (diagnostic) One point is added to the score for each month a client waits.	The three regional CES committees use the following scale to prioritize applications for assistance for nonstandard equipment, where 1 represents the highest priority and 5 represents the lowest priority. Eligible applications are considered in terms of these priorities and placed on a waiting list, pending the availability of funds. Applications rating 1 to 3 are placed on the high priority waiting list; 4 and 5 are placed on the low priority waiting list.	Although a person may be eligible for assistance under the TIME scheme, it does not guarantee that a particular aid or item of equipment will be provided. This decision is dependent on the priority of the application and the availability of funds. To ensure clients most in need are assisted, each prescription item will be prioritized by a set of criteria stated in the policy document (e.g., Category 1—life support and safety devices).	Priority is given in descending order: —Highest priority given to equipment that will keep applicant out of hospital —Replacement of unsafe or damaged equipment —Equipment service and repair —Ordinary applications —Applications for wheelchairs and other high-cost items are weighted against established criteria to decide priority.

Equipment Covered by the Program	Equipment categories are defined in the policy guidelines. Equipment covered includes devices for mobility and seating, environmental control, communication needs, computer access, medical monitoring, sensory function and transfer. Policy guidelines outline criteria for equipment included and excluded.	Electronic communication aids, electronic voice aids, environmental control units, wheelchairs and scooters	Communication aids, cochlear implant speech processor, positioning equipment, respiratory appliances, seating, transfer aids, wheeled mobility devices	Communication aids, mobility aids	Electric beds, pressure management overlays, communication devices, doorways, mobility devices: manual wheelchairs, power scooters, power wheelchairs, children's buggy pusher, children's manual tricycle, children's manual castor cart, children's power castor cart	Mobility aids, specialized seating and positioning equipment, communication aids, transfer devices	Communication aids, personal call alarms, pressure care, specialized items, wheelchairs and scooters	Adjustable bed, communication aid, patient hoist and sling, manual wheelchair, scooter, wheelchair, power wheelchair, modifications to seating controls, etc., pressure redistributing mattress and seat cushion
Local or Centralized Processing	Local area health services are responsible for PADP, with New South Wales Health responsible for the monitoring and evaluation of the area health services.	Department of Human Services manages the budget and allocations to local regional Victorian Aids and Equipment Program service providers. Service providers manage program and determine priorities of funding applications.	Disability Services Commission manages the budget allocated to local service providers who in turn manage the distribution of funds among the disability types that their organization serves. Service providers are, for example, state-funded hospitals, Cerebral Palsy Association, etc.	Queensland Health Department manages the overall budget and four local MASS service centers deliver the client services.	Processing is centralized through ILEP.	The three (local) regional ces outlets are based at: North West–Burnie Community Health Centre, Jones Street North–Launceston General Hospital South–Repatriation Centre, Hobart	Each district is responsible for the provision of TIME scheme services in accordance with their service agreements. There are seven local TIME scheme service providers. These are Darwin Urban, Darwin Rural, East Arnhem, Katherine, Barkly, Alice Springs Urban, and Alice Springs Rural.	Applications processed centrally in the ACTESS office at Canberra Hospital, Australian Capital Territory.
Managing Authority	New South Wales Health and Area Health Services	Department of Human Services	Disability Services Commission	Queensland Health	Disability Services	Department of Health and Human Services	Department of Health and Community Services	Aged Care and Rehabilitation Service, Australian Capital Territory Health

Australian Commonwealth Funded Schemes for the Older Person

The Australian government contributes funding for assistive technology and services for some people with disabilities. The funding is provided through the Department of Health and Ageing *(http://www.health.gov.au)* and is distributed through schemes that are common to all states and territories throughout Australia. The government-funded schemes are aimed at the frail older person and are generally for the provision of care and accommodation rather than for assistive technology. The eligibility of a person with a disability as distinct from a frail older person to benefit from a funding program is usually an "also" statement grafted on to the definition of a particular scheme.

There are four commonwealth-funded schemes, two that relate to nursing home care and two that relate to funding packages aimed at maintaining frail older people and people with disabilities in the community. Community Aged Care Packages (CACPs) are designed to enable older people who are assessed as eligible for low-level residential (or hostel) care to alternatively remain living in the community. Under the CACP program, a range of services can be provided to the individual, but assistive technology is not included. Extended Aged Care in Home (EACH) packages are similar to CACPs; however, they are targeted at clients who need a high level of care. They were created so that funding can be allocated more efficiently between clients who need high- and low-level care. EACH packages equate to the high-care residential nursing home situation and it is stated in the guidelines that program funds can be used to provide assistive technology.

Australian Department of Veterans' Affairs—Rehabilitation Appliances Program

The DVA exists to serve members of Australia's veteran and defense force communities, war widows and widowers, and widows and dependents, through programs of care, compensation, commemoration, and defense support services. The Rehabilitation Appliances Program (RAP) is one of the support services offered by the DVA. It is administered by the DVA and provides aids and appliances to eligible members and their dependents of the veteran community to help them maintain their independence as they grow older. This includes war veterans, members of the Australian Defence Force, former members of the Australian Defence Force, cadets, and war veterans from the United Kingdom and other Australian allies, in some cases. The DVA has major offices in all state capitals and 26 Veterans' Affairs Network offices throughout Australia. Appliances provided under this program must meet a clinical need and must be the simplest, most effective, and least costly equipment that will suffice. Box 5-2 lists typically funded items under the Australian RAP program. DVA funding for appliances is

---

BOX 5-2   Fundable Rehabilitation Appliances Program Equipment/Items

Alarm system/communication appliances/assistive listening devices
Bed adjustable (mechanical/hydraulic/electrical)
Communication aids (electronic)
Computer (personal)
Environmental control unit
Hearing aids
Low-vision appliances
Personal response systems
Scooter (electric)
Voice prosthesis
Wheelchairs (electric and manual)

For further guidelines refer to the RAP Schedule of Equipment. This can be obtained on-line at *http://www.dva.gov.au/health/rap/rap.htm.*

---

eligibility tested, and if a person with a disability is eligible for either of the funding schemes the person is generally excluded from using state-based schemes.

Australian Motor Vehicle Compulsory Third Party Personal Injury Insurance

Each state/territory in Australia has a motor vehicle insurance commission designed to provide compensation for people who are injured and become disabled as a result of road accident trauma. Settlements received by people in this situation should be designed with the provision of assistive technology as one of the essential compensatory strategies for the loss of function by the injured person. The insurance commissions or their representatives are listed in Table 5-5, along with the respective Web sites. Australia wide, Motor Vehicle Third Party Personal Injury Insurance is compulsory; it is commonly known as Compulsory Third Party Insurance.

Australian Government Education Departments

In Australia, the delivery of education services is a state government responsibility. Education departments in each state provide some assistance to students who need assistive technology to pursue their educations. The programs have tended to develop in isolation and therefore differ in detail from state to state. However, the programs generally concentrate on providing assistive technology that is essential for the student's education, thus limiting the availability or use of assistive technologies (such as communication aids) more broadly in the community. It is recommended that those interested in pursuing this avenue of funding for assistive technology seek further information from the particular state's education department.

TABLE 5-5	Motor Vehicle Compulsory Third-Party Insurance Funding for Assistive Technologies in Australia	
Jurisdiction	Program	Web Link
Western Australia	Insurance Commission of Western Australia	http://www.icwa.wa.gov.au/icwa/ic_menu_list.shtml
South Australia	Motor Accident Commission Allianz Australia is the sole claims manager acting on behalf of the Motor Accident Commission of South Australia.	http://www.allianz.com.au/allianz/CICT+SA.html
Queensland	Motor Accident Insurance Commission (MAIC)– Allianz Australia is the sole claims manager acting on behalf of the MAIC Queensland.	http://www.allianz.com.au/allianz/CICT±QLD.html
Victoria	Transport Accident Commission	http://www.tac.vic.gov.au/jsp/content/Navigation Controller.do;jsessionid=MGOLMNDPMBIA?areaID=25
NSW	Motor Accidents Authority	http://www.maa.nsw.gov.au/index.aspx
Northern Territory	Motor Accidents (Compensation) Act	http://notes.nt.gov.au/dcm/legislat/legislat.nsf/0/960af 9d56ee9b5d969256e5c00095824?OpenDocument
Tasmania	Motor Accidents Insurance Board	http://www.service.tas.gov.au/Search/PhraseSearch.asp? Task=Applications&DisplayHeading=Motor+vehicle+ insurance
Australian Capital Territory	Third Party Insurance–Australian Capital Territory	http://www.nrma.com.au/pub/nrma/motor/ctp/act/ index.shtml

The Australian Disability Discrimination Act 1991 includes a document entitled "Disability Standards for Education 2005" *(http://www.dest.gov.au/sectors/school_ education/programmes_funding/forms_guidelines/disability_ standards_for_education.htm)*. This Australian government standard outlines the obligation that educational institutions have to provide equal access to education for a person with a disability. This standard does not directly discuss assistive technology or funding for devices, but it does clearly state the need for the application of both the hard and soft forms of such technologies to ensure access to education for students with disabilities.

PRIVATE SOURCES OF FUNDING

In addition to public funding sources, there are private sources of funding. These vary by country. Examples of U.S. sources are identified in Box 5-1. Private sources of funding in Canada are shown in Table 5-1. Other Australian sources of funding include nongovernment schools, charitable sources (lotteries, service clubs [e.g., Rotary, Lions, Variety]), philanthropic organizations, private health insurance, and worksafe programs. The availability of these programs, the specific coverage, and the eligibility criteria vary across the country.

Self-Funding

Personal sources of funding include out-of-pocket cash paid by the consumer, private trust funds, and loans. Because of the cost of assistive technology equipment and services, paying cash could be a hardship on the consumer. Sometimes this is the only alternative, however. Some individuals have

trust funds set up where money received from a legal settlement is kept to provide for the equipment and services they may need, including assistive technologies. Individuals who use personal funds to purchase assistive technology may be eligible for a deduction or credit on their taxes and should consult with a tax accountant.

In the United States and some other countries low-interest loans are also available for the purchase of assistive technology. These programs are a major initiative of the Assistive Technology Act, which sought to broaden the availability of low-interest loan programs throughout the country. In procuring a loan, the consumer shares the responsibility of paying for the equipment, which may increase the consumer's involvement in the process (Reeb, 1989). The Easter Seal Society has recently set up a national loan fund to help persons with disabilities purchase assistive technologies. The loan fund was made possible by a U.S. Department of Education grant. Up to 75% of the equipment costs can be financed. The maximal amount that can be financed is $3200. Some manufacturers and vendors also provide low-interest loans. A consumer in need of a loan should check with these sources as well.

Private Health Insurance

Private health insurance is the source of approximately 35% of all health expenditures in the United States (government and direct private payments comprise the other sources) (U.S. Dept. of Commerce, Bureau of the Census, Statistical Abstract of the United States, 2006, Table 118, p. 98). Most often, insurance is an employment fringe benefit, although individuals also can purchase an insurance policy on their own. Although insurance policies may vary considerably, benefits such as durable medical equipment are almost always included. Very often, rehabilitation therapies such as occupational therapy, physical therapy, and speech-language pathology services also will be covered. When assisting an individual with insurance, the ATP will have to ensure that the item or service being sought fits within one or more of the covered services of the policy and that no coverage exclusions or limitations apply. This information will be found in the benefits booklet that is provided with the policy, which details the scope of coverage and exclusions as well as co-payments, deductibles, preferred providers, if any, and appeal procedures. As in public health insurance, funding by private health insurance companies is based on a medical diagnosis and justification of medical necessity. Most private forms of health insurance require the use of current procedural terminology (CPT) codes for billing (see section on billing and coding later in this chapter).

Private health insurance is also a potential source for funding assistive technology devices and speech-language pathology and occupational and physical therapy services beyond what is publicly funded in Canada. Private health insurance is often used to "top-up" benefits when funded amounts are inadequate (e.g., too few hours of training for an augmentative communication device) or when there is a co-payment.

OTHER SOURCES OF FUNDING

There are alternative sources for funding that do not fall under the categories of public or private agencies (see Box 5-1). These sources include service clubs, private foundations, and volunteer organizations. There are various community service clubs (e.g., Kiwanis, Rotary Club) that may be a source of funding for a local individual who has no other means of funding. Service clubs are more likely to provide funding if one of their goals is to help certain disability groups or if the consumer is a member of the club or personally knows someone who is a member. Examples are two funds created by the Muscular Dystrophy Association that allow individuals with neurodegenerative diseases such as MD or ALS to receive up to $2000 to facilitate access to a speech-generating device and up to $2000 to facilitate access to a mobility device.

There are foundations related to a specific disability group that directly supply equipment and services to individuals with that particular disability. Other disability-related foundations provide partial funding or assist the consumer in obtaining funding. The American Federation for the Blind provides low-interest loans, for example, to individuals who are visually impaired and need to purchase equipment (Matheis et al, 1991). There are also a number of volunteer organizations (e.g., Telephone Pioneers of America) that may contribute by fabricating a custom device. Usually the labor is provided and the consumer pays for the cost of materials.

Similar benefits are provided by the Canadian National Institute for the Blind.

FUNDING PROCESS AND GUIDELINES FOR PROCURING FUNDING

To obtain funding for assistive technology devices services, individuals with disabilities must follow the procedures and guidelines established by each program for which they are eligible and that covers the items being requested. ATPs play a crucial role in this process. Most often it is the ATP who must make the case for funding by conducting assessments, preparing reports, gathering prescriptions and other documentation, and communicating with equipment suppliers and funding program staff. If there is a trial period, the ATP will generally supervise it and report the results to establish the potential benefit of the device. ATPs also are the primary liaison between the client, the supplier, and the funding sources. If funding is denied, ATPs are often called on to coordinate appeals, which may involve representation of the client or soliciting and then working with a professional advocate who will pursue the appeal on the client's behalf. Although most of these tasks are not compensated, funding has to be pursued, ATPs have to do it, and it has to work for the consumer to receive the services and devices.

A complicating factor is that consumers may be eligible for multiple sources of funding, each of which may have different rules and procedures. This is particularly true because funding and benefits programs have been created to serve very specific purposes, yet health services are able to serve broader goals. Thus, the same services may be covered by multiple programs (e.g., occupational therapy will be covered as a special education–related service and a health benefit within health insurance) or by Medicaid (in the United States). It also is not uncommon for individuals to have multiple sources of health care coverage (e.g., private health insurance and Medicaid or Medicaid and Medicare). Coordinating the benefits of these programs is important to ensure maximum benefit to the consumer.

Over time, the ATP may be called on to seek funding for the same client and for the same item or service multiple times. Funding will be sought to pay for the initial assessment, for purchase of a device, for payment for training and other services; for repairs or modifications to the device; for periodic reassessment of needs; and ultimately for device replacement. Most programs that pay for equipment purchase or rental also will pay for equipment repair and, as necessary, replacement.

Soft technology services such as training are important for many types of assistive technologies, both for the device user and caregivers. Funding for these services, however, is not always covered, even if device purchase is covered. Obviously, the provision of a device without these services can have adverse consequences for the individual. The ATP may be called on to identify alternative sources for these services, such as training offered by supplier sales representatives.

The several points during the service delivery process at which funding may need to be pursued are shown in Figure 4-2. To the novice ATP, funding programs can appear as a dense or even impenetrable web, but the funding process is navigable. Care and attention to detail are required, but this is not different from the general obligations of the ATP in all his or her professional activities.

◼ IDENTIFYING THE FUNDING SOURCE

The various funding sources are described earlier in this chapter and in Chapter 1. This section provides guidelines for navigating the U.S. process of obtaining funding. This process also applies in broad terms to other countries. In general, consumers will know what programs they are eligible for. If they are eligible for Medicaid, Medicare, private insurance, or Tricare, they will possess a wallet card stating their eligibility. (Suppliers may require photocopies of both sides of this card to be submitted along with the other documentation to support a funding request.) Those who are veterans will know they are eligible for DVA services. Children with disabilities are likely to already have been identified and referred to the early intervention or special education systems. The only program where an ATP is likely to be a valuable asset regarding initial program eligibility is vocational rehabilitation. The client's ability to demonstrate a potential to work may be dependent on access to assistive technology, and it will be the ATP's evaluation and report that both identifies that need and establishes eligibility for the broader range of vocational rehabilitation services. From this list of potential funding programs, the ATP must begin to coordinate the justification and documentation process. Specific evaluations and reports may be required by each program. Great care must be taken to prepare written reports to ensure that the standard of need for each program or unique program vocabulary is stated. For example, each of the agencies that provide funding for assistive technologies may have a different standard of need. Educational agencies will fund assistive technology that provides a student with access to education. Medicare and Medicaid only fund durable medical equipment that is medically necessary, such as wheelchairs and seat cushions. In state vocational rehabilitation agencies, there is a standard that the assistive technology must significantly contribute to the individual's ability to be productive at work for it to be funded. The role of the ATP is to know which programs are likely to fund the particular types of services and devices that are required by an individual consumer. These can then be matched to the benefits provided by the programs for which the consumer is eligible. Assistive technology equipment suppliers are aware of the funding sources that can be used for reimbursement

of their products, and they can be useful sources of information to the ATP and the consumer. ATP reports describing "needs" must be written with care and written with the expectation the reviewer will be looking for vocabulary that is consistent with the reviewer's program's purposes.

Dealing with the multiple public or private agencies is a challenge. Procedures for obtaining funding for assistive technologies, levels of funding, and staff familiarity with the scope of and need for assistive technology and related services vary from agency to agency. For example, some funding agencies require that equipment and services be purchased from an approved list of vendors. Other funding agencies require approval for services and equipment before implementation. It is the responsibility of the consumer and the ATP to locate for each agency the regulations that apply to assistive technology and pursue funding on the basis of those regulations. Another important consideration is the principle of "payer of last resort," which requires a specific sequencing of multiple benefits or funding programs. The Medicaid program is identified by statute as the payer of last resort in relation to other health benefits programs. For this reason, if a consumer has both Medicaid and Medicare or Medicaid and private health insurance, the procedures related to obtaining payment from Medicare or from the private insurance must be followed first before a claim can be submitted to Medicaid. In general, the procedure for sorting the relationship between multiple funding programs is called "coordination of benefits." Another characteristic of benefits and funding programs, particularly those that provide health benefits, is that they compartmentalize coverage. Specific services will be provided, such as durable medical equipment, occupational therapy, physical therapy, or speech-language pathology. However, not all these services may be covered. Thus, a program may pay for an item of durable medical equipment but not cover the assessment to establish need for the item or training in its use. These limitations force the ATP to be alert for alternative sources of funding so that all the person's needs can be met.

As a practical matter, an ATP may not only be interacting with multiple funding programs for the same item or service if a person has dual eligibility and both programs cover the service but also may be working to secure multiple items or services for the client at the same time. The following case study provides an example of a person with multiple funding programs and multiple needs.

To simplify the process of obtaining funding, it is recommended that a funding strategy be developed for each consumer. Beukleman and Mirenda (2005) identify five steps in developing such a strategy:

1. Survey the funding resources that are available to the individual.
2. Identify various funding sources for the various activities of an intervention (i.e., assessment, equipment, and training).

CASE STUDY

FUNDING FOR MIRANDA

Miranda is 14 years old and a freshman in high school. She has cerebral palsy and uses a wheelchair for mobility. She is also nonverbal. Her teacher referred her to the assistive technology center for an augmentative communication evaluation. During the needs assessment, it was discovered that Miranda was also in need of a new seating and mobility system. Her mother also expressed a desire for Miranda to be more independent at home and to be able to turn the TV and her stereo system off and on. Miranda has a range of assistive technology needs, and it became apparent to the ATP that funding for Miranda was going to have to come from multiple sources. Given the information that was shared during the needs assessment, the ATP completed a personal funding worksheet for Miranda. The ATP will seek funding from the state Medicaid system for the seating and mobility system, from the school system for an augmentative communication device, and from Miranda's personal resources for an electronic aid to daily living (EADL) to turn her TV, stereo, and appliances off and on. Her father is also involved in the local Rotary Club and that may be another source of funding for the EADL.

The use of a personal funding worksheet such as the one shown in Box 5-3 is helpful.

3. Prepare a funding plan with the consumer and the family members.
4. Assign responsibility to specific individuals for pursuing funding for each aspect of the intervention.
5. Prepare necessary documentation for the funding request. Be sure to make all requests in writing so that a written record is available if an appeal is necessary.

Keeping current on funding information is time consuming but absolutely essential for the ATP. Every state has a technology assistance project (see Chapter 1) that disseminates information on funding resources and strategies. For contact information, refer to the Rehabilitation Engineering and Assistive Technology Society of North America Technical Assistance Project Web site *(www.resna.org). Assistive Technology: A Funding Workbook* (Morris and Golinker, 1991) also provides information on funding resources and strategies. The independent living centers found in each state are another source of funding information and advocacy. Networking with other assistive technology professionals at conferences, by listservs, and over the phone are other invaluable resources.

■ JUSTIFYING FUNDING FOR ASSISTIVE TECHNOLOGY SERVICES AND DEVICES

Third-party payers require adequate documentation and proof of need before they will approve funding for assistive technology services or equipment. The essential question funding sources want answered is how this technology will improve the individual's functioning. Whether it is a medical, vocational, or educational need, there are essential components that should be included in any written justification. Golinker and Mistrett (1997) identify components to address when justifying a medical need for a device, but these elements can apply to other justifications as well. These components are summarized as follows:

1. A description of the specific functional limitation that the device and service addresses
2. A detailed description of the device, including features, accessories, and customization
3. A specific description of the effect of the device or service (e.g., how it will alleviate or ameliorate the functional limitation)
4. A description of the evaluation process, how the recommendation was arrived at, and what other alternatives were considered
5. An explanation of why the device being recommended is the least costly equally therapeutically effective solution
6. A description of the expertise of the ATP (or interdisciplinary team) recommending the services or equipment, including general professional experience and specific experience in assistive technology services

A specific criterion for funding under Medicare, Medicaid, and private health insurance is **medical necessity.** This requires that the justification include "identification of a medical diagnosis, or condition, that is specifically coupled to the functional impairment being addressed by the device" (Golinker and Mistrett, 1997, p 217). A physician's prescription is required for devices that are medically necessary. Appendix 5-1A provides an example of a form to use to justify funding for augmentative communication devices and Appendix 5-1B shows an example of a justification form for seating and wheeled mobility systems.

When funding is being pursued through a vocational rehabilitation agency, it is important that the written justification specify how the device will enhance the individual's ability to function in a work setting. For assistive technology services and equipment to be considered, they need to be part of the consumer's IPE. Similarly, when funding is being pursued through special education, the justification needs to address how the equipment will give the child access to a free and appropriate education in the "least restrictive environment." All assistive technology services and equipment must address goals written in the child's IFSP for children from birth to 2 years old or in the IEP for children aged

BOX 5-3 **Personal Funding Worksheet**

Client: _____

Type of intervention (e.g., augmentative and alternative communication devices, mobility): _____

Funding Source	Assessment/ Recommendations	Equipment Purchase	Training	Follow-up and Follow-along
Medicare				
Medicaid				
Children's Medical Services				
Developmental services				
Tricare				
School				
Vocational rehabilitation				
PASS				
VA				
Self-funding				
Private health insurance				
Workers' Compensation				
Community organizations				
Other				

Modified from Beukelman DR, Mirenda P: *Augmentative and alternative communication, management of severe communication disorders in children and adults,* Baltimore, 2005, Paul H Brookes.

3 to 21 years. For children in school, an additional comment is appropriate. Many health services also are school-related services. Typically, schools provide these services. If a child needs more health services than a school offers, health services programs such as Medicaid or insurance will be sought as a supplemental benefit. For Medicaid-eligible children, Medicaid will often pay the school for its provision of certain related services that also are covered by Medicaid, such as audiology, occupational therapy, physical therapy, speech-language pathology, and nursing services.

It is likely that the staff person reading the funding justification has never met the consumer and may not have had any experience with a person with a disability or with assistive technology. It is important that the justification be easily understood and that it clearly depict who this person is, what the needs are, and how the system can help. It may be helpful to include a picture or videotape of the consumer with the system being recommended.

■ APPEALING THE FUNDING DENIAL

At any point in the funding process, a denial for funding may be received. When requests for funding have been

denied, it helps to be persistent and to submit an appeal for the denial. It is through this persistence that funding sources may eventually include assistive technologies as a regular part of the support they provide.

Every funding agency has an **appeals process** whereby the client, ATP, family member, or a professional advocate can appeal a funding denial. The first step taken is to determine the procedure for an appeal and the time limitations related to appeals. The next step is to find out why the request was denied. Almost all funding programs will provide an explanation to the client in writing. By knowing the reason for denial, all persons working to help the client can develop an appeal plan. It will be based on a comparison of the denial reason to the facts, to the scope of benefits offered by the program, including program definitions and guidance, and wherever possible, to a comparison of the funding program's past actions when the same item or service was sought. In short, an appeal plan allows for the development of a specific statement of why the denial is wrong and why it should be reversed. It also will allow for identification of any missing information or clarifying statements to supplement what already has been submitted. Implementation of the plan will be an appeal that specifically addresses the denial reason and thus decreases the likelihood of the appeal being denied as well.

Sometimes a request is denied because a piece of information was inadvertently omitted, such as a billing code, and resubmission of the request with the necessary information is all that is needed. Or, the denial may have been made because the agency believes that the plan or policy does not include such a benefit, or it may be based on the fact that the provider does not think that the request meets the criteria for funding.

Mendelsohn (1996) discusses typical grounds for appeal and the format that appeals may take. The purpose of an appeal is to convince the funding agency that the denial was erroneous and to have the decision reversed. The appeal should be made in writing to the funding source. It should explain why the denial for funding was inappropriate and provide any additional information that may have been omitted in the initial request (Golinker and Mistrett, 1997). During the appeals process it may be necessary to ask for assistance from a skilled advocacy layperson or an attorney.

■ BILLING AND CODING FOR SERVICES

Preparing the billing form correctly and using the proper codes on billing forms are necessary to ensure payment. Medical payers require that the provider use diagnosis codes and procedure codes when services are billed. **Diagnosis codes** are used to describe the person's condition or the medical reason for the services being requested; it is this condition that is the key to establishing medical necessity. The most widely used diagnosis coding system in the United States is *The International Statistical Classification of Diseases and Related Health Problems*, tenth revision (World Health Organization, 1992).

In the United States **procedure codes** are used to describe the services that the provider implemented or the equipment delivered and that are being billed. The Health Care Financing Administration (HCFA) Common Procedure Coding System (HCPCS) is the most commonly used procedure coding system. It has three levels: (1) the American Medical Association's physician's CPT is referred to as Level I HCPCS, (2) Level II HCPCSs are the HCFA-developed alphanumerical codes, including codes for durable medical equipment, prosthetics, orthotics, and supplies, and (3) Level III HCPCSs are local codes created as needed by Medicare and other carriers (Acquaviva, 1998). Example CPT codes relevant to assistive technology devices and services are shown in Box 5-4.

The CPT codes are a set of five-digit codes that pertain to the medical service or procedure performed by physicians and other service providers. The CPT Editorial Panel of the American Medical Association establishes the CPT codes, which have become the industry standard for reporting, and updates them on an annual basis. There is a physical medicine and rehabilitation section of the CPT codes under which

---

BOX 5-4　Example CPT Codes Used for Assistive Technology Devices and Services in the United States

92605: Evaluation for prescription of non-speech-generating augmentative and alternative communication device

92606: Therapeutic service(s) for the use of non-speech-generating-device, including programming and modification

92607: Evaluation and prescription for speech-generating augmentative and alternative communication device, face-to-face with the patient; first hour

92608: Evaluation and prescription for speech-generating augmentative and alternative communication device, face-to-face with the patient; each additional 30 minutes

92609: Therapeutic services for the use of speech generating device, including programming and modification

97504: Orthotics fitting and training

97353: Self-care/home management

97535: Self-care, home management training

97542: Wheelchair management and propulsion

97537: Community/work reintegration training

97755: assistive technology assessment

97761: Prosthetic training, upper and/or lower extremity(s)

97762: Checkout for orthotic/prosthetic use, established patient, each 15 minutes

97760: Orthotic management

---

occupational, physical, and speech therapy can bill for certain procedures that may encompass assistive technology intervention. The codes in this section are defined in 15-minute segments. For example, an occupational therapist who has instructed a consumer with a visual impairment on the use of sensory aids to increase independence in self-care can bill using CPT code 97535 ("Selfcare/Home management training [e.g., ADLs and compensatory training, meal preparation, safety procedures, and instruction in the use of adaptive equipment direct one-on-one contact by provider, each 15 minutes"). Practitioners may use codes in any section of the CPT as long as the service is within the scope of practice for the practitioner (Acquaviva, 1998). A new code specific to assistive technology has been drafted and is in the process of getting approved as an addition to the CPT codes.

■ PAYMENT PRACTICES

The traditional method of payment for health care has been **fee for service.** Under this method of payment, providers are paid a certain rate per unit of service (American Occupational Therapy Association [AOTA], 1996). As a result of skyrocketing health care costs in the United States, however, payment practices in the health care field have changed significantly over the last decade. **Managed care** has emerged as a means of controlling health care costs.

The term managed care is used to describe "any method of health care delivery designed to reduce unnecessary utilization of services, and provide for cost containment while ensuring that high quality of care or performance is maintained" (Rognehaugh, 1998, p. 134). Managed care plans are now a major part of private health insurance offerings, as well as part of publicly funded insurance programs such as Medicare, Medicaid, Workers' Compensation programs, and CHAMPUS.

Several measures are used by managed care plans to limit either provider payments or enrollee use of services. The primary cost-cutting mechanism used in managed care is capitation. Negotiating with providers for a prepaid amount gives providers a direct stake in controlling their costs. In this arrangement the managed care organization (MCO) agrees to pay the provider a set amount of money on a per-member basis in exchange for the provider's assuming responsibility for furnishing all or certain health services to a patient for a specified period of time (AOTA, 1996). The provider takes the risk that the capitation rate will be sufficient to cover all the costs of care for the members. An enrollee in the MCO's plan is restricted to using providers that have a contractual agreement with the MCO.

Other measures used by MCOs to control costs include precertification or preauthorization, mandatory second opinions, case management, and use of a third-party administrator (AOTA, 1996). For ATPs, the implications of managed care are many. Primarily it makes it difficult or impossible to get paid for services if the ATP does not have a contract with an MCO or is not part of a group that contracts with an MCO. The ATP also should determine whether the provider requires preauthorization or second opinions before carrying out any services with the consumer. Case managers are being used more often, particularly in situations where the individual has had an injury or accident resulting in a long-term disability.

Most case managers in the United States are nurses who may have limited experience with assistive technology. The case manager is a gatekeeper who controls access to the services that are provided to the individual, including assistive technology. One way for ATPs to learn more about case management and conversely to educate case managers about assistive technology is through the Case Management Society of America (CMSA) and its on-line forums, which can be accessed at the CMSA Web site *(www.cmsa.org)*.

Consumers and ATPs need to continually be involved in educating funding sources and advocating for the inclusion of assistive technology equipment and services in agencies' policies. As discussed in Chapter 4, ATPs need to expand their documentation of the benefits and outcomes of assistive technology. This documentation provides helpful information when advocating for increased allocation of funding by public and private agencies.

■ SUMMARY

The various sources of funding for assistive technology services and equipment are described in this chapter. Sources of funding for assistive technology are either public or private and include programs such as Medicare, Medicaid, vocational rehabilitation, education, private health insurance, low-interest loans, and grants. The ATP should be knowledgeable about the different funding sources and the process for successfully obtaining funding. This includes identifying the appropriate funding source for the consumer, writing a funding justification, billing and coding for assistive technology, and appealing denials as needed. Furthermore, it is important that the ATP advocate at the public policy level for increased coverage of assistive technology services and equipment.

Study Questions

1. List the major steps in identifying a funding source for a particular assistive technology device or service.
2. What are the major categories of funding for assistive technology devices?
3. What are the major assistive technology funding sources typically available for a child who is in an educational program and needs an augmentative communication device?
4. What are the most likely funding sources for support of assistive technology devices and services for an adult who sustains a head injury at the age of 25 years?
5. Compare funding sources for assistive technologies in the United States, Australia, and Canada. What features are common and which are different?
6. Describe two distinct funding sources and identify at least one criterion that must be met by the consumer to be eligible for funding of assistive technology services from each source.
7. What are the types of personal funding?
8. What restrictions are typically placed on private insurance funding of assistive technology devices and services?
9. What is the source of the benefits available under Workers' Compensation?
10. What are the major challenges in identifying the most likely funding source for a given situation?
11. Define the term "medical necessity."
12. When writing a medical justification for a device for a consumer, what elements should be included?

13. What are CPT codes, and how can they be used in securing funding for assistive technology services and devices?
14. List three types of alternative funding sources for assistive technology devices and services.
15. What are the five steps recommended for developing a funding strategy?
16. Describe the two types of billing codes commonly used in health care.
17. What is managed care, and how does it affect assistive technology service delivery?
18. What is meant by the term capitation? What are the implications of capitation for assistive technology service delivery?
19. What are the major steps taken to appeal a funding denial?
20. How can consumers and ATPs work together to inform funding sources of the needs for assistive technology services and devices?

References

Acquaviva J, editor: *Effective documentation for occupational therapy*, ed 2, Bethesda, MD, 1998, American Occupational Therapy Association.

American Occupational Therapy Association Managed Care Project Team: *Managed care: an occupational therapy sourcebook*, Bethesda, MD, 1996, The Association.

Beukelman DR, Mirenda P: *Augmentative and alternative communication, management of severe communication disorders in children and adults*, ed 3, Baltimore, 2005, Paul H Brookes.

Burton J: Workers' compensation, twenty-four-hour coverage, and managed care, *Work Comp Mon* 9:11-21, 1996.

Golinker L, Mistrett SG: Funding. In Angelo J: *Assistive technology for rehabilitation therapists*, Philadelphia, 1997, FA Davis.

Matheis D et al: *The buck starts here ... a guide to assistive technology funding in Kentucky*, Frankfort, KY, 1991, Department of the Blind.

Mendelsohn S: Funding assistive technology. In Galvin JC, Scherer MJ, editors: *Evaluating, selecting, and using appropriate assistive technology*, Gaithersburg, MD, 1996, Aspen Publishers.

Morris MW, Golinker LA: *Assistive technology: a funding workbook*, Arlington, VA, 1991, RESNA Press.

Reeb KG: *Assistive financing for assistive devices: loan guarantees for purchase of products by persons with disabilities*, Washington, DC, 1989, Electronic Industries Foundation.

Rognehaugh R: *The managed care health care dictionary*, ed 2, Gaithersburg, MD, 1998, Aspen Publishers.

U.S. Department of Commerce, Bureau of the Census: *Statistical abstract of the United States*, 2006, Table 118, p. 98.

World Health Organization: *The International statistical classification of diseases and related health problems*, 10th revision, Geneva, 1992, World Health Organization.

Sample Forms for Documenting Consumers' Equipment Needs

▧ APPENDIX 5-1A

Communication Prosthesis Payment Review Summary

Instruction

1. PATIENT INFORMATION
   > Name—Patient's complete name
   > Address—Patient's home address
   > Birthdate—Month/day/year
   > Health Insurance Number—Appropriate number for coverage
   > Medical Diagnosis—Document medical diagnosis (ICD-9-CM) for the patient
   > Speech-Language Diagnosis—Document Speech-Language diagnosis (ASHACS) for patient

2. FACILITY INFORMATION
   > Facility—Wherre the patient is receiving treatment
   > Address/Phone Number—Facility address and phone (with area code)
   > Physician/Specialty—Physician in charge of this case
   > Speech-Language Pathologist—SLP working with patient

3. DEVICE INFORMATION
   > Item Description—General description of device being recommended
   > Manufacturer—Maker of the device
   > Distributor/Dealer—Local source of supply, including service and training

4. PATIENT'S PHYSICAL STATUS
   > Check the square that characterizes the patient's current physical condition per medical/clinical documentation or personal observation
   > Adequate/inadequate rating related to physical patameters only as they apply to the use of the specific communication device
   > Nonessential rating indicates status is not related to the use of the device for this patient.

5. PATIENT'S COGNITIVE PREREQUISTES
   > Check the appropriate square that best describes the patient's current status.
   > If applicable, provide the name of the testing instrument and the scores obtained

6. SELECTION OF AUGMENTATIVE COMMUNICATION DEVICE
   a. Current Means—Describe how this patient currently communicates and why it is not the best method of choice.
   b. Other Devices—List other devices considered for this patient and why they would not be applicable.
   c. Rationale—What characteristics of this device influence the determination that it was the best choice, e.g., portability, size, symbols, service, or training.
   d. Indicators—Has the patient had an opportunity to use the device? How long? Rental? What was observed, e.g., increased initiation of ADLs

7. PROGNOSIS
   a. Communication Ability—Will the patient's ability to communicate basic needs, such as health and safety information, be improved?
   b. Independence—Will the patient's independence increase with the use of the device?
   c. Placement—Will the community placement be affected? Example: group home vs. nursing home.
   d. Academic Ability—Will the patient's ability to learn and retain new information change?
   e. Vocational Training—Will the patient's ability to advance in vocational rehabilitation improve?

8. COMMENTS—Give any comments unique to this device or what it will offer for this individual that would help in determining payment. Use space provided on the reverse side of the summary form.

PLEASE HAVE THE SUMMARY SIGNED AND DATED BY THE PHYSICIAN AND THE SPEECH-LANGUAGE PATHOLOGIST.

Communication Prosthesis Payment Review Summary

1. PATIENT INFORMATION

Name _____

Address _____

City _____ State ____ Zip _____

Birthdate _____ Health Ins. # _____

Medical Diagnosis _____

Speech-Language Diagnosis _____

2. FACILITY INFORMATION

Facility _____

Address _____

City _____ State ____ Zip _____

Telephone _____

Physician _____

Specialty _____

Speech-Language Pathologist_____

3. DEVICE INFORMATION

Item Description _____
_____

Manufacturer _____

Distributor/Dealer _____

4. PHYSICAL STATUS PER DOCUMENTATION

(Check Appropriate Square)

	Adequate	Inadequate	Nonessential
a. General medical status	☐	☐	☐
b. Respiratory	☐	☐	☐
c. Hearing	☐	☐	☐
d. Vision	☐	☐	☐
e. Head control	☐	☐	☐
f. Trunk stability	☐	☐	☐
g. Arm movement	☐	☐	☐
h. Ambulation	☐	☐	☐
i. Seating/positioning for use of device	☐	☐	☐
j. Ability to access the device (switches, etc.)	☐	☐	☐

Summary _____
_____
_____
_____
_____

5. COGNITIVE PREREQUISITES

(Check Appropriate Square)

	Present	Absent
a. Attempts to communicate with consistent response mode	☐	☐
b. Functional yes/no	☐	☐
c. Understands that communication will cause an action to occur	☐	☐
d. Understands that symbols (i.e., words, pictures, Bliss, sign) stand for verbal communication	☐	☐

	Guarded	Poor	Absent
e. Prognosis to develop intelligible speech	☐	☐	☐

	Present	Absent	Unknown
f. Demonstrates memory retention of verbal instruction	☐	☐	☐

g. Names of standardized tests and scores (if applicable)

Spelling _____ _____

Reading _____ _____

Cognition _____ _____

6. SELECTION OF DEVICE

a. Patient's current means of communication: _____
_____

b. Other devices considered and rationale for elimination:
_____
_____

c. Rationale for selection of specific devices: _____
_____

d. Indicators for success with recommended devices: _____

7. PROGNOSIS

a. Communication ability: _____
_____

b. Independence within environment: _____

c. Placement in less restrictive environment: _____

d. Academic ability: _____

e. Vocational training/retraining: _____

Physician _____ Speech-Language Pathologist _____
(Signature/Date) (Signature/Date)

1988 Specialized Product/Equipment Council (SPEC)

Communication Prosthesis Payment Review Summary

8. ADDITIONAL COMMENTS

DEVELOPED BY
SPECIALIZED PRODUCT/EQUIPMENT
COUNCIL (SPEC) 1988

APPENDIX 5-1B

Funding Justification Letter for Seating and Mobility Systems

---

Date:

To whom it may concern:

Attached please find a detailed assessment, medical justification and equipment recommendation for

_____ (First Name) _____ (Last Name)

who was referred to us for _____

He/she presents as a _____ year old with a diagnosis of _____

He/she weighs _____ lbs., is _____ inches tall, and requires a wheelchair for

_____

_____

He/she presently uses _____ , which is _____ years old.

Observation of seated posture in this equipment shows:

_____

_____

The problems(s) with this equipment is (are):

_____

_____

Our assessment revealed:

_____

_____

He/she requires a: Seat height of: _____ inches

Frame depth of: _____ inches

Frame width of: _____ inches

Our recommendation is that the following equipment be provided:

_____

_____

We expect the following outcomes

1. _____
2. _____
3. _____
4. _____

Other family members present:

Evaluator Name: _____

Evaluator Title: _____

Facility: _____

Physician Name: _____

Physician Title: _____

Facility: _____

RTS Name: _____

RTS Title: _____

Company: _____

If you have any additional questions, please feel free to call me at: _____

Source: www.rehabcentral.com

Justify Mobility/Seating

Mobility system and seating chosen and why:

	Mfg	**Model**	**Size**
Manual	_____	_____	_____
Power	_____	_____	_____

Environment where equipment will be used:

Home ○ Full time ○ Part time **School/Work** ○ Full time ○ Part time
Community ○ Full time ○ Part time **Institution** ○ Full time ○ Part time

Other: _____

Drive system for powered w/c: _____

Small turning radius needed for environmental access? ○ Yes ○ No
Narrow width needed for environmental access? ○ Yes ○ No

Mobility system: ☐ Folds side/side ☐ Breaks apart ☐ Back folds down onto seat only
☐ Doesn't fold at all ☐ Has quick-release axles

Available adjustment/growth:

Frame depth: ____ inches   Seating depth: ____ inches

Frame width: ____ inches   Seating width: ____ inches

Further growth achieved by:

☐ Purchase of frame parts ☐ Adjustment ☐ Replacement of seating

---

Mobility Base

Lighter weight required: ☐ To allow self-propulsion ☐ To allow lifting ☐ Family preference
Other: _____

Heavy duty required for: ☐ User weight greater than 250 lbs. ☐ Extreme tone problems
☐ Overactive user ☐ Broken frame and/or components on previous chairs
☐ Multiple power seat functions
Other: _____

Portability required for: ☐ Increased community access
Other: _____

Seat height specified for:

☐ Foot propulsion ☐ Transfers ☐ Accomodation of leg length ☐ Table/desk access
Other: _____

Variable wheel placement required for:

☐ Improved hand access to wheels ☐ Improved stability
☐ Changing angle in space for assistance with postural stability
☐ 1-arm drive access ☐ Stability (amputee placement)
Other: _____

Angle adjustable back: _____ **degrees**

Required for: ☐ Postural control ☐ Control of spasticity ☐ Accommodation of limited ROM
Other: _____

Reclining back: _____ **degrees** ○ **Manual** ○ **Power**

Required for: ☐ Pressure relief ☐ Transfers ☐ Clothing or diaper changes, catheterization
☐ Head positioning ☐ Repositioning ☐ Relief from gravity
☐ Rest periods ☐ Accommodation of limited ROM
Other: _____

Backward tilt: _____ **degrees** ◯ **Manual** ◯ **Power**

  Manufacturer: _____

    Required for: ☐ Facilitation of postural control   ☐ Repositioning   ☐ Pressure relief

                ☐ Head positioning   ☐ Management of spasticity   ☐ Transfers

                ☐ Relief from gravity   ☐ Rest periods   ☐ Control of lower extremity edema

                Other: _____

Foreward tilt: _____ **degrees** ◯ **Manual** ◯ **Power**

Required for facilitation of:

                ☐ Head control   ☐ Trunk extension   ☐ Upper extremity movement/contol   ☐ Transfers

                Other: _____

  Arm style: ☐ Fixed   ☐ Removable   ☐ Flip back   ☐ Fixed height

              ☐ Swing-away   ☐ Adj. height   ☐ Adj. angle   ☐ Desk length

              ☐ Full length   ☐ Special height   ☐ Custom length   ☐ Reinforced

              ☐ Flip back/locking   ☐ Reclining

    Required for: ☐ Change of height/angles for variable activities   ☐ Durability

                ☐ Improved wheel access   ☐ Push-ups/transfers

                ☐ Upper extremity support   ☐ Support for UE support surface

                Other: _____

Foot/leg support: ☐ Elevating (Power)   ☐ Elevating (Manual)   ☐ Articulating   ☐ Angle adj. foot

                    ☐ Swing-away   ☐ Fixed   ☐ Angle adj. knee   ☐ Lift off

                    ☐ Depth adj. foot   ☐ Swing under   ☐ Heavy duty   ☐ Recessed calf panel

                    ☐ Rotational hanger bracket(s)   ☐ Flip-up footplate

    Required for: ☐ Comfort   ☐ Reduce swelling   ☐ Accommodation of ROM

                ☐ Durability   ☐ Transfers   ☐ Suppport

                ☐ Proper foot placement   ☐ Proper knee flexion angle   ☐ Proper leg placement

                Other: _____

  Wheels: _____

Axle adjustment: ◯ None   ◯ Semi adj.   ◯ Fully adj.

  Handrims: _____

  Casters/forks: _____

    Required for: ☐ Durability   ☐ Access for propulsion

                ☐ For ease of maintenance (no flats)   ☐ Use over rough terrain

                ☐ Angle adjustment for postural control   ☐ Grasp

                ☐ Seat height adjustment   ☐ Decreased pair from road shocks

                ☐ Decreased spasms from road shocks

                Other: _____

  Push handles: _____

                ☐ Extended or angle adjustable

    Required for: ☐ Caregiver access   ☐ Caregiver assist

                Other: _____

Brake extensions: _____

    Required for: ☐ Access   Other: _____

  Antitippers: _____

    Required for: ☐ Safety   Other: _____

  Bag & pouch: _____

    Required to hold: ☐ Medicines   ☐ Clothing changes   ☐ Diapers

                   ☐ Orthotics   ☐ Special food   ☐ Catheters   ☐ Ostomy supplies

                   Other: _____

Required for: ☐ Safety   ☐ Long distance driving
              ☐ Operation of power seat functions
              ☐ Compliance with transportation
              Other: _____

Swingaway/retractable joystick: _____
Required for: ☐ Allow table access   ☐ Allow special placement
              Other: _____

Base chosen accommodates: _____
              ☐ Required seating   ☐ Needed joystick style/size
              ☐ Switches needed for driving or seat function
              ☐ Computer access   ☐ ECU capability   ☐ Communication device
              ☐ Add-on power tilt   ☐ Add-on power recline
              ☐ Add-on power elevating leg rests   ☐ Add-on power seat elevator
              Other: _____

Overall comments on mobility equipment:

_____
_____

Seating and Accessories

Seat cushion: _____

Seat support: _____
Required for: ☐ Comfort   ☐ Pressure relief
              ☐ Ease of use   ☐ Low maintenance
              ☐ Increased stability ☐ Accommodation of ROM/asymmetries
              ☐ Control of posture/alignment
              Other: _____

Back cushion: _____

Back support: _____
Required for: ☐ Accommodation of ROM/asymmetries
              ☐ Comfort   ☐ Pressure relief   ☐ Support
              ☐ Improved swallowing/respiration   ☐ Control of posture/alignment
              ☐ Ease of use   ☐ Low maintenance   ☐ Increased stability
              Other: _____

Interfacing seat: _____

Interfacing back: _____
Required for: ☐ Growth and/or angle adjustments
              ☐ Wheelchair folding   ☐ Disassembly for cleaning
              Other: _____

Head rest: _____
Required for: ☐ Optimal positioning
              ☐ Support during tilt/recline   ☐ Improving vision
              ☐ Safety   ☐ Placement of switches
              ☐ Accommodation of ROM   ☐ Control of posture/alignment
              ☐ Improved feeding/swallowing/respiration
              Other: _____

Anterior chest support: _____
Required for: ☐ Safety   ☐ Support   ☐ Stability   ☐ Alignment
              ☐ Accomodation of TLSO   ☐ Added abdominal support
              ☐ Assistance with head position/alignment
              ☐ Assistance with shoulder control/alignment
              Other: _____

Lateral trunk supports: _____

Required for:
- ☐ Swing-away for transfers
- ☐ Accommodation of asymmetries/decreased ROM
- ☐ Support   ☐ Alignment
- ☐ Improved head and UE function
- ☐ Contoured for more support
- ☐ Safety
- ☐ Control spasticity

Other: _____

Lateral hip support: _____

Required for:
- ☐ Removable for transfers
- ☐ Support   ☐ Control of spasticity   ☐ Alignment   ☐ Safety
- ☐ Accommodation of asymmetry/ROM
- ☐ Contoured for more support

Other: _____

Lateral knee support: _____

Required for:
- ☐ Removable for transfers
- ☐ Accommodation of asymmetry/ROM
- ☐ Control   ☐ Alignment

Other: _____

Medial and/or anterior knee support: _____

Required for:
- ☐ Removable/flip down for independence
- ☐ Accommodation of asymmetry/ROM
- ☐ Alignment   ☐ Control of position
- ☐ Control of spasticity

Other: _____

Foot positioners: _____

Required for:
- ☐ Accommodation of asymmetry/ROM
- ☐ Alignment   ☐ Safety   ☐ Stability
- ☐ Control of position   ☐ Control of spasticity

Other: _____

Pelvic belt/bar: _____

Required for:
- ☐ Pad for comfort/protection over bony prominences
- ☐ Safety   ☐ Alignment   ☐ Independent use
- ☐ Maintainence of pelvic position
- ☐ Special pull angle to control rotation

Other: _____

UE support surface: _____

Required for:
- ☐ Support   ☐ Work surface   ☐ Control of upper extremity position
- ☐ Improves shoulder/head position
- ☐ Placement of communication aids
- ☐ Protection of flailing upper extremities

Other: _____

Overall comments on seating equipment: _____

_____

_____

_____

_____

_____

_____

_____

_____

PART 3

The Activities: General Purpose Assistive Technologies

CHAPTER 6

Seating Systems as Extrinsic Enablers for Assistive Technologies

For a user of assistive technologies, a prerequisite to any interaction or activity is a physical position that is comfortable and that promotes function. The primary purpose of seating devices is to maximize a person's ability to function in activities across all performance areas (self-care, work or school, play or leisure); for this reason, they are considered to be general-purpose extrinsic enablers.

The first part of this chapter describes the needs served by seating systems, evaluation of individuals for seating, and biomechanical principles related to seating. The remainder of the chapter provides in-depth information on each of the three categories of seating needs, including related principles and the technologies used for intervention. Seating components are typically interfaced with some type of mobility base. For purposes of this text, however, these two systems are separated. Mobility is viewed as a specific-purpose extrinsic enabler (see Chapter 12).

OVERVIEW OF NEEDS SERVED BY SEATING

Three distinct areas of seating intervention have emerged, each serving a particular consumer need. These three categories of seating intervention are (1) seating for postural control, (2) seating for tissue integrity, and (3) seating for comfort (Geyer et al, 2003).

The needs of children and adults with cerebral palsy and other neuromuscular disorders have led to the development of seating interventions for postural control and deformity management. These individuals typically have abnormal muscle tone, muscle weakness, primitive reflexes, or uncoordinated movements that impair their ability to maintain an upright posture in a wheelchair. Their impaired motor control affects their ability to participate in activities of daily living, can compromise their general health status, and can result in skeletal deformities.

The principles that guide seating design and selection for individuals with cerebral palsy are also relevant to individuals with other neurological disorders resulting in impaired motor control, such as cerebral vascular accident and traumatic brain injury. One commonality across all these groups is the dynamic nature of their seating needs over time. Individuals whose motor control impairment results from trauma usually realize improvements in motor function with recovery. In other situations, individuals lose motor control as a disease progresses. Children grow and develop motor skills. The seating system that is designed for individuals in

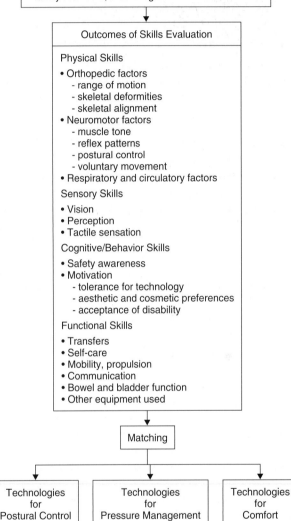

BOX 6-1   **Potential Outcomes of Proper Seating and Positioning**

Facilitation of optimal postural control to enable engagement in functional activities
Provision of an optimal balance between stability and mobility in the seated position
Maintenance of neutral skeletal alignment
Prevention of skeletal deformities
Maintenance of tissue integrity
Maintenance of a position of comfort
Decreased fatigue
Enhance respiratory and circulatory function
Facilitate caregiver activities

these groups must be flexible so that it can accommodate their changing needs. The primary population served by the category of seating interventions for pressure management is individuals with spinal cord injury. These individuals can have partial or complete paralysis and reduced or absent sensation below the level of their lesions. As a result, they are susceptible to breakdown of the tissue over bony prominences on weight-bearing surfaces. Individuals with multiple sclerosis, those with muscular dystrophy, the elderly, and others who have limited mobility and therefore a reduced ability to relieve pressure from weight-bearing surfaces also benefit from technologies in this category. Postural management to achieve even pressure distribution is a further need of this group.

The third category of seating addresses the need to improve an individual's level of physical comfort through postural accommodation. Persons in this category may or may not use a wheelchair on a regular basis and typically have normal or near-normal sensation; however, any prolonged sitting causes discomfort from which they are unable to obtain relief. Therefore they have unique needs and are not completely served by either category described above. Specialized seating can help to alleviate this chronic discomfort and maximize function. Box 6-1 shows some of the potential outcomes of seating intervention for these populations.

■ EVALUATION FOR SEATING

The process of assessing individuals for the purpose of recommending seating technologies requires a systematic method that includes consideration of many factors. The discussion of design of an assistive technology system in Chapter 2 gave a general framework to guide assessment. The purpose of this section is to provide a framework for evaluating consumers specifically for seating. Figure 6-1 outlines a framework to guide the assistive technology practitioner (ATP) through the decision-making process and ultimate selection of seating and positioning technologies that match the needs and skills of the user.

Figure 6-1   Framework for seating and positioning decision making.

As with other areas of assistive technology, the process of delivering seating services is a transdisciplinary effort involving the skills of several professionals. Occupational and physical therapists typically provide expertise in neuromotor function, human development, and knowledge of disabilities. A physician documents the medical status and prognosis of the consumer and the medical justification for the seating system. The physician can also indicate whether surgery or other medical procedures are planned and what effects these procedures may have on the consumer's seating. Assistive technology suppliers often provide knowledge of available technologies and their application to meet specific goals. Sometimes a rehabilitation engineer provides this service. In cases where the consumer's need cannot be met by commercial products, the rehabilitation engineer or seating technician can design and build a custom system.

Needs Identification

Figure 6-1 lists the desired outcomes of the identification of needs. It is important to determine exactly what an individual's specific needs are regarding seating. From the identified needs, goals to be addressed by the seating intervention are developed. It is the ATP's responsibility to facilitate the identification and prioritization of these goals. Design of a seating system sometimes involves compromising the various goals. For example, desired biomechanical alignment may not be possible for a person with severe postural deformities when the resulting properly aligned position is too uncomfortable. Any assessment with the goal of identifying seating needs and recommended technology starts with discussion of the occupations the user wants and needs to complete while using the seating system. A general measure such as the Canadian Occupational Performance Measure (Law et al, 1997) provides a systematic means of discussing key occupations in the area of self-care, productivity, and leisure. There are some measures that are specific to seating and wheeled mobility, including the Functioning Everyday in a Wheelchair measure (Mills et al, 2002). The Wheelchair Outcome Measure (Miller, Mortenson, and Garden, 2006) is a new measure that considers function in self-care, productivity, and leisure specifically from the view of an individual who uses seating and mobility devices.

The level of assistance an individual requires to use the seating system is an important consideration in the assessment. Consideration must be given to whether an individual can transfer to the system and fasten any straps independently when he or she expects to use the seating system independently. The complexity of the system and the ease of access influence the demands placed on an individual providing assistance with a transfer.

Functional skills, including transfers to and from different surfaces (e.g., bed to wheelchair, car to wheelchair), self-care skills (e.g., feeding, dressing), wheelchair mobility, written and verbal communication skills, and bowel and bladder care should be evaluated. Equipment the person will use while in the seating system needs to be taken into consideration. For example, respiratory equipment and augmentative communication devices are frequently mounted on the wheelchair and need to be in a position that is functional for the user.

It is important that the individual's ability to perform functional activities be evaluated both in the existing system and in a simulation of the proposed system. By observing the consumer performing functional activities from his or her existing system, the ATP learns two things. First, the ATP can determine the consumer's level of independence and areas where function is impeded. The ATP can also learn what strategies the individual currently uses to complete functional activities. By using the methods described below, the ATP can then simulate different positions with the consumer. The ATP can have the individual perform functional tasks while in these simulated positions. Changing the sitting position will affect the person's ability to perform certain activities. It is important to select a system that maximizes the person's function and does not interfere with the use of strategies that have proven to be beneficial. For example, a teenager who uses an abnormal asymmetrical tonic neck reflex to operate a single switch should not be prohibited from doing so unless another movement can be found that accomplishes this task. It will sometimes be necessary to trade an ideal seated posture for a posture that allows the individual to be more functional.

Human Factors

Physical Skills or Mat Assessment. The physical evaluation includes assessment of orthopedic factors, postural control, and respiratory and circulatory factors (see Figure 6-1). It is recommended that evaluation of physical skills take place with the person both in a sitting position and supine on a flat surface such as a mat.

Orthopedic Factors. Orthopedic evaluation involves measurement of joint range of motion and assessment of skeletal deformities and skeletal alignment to determine optimal angles for sitting. Obtaining information regarding limitations in range of motion and deformities is necessary to determine whether the goal of the seating system will be to prevent deformities, correct deformities, or accommodate deformities (Trefler, Hobson, and Taylor, 1993).

Starting with the consumer supine on the mat, mobility of the lumbar spine and pelvis are assessed, followed by *range of motion measurements* of the hips, knees, ankles, upper extremities, and neck. Joint angle and body measurements as shown in Figure 6-2 should also be made at this time. Alignment of the individual's head, shoulders, and trunk with the pelvis is determined next. Range of motion and skeletal alignment should also be assessed with the individual in a sitting position to determine how the body parts are affected by gravity. Bergen, Presperin, and Tallman (1990) describe in detail a process for measuring joint angles and assessing skeletal alignment.

It is important to determine whether any skeletal deformities present are fixed or flexible. In a **fixed deformity,** permanent changes have taken place in the bones, muscles, capsular ligaments, or tendons that restrict the normal range of motion of the particular joint. Fixed deformities affect the skeletal alignment of the other joints and typically require a

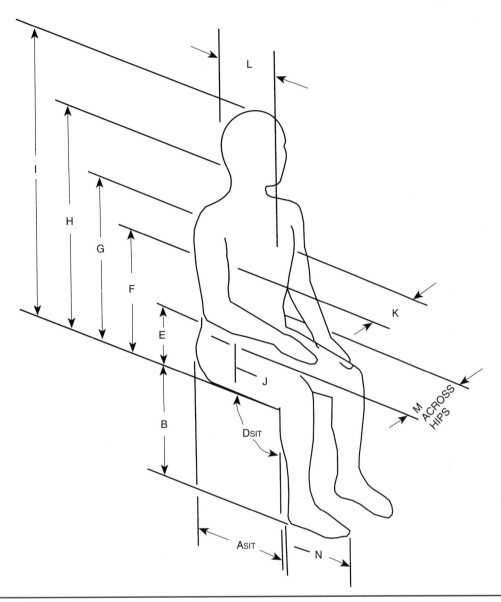

Figure 6-2   Joint angle and body measurements taken during the evaluation. A_{Sit} (R and L), behind hips/popliteal fossa; B (R and L), popliteal fossa/heel; D_{SIT}, knee flexion angle; E, sitting surface/pelvic crest; F, sitting surface/axilla; G, sitting surface/shoulder; H, sitting surface/occiput; I, sitting surface/crown of head; J, sitting surface/hanging elbow; K, width across trunk; L, depth of trunk; M, width across hips; N, heel/toe. (From Bergen AF, Presperin J, Tallman T: *Positioning for function: Wheelchairs and other assistive technologies*, Valhalla, NY, 1990, Valhalla Rehabilitation Publications.)

seating system that is designed to accommodate the deformity. Often, increased tone and muscle tightness cause persons to assume certain postures, and they may appear to have a deformity. With externally applied resistance (passive stretch) in the opposite direction, however, it is possible to move the joint and reduce the deformity. The person is then considered to have a **flexible deformity** at that joint. Depending on the situation, the seating system may be designed to correct a flexible deformity. Specific deformities and their effects on sitting posture are described in the section on seating principles for postural control.

Some individuals have had surgery to correct one or more deformities. The ATP should be aware of any surgery the consumer may have undergone and be knowledgeable about the implications it has for seating intervention. In other cases, the team may decide during the evaluation that surgical or orthotic intervention should be considered before seating intervention takes place. If this is the situation, referral to the appropriate medical professional is necessary. Letts (1991) examines surgical interventions related to the seated position. *Postural Control.*   The user's *postural control* is a key element to assess, particularly for children developing motor control, individuals recovering motor function after a neurological injury such as traumatic brain injury, or someone losing motor control as a consequence of a progressive illness. Two important aspects should be considered: the individual's ability to control the posture in a sitting position (i.e., how much support is required to maintain a comfortable sitting position with a reasonable amount of effort) and the response to various positional changes. The most effective way to assess these aspects is with the client seated on a mat.

The ability of an individual to control his or her posture during sitting is determined with the client seated on a mat with the feet supported. The client's sitting ability is described by the amount of support required to maintain a seated position. Hands-free sitters are those who do not need to use their hands to support themselves to maintain sitting, whereas hands-dependent sitters do need to use their hands. These individuals could not perform a seated activity using the hands without some type of external support. A dependent sitter does not have sufficient motor control to support himself or herself in sitting at all. Postural control tends to be less than in those in the other two categories.

Postural control typically develops in a cephalocaudal direction, although recovery of postural control after traumatic brain injury does not necessarily proceed in this fashion. The amount of external control required to assist an individual to maintain a seated position is an important determination. Kangas (2000) recommends provision of the minimal amount of external support. Support may vary with the activity. Less support may be needed when the individual is engaged in a sedentary activity such as watching television. Alternatively, more support is needed when the individual is using his hands for an activity and the focus of attention is on the activity. The individual should not need to divert attention to the maintenance of posture when engaged in an activity.

Finally, the ATP needs to determine the individual's response to various postural changes. Primarily, the ATP should assess the effect of changes of pelvic position on the client's postural control. What happens when the pelvis is positioned in a neutral, anterior-tipped or posterior-tipped position? Similarly, what effect does change of spinal alignment or lower limb position have on postural control? The client's response to these position changes will influence the configuration of the seating system and whether any dynamic elements need to be provided.

Respiratory and Circulatory Factors.   The person's *respiratory* status and *circulation* are other factors addressed during the evaluation. With skeletal deformities, pulmonary and cardiac function can be compromised. It is important to know whether certain positions enhance or limit respiration. Circulation, particularly in the lower limbs, needs to be considered as well. Some individuals may have a condition that predisposes them to circulatory problems; particularly for these consumers, positions that impair circulation should be avoided.

CASE STUDY

JILLIAN

Jillian is a happy 5-year-old girl with cerebral palsy resulting in severe motor impairment. Jillian is nonverbal and uses a smile or an eye blink to indicate yes. She is very alert and aware of her environment. She will be attending kindergarten in the fall. She does not have a wheelchair and has never been evaluated for a seating system. Her parents carry her from place to place or use an umbrella stroller for her as needed. She receives therapy with a neurodevelopmental treatment approach three times a week. When they made the initial phone referral, Jillian's parents stated to you that they have put off getting a seating system for Jillian because they did not want her to "look handicapped." With Jillian soon to be attending school, they have decided it is time to get her a wheelchair and seating system.

Jillian has mixed tone. Her lower extremities, particularly her ankles, have increased tone. The tone in her upper extremities is increased as well. Her trunk and neck are hypotonic. She exhibits a startle reflex and the symmetrical tonic neck reflex. She does not have any apparent orthopedic deformities. She is unable to keep her head up for any length of time unless she is reclined back slightly. Jillian can use a switch with her right hand when her head is held upright. She can also use the touch screen on the computer, but she needs help with sitting. Jillian is dependent for mobility and all other functional activities.

QUESTIONS

1. From the information you have so far, what might be the goals of seating for Jillian?
2. Write a list of interview questions you would ask of her parents and therapists.
3. How would you proceed with a seating evaluation for Jillian?
4. On the basis of the information you have about Jillian at this time, what technological approaches would you consider for her and why? What type of positioning accessories would you consider and why?
5. List potential funding sources for Jillian's seating system. How would you justify her system to the funding source (refer to Chapter 5)?

Sensory and Perceptual Skills

Vision and visual perception, as discussed in Chapter 3, contribute to a person's balance and sitting posture, and deficits in these areas need to be considered during the evaluation. The configuration of the seat can affect the user's line of vision. For example, an individual with poor postural control who is unable to maintain spinal extension with consequent neck flexion may not be able to maintain the head in an upright position if the seat to back angle is set at 90 degrees. The user's line of vision will be downward in this seating configuration. A person's awareness of body position *(proprioception)* in space also influences body posture.

Tactile sensation is another factor to consider. Some individuals may react defensively to the touch of certain textures or positioning components on the body. Other individuals lack tactile sensation, which can contribute to skin breakdown. The ATP should determine whether there is any known decrease in sensation, particularly in the buttock area, and whether there is a history of pressure ulcers. The condition of the person's skin on weight-bearing surfaces (including areas on the trunk that are braced by lateral supports) should be checked for evidence of skin breakdown, circulation, color, smoothness, sensation, and moisture (Tredwell and Roxborough, 1991).

Cognitive Skills

Cognitive skills such as problem solving and motor planning are not as much of an issue in seating as in mobility. However, there are a few areas that require consideration. Individuals with poor safety judgment may not be aware of the need to keep a positioning belt fastened, and special considerations may be necessary. When the seating system is complex, understanding the client's cognitive abilities will aid the decision to teach the client or the caregiver about the proper use of the system. Knowing the individual's language and communication skills (see Chapter 11) will help determine how the ATP gathers information during the evaluation. For example, if a person relies on an augmentative communication device or on yes/no responses, these modes of communication should be used during the evaluation process. If it is known that the consumer is not reliable in his or her responses, then the ATP should seek assistance from a caregiver in interpreting the consumer's responses to the seating system.

Psychosocial Factors

The meaning that technology holds for the individual is an important factor to explore with the user, although it is more significant for the mobility component of a seating and mobility system. Many clients prefer technology that does not draw attention to a disability. This preference will be a factor in the selection of a seating system. Esthetics is an important factor in acceptance and rejection of the technology (Pape, Kim, and Weiner, 2002). Behavioral problems, such as an agitated person who throws himself against the back of the chair, can also present a safety problem that needs to be addressed. Working together with the consumer and the caregiver to address these concerns is essential.

Environmental Considerations

Physical Context.   The seating assessment should determine in which environments the seating system will be used (e.g., home, school, workplace, and vehicle and whether it is necessary for the system to be used in different environments). Knowledge of where the seating system will be used helps the ATP determine whether the system will be removed and reinstalled in the mobility device or other devices. For instance, an individual who transfers to the car seat when traveling from home to school will remove the seating system when the mobility device is stored in the vehicle and replace it on arrival at the destination. Many seating devices designed for young children are intended to pair with different bases (e.g., the system may be used in a stroller, high chair, or floor sitter).

The ATP should determine the extent to which the seating system will be used outdoors. Temperature is an important factor to consider when designing a seating system. Extreme heat or cold will affect the function of many materials, limiting their ability to meet the goals set for use of the system. A more complete discussion of the effect of temperature on materials used in seating systems follows. Exposure to light sources may affect some materials used to cover a system component, altering its properties and again, affecting the function of the system.

Social Context.   The ATP must know who is available to assist the consumer with the use of the system when it is used in multiple settings. This knowledge influences the instruction given to the users of the system and influences considerations with respect to the weight, complexity, and maintenance of the system. Many ATPs who recommend seating products have seen situations where a simple seat cushion is placed backward in a mobility device, causing great discomfort to the user. The risk of misuse is much greater with complex seating systems. Consequently, the ATP must ensure that the user and any caregivers are familiar with proper use of the seating system. Adequate instruction is key to preventing misuse of the system.

Individuals who routinely lift and carry a seating system must be able to do so without risk of injury. Materials used to construct seating systems have changed in recent years, in part to decrease the weight. However, some custom-made systems, such as foam in place, which will be discussed below, can be quite heavy. Maintenance of the system is another consideration. Air-filled cushions require careful attention to ensure that they are properly inflated and free of punctures. As mentioned above, the properties of some materials are affected by extremes of temperatures, so whoever is responsible for maintenance of the system must take care to avoid damage to it in this manner. In some situations, the system that is most ideal for the client cannot be recommended because of the ability of the caregiver to use and care for it.

Institutional Context.   Funding implications are a key institutional consideration. General considerations with respect to funding were described in Chapter 5. The ATP needs to remain current on funding requirements when recommending seating products. Another type of legislation has unique implications for seating products: the use of restraints. Certain legal jurisdictions have legislation that regulates the use of restraints with individuals residing in institutional settings. The intent of this legislation is to limit inappropriate use of restraints, such as tying an individual into a chair simply to prevent him or her from moving around, when safety is not an issue. This legislation has implications for the use of straps, pelvic belts, and sub–anterior-superior iliac spine (ASIS) bars that are used in seating systems for positioning and safety reasons. The ATP should be aware of whether these types of legislation affect the ability to incorporate positioning belts, and so forth, in a seating system.

Matching Device Characteristics to a Consumer's Needs and Skills

The information that has been gathered regarding needs and skills provides a profile of the user. It can then be determined which of the three categories in Figure 6-1 matches the consumer's profile, which allows identification of potential technologies and evaluation of their effectiveness in meeting the consumer's needs.

The next step is to actually simulate with the consumer one or more of the alternatives. The ATP can observe the effects of changes in body position and materials by having the consumer try variations of the positioning system. Trial positioning is also helpful for assessing the person's ability to use control interfaces such as the joystick of a power wheelchair. Changes in position can be made to see whether there are beneficial or adverse effects on the person's ability to control a device or perform other functional skills. Simulation makes it easier to document the need for and effectiveness of a particular system so that funding can be obtained. If specific cushions or positioning components are being considered for a consumer, it helps to have him or her try the actual product and determine whether he or she likes it. In some instances it may be desirable for the consumer to take the system home for a trial period, which allows the person to use the system over a longer period and in his or her natural environment.

There are several critical questions that can help the ATP evaluate the effectiveness of the technologies that have been simulated and to select an appropriate seating system for the consumer. These questions, which summarize the needs evaluation, the skill assessment, and the simulation, are shown in Box 6-2. The primary concern is whether the simulated seating system meets the goals identified during the needs assessment. The ATP should consider the extent to which the system achieves desired goals with respect to positioning, support of function, and comfort. The caregiver's ability to lift, carry, and maintain the seating system is a further factor to consider. A system that does not meet these goals to the satisfaction of the client of the caregiver will not be used.

BOX 6-2 Critical Questions for Evaluating Seating Technologies

Does the seating system as simulated meet the consumer's goals and needs (e.g., postural control, deformity management, pressure relief)?

Does the seating system provide stability and allow for maximal performance in functional activities (e.g., transfers, weight shifts, activities of daily living)?

Is the seating system comfortable for the consumer?

Is the seating system durable enough to meet the consumer's needs for a reasonable period?

Is the seating system sufficiently flexible to meet the consumer's changing needs (e.g., change in functional abilities, growth changes)?

Are there resources available to ensure appropriate maintenance of the seating system?

Can the consumer or third-party payer finance the cost of the seating system?

■ BIOMECHANICAL PRINCIPLES

To design and implement seating systems effectively for consumers with disabilities, it is important to understand how the laws of physics govern the actions and effects of the mechanical elements of the postural control system. These principles are embodied in *biomechanics,* the study of body position and movement. This section presents the major concepts of biomechanics, which are fundamental to an understanding of seating and positioning systems for persons with disabilities.

Kinematics: Study of Motion

When seating systems are designed, the position of the consumer, the position of the seating system components, and their movements should be considered. The term *kinematics* describes movement. The term *displacement* is used to define the position of a body in space; a change in displacement results in a new position. For example, in a postural support system, one goal is to bring the trunk to a midline position. This action may require a *displacement* from the rest position to midline by application of an external lateral trunk support. The rate of change in displacement is called *velocity.* It is also important to know how fast the velocity is changing (increasing or decreasing); this change is called *acceleration.* One of the most common accelerations is that of gravity. The term *gravity* actually refers to the acceleration of an object toward the center of the earth. Acceleration of an object is directly related to the force generated by the object's movement.

There are two fundamental types of displacement: linear and rotational. When all parts of a body move in the same direction, at the same time, and for the same distance, the movement is **linear** (Low and Reed, 1996). For example, a person generates translational movement when walking.

Displacements caused by external positioning components can also be translational. If the direction, distance, and time of the movement occur simultaneously, but the movement is through an angle instead of in a straight line, the movement is called **rotational.** Rotational movements occur around an axis called the **fulcrum.** The majority of body movements are rotational, such as hip or elbow flexion and shoulder flexion or extension. Some positioning components cause rotational displacements (e.g., reclining the back of a wheelchair causes rotation at the pelvis and hip).

Kinetics: Forces

Force is a major element in biomechanics and seating for individuals with disabilities. **Force** is anything that acts on a body to *change* its rate of acceleration or alter its momentum (Low and Reed, 1996). It is described by both magnitude and direction (Sprigle, 2000). Forces always occur in equal and opposite action-reaction pairs between bodies, although it is often convenient to think of one body being in a force field. Forces can be applied to the body internally or externally. Internal forces are generated inside the body, such as muscle contractions that cause movement of the joints. Externally applied forces come from outside the body and act on it in some way, such as the forces applied by a support surface and components of a seating system such as lateral supports. The force resulting from the acceleration of gravity is another external and ever-present force that acts on the body and influences its posture and movement (Sprigle, 2000). This force on the body acts along a line called the **gravitational line,** and its effect is localized around a point in the body called the **center of gravity.** The force of the earth's gravitational field tends to pull the body toward the center of the earth and must be accounted for in designing a seating system. The center of gravity changes as posture changes from standing to sitting and in different sitting positions.

Four properties of force, which ultimately determine its result, are magnitude, direction, line of application, and point of application. *Magnitude* is the amount or size of the force measured in newtons, pounds, or kilograms. Forces are applied in some *direction,* either pushing or pulling, and are applied along a particular **line of application.** The force acts at a particular point on the body, called the *point of application* (Low and Reed, 1996).

Types of Forces.

There are three different types of force. Each of these types produces different effects on the body, and it is important to understand these differences when designing seating and positioning systems. **Tension** forces act in the same line but away from each other (pulling apart), such as the force applied on the antagonist muscle during contraction of the agonist muscle. **Compression** occurs when forces act toward each other (pushing together), such as the force of the vertebrae on the disks in the spinal column. **Shearing** occurs when the forces are parallel to each other (sliding across the surfaces), such as the movement that occurs as the head of the femur moves across the acetabulum during hip movement. Each of these types of forces can also be applied externally to the body, such as the force exerted by a seating surface on the ischial tuberosities (compression), the force exerted by lateral supports to extend the trunk (tension), or the force exerted on the tissues in the buttocks when a seat back is reclined (shearing).

Stress.

Stress is the resulting molecular change inside biological (e.g., soft tissue and bone) or nonbiological (e.g., metals, plastics, or foams) materials. Stress is caused by the same three types of forces—tension, compression, or shear—and can result in damage to the biological tissue or other material if it is prolonged. For example, a shear force applied to a foam seat cushion can result in tearing of the foam. This is a change in the molecular structure of the foam caused by an externally applied force. Likewise, a piece of connective tissue that is subjected to severe or prolonged compression loading by sitting (e.g., under the ischial tuberosities) may be damaged by crushing of the tissue. This externally applied force results in compression inside the tissue, causing a change in the structure of the biological material.

Pressure.

Every force is applied over a surface area. For example, with a postural support system, the force of each component is applied to an area of the body. It is important to determine the effect of each of these forces, and the concept of pressure is important. **Pressure** is defined as force per unit area, which means that a force applied over a very small area generates more pressure than the same force applied over a larger area. Imagine a 10-pound cat lying on a surface such as your stomach. The force generated by the cat is applied over the entire surface of its body and the pressure is uniform. Now imagine the same cat standing on your stomach. The force of the cat is the same, but the pressure at each of the cat's paws is much greater (and it hurts more) because the area of application (the paw) is much smaller than when the force is distributed over the whole surface area of the cat. This basic concept of distributing pressure by increasing the area of application is applied extensively in seating and positioning systems.

Newton's Laws of Motion.

The English scientist Sir Isaac Newton formulated three laws relating to forces on bodies at rest and in motion. *Newton's first law* states that a body at rest tends to remain at rest and that a body in motion in a straight line tends to remain in motion unless external forces act to change either of these states. In other words, a body likes to continue what it is doing, moving or resting. This law defines inertia, which is equal to the force required to accelerate an object. *Newton's second law* relates three parameters: the mass of a body, the change in velocity (acceleration), and the forces acting on that body. The force is equal to the mass (in kilograms) multiplied by the acceleration of the body (Force = Mass × Acceleration), which means that the greater the force, the greater the acceleration, or conversely, the greater the mass for the same force, the smaller the acceleration. The force of gravity is the mass of the object multiplied by the acceleration of gravity. This force is commonly referred to as the *weight* of an object, and it is the reason that an object weighs less on the moon, because the gravitational acceleration there is less than that on the earth.

Newton's third law is the one most applicable to seating and positioning systems. This law states that if one body exerts a force on another, there is an equal and opposite force, called a reaction, exerted on the first body by the second (Low and Reed, 1996). This law is applied to seating systems with the assumption that every force exerted by the human body while sitting in a wheelchair or a seating system is balanced by an opposite force exerted by the sitting surface on the person (Sprigle, 2000). The force generated by the body is equal in magnitude and opposite in direction to the force generated by the seating system, which is often referred to as **equilibrium.** When a body is at rest and all internal and external forces are balanced, the body is in a state of *static equilibrium.* When forces are balanced around a body during movement, resulting in a constant velocity, it is described as *dynamic equilibrium.* Both types of equilibrium are important in seating and positioning systems.

Friction. Throughout this discussion, it has been assumed that ideal circumstances exist. For example, a shear force applied to a body causes it to move across a surface, and ideally it encounters no resistance to movement from that surface. In reality, of course, this is not true because **frictional forces** exist between two bodies in contact moving in opposite directions (Sprigle, 2000). Two types of friction are defined: static friction and dynamic friction. *Static friction* is that force that must be overcome to start a body in motion. Static friction is proportional in magnitude to the perpendicular (compression) force holding the two bodies together. Static friction is independent of the area of contact between the two bodies. Once motion is initiated, the resistive force is generally smaller, and it takes less force to keep the bodies moving relative to each other than to start movement. Friction during movement is called *dynamic friction.* Both these frictional forces are affected by surface conditions such as moisture, heat, texture, and lubricants, and both are important considerations in the recommendation and design of seating surfaces.

Sitting Posture and Center of Pressure

Stability and mobility are two related dimensions of seated postural control. **Stability** allows an individual to maintain an upright seated position while mobility allows movement that enables function; for example, **mobility** allows the individual to lean forward to reach to shake a friend's hand. Seating interventions for postural control must achieve an optimal balance between stability and mobility.

Two constructs are important to consider when discussing postural control: center of gravity and center of pressure. The location of the center of gravity is fairly well defined in standing. Its location is described as passing through the mastoid processes of the jaw, a point just in front of the shoulder, a point just behind the center of the hip joints, a point just in front of the center of the knee joints, and approximately 5 to 6 cm in front of the ankle joints (Figure 6-3). In this posture the pelvis is in a neutral position and there is a natural lordosis of the lumbar spine (Zacharkow, 1988). The location in sitting is more difficult to determine, but it is usually considered to be lower, with the buttocks and thighs forming the base of support. The individual must maintain the center of gravity over the base of support to maintain an upright posture in either sitting or standing. Seating interventions for postural control assist the client to keep the center of posture within the limits of the base of support.

It is not practical to measure or monitor the center of gravity in the clinic. The center of gravity is defined by three-dimensional coordinates. The **center of pressure** is described only in the horizontal plane, which makes it a much more clinically useful outcome. Its location in the frontal and lateral planes can be identified and monitored in the clinic by using a pressure mapping system. These systems use various technologies to monitor the pressure between the individual and a support surface (i.e., between the client's buttocks and thighs and the seat cushion). They are most commonly used to show pressure distribution when pressure-relief cushions are evaluated, so their function will be described in greater detail in that section.

As mentioned above, the aim of postural control in seating intervention is to provide the client with a functional upright position (i.e., provide enough support to enable him or her to retain a seated position but also to enable sufficient movement to promote function in sitting). Monitoring of the center of pressure during quiet and active sitting is one way to evaluate the outcome of specific seating interventions. Discussion of the center of pressure is a relatively recent occurrence in the literature. The ideal location of the center of pressure is midway between the ischial tuberosities. Dunk and Callaghan (2005) found that the location of the center of pressure in the frontal plane varied between men and women. They studied various sitting postural parameters of university students engaged in computer activities while sitting on different office chairs. They found that the center of pressure was behind the center of mass of the chair for men and ahead of it for women. This finding has interesting implications for seating intervention, although it has not been explored.

Parkinson, Chaffin, and Reed (2006) describe the **stability zone** or limit, which they define as the balance limits for a

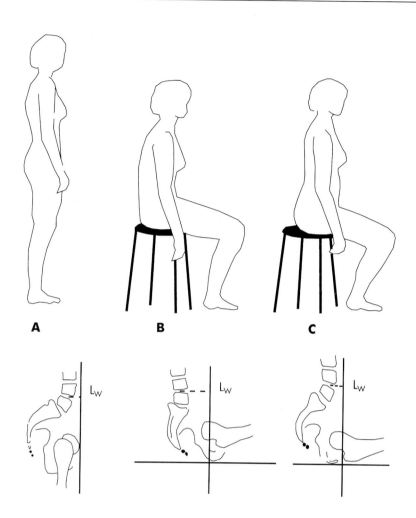

Figure 6-3 **A,** Line of gravity in erect upright standing. **B,** Relaxed unsupported sitting resulting in backward tilt of the pelvis and flattening of the lumbar lordosis. **C,** Erect sitting with reduction in backward pelvic tilt and increased lordosis. L_W, Lever arm. (From Frankel VH, Nordin M: *Basic biomechanics of the skeletal system,* Philadelphia, 1980, Lea & Febiger.)

person in either sitting or standing. A seat back and laterals or armrests will affect the stability limits in sitting. The authors initially hypothesized that the stability was limited laterally by the ischial tuberosities and posteriorly by the coccyx in the absence of these system features. The thighs provide support when the individual is reaching forward. Age, strength, and range of motion were identified as additional factors that affected the stability zone. They quantified the center of pressure during a lateral reaching task with a sample that included both young and older individuals and subjects with a body mass index range from underweight to obese. The greater trochanter, rather than the ischial tuberosities, was found to be more indicative of the stability zone because subjects shifted their weight laterally as they reached. Stability during reach was also affected by age, reach direction (lateral and forward reach were greater than rearward), and hip breadth (Parkinson, Chaffin, and Reed, 2006).

The center of pressure is an interesting phenomenon that has been explored recently, primarily in a nonclinical population. The studies described above suggest that differences exist in parameters related to center of pressure between men and women (Dunk and Callaghan, 2005), body mass,

and age (Parkinson et al, 2006). These studies did not include individuals with disabilities, so the implications of the findings to this group are not clear. Further study is needed to explore the relationship between center of pressure and function and the effect of various seating interventions on this relationship.

■ PRINCIPLES OF SEATING FOR POSTURAL CONTROL

Children and adults who have irregular tone, muscle weakness, abnormal reflex patterns, shortening of a muscle group, or skeletal deformity are likely to require external positioning devices to control their posture and prevent deformities. Within this category some individuals have mild impairment and require only minimal support, whereas other individuals have severe physical impairment and require extensive postural support. The components making up a seating system can provide support to the body to improve skeletal alignment, normalize tone, prevent deformities, and enhance movement.

Guidelines for Postural Control

The most important principle related to postural control is that proximal stabilization, near the center of the body, facilitates movement and control of the head and the extremities (e.g., function). During normal development, the infant achieves stability in the proximal joints before using the distal limbs for manipulation. For example, before a baby can successfully reach out and grab a toy while sitting, he must have mastered the ability to maintain a balanced sitting posture (Bertenthal and Von Hofsten, 1998; Hadders-Algra, Brogen, and Forssberg, 1998; Hadders-Algra et al, 1999; Savelsbergh and Van der Kamp, 1994). Otherwise the hands must be used to maintain balance, which limits their use for manipulation. Seating for postural control provides external positioning components for the individual who does not have internal mechanisms to control body posture. Tredwell and Roxborough (1991) present a classification scheme (Box 6-3) that is useful in describing the amount of control a person exhibits in sitting. Each category is matched with a brief description of the recommended degree of support provided by the seating system.

When any type of external support is provided, care needs to be taken so that the individual is not excessively positioned. We need to keep in mind that sitting is a *dynamic activity*. We often associate sitting with relaxation and lack of activity and movement, when in fact many activities are performed while sitting, such as writing, driving, talking on the phone, and typing. Even during quiet sitting an individual frequently shifts weight to maintain comfort. It is not uncommon to see individuals "properly" positioned to the point that they are no longer able to use the motor movements they have used in the past to complete functional tasks. The *fewest* restraints necessary to optimize function should be used (Kangas, 2000).

In this section we present a set of general guidelines for proceeding with the development of a postural seating system for an individual.

BOX 6-3   **Levels of Postural Control in Sitting**

THE HANDS-FREE SITTER

Can sit for prolonged periods without using the hands for support

Seating system is designed primarily for mobility, to provide a stable base of support, and to be comfortable

THE HANDS-DEPENDENT SITTER

One or both hands are used to maintain support while sitting

Seating system is designed to provide pelvic or trunk support to free the person's hands for functional activities

THE PROPPED SITTER

Lacks any ability to support self in sitting

Seating system provides total body support

Pelvis and Lower Extremities.

We have described the important role of the pelvis in relation to the center of gravity and sitting. The pelvis is a key point of control, and its position affects the posture of the rest of the body. Therefore, alignment and stabilization of the pelvis is normally the first area addressed in positioning an individual. A position with the pelvis in neutral or in a slight anterior tilt is desired (Mayall and Desharnais, 1995). The pelvis should be level and in midline.

Research examining the role of pelvic stability in the facilitation of function supports the assertion of starting with the pelvis when an appropriate seating system in being determined. Two studies investigated the effect of two methods of pelvic stabilization: a regular lap belt, typically using hook and pile fastening versus a rigid pelvic stabilizer (a sub-ASIS bar in one case and the Embrace Pelvic Positioner [Body Tech NW, Mukilteo, Wash.; *http://www.dresch.org/web/BodyTechNW.com/*] in the second) on function of children with cerebral palsy (Miller Polgar et al, 2000; Rigby et al, 2001). Both these studies compared daily function, as perceived by the participants and their families, when using the typical lap belt versus the rigid pelvic stabilizer. Results were comparable in both, with better function found with the rigid pelvic stabilizer. Significant differences were found on the Canadian Occupational Performance Measure (Law et al, 1997) before and after implementation of the rigid pelvic stabilizer. The results of these studies are limited by the small sample size, but the convergence of their findings provides evidence for the practice of controlling the pelvis in seating for postural control.

A position with the hips flexed at approximately 90 degrees is recommended for most individuals (Bergen, Presperin, and Tallman, 1992; Trefler, Hobson, and Taylor, 1993; Tredwell and Roxborough, 1991). This angle of hip flexion helps to inhibit extensor tone and reduces posterior tilt of the pelvis, thus keeping the individual positioned back in the seat. In some instances it is necessary to increase the amount of hip flexion (thus reducing the angle to less than 90 degrees) to further inhibit extensor tone. On the other hand, in some instances 90 degrees of hip flexion is not achievable (because of deformity) or is not the most appropriate position. Some individuals are not able to maintain an upright position when placed in a position of 90 degree hip flexion. Similarly, tight hamstrings may prevent achievement of 90 degrees at the knees. The ATP needs to determine the effect of deformities and muscle tone on both function and comfort in the sitting position, during a mat assessment, to determine the most appropriate position of the pelvis, hips, and lower extremities. Asymmetrical postures that may be present in the pelvis and hips include pelvic obliquity, pelvic rotation, pelvic tilt, and windswept hips. These postural asymmetries are often interrelated. They may be flexible postures or fixed bony deformities that restrict the mobility of the pelvis and limit the attainment of the recommended pelvic position.

An individual with a **pelvic obliquity** has one side of the pelvis higher than the other when viewed in the frontal plane (Figure 6-4, *A*). The obliquity is named for the side

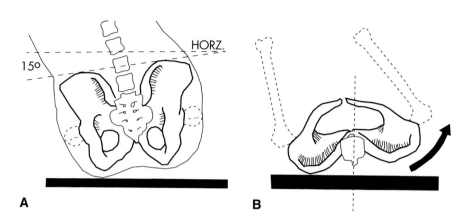

Figure 6-4 **A,** Pelvic obliquity viewed in the frontal plane. **B,** Pelvic rotation. (From Siekman A: The biomechanics of seating: a consumer's guide, *Action Dig* March/April:8-9, 1992.)

that is lower; for example, with a left pelvic obliquity the left side is lower than the right. This deformity is often accompanied by **pelvic rotation,** where one side of the pelvis is forward of the other side (Figure 6-4, *B*). **Windswept hip deformity** manifests itself with one hip adducted and the other hip abducted. This deformity has usually been found to be the end stage of a sequence that proceeds as follows: hip subluxation and dislocation, pelvic obliquity, scoliosis, windswept hip deformity. Typically, all these components are present in this deformity. The hip on the high side is typically dislocated, and the opposite hip may or may not be dislocated (Letts, 1991). When fixed deformities such as these are present, the seating system should be designed to accommodate them rather than to attempt to correct them (Mayall and Desharnais, 1995).

Support to the pelvis can be provided under, behind, in front, or from the sides. At the very least, a firm seating surface for the individual to sit on will level and stabilize the pelvis. Individuals with moderate to severe involvement typically need more support for stabilization. This support can be provided by contours around the buttocks and up

into the lumbar area. Alteration of the seat to back angle may be required when the individual has severe extensor tone. During the mat assessment, with the person in sitting, the therapist should move the client through different hip ranges to determine which hip angle achieves the most functional muscle tone. This optimal angle can then be replicated in the seating system, bearing in mind that the actual angle of the hip (femur to acetabulum) will be more acute than the seat to back angle of the seating system. A seat with a preischial block is another option used to control excessive extensor tone (Figure 6-5). With this approach, a depression is made in the cushion to accommodate the pelvis and to stop forward movement. Supports to prevent lateral shifting of the pelvis or external rotation of the hips can be provided either by contouring the seat to provide channels that position the thighs or with some form of lateral support at the pelvic level. To support the pelvis from the front, various types of pelvic positioning belts or knee blocks are used. The placement of the belt is important to effectively maintain pelvic position. Depending on the person's pelvic mobility, comfort, and positioning needs, the pelvic positioning belt is placed at an angle ranging from 45 to 90 degrees to the seating surface, as shown in Figure 6-6. In most cases, a belt with an angle of pull at 45 degrees sufficiently maintains the pelvis in position. If there is excessive hip extension or a need for anterior pelvic mobility, positioning the belt at a 90-degree angle of pull is more effective. Pelvic positioning belts can be soft and flexible (e.g., webbing or padded vinyl) or rigid when more support is required. A rigid pelvic positioning device, also called a sub-ASIS bar (Figure 6-7), is typically a close-fitting, padded metal bar that is attached to the wheelchair frame or seat insert to position the pelvis below the individual's ASIS. It is designed to be used in conjunction with a complete seat and back system for individuals who require greater control to maintain the neutral position of the pelvis and to prevent pelvic rotation. Similarly, handling of the client to determine the effect of pressure, or control, around the pelvis (e.g., at the ASIS or posterior-superior iliac spine) will help determine optimal placement of any pelvic stabilizing devices.

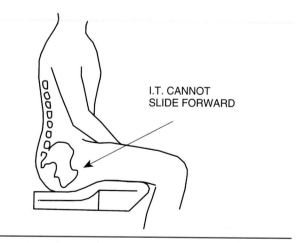

I.T. CANNOT SLIDE FORWARD

Figure 6-5   Antithrust seat. (From Bergen AF, Presperin J, Tallman T: *Positioning for function: wheelchairs and other assistive technologies,* Valhalla, NY, 1990, Valhalla Rehabilitation Publications.)

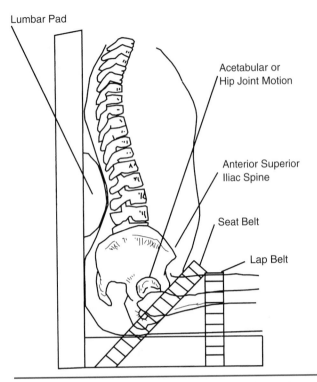

Figure 6-6   Pelvic positioning belts can be applied at 45 degrees (seat belt) or at 90 degrees (lap belt). (From Church G, Glennen S: *The handbook of assistive technology,* San Diego, 1992, Singular Publishing Group.)

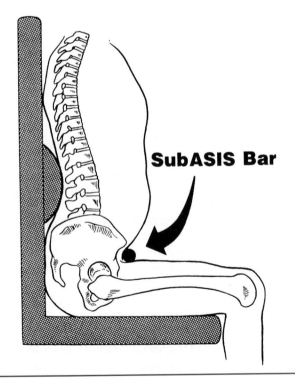

Figure 6-7   Sub-ASIS bar. (From Margolis SA, Jones RM, Brown BE: The subASIS bar: an effective approach to pelvis stabilization in seated positioning, *Proceedings of the RESNA Eighth Annual Conference,* pp 45-47, June 1985.)

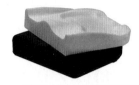

Figure 6-8   Example of sculpted foam cushion to maintain pelvic and femur alignment. (Courtesy Invacare Corp., www.invacare.ca.)

Adequately positioning the lower extremities helps to maintain the pelvic and hip positions. The positions of the legs and feet affect the position of the pelvis and therefore need to be addressed simultaneously. It is recommended that the legs be positioned so that the femurs are neutral with respect to abduction and adduction and rotation and with approximately 90 degrees of knee flexion, although there are some exceptions that will be noted below. Some form of sculpting is frequently used in the seat to keep the femurs in a neutral position and to limit adduction and internal rotation (Figure 6-8). A frequently encountered problem in the lower extremities is hamstring tightness, which may or may not result in flexion contractures of the knees. Recall that these muscles are closely related to the position of the pelvis. Attempts to position the individual to stretch these muscles and reduce the flexion contracture only result in posterior pelvic tilt and a sliding forward in the chair into a sacral sitting position. Instead, it is best to accommodate this problem by modifying the seating surface (shortening the seat depth or undercutting the front edge) so that the legs are allowed to flex under the seating surface. This maintains the correct pelvic position. If there is fixed knee extension, the lower leg must be completely supported with pads or troughs that match the range of motion in the knee.

Support for the feet is important for maintaining hip and knee position, for preventing deformities in the ankles, and for distributing pressure. If the feet are left to hang or are positioned too low, pressure increases under the anterior thigh area, which can cut off blood flow. Positioning the feet too high places excess pressure on the ischial tuberosities and the sacrum, which can cause formation of a pressure ulcer. It is recommended that the feet be positioned flat and with 90 degrees of ankle flexion (Mayall and Desharnais, 1995). Support surfaces for the feet can be one or two platforms and in different sizes, depending on the person's needs. Increasing the thickness of the foot support under the shorter leg serves to accommodate unequal lower leg length. Foot platforms can be angled to accommodate fixed plantar flexion contractures of the ankle. Various strapping systems can be used to maintain the desired ankle position, including straps over the top of the foot, behind the heel, and enclosing the ankle (Figure 6-9).

Trunk.   Once the desired position in the pelvis and lower extremities has been obtained, the trunk is considered. An upright position with the trunk aligned in midline is desirable.

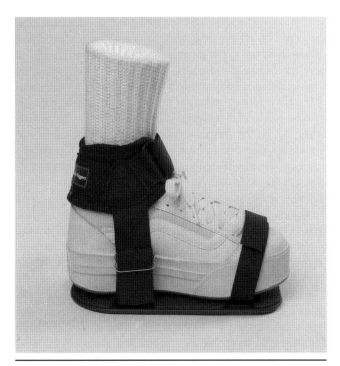

Figure 6-9   Example of an ankle positioning system that attaches to the footplate of a wheelchair. (Courtesy Bodypoint designs, Inc., www.bodypoint.com.)

This position may not be attainable if the individual has fixed deformities. Possible spinal deformities are (1) scoliosis, (2) lordosis, (3) kyphosis, or (4) a combination of these. **Scoliosis** of the spine occurs when there is lateral curvature or rotation of the vertebral column. Scoliotic curves are further defined according to the anatomical site in the vertebral column that is involved, that is, cervical, thoracic, or lumbar. Compensatory (or secondary) curves develop as a result of the head's attempting to maintain its upright position (Figure 6-10, *A*) (Cailliet, 1975). Figure 6-10, *B,* shows an uncompensated curve with the spine unbalanced and the head lateral to the center of gravity. Rotation of the vertebrae is also frequently found in scoliosis and can cause greater respiratory difficulty than lateral curving (Cailliet, 1975).

The amount of trunk support required depends on how much control over the trunk that the individual has. As in the pelvis, trunk support can be provided from behind, at the side, or in front. The amount of support provided from behind is related to back height and contouring. The height of the back can be varied, depending on the amount of upper body support needed. Someone who requires minimal support can use a lower backrest height, whereas a higher backrest is necessary for the individual with a need for greater support. Contouring allows us to accommodate the individual's body shape and provide optimal support. If the person has a kyphosis, the back needs to be recessed so that he or

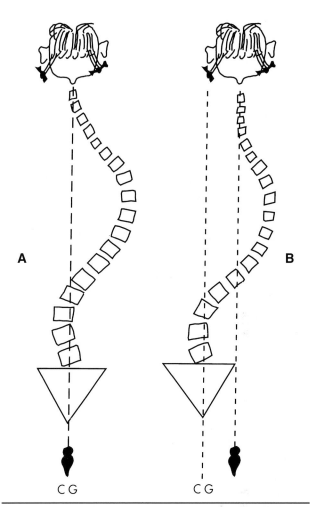

Figure 6-10   **A,** Development of compensatory curve in scoliosis. **B,** Uncompensated scoliotic curve. CG, Center of gravity. (From Cailliet R: *Scoliosis: diagnosis and management,* Philadelphia, 1975, FA Davis Co.)

she is not pushed forward in the seat. For a lordosis, lumbar support can be added to bring the seat back in contact with the person. In cases where the shoulders are retracted, wedged blocks can be added to the back to position the shoulders forward.

When a person has difficulty maintaining a midline position (side to side) of the trunk, lateral support is provided (Figure 6-11). The positioning of the lateral supports depends on how much control the person has. Lateral supports placed high on the trunk and close to the body provide greater control than those placed lower on the trunk (Mayall and Desharnais, 1995). Because the forces placed on the body by the lateral supports can be great, care should be taken in placement of these components and selection of materials (well padded) to prevent tissue damage. If there is scoliosis, the application of force at three positions on the body is one means to attempt to limit the progress of the scoliosis, although there is limited evidence to support or refute this use. This three-point system uses

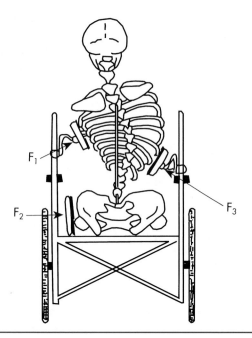

Figure 6-11   Three-point system of control for reducing the effects of scoliosis. (From Nwaobi OM: Biomechanics of seating. In Trefler E, editor: *Seating for children with cerebral palsy: a resource manual,* Memphis, 1984, University of Tennessee.)

the principles of equilibrium of forces to stabilize and align the trunk. As shown in Figure 6-11, one pad is applied under the apex of the curve on the convex side *(F₃)*, with two other pads opposing it to provide resistance (*F₁* and *F₂*). One of these pads is placed up high under the armpit and the other point is on the pelvis (Trefler, Hobson, and Taylor, 1993).

Tilting the seating system back slightly can eliminate some of the effects of gravity for individuals with spinal deformities, low tone, decreased strength in the trunk, or poor head control and can also help the individual maintain a more symmetrical posture. The force of gravity is reduced in the tilt position, making it easier to maintain the trunk in midline and increasing the comfort of the laterals. The positive effects of tilt on trunk position must be evaluated by the limitations this position can place on function. Vision, the ability to eat, use of equipment on a tray, and social engagement are just some activities that can be compromised when the wheelchair seat is tilted.

When control is required to prevent forward trunk flexion, anterior supports can be used. This type of support is necessary for individuals who need to be in an upright position for a functional or therapeutic activity but who do not have the ability to maintain this position independently. The most common approaches used are straps, chest panels, and rigid shoulder supports. One simple approach is to use straps that are attached to the seat back below shoulder level, come up over the shoulders, and attach to the seating system near the hips (Figure 6-12, *A*). The chest restraint must be well maintained because it poses a safety concern if the lower attachment becomes loose, allowing the strap to constrict around the neck (Trefler, Hobson, and Taylor, 1993). Another approach is a solid chest panel in a butterfly, **X**, or **I** shape with straps that attach to the seating system as above (Figure 6-12, *B*). The final approach is to use rigid shoulder components (Figure 6-12, *C*) that come over the clavicle and hold the shoulder girdle back against the seating system. These components should be adjustable and well padded to ensure stabilization without excessive pressure.

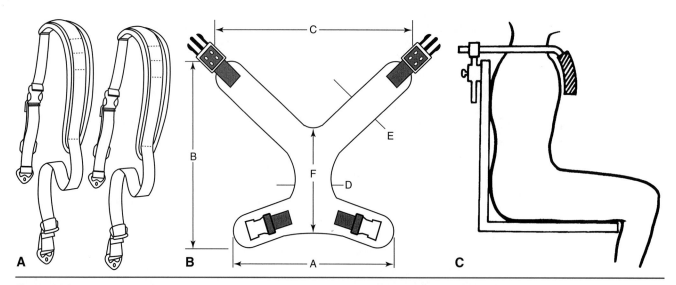

Figure 6-12   **A,** An example of a chest strap that attaches to the seat back below shoulder level, comes up over the shoulders, and attaches to the seating system near the hips. (Courtesy Bodypoint Designs, Inc., www.bodypoint. com.) **B,** Solid chest panel in an X design. (Courtesy Daher Manufacturing, Inc., www.daherproducts.com.) **C,** Rigid shoulder supports. (From Bergen AF, Presperin J, Tallman T: *Positioning for function: wheelchairs and other assistive technologies,* Valhalla, NY, 1990, Valhalla Rehabilitation Publications.)

Head and Neck.   With the pelvis, lower extremities, and trunk positioned, head and neck positions are considered next. The position of the head is important in inhibiting abnormal reflexes and maximizing the visual skills of the individual. In some cases a headrest is necessary only part of the time, for example, when the individual becomes fatigued or during transportation. The most common problems leading to the need for positioning of the head include hyperextension of the neck, weak neck musculature, lateral neck flexion, and neck rotation. In addition, support may be required to right the head when the person has been reclined. As in the positioning of other body segments, posterior, anterior, or lateral components are used for support. Figure 6-13 shows examples of components for each of these types of support. Posterior support can range from a high backrest (for those requiring minimal support) to headrests of different types. With any posterior head support, it is important to avoid triggering extension or pushing the head forward into flexion. Anterior support is typically provided by headbands, which are used in conjunction with posterior head supports. Elastic materials or pulleys provide

a dynamic type of support. These allow movement of the head within a limited range. Lateral supports can be incorporated into a headrest or provided as separate components. They can be applied at the temporal area, at the neck, or at the side of the face just in front of the ear.

Upper Extremities.   Support of the upper extremities is an essential component of the seating system. A lack of support for the arms can adversely affect head and neck position. Additionally, arms that are left to hang can sustain injury if caught on something or can acquire subluxation of the glenohumeral joint of the shoulder. Using an upper extremity support surface, such as a lap tray, helps with positioning of the head and neck, reduces the likelihood of damage to the arms and shoulder joints, and places the hands in a midline position that facilitates bilateral manual activities. The height of the lap tray depends on the needs of the consumer. Commonly the tray is mounted so that it allows the forearms to rest on it with the elbows bent at a 90-degree angle. For individuals with spasticity, a tray mounted higher will help to reduce upper extremity tone

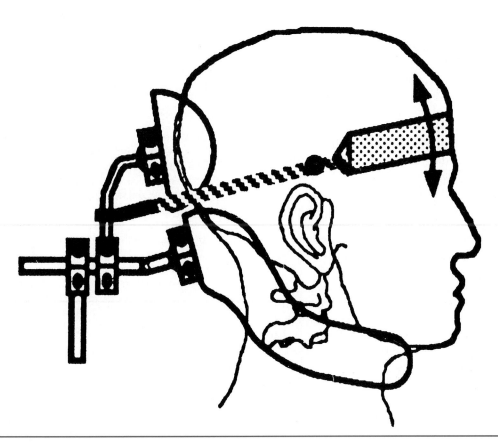

Figure 6-13   Head positioning components include headrest, lateral supports, and headband. One or more of these components are included in head supports. (Courtesy Whitmyer Biomechanix, Inc.)

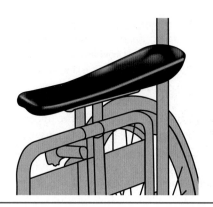

Figure 6-14   Arm trough. (Courtesy Otto Bock, www.ottobockus.com/products/r_wheel.htm.)

(Trefler, Hobson, and Taylor, 1993). Some individuals do not want a lap tray but still require positioning of the upper extremities. For these situations, individual arm troughs (Figure 6-14) mounted to the armrests of the wheelchair are available, which provide channeling and support for the arms.

■ PRINCIPLES OF SEATING FOR TISSUE INTEGRITY

A second major goal of seating interventions is pressure management. The emphasis in this area is to manage sitting pressure and maintain the skin in a healthy condition so that pressure ulcers are prevented. A **pressure ulcer** is a lesion that develops as a result of unrelieved pressure to the area and that results in damage to underlying tissue (Bouten et al, 2003). Pressure ulcers usually occur over bony prominences, with the sacrum, coccyx, ischial tuberosities, trochanters, external malleoli, and heels being the areas most commonly affected. These lesions have also been referred to as decubitus ulcers, bed sores, pressure sores, and dermal ulcers. Because pressure is the major factor influencing the development of these lesions, it is recommended that the term *pressure ulcer* be used to describe them (National Pressure Ulcer Advisory Panel, 1992).

Much research has been conducted attempting to determine the various factors that contribute to the development of pressure ulcers and to identify tools and strategies for preventing their occurrence. However, it is difficult to isolate all the variables that affect individuals as they go through their daily lives and to make substantive conclusions for a population as a whole on the basis of this research. Each person must be considered individually, and a comprehensive program of risk assessment and prevention must be developed to address his or her needs. The ATP needs to be aware of the role of seating, as well as all the other variables, to prevent pressure ulcers.

CASE STUDY

ALEX

Twenty years ago, at the age of 22 years, Alex sustained a spinal cord injury in a single-car accident. The lesion was at T1-T2, leaving him completely paralyzed below that level. After his initial hospitalization and adjustment to his disability, he returned to college and completed a master's degree in vocational counseling. He has a successful private practice as a vocational counselor, which has kept him very busy. So busy in fact that he did not pay attention to his skin and ended up with a small pressure sore on his left ischial tuberosity. After weeks of medical treatment and hours spent in bed allowing the ulcer to heal, he is ready to get back to working full time again. His doctor has referred him to the ATP for evaluation for a seating system that will manage his pressure. The physician's report states that scoliosis is also beginning to develop.

Alex currently has a lightweight manual wheelchair with a sling back and a 2-inch foam cushion with a knit cover placed on top of the sling seat. He is independent with mobility by using his upper extremities. He transfers in and out of the wheelchair to all surfaces independently, including to and from his car. He is independent in all self-care activities. He is married, and his wife is responsible for all home management activities. He does admit that he has gotten into the habit of hooking his left arm behind the wheelchair push handle for stability during certain activities. He did not realize that this could be the cause of some of his problems.

QUESTIONS

1. On the basis of the information given, what might be the goals of seating for Alex?
2. Write a list of questions to ask of Alex during the initial interview.
3. How should the ATP proceed with a seating evaluation for Alex?
4. On the basis of the information given, what technological approaches should be considered and why? What types of positioning accessories should be considered and why?
5. List potential funding sources for Alex's seating system. How could his system be justified to the funding source (see Chapter 5)?

Incidence and Costs of Pressure Ulcers

Individuals who remain in bed for prolonged periods of time or who use a wheelchair and have limited ability to reposition themselves are at risk for development of pressure ulcers. In particular, individuals with spinal cord injury are at a high risk because they lack sensation and have limited movement below the level of the lesion. It is estimated that approximately one third of individuals with spinal cord injury will encounter some type of tissue breakdown during their lifetimes (Krause et al, 2001) and that approximately 25% of the health care costs associated with the consequences of a spinal cord injury are related to a pressure ulcer (Krause et al, 2001). Other populations with a high incidence of pressure ulcers include individuals with hemiplegia caused by stroke, multiple sclerosis, cancer, the elderly, and individuals who have had a femoral fracture.

Chen, DeVivo, and Jackson (2005) examined pressure ulcer prevalence in persons with spinal cord injury who were followed up through the National Spinal Cord Injury Database over the past two decades. Their sample included 3361 community-dwelling individuals with spinal cord injury who were followed up by nine centers participating in the Model Spinal Cord Injury Systems project. These nine centers were chosen because they collected continuous data throughout the duration of the study. The authors explored the relationship of risk factors and prevalence of pressure ulcer over time following the injury. Thirty-three percent of the sample had a pressure ulcer on entry to the study. It was found that the risk of pressure ulcer was relatively stable in the first 10 years following the injury. There was also a significant prevalence of recent pressure ulcers, which was not fully explained by other factors. Older subjects (50 years and older) were more likely to have a pressure ulcer. Other significant risk factors included male sex, African-American race, single marital status, education less than high school, and presence of other comorbid medical conditions (Chen, DeVivo, and Jackson, 2005).

In addition to the costs for medical care, there are social costs, which have a greater effect (Krouskop et al, 1983). Krouskop et al (1983) identify these costs as including (1) time lost from work, which affects the person and his or her family, (2) time lost from school, (3) time away from family, which can affect the person's social development, and (4) loss of personal independence and productivity, which results in decreased self-esteem and self-worth.

Origins of Pressure Ulcers

Many factors contribute to the development of pressure ulcers; these are shown in Figure 6-15. External forces applied to a localized area are considered to be the primary cause. With application of external pressure, the normal flow of blood and oxygen to tissue in that area is reduced. If this situation is sustained, changes occur in the tissue cells, and these changes eventually lead to death of the cells. Individuals who have limited movement and lie in bed or sit in a wheelchair for prolonged periods generate compression forces that reduce the blood supply to the tissues and make them prone to pressure ulcers. Pressure ulcers are most common over weight-bearing, bony prominences because the force at these sites is greater than at other locations covered by subcutaneous tissue.

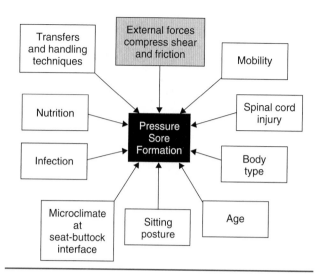

Figure 6-15 Factors that contribute to pressure ulcer development.

The amount of external pressure sufficient to restrict the blood flow enough to cause tissue damage has been a point of discussion over the years. The average blood pressure in capillaries ranges from 12 mm Hg in the venous limb to 32 mm Hg in the arteriolar limb (Landis, 1930). External pressure on the weight-bearing surface that exceeds these pressures produces obstruction of the capillaries. When sitting pressures of subjects on various types of surfaces were measured, it was found that the pressure generated by each surface under the ischial tuberosities greatly exceeded capillary blood pressure (Kosiak et al, 1958). A contoured, alternating pressure chair was the only surface that provided intermittent reduction (in the down position) of pressure to levels in the range of capillary blood pressure. Because most of the seating surfaces in this study generated pressures that exceeded capillary pressure, investigators were led to question whether that is the primary cause of pressure ulcer formation or whether other factors are involved.

The duration of pressure is a significant variable in the development of pressure ulcers. Kosiak (1959) determined that there is an inverse relationship between the amount of pressure sustained and the time over which it is applied. In a study involving dogs, Kosiak found that a pressure of 600 mm Hg produced ulceration in approximately 1 hour and a pressure of 150 mm Hg produced ulceration in 12 hours. The results of this study are shown in Figure 6-16, *A*. Microscopic tissue changes were found after application of as little as 60 mm Hg of pressure over 1 hour. This finding is consistent with the theory that exceeding the capillary pressure deprives the cells of enough important nutrients to cause damage at some level.

Time as a variable in pressure ulcer development is taken into consideration with the broad guidelines developed by Reswick and Rogers (1976). These guidelines, based on

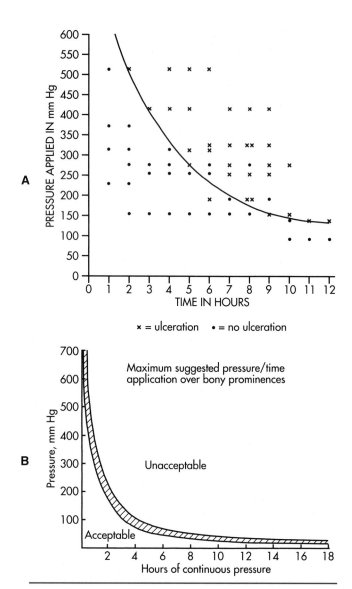

Figure 6-16   **A,** Relationship between applied pressure and time. Most points above the curve result in ulceration. (From Kosiak M: Etiology of decubitus ulcers, *Arch Phys Med Rehab* 42:19-29, 1961.) **B,** Allowable pressures versus time of application for tissue under bony prominences. (From Reswick JB, Rogers JE: Experience at Rancho Los Amigos Hospital with devices and techniques to prevent pressure sores. In Kenedi RM, Cowden JM, Scales JT, editors: *Bedsore biomechanics,* Baltimore, 1976, University Park Press.)

formation of pressure ulcers as well. Shear forces are generated when two surfaces move across each other in opposite directions, for example, when an individual slides his hips forward in a wheelchair and assumes a sacral sitting posture. In this position the skin remains in contact with the seat surface and the superficial fascia is interlocked with the skin. The deeper portion of the superficial fascia, however, is mobile and slides forward. The blood vessels in this area are stretched and angulated, which causes occlusion. Resulting tissue damage is at a deeper level and typified by a large area of undermining around the base of the ulcer (Reichel, 1958). Bennett et al (1979) believe that it is the combination of pressure and shear that is so effective in occluding blood flow. They found that, when sufficient shear was present, only half as much pressure was needed to cause occlusion. Unfortunately, because of the difficulty in measuring shear, there is still uncertainty regarding the extent to which shear contributes to the development of pressure ulcers.

Friction, the force between two surfaces at rest or in motion, is another component of shear and the development of pressure ulcers. Friction leads to injury and ulceration of the surface of the skin. A typical friction injury to the skin occurs when it moves across a rough surface such as bedding. Dinsdale (1974) found that the skin's susceptibility to pressure ulcer development is increased with friction. When pressure alone was applied, 290 mm Hg was required to produce ulceration. With the application of pressure *and* friction, ulcerations were produced with pressure levels as low as 45 mm Hg. Moisture, heat, or properties of materials such as clothing can increase frictional forces.

Other Factors That Contribute to Pressure Ulcer Development

Some individuals can be exposed to the mechanical forces of pressure and shear without pressure ulcers developing, whereas others have very little tolerance to these mechanisms. Although compression and shear forces are typically considered to be the chief causes of pressure ulcers, there are several other factors that contribute to skin breakdown and cause some individuals to be more susceptible than others.

Mobility.   Moving to relieve pressure over an area is how the body typically responds to prevent tissue damage. Nondisabled subjects make side-to-side weight oscillations several times per minute while sitting (Tredwell and Roxborough, 1991). Normally, when there is a lack of oxygen and chemical irritation, pain signals from the nerve endings trigger postural changes and there is little tissue damage. Individuals who lack normal sensation, such as those who have sustained a spinal cord injury, are unable to recognize and respond to these pain signals and are particularly susceptible to development of pressure ulcers (Chen et al, 2005).

years of clinical experience with individuals who have spinal cord injury, establish allowable amounts of pressure that tissue surrounding bony prominences can endure over certain periods. They recommend that pressures on the ischial tuberosities remain in the range of 30 to 60 mm Hg, as shown in Figure 6-16, *B.* Tissues that are not susceptible to the internal pressure exerted by bony prominences can tolerate higher skin surface pressures or lower pressures for longer periods.

Up to this point the effects of sustained perpendicular (compression) pressure forces on tissue have been discussed. Parallel (or shear) forces play a significant role in the

Individuals whose ability to reposition themselves or whose activity is limited to bed or chair should be assessed for the risk of pressure ulcer development. There are scales available that determine the magnitude of risk by measuring the degree to which mobility and activity levels are limited. Two commonly used scales that assess these factors are the Norton Scale (Norton, McLaren, and Exton-Smith, 1975) and the Braden Scale (Bergstrom et al, 1987). In addition to mobility, these scales also assess other factors that place a person at risk for development of pressure ulcers, such as incontinence, impaired nutritional status, and altered level of consciousness. Individuals should be assessed with a validated systematic risk assessment tool on admission to acute care and rehabilitation hospitals, nursing homes, home care programs, and other health care facilities and at other periodic intervals. Identified risk factors can be reduced through intervention, and the development of pressure ulcers might be prevented.

Spinal Cord Injury.   As discussed above, loss of sensation and limitations in mobility put individuals with spinal cord injury at great risk for development of pressure ulcers. In addition, some researchers speculate that other changes in the body that result from the denervation caused by the spinal cord injury increase a person's susceptibility to pressure ulcers. In a study of normal and paraplegic rats, no differences were found in their susceptibility to pressure (Kosiak, 1961). Constantian (1980) concludes that there is not adequate objective evidence that individuals with denervated tissue are predisposed to the development of pressure ulcers nor that denervated tissue heals more slowly or differently than skin with normal enervation. On the other hand, there is evidence that after spinal cord injury there may be tissue alterations (e.g., loss of collagen, abnormal vascularity, tone changes) and changes in hormonal response to stress that place a person more at risk for development of pressure ulcers and that impair the normal healing process (Patterson et al, 1992; Pfeffer, 1991; Whimster, 1976).

Differences in circulatory tissue perfusion between persons who have a spinal cord injury and those who do not have been documented (Patterson et al, 1992). With externally applied pressures of 32 mm Hg, it was found that the partial pressure of oxygen (an indicator of the perfusion of the tissue) was significantly lower in spinal cord–injured subjects than in subjects without a disability. To evaluate the *response* of the peripheral circulation to externally applied pressure, Patterson et al (1992) cycled the pressure loads on and off. Although oxygen perfusion was lower during both on and off periods for the persons with spinal cord injuries, it was only during the on period that these differences were statistically significant. At higher external pressures (75 mm Hg), the differences in oxygen perfusion for the two groups were not statistically significant. The difference between the two groups at the lower pressure was attributed to a lack of vascular autoregulation in the subjects with spinal cord

injuries (Patterson et al, 1992). Autoregulation requires a minimal difference between internal pressure and external pressures. At 75 mm Hg autoregulation cannot occur because the external pressure is near the arterial pressure. Measurements of blood volume showed significant differences between the two groups at both external pressures. This study indicates that there are tissue perfusion changes in spinal cord injury that significantly impair the response to external pressure loads.

Measurement of these factors that may affect the development of pressure ulcers is improving but remains difficult, which makes it difficult to specify their particular effects on pressure ulcer development. However, it is likely that there are intrinsic changes in the body as a result of spinal cord injury that cannot be ignored. These changes may result in tissue with different properties and a reduced tolerance to external pressure.

Body Type.   The body type of the individual has some effect on pressure distribution. A thin person has less subcutaneous fat to act as padding, and therefore forces per unit area of the skin are increased. An overweight individual has more padding over which to distribute pressure. However, it may be more difficult for the overweight individual to perform pressure relief exercises. Caregivers may also have more difficulty moving an overweight individual, which may make shearing and friction forces a greater possibility.

Nutrition.   Inadequate nutrition is often associated with weight loss and muscular atrophy, both of which reduce the amount of tissue between the seat surface and the bony prominences. Inadequate dietary intake, which results in anemia, decreased protein levels, and vitamin C deficiency are also known to interfere with the normal integrity of the tissue (Berecek, 1981; Breslow, 1991) and have been linked not only to pressure ulcer development but also to delayed healing. An increased intake of protein and calories has been shown to improve the healing rate of pressure ulcers (Breslow, 1991).

Infection.   Torrance (1983) identifies three reasons why infection may contribute to pressure ulcer development. First, fever caused by infection increases the metabolic rate, which increases the demand for oxygen, which in turn endangers areas that are ischemic. Second, severe infection can also affect the nutritional balance of the body. Finally, localized bacteria increase the demand on metabolism in a localized area.

Age.   As people age, the skin loses some of its elasticity and muscles atrophy, which increases vulnerability to friction or shearing. Vascular and neurological diseases associated with aging (e.g., diabetes, renal disease) affect the circulation and may also increase an individual's susceptibility to skin breakdown.

Sitting Posture.   Posture and deformity can affect the pressure distribution of the seat/buttock interface and can potentially contribute to skin breakdown. Two specific postures that pose a risk for pressure ulcer formation are pelvic obliquity and sacral sitting. Pelvic obliquity, which was discussed in detail in a previous section, results in increased pressure and shear under the affected lower ischial tuberosity and the posterior aspect of the lower greater trochanter (Hobson, 1989; Zacharkow, 1984, 1988). The loss of lumbar lordosis when sitting is another risk factor. This position occurs as a result of limited hip mobility for flexion or decreased spinal mobility for extension (Zacharkow, 1984). Consequently, a sacral sitting posture is typically assumed, which results in significant amounts of pressure being placed on the sacrococcygeal region.

Microclimate at the Seat/Buttock Interface.   The microclimate between the body and the seating surface is a critical factor that is often overlooked. The temperature of the skin and the presence of moisture both affect the formation of pressure ulcers. An increase in skin temperature of 1°C is accompanied by a 10% increase in the metabolic demands of tissue (Fisher et al, 1978; Stewart, Palmieri, and Cochran, 1980). In tissue that already has limited oxygenation as a result of pressure, the potential for breakdown is exacerbated. Moisture, from perspiration or incontinence, also increases the risk of skin breakdown for a number of reasons. Wet skin is weaker than dry skin and therefore more likely to incur damage as a result of compression and friction (Stewart, Palmieri, and Cochran, 1980). Additionally, moisture increases the potential for bacterial growth and infection. Keeping the skin clean and dry is important for these reasons.

The material of the seat cushion and its cover can alter the temperature and the amount of moisture at the seat/buttock interface. Foam cushions have been found to cause an increase in skin temperature, whereas water-filled cushions reduced skin temperature (Fisher et al, 1978; Stewart, Palmieri, and Cochran, 1980). Excessive moisture can also be a problem that varies with the cushion, its cover, and the user. Gel and water cushions have been found to increase the amount of humidity at the seat/buttock interface by 23% and 20%, respectively (Stewart, Palmieri, and Cochran, 1980). Selecting cushion materials and coverings that reduce temperature and moisture accumulation is discussed later in this chapter.

Transfers and Handling Techniques.   Abrasions or ulcerations can be caused by hitting objects or sliding across a surface during transfers. Whether the individual transfers independently or has someone providing assistance, care should be taken to prevent abrasions. The same holds true for mobility in bed. Pulling an individual across the bed sheets can cause abrasions or ulcerations from the friction. Caregivers should be reminded to lift an individual to move him or her in bed instead of sliding the individual across the bedding.

The development of pressure ulcers is a complex process, and there is still much to be learned about the exact mechanisms involved. Identifying factors that predispose an individual to pressure ulcers will help in developing a comprehensive pressure ulcer prevention program. A program for preventing pressure ulcers should include (1) a wheelchair and seating prescription for pressure distribution, postural alignment, and stability, (2) a pressure relief program, (3) dietary instruction and adequate nutrition, (4) instruction in proper transferring and lifting techniques, and (5) maintenance of good personal hygiene and skin care (McDonald, 2001). The development and implementation of the prevention program should be considered a continuing team effort involving the consumer, his or her therapists, and medical personnel.

Pressure Measurement

Pressure ulcers result from sustained compression of soft tissues, particularly under bony prominences. The predominant hypotheses concerning the pathogenesis of pressure ulcers include localized tissue ischemia, sustained deformation of the cells, impaired nutritional flow to the cells, reperfusion injury, and inadequate drainage of cellular waste products (Lander Ganz and Gefen, 2004; Stekelenburg et al., 2006). Lander Ganz and Gefen demonstrated that the pressure measured at the deep tissue level was significantly greater than that measured at the surface interface, although they could not predict a specific relationship. The prevalence of pressure ulcers and the resulting costs underscore the need to measure the forces applied to the muscle in an attempt to prevent prolonged exposure to high loads. Many sophisticated pressure measurement systems have been developed, including near infrared tissue spectrophotoscopy, Raman spectrography, and in-dwelling sensors. However, these systems are not feasible in the clinical situation.

In the clinic, pressure mapping systems are the primary means of quantifying pressure. These systems quantify pressure at the buttock/seat interface, allowing a comparison among various cushions. In measuring sitting pressure, it can also be determined whether the individual has any evidence of asymmetry in sitting and what influence changing the configuration of the seating system has on correcting the asymmetry. Many commercial pressure measurement systems are available for commercial and research use. These technologies are constantly improving, but issues remain with consistency of the measurement and lack of agreement around best practices for pressure measurement protocol. The three most common pressure mapping systems are the Force Sensing Array (Vista Medical; *www.pressuremapping.com*), F-Scan (Tekscan) (*www.tekscan.com*), and Xsensor (Xsensor

Technology Corporation, *www.xsensor.com*). Each of these systems uses a flexible matrix of pressure sensors that provide a map of the distribution of pressure at the interface between the seat cushion or back and the client's body. These sensors are arranged in a grid pattern on the pressure mat. The number of sensors and their sensitivity varies across the different systems and should be taken into consideration when considering the purchase of a system. They vary in the technology used to measure pressure. These technologies include capacitance sensors that measure the ability to store an electrical charge, piezo-resistive sensors that measure the change in resistance when force is applied, and electrically conductive sensors that measure the change in current flow. Two properties influence the reliability of the pressure measurements: creep and hysteresis. Creep refers to the stability of the pressure reading over time. Hysteresis refers to the change in pressure reading as the device is loaded and unloaded (e.g., as the client sits on the cushion). Each of these systems corrects for these two variables in their software, but these properties still influence the reliability of the measurement systems to varying degrees, which needs to be taken into consideration when these systems are used clinically.

The output from each of these systems is generally similar, although care must be taken when the results of research or measurements obtained by use of the different systems are compared. As will be seen below, these systems differ in their performance. All the systems provide a visual output (Figure 6-17) that allows a quick inspection of the

pressure distribution. The visual output may show pressure distribution with a color display or as peaks and depressions. The actual pressure value for each cell can be displayed as well. Data are captured continuously at varying sampling rates. The system will provide data on peak and mean pressure, number of sensors activated, minimum and maximum pressure, and the location of the center of pressure. Some systems have the capacity for a split screen that displays the pressure map on one side and a video recording on the other. Another useful feature is the ability to define a particular area of the pressure map for which the system will generate pressure statistics. The breadth of information that these systems provide is both useful and a distraction. Although data showing peak and mean pressure seem easy to interpret, there is little consensus on what is desired pressure at the seat/buttock interface. Different ways of interpreting these data will be discussed below in the discussion of a pressure mapping protocol.

Ferguson-Pell and Cardi (1993) completed an evaluation of three computer-based pressure mapping systems. Although this work evaluated technology that is dated, it continues to influence thinking about pressure measurement systems as it applies a systematic protocol, involves both consumers and users, and identifies key parameters that must be considered in both the selection of a pressure mapping system and interpretation of the resulting data. The three systems that were evaluated included: the Force Sensing Array (Vista Medical), with a 15 × 15–cell array of force-sensing resistors, the Talley Pressure Monitor (TPM, Progressive Medical), consisting of an array of bladder-type sensors, and the Tekscan Seat (Tekscan Inc.), with an array of 2056 force sensors. With these systems, Ferguson-Pell and Cardi (1993) carried out "bench tests" to determine the properties of the sensors under controlled loads. The measurement variables of interest were accuracy, linearity and reproducibility, hysteresis, and stability (Ferguson-Pell and Cardi, 1993). In other words, they measured the relationship between the pressure measured by each system and a known applied pressure, creep, and hysteresis. These were examined with planar and contour loads under laboratory conditions and across four different pressure relieving cushions, with five wheelchair users as subjects. The four cushions used to evaluate the performance of each of the pressure mapping systems included (1) foam, (2) gel, (3) hybrid (Jay), and (4) air filled (ROHO). The actual results of this work are less critical today because of the changes that have occurred in both measurement systems and cushion technology. However, this study remains an important one because of its use of a systematic research protocol and identification of critical factors that influence the reliability of pressure mapping systems.

A recent study involved a similar comparison of more current pressure mapping technologies (Hadcock et al., 2002). Incremental loading, low threshold, and stability

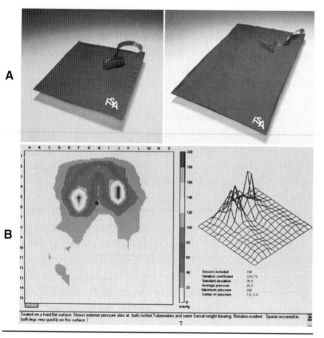

Figure 6-17   Pressure measurement system. **A,** Map with an array of sensors. **B,** Sample display of an individual's pressure distribution profile (Courtesy Vista Medical, www.pressuremapping.com.)

(creep) of the F-scan FSA and Xsensor systems were evaluated under static and dynamic conditions by using planar and curved surfaces. The curved surface was cylindrical; quite different from a contoured seating surface, so the results of this aspect of the study must be interpreted with caution for the purposes of seating intervention. This study involved bench testing and did not include measurement with any wheelchair users. The results on a flat surface indicated that the FSA system was the most accurate, followed by the Xsensor and the F-scan. Creep was similar for the Xsensor and F-scan (17.62% and 17.23%, respectively) systems, and both were better than the FSA system (19.54%) (Hadcock et al., 2003). The Xsensor was better at detecting pressures under light loading conditions.

The studies by Ferguson-Pell and Cardi (1993) and Hadcock et al. (2003) provide some evidence for the difference in performance across pressure mapping systems. In addition to the performance characteristics evaluated in these studies, the selection of a system will depend on familiarity with the technology, the specific purpose (e.g., clinical evaluation versus research), and the functionality of the systems as they meet the needs of the user.

A second major issue with respect to pressure mapping is the identification of an accepted protocol for clinical use. There is no compelling evidence in the literature to suggest a particular number above which a pressure ulcer will certainly develop. Consequently, pressure mapping in the clinical situation is used to make comparisons among various cushions so that the clinician can rank the cushions for their ability to distribute pressure as measured by the pressure mapping systems. Swaine (2003) has developed a protocol for both obtaining and interpreting pressure measurements that is becoming more prevalent internationally. Swaine describes a consistent setup of the equipment and cushions to be evaluated, an initial check of the equipment, length of recording time, palpation of bony prominences, and documentation. She also suggests that interpretation of the results is based on peak pressure, the area of the client's buttocks that are in contact with the pressure mat, and any asymmetries of pressure distribution.

Swaine's work provides a useful basis for clinicians using pressure mapping to determine the optimal cushion for their clients' needs. Caution is still advised because questions remain about a protocol and the interpretation of the data. For example, Swaine (2003) suggests that peak pressure is determined by taking the average of the four highest sensor cells around a bony prominence, whereas Dunk and Callaghan (2005) take the average of all sensors within 10% of the cell, measuring the highest peak pressure. Swaine recommends that clients sit on a cushion for 8 to 10 minutes, whereas Stinson, Porter, and Eakin (2002) suggest that 6 minutes is sufficient. Pressure gradient rather than absolute pressure has been suggested as a better indicator of risk for development of a pressure ulcer, but there is no consensus on what constitutes an acceptable gradient. These concerns suggest that, although pressure mapping remains a very useful tool its augment clinical judgment, it does not replace it.

Behavioral strategies to reduce the risk of development of pressure ulcers were identified earlier. Two main technologies exist to manage pressure for persons who use wheelchairs: pressure relief cushions and tilt and recline components on wheelchairs. The latter will be discussed in Chapter 12. Numerous studies have measured characteristics and properties of a variety of pressure relief cushions. The majority of investigations have used tissue interface pressure as the basis for comparing these products. Some studies have also compared changes in transcutaneous oxygen tension and capillary blood flow. Although it has been shown that seating technologies play a significant role in pressure ulcer prevention by reducing the mechanical load on the tissue, there is no evidence that one type of pressure-reducing device works better than all others under all circumstances (Brienza et al, 2001; Conine et al, 1994; DeLateur et al, 1976; Ferguson-Pell et al, 1986; Garber, Krouskop, and Carter, 1978).

■ PRINCIPLES OF SEATING FOR COMFORT

This section considers seating and technologies that address that comfort. There are three distinct populations who can benefit from seating technologies for comfort: (1) wheelchair users who have sitting discomfort and pain (e.g., individuals with postpolio syndrome, amyotrophic lateral sclerosis, and multiple sclerosis), (2) the elderly, and (3) individuals with low back pain, which can keep them from effectively performing their jobs. For individuals in any one of these populations, discomfort in seating can lead to a decreased ability to participate in activities of daily living. In cases of severe discomfort, the individual may be restricted to bed rest for some or all of the day, which further reduces the individual's ability to function and can lead to medical problems as well. There are unique technologies for each of these populations, but the commonality is that they enhance comfort in the seated position.

In comparison to the other two categories of need, the technologies available to meet the comfort seating needs of individuals fall far short. There are a number of reasons for this. One is that equipment that is deemed necessary for comfort typically is not paid for by third-party funding sources because it is not considered a medical necessity. Another reason is that there is very little agreement among researchers on how to define and assess comfort and discomfort (Hobson and Crane, 2001). Although much research has been done to assess comfort, it is a difficult variable to objectively measure because it can be highly subjective and involve multiple factors. A cushion that is described as comfortable by one individual may feel uncomfortable to another.

Researchers have also been unsuccessful in tying discomfort to quantitative measures such as posture, muscle fatigue as indicated by electromyographical measurements, or seat interface pressure (Hobson and Crane, 2001). The lack of outcomes relating to the effectiveness of seating products said to promote comfort makes it necessary for clinicians to use a trial-and-error approach to recommending equipment for the consumer. This can be costly and is often not funded by third-party sources. In turn, without funding at the clinical level for such products, there is no financial incentive for manufacturers to address this unmet need. It is necessary that those involved in this industry determine the best way to assess the many factors of discomfort and comfort. Only then can the efficacy of the current technologies for this population be carefully evaluated and new technologies be developed.

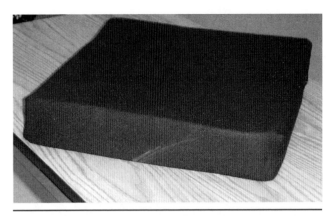

Figure 6-18   Planar foam cushion.

TECHNOLOGIES FOR SEATING AND POSITIONING MANAGEMENT

There is considerable overlap between the technologies used to address goals related to postural control, tissue integrity, and comfort. Further, many clients require seating that addresses two or more of these goals. Seating technologies in general will be discussed, with identification of their specific application to these goals where appropriate. This section is divided into two components: the design and the construction of the seating system and the properties of the materials used to construct it. The evaluation process described at the beginning of this chapter guides the selection of the most appropriate system. The client should be allowed a trial period of use of the system because comfort and functional issues will become evident with use of the system over time.

Design and Construction of Seating Systems

The design of the seating system refers to the degree of contouring present in the seat and back and the degree of adjustability that is present in the components. These technologies range from systems that are relatively flat, without any contouring to match the shape of the body segments they support, to custom-contoured systems that are constructed to match as closely as possible the body contours of the user. Prefabricated technologies are available so that the ATP no longer needs to construct the components in the seating system.

Planar.   **Planar** technologies are flat surfaces that support the body only where it easily comes in contact with the body, such as at bony prominences. In general, they are appropriate for individuals who require minimal support. Other positioning components can be added to this basic structure if additional support is required. Planar foam cushions, as shown in Figure 6-18, are designed from flat blocks of foam, which

can be highly adaptable. These blocks can be fabricated with one layer of a selected thickness (up to 4 inches) and selected density of foam, or they can be fabricated from multiple densities and varying thicknesses of foam (Hobson, 1990). In the latter case, for example, a piece of a stiff foam that is 1 to 2 inches thick might be used on the bottom to provide a stable base and a $^3/_4$- to 1-inch-thick piece of soft foam could be placed on top for pressure relief. Planar foams can also be adapted by cutting out (e.g., under the ischial tuberosities) or building up areas as necessary for pressure distribution or postural management.

Prefabricated.   Prefabricated planar components are made in standard sizes to fit a wide range of individuals. The back and seat surfaces are generally plywood or molded plastic pieces to which foam has been attached. Lateral supports and an abductor for pelvic and hip support can be attached with hardware to the basic seat, and lateral supports for trunk stability can be attached to the back section (Figure 6-19) (Adaptive Engineering Lab, Inc., *www.aelseating.com*). The seat and back are attached to the wheelchair frame with interfacing hardware once the upholstery has been removed. Much of the hardware that interfaces the various components can be adjusted for angle, width, and depth. The advantage of having adjustable components is that they allow the system to be modified for growth or postural changes.

Custom Fabricated.   Custom-fabricated planar systems are made of similar materials and design as prefabricated systems, but the dimensions of the seating surface and components are customized to fit the individual. These systems can be fabricated on site directly with the consumer, or specifications of the consumer's measurements can be sent to a manufacturer for fabrication. The density of the foam pieces can also be selected to accommodate the needs

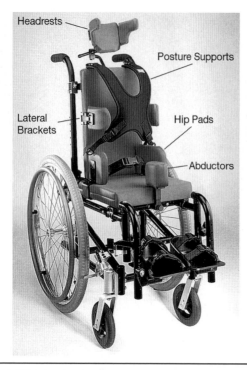

Figure 6-19   Planar seating system with positioning components. (Courtesy Adaptive Engineering Lab, Inc., www.aelseating.com.)

of the individual. Lateral supports, headrests, and other components are added to the basic foam and plywood (or plastic) structure. This approach can be highly labor intensive and is being replaced at many facilities as a result of the advent of a large array of off-the-shelf technologies.

Standard Contoured Modules

Contoured technologies are useful for individuals with moderate seating and positioning needs for postural management or who are at low risk for pressure ulcer development. These technologies use curved surfaces that more closely match the shape of the human body. The amount of contact that the body has with the seating surface is increased by contouring the seating surface to the person's body, providing increased support and control. Further, a generic contoured cushion will distribute pressure across the seating surface and will fit people within a certain size range. This approach is also generally less costly than a custom-contoured cushion. The Matrix is one example of a standard contoured cushion (Figure 6-20) (Invacare, *www.invacare.ca*).

Custom Contoured

The cushion that provides the greatest amount of body contact and therefore the most support is one that has been shaped, or custom contoured, to the individual's body. A number of technologies are available to achieve a custom-contoured system. One example is shown in Figure 6-21. These types of systems differ primarily in terms of the fabrication techniques used and whether the fabrication is completed on site or in a central location. The disadvantages of custom-contoured support surfaces include the following: transfers to and from the system are more difficult; the system is static and has no dynamic properties, thus limiting the individual to one fixed position; and there is limited ability within the system to allow for growth of the individual.

Foam in place systems allows the ATP to fabricate a custom-contoured cushion on site. The client is placed in a frame that has a flexible covering over one side. This covering is matched to the shape of the person, and he or she is positioned in the most desirable seated posture. The foam materials are then added to the frame and allowed to expand to contour to the person's shape. The person is removed from the frame, and the foam is allowed to harden for several hours. Once the foam hardens, the flexible covering

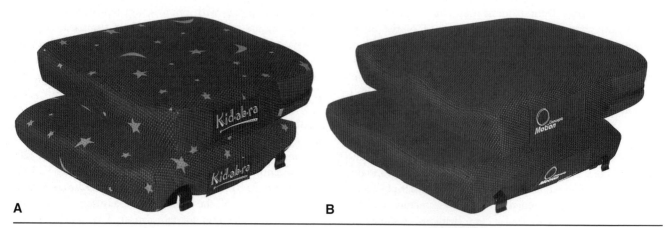

Figure 6-20   Matrix cushion. **A,** Child's version. **B,** Adult version. (Courtesy Invacare Corp., www.invacare.ca.)

This sheet is then sent to a central fabrication facility, along with other recommendations related to foam density, special construction related to pressure relief (e.g., use of different foams), and required accessories such as laterals and strapping systems. The Shape Sensor system by Invacare *(www.invacare.com)* is an example of this technology.

Prefabricated Adjustable Backs

Prefabricated adjustable backs have become available in recent years. These products provide a large degree of adjustability that can be accomplished in the clinical setting. The Infinity Back is an example of an adjustable back. The ATP can make adjustments on the basis of an optimal seated position determined by a mat assessment. These backs allow the clinician to adjust height, depth, width, back angle, and placement of the laterals. Some of these systems allow the ATP to create a biplanar back in which the upper and lower segments of the back are set at different angles. This configuration is often used to provide specific postural control. Although the pivot point can be placed at any spinal level, when placed at the level of the posterior superior iliac spine, it can assist with control of the pelvis. Studies have investigated the effect of pelvic stability on function (Miller Polgar et al, 2000; Rigby et al, 2001;), but there have been no clinical studies that have evaluated the effect of this particular back configuration on postural control and subsequently function.

■ PROPERTIES OF MATERIALS USED TO CONSTRUCT SEATING SYSTEMS

An understanding of the properties of the materials used in seating technologies will assist in the selection of appropriate cushions. Sprigle (1992) identifies and describes five properties of cushion materials: (1) density, (2) stiffness, (3) resilience, (4) dampening, and (5) envelopment.

Density of a material is the ratio of its weight to its volume. A greater density generally means a more durable material, but not always. Low-density materials will fatigue faster than high-density ones under the same loading conditions. **Stiffness** of a material describes how much it gives under load. In a cushion, this is the distance that the person sinks into the cushion. Soft materials may bottom out, but failure to compress can also lead to an increase in seating pressures and tissue breakdown. The International Standards Organization standards also describe lateral and forward stiffness that describes the response of the cushion to a lateral force. It is easier to slide on a cushion with low stiffness, but the shearing forces are higher, resulting in a cushion with less stability. **Sliding resistance** is a cushion property related to friction. A cushion with high resistance

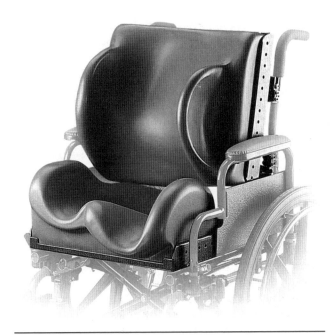

Figure 6-21   Custom-contoured seating system. (Courtesy Invacare Corp., www.invacare.com.)

is removed. Further shaping of the foam can be completed by hand at this time. The foam is encased in a fabric cover. The foam can then be attached to a solid backing (usually plywood or plastic) and mounted to the wheeled base. This approach can be used on site, and a cushion can be completed in about 12 hours.

A *vacuum consolidation* process seats the client on a latex bag filled with beads (Lemaire et al, 1996). This bag is placed on top of a wheelchair or fitting chair. The ATP assists the client to achieve an optimal position to support goals of function, pressure relief, or comfort. The latex bag is then manipulated to conform to this position and the vacuum is used to draw the air out of the bag, consolidating the enclosed beads. At this stage, the cushion can be fabricated either on site by a foaming procedure or sent to a central manufacturer for remote fabrication.

Seating simulators use technology that allows the ATP to map the client's body contours, which are then digitized. Computer-aided manufacturing technology is then used to fabricate the cushion or back. The process of determining the optimal cushion or back shape is similar to that described for vacuum consolidation. A simulator chair is used that allows multiple adjustments to manipulate seat depth, seat to back angle, and other common wheelchair configurations. An initial baseline reading is taken without the client seated in the simulator. Once the client is comfortably positioned in the chair, mechanical plungers are positioned to simulate the optimal seated position of the client. This information, along with the baseline reading, is transferred to a pressure-sensitive data recording sheet.

limits how much the user slides, helping to support upright posture, but consequently makes transfers more difficult.

Resilience is the ability of a material to recover its shape after a load is removed or to adjust to a load as it is applied. Short-term resilience is the immediate recovery when a load is altered, such as when someone shifts weight on a seat cushion. Long-term resilience is the overnight recovery of a cushion that has been loaded and then unloaded. **Dampening** is the ability of the cushion to soften on impact; it is best observed by dropping a relatively heavy object on the material. If the object sinks into the material, then dampening is occurring. If it bounces off, or if the material does not react to the object, then the material is poorly dampened. This is the "shock absorber" feature of cushion materials and is important in minimizing the transmission of forces from the ground to the individual as they travel over rough surfaces or obstacles. **Envelopment** is the degree to which the person sinks into the cushion and the degree to which the cushion surrounds the buttocks. Good envelopment promotes stability and helps reduce peak pressures. **Recovery** refers to the degree to which a cushion returns to its preloaded state when a load is removed.

Classification of Cushion Technologies

Sprigle, Press, and Davis (2001) describe uniform terminology for classification of the material used to construct wheelchair cushions. They described the following categories of cushions: (1) made from cellular materials, (2) containing fluid, and (3) other constructions.

Cushions Made From Cellular Materials.   This category includes cushions made from "foam," "flexible matrix," "viscoelastic foam or matrix," and "nondeforming foam or matrix" (Sprigle, Press, and Davis, 2001, pp. 451-2). Over the years, foams have been the material most commonly used in the fabrication of cushions. Polyurethane or latex foams come in a variety of thicknesses and densities and are often characterized by their cell structures. There are two commonly used cell structures for foams: open cell and closed cell. Open-cell foams have interconnected, perforated membranes that permit airflow between the cells and result in better ventilation (Tang, 1991). This type of foam is often less dense because of the air captured in the open cells. Open-cell foams absorb fluids, which makes them difficult to clean. Closed-cell foams are composed of individual structures encased in a membrane. These foams are generally less compliant than open-cell foams, and airflow is restricted. Examples of these foams include polyurethane and latex (open cell) and ethafoam (closed cell).

Foam cushions are typically lightweight and inexpensive. Foams compress with the application of weight, which results in good envelopment. The amount of compression depends on the stiffness of the foam. Although soft foam will compress and allow the person to sink in more, a foam that is too soft might bottom out. Because foams have a tendency to trap heat near the body, their thermal features are considered to be poor. In general, the short- and long-term resilience of foam is good, but again this varies depending on the structure and density of the foam. The two main disadvantages of using foam are that it (1) is prone to deterioration from light and moisture and (2) has a tendency to loose its resilience over time. Replacement of the foam depends on the type of foam and how much time the user spends sitting on the cushion.

Viscoelastic Foam or Matrix.   Viscoelastic foams were originally developed by the National Aeronautics and Space Administration for space travel. These foams, because of their high viscosities, tend to resist deformation if pressed quickly, but they will accommodate slowly to a constant load. They also have memory, which delays their return to the original shape. This time-dependent property is the most distinguishing feature of this type of foam (Sprigle, Press, and Davis, 2001). Viscoelastic foam also has good thermal properties and good envelopment. The resilience and dampening properties are variable depending on the density and other properties (Sprigle, 1992). Sunmate (*www.sunmate cushions.com*), T-foam, and Tempur-Med (*www.tempurcanada.com*) are examples of this type of foam (Figure 6-22).

Flexible Matrix.   Honeycomb cushion material is made from an array of thermoplastic elastomers. The material consists of layers of interconnected open cells that flex when pressure is applied. The flexibility of the cells results in a cushion that conforms to the user's body shape, providing pressure relief. These cushions have good resiliency. The open cells allow air to flow through, which keeps the cushion cooler and prevents moisture. Cushions that use flexible

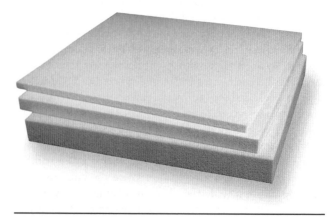

Figure 6-22   Examples of Viscoelastic foam. Sunmate foam. (Courtesy Sunmate, www.sunmatecushions.com.)

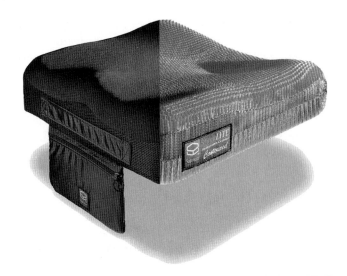

Figure 6-23   Flexible matrix technology, Stimulite cushion. (Courtesy Supracor Inc., www.supracor.com.)

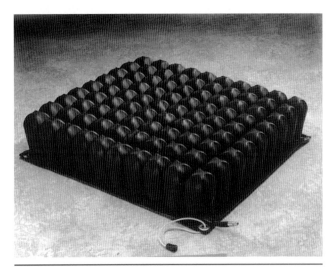

Figure 6-24   The ROHO High Profile air-filled cushion. (Courtesy Crown Therapeutics.)

matrix technology have both planar and contoured versions. Stimulite by Supracor *(www.supracor.com)* (Figure 6-23) is an example of a cushion with a flexible matrix technology.

Cushions Containing Fluid

Air Filled. Air-filled cushions consist of a sealed receptacle that holds air. The cushion may be configured to allow the air to circulate within the whole receptacle, or it may be divided into compartments to better control the air flow. Air-filled cushions distribute pressure from high-pressure areas, such as the ischial tuberosities, to areas where there is less pressure. These cushions have good long-term and short-term resilience. The pressure-relieving properties of this type of cushion are typically good; however, the ability of this cushion to envelop the user and thus its effectiveness are dependent on the amount of inflation. An air-filled cushion that is overinflated will not envelop the buttocks and will result in increased pressure at bony prominences and reduced sitting stability. Underinflation of the cushion can result in the air being pushed away from the high-pressure areas, allowing them to "bottom out" against the hard sitting surface of the seat. Persons who lack sensation may not be able to feel whether the cushion is underinflated.

Commonly used air-filled cushions are the ROHO and Bye Bye Decubiti. The ROHO cushion (Crown Therapeutics, *www.crownthera.com*) consists of a number of rubber-balloon cells that are interconnected at the base to allow for airflow among cells (Figure 6-24). It is available in a number of configurations, including a high and low profile (4- and 2-inch cells, respectively) and various inflation configurations. The multiple compartments allow the air to be regulated in each compartment separate of the other compartments. Air-filled cushions are generally lightweight, and the materials they are made of do not deteriorate over time.

A main disadvantage to these cushions is that they must be properly inflated, with consistent monitoring of the inflation to provide maximal benefits. Puncture and tears also occur, which influence their function. However, there is some evidence to support the superior pressure-relieving properties of an air-filled cushion over other pressure relief (Koo, Mak, and Lee, 1996; Shechtman et al, 2001).

Viscoelastic Fluid. A viscoelastic fluid is relatively stiff, yielding to small forces (Sprigle, Press, and Davis, 2001). The elastic component refers to the fluid's ability to store energy (Sprigle, Press, and Davis, 2001). The viscous property refers to the degree to which fluid molecules move across each other. A highly viscous fluid will not flow easily because the molecules do not easily slide across each other. A low-viscosity fluid or nonviscous fluid (such as water) will flow easily (Figure 6-25). High viscosity means

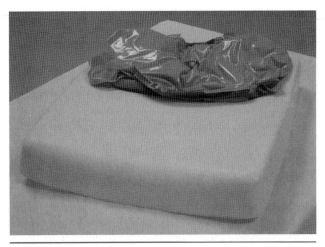

Figure 6-25   Example of viscoelastic fluid cushion, J Extreme.

that envelopment is poor and short- and long-term resilience is poor. These cushions have good dampening and thermal properties (they conduct heat away from the body) and provide a more stable base than does an air cushion. However, they are affected by temperature and will freeze in cold weather. In addition, some gels that are encased in a large bladder can shift, allowing the user to sit on the hard support surface. Cushions with this construction must be kneaded to ensure that the distribution of the gel is uniform to prevent contact with the support surface.

Alternating Pressure Cushions. Research (Kosiak, 1959; Reswick and Rogers, 1976) has documented a relationship between the amount of pressure applied and its duration and the development of pressure ulcers. In a study described earlier, it was found that the alternating pressure cushion was the only seating surface to intermittently bring pressures within the range of capillary blood pressure (Kosiak et al, 1958). All the cushions described thus far are static cushions, which have been designed on the premise that (1) they redistribute pressure over the sitting surface and (2) the individuals using them also need to follow through with pressure relief activities. Alternating pressure devices are designed on the basis that weight-bearing surfaces can tolerate high pressures for a time if alternated with increments of no pressure.

The principle of intermittent pressure relief is implemented in commercially available cushions by use of an oscillating pump to alternately inflate bellows arranged in rows (Hobson, 1990). Each individual elastomeric bellow (typical cushions have arrays of 48 arranged in eight rows of six) can be inflated individually or in groups. Generally, rows are inflated together. One approach couples every third row of the array of bellows. During operation, two of the coupled rows are inflated and one is deflated, which relieves pressure over one third of the seating surface; then the next third of the array is deflated, and so on. An alternative approach automatically cycles only the back four rows (out of eight total) under the ischial tuberosities. Each row is sequentially inflated and deflated to provide intermittent pressure relief to local tissue. These cushion systems use a recycling air pump powered by a battery to inflate the bellows. If the pressure pump should fail to operate in these systems (e.g., the battery becomes discharged), the cushion can still be used as an air-filled cushion. Because of the added weight, the need for recharging of the battery, and the cost, these seating devices have not been as widely distributed as other cushion types.

Hybrid Cushions. Hybrid cushions consist of a combination of the materials described above. The most typical combination is a closed-cell foam base with a membrane that contains gel, viscous fluid, or air that is placed on top or

inserted in a cutout. This method provides a combination of good envelopment, good thermal properties, pressure relief (because of the flotation materials), and good support and dynamic properties, which are provided by the foam base (Sprigle, 1992). The series of Jay cushions are commonly used hybrid cushions that consist of a combination of a standard-contoured, high-density foam base with a gel-filled pad that sits atop the foam base. The pad can be purchased in different configurations, such as an overfilled pad or pads with the gel sectioned off into quadrants, which prevents the pooling of gel into certain areas. The Cloud cushion from Ottobock *(www.ottobock.com)* (Figure 6-26) is an example of a hybrid cushion that has a foam and air-holding membrane that sits on top of a standard-contoured foam base. The overall properties of these types of cushions depend on the type of container and on the properties of the foam base.

Cushion Covers

Selection of a cover for a seat or back cushion can be as important as the determination of the material used to make the cushion because an improper cover can negate some of the benefits of that material. The cover selected should conform integrally to the cushion's contours, particularly in nonplanar systems. It should not interfere with the envelopment properties of the cushion nor add to shearing and friction. A cover that is too tight will prevent the client from sinking into the contours of the cushion. One that is too large will wrinkle, creating additional pressure points.

The ATP should know how the fabric handles moisture, either as a result of incontinence or perspiration. Most cushions will be used in hot, humid conditions for at least part of the year, so perspiration is an issue even when incontinence

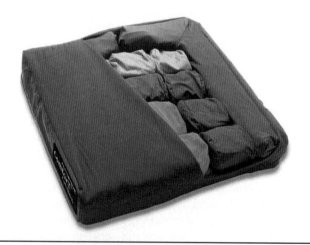

Figure 6-26 Example of a hybrid cushion. (Courtesy Otto Bock, www.ottobock.com.)

is not a concern. Many technical fabrics, blending Lycra and polyester, wick moisture away from the body, which is an important consideration when prevention of pressure ulcers is a goal. The cushion cover should be easy to remove and clean.

SEATING FOR PRESSURE DISTRIBUTION AND POSTURAL SUPPORT

Individuals who are at risk for development of pressure ulcers can benefit from proper positioning in the wheelchair as well. In fact, it is recommended that positioning be addressed first because postural alignment often results in changes in pressure distribution (Minkel, 1990). Through postural alignment, pressure can be distributed more evenly; postural deformities, such as pelvic obliquity, scoliosis, and kyphosis, can be prevented; back pain can be alleviated; and stability can be increased. These changes will influence the individual's mobility, energy expenditure, and function.

Many of the principles described regarding sitting posture and postural control apply to individuals at risk for pressure ulcer development as well. Some of the technologies for postural control are beneficial for persons with spinal cord injuries, and new technologies that specifically address the needs of this population have been developed. Some basic strategies for positioning for postural management for this population are described.

A cushion, without a firm base, placed in the seat will not totally eliminate the hammocking effect, and eventually the sling seat stretches further and the cushion conforms more to the sling. Simply installing a solid seat can minimize the hammocking effect of the sling upholstery. Solid seats can be made from a 3/8-inch sheet of plywood, or plastic seats can be purchased from many cushion manufacturers. Any of the cushions described earlier can then be placed on the solid seat. The upholstery back of the wheelchair does not provide lumbar support and promotes a sacral sitting position with kyphosis of the spine. The upholstery back can be replaced with a solid, contoured back that is commercially available (e.g., Varilite Evolution Back or J2 Back) (Figure 6-27 shows an example of a commercially available back) or custom made of foam. The seat back should be assessed for appropriate height and seat-to-back angle. It is recommended that the back be reclined approximately 15 degrees to help stabilize the trunk and prevent forward loss of balance. The back height is determined by the amount of support needed by the individual. Many persons with paraplegia have adequate trunk strength and wish to preserve mobility (particularly for sports), so they prefer lower backs on their wheelchairs and prefer not to use trunk-positioning components. Persons with C4, C5 quadriplegia, with less trunk control, can benefit from a higher seat back that supports all

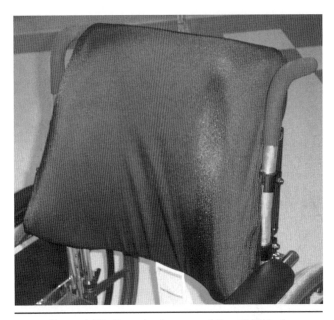

Figure 6-27   Example of a commercially available back.

or part of the scapulae, and those with C1 to C3 spared will require headrests.

Technologies to Enhance Sitting Comfort for Wheelchair Users

In a study that assessed the satisfaction of wheelchair users, comfort was rated as the most important variable for a wheelchair seating aid (Weiss-Lambrou et al, 1999). At the same time, comfort was rated as the least satisfying variable among these wheelchair users. The reasons stated for dissatisfaction related to comfort included seat cushions that caused pain and discomfort, fatigue, uncomfortable headrests and thoracic supports, sliding in wheelchair seat caused by discomfort, and poor posture as a result of unsuitable installation. Comfort is also related to the contact surface between the seating system and the person. For example, materials that provide good air exchange, maintain an even temperature, and control moisture are more likely to provide a comfortable sitting climate.

Wheelchair users who have discomfort and chronic pain need seating systems that allow them to relieve the discomfort and participate fully in activities of daily living. These needs are best addressed after a thorough mat assessment that identifies the user's most comfortable seated position and the combination of technologies identified above that best addresses comfort needs. (Mobility technologies that provide users with the ability to adjust their positions in the wheelchair will be discussed in Chapter 12).

Technologies That Increase Ease of Sitting for the Elderly

People are living longer, which means that the number of well elderly and those in need of supervised care is growing considerably. As an individual ages, mobility may be reduced as a result of acute illnesses or trauma, such as stroke, hip fracture, or progressive conditions such as arthritis. Consequently, it is likely that the amount of time the individual spends sitting increases. The goal of seating in this category depends on the individual's needs and skills, as it does for the other categories. Just as there is a range of needs for the elderly population, there is also a range of seating technologies. Seating technologies for the aging population can be matched to the level of functional mobility the individual has: (1) ambulatory (2) mobile, nonambulatory, and (3) dependent mobile (Fernie and Letts, 1991). Chairs are needed that promote comfort, safety, ease of ingress and egress, and propulsion if necessary.

■ SUMMARY

This chapter has shown the potential outcomes that can be achieved through seating in three primary areas of need: postural control, tissue integrity, and comfort. Procedures for evaluation and matching of device characteristics to the individual's needs were presented. Basic principles of biomechanics frequently used in seating and positioning were discussed. Different types of seating technologies and cushion classifications were described, along with their application to the three primary goals of seating.

Study Questions

1. Describe the three primary goals of seating intervention. What are the key elements of a mat assessment? Describe each of these.
2. Describe three additional factors that the ATP should consider when designing a seating system.
3. Describe the influence of the physical, sociocultural, and institutional contexts on design of a seating system.
4. What are the three types of force? Why are they relevant to seating and positioning?
5. What is meant by the *center of pressure,* and how does it relate to seating and positioning systems?
6. Describe the basic premises underlying seating intervention for postural control.
7. Why is the pelvis the starting point when seating for postural control? Describe the major approaches used to obtain alignment and control of the pelvis.
8. Describe the three spinal deformities that may occur.
9. List three methods used to support the trunk in postural control seating systems, and describe when each method is indicated.
10. Describe how the head can be positioned posteriorly, anteriorly, and laterally. What factors lead to the use of each of these?
11. What is the major cause of pressure ulcer development? What are other factors that contribute to the development of pressure ulcers?
12. Define hysteresis and creep. Describe how each of these affects the reliability of pressure map measurements.
13. Describe Swaine's pressure mapping protocol. Describe the output of pressure mapping systems. Discuss two controversial aspects of pressure measurement.
14. What is a honeycomb cushion? What advantages does it have over other approaches?
15. How do viscoelastic fluid-filled and foam cushions differ? List an advantage and disadvantage of each.
16. What are the primary populations for whom comfort is the major goal in developing a seating system?
17. Identify the reasons why there are limited technologies available for populations for whom comfort is the major goal.

References

Bennett L et al: Shear vs pressure as causative factors in skin blood flow occlusion, *Arch Phys Med Rehabil* 60:309-314, 1979.

Berecek KH: Etiology of decubitus ulcers. In Horsley JA, editor: *Preventing decubitus ulcers,* New York, 1981, Grune & Stratton.

Bergen AF, Presperin J, Tallman T: *Positioning for function: wheelchairs and other assistive technologies,* Valhalla, NY, 1990, Valhalla Rehabilitation Publications.

Bergen AF, Presperin J, Tallman T: Planning intervention, *Team Rehabil Rep* 3:38-41, 1992.

Bergstrom N et al: The Braden Scale for Predicting Pressure Sore Risk, *Nurs Res* 36:205-210, 1987.

Bertenthal B, Von Hofsten C: Eye, head and trunk control: the foundation of manual development, *Neurosci Biobehav Rev* 22:515-520, 1998.

Bouten CV et al: The etiology of pressure ulcers: skin deep or muscle bound? *Arch Phys Med Rehabil* 84:616-619, 2003.

Breslow R: Nutritional status and dietary intake of patients with pressure ulcers: review of the research literature 1943 to 1989, *Decubitus* 4:16-21, 1991.

Brienza D et al: A randomized control trial to evaluate pressure-reducing seat cushions for elderly wheelchair users. *Adv Skin and Wound Care* 14: 120-129, 2001.

Cailliet R: *Scoliosis: Diagnosis and management,* Philadelphia, 1975, FA Davis.

Chen Y, DeVivo MJ, Jackson AB: Pressure ulcer prevalence in people with spinal cord injury: Age-period-duration effects, *Arch Phys Med Rehabil* 86:1208-1213, 2005.

Conine T et al: Pressure ulcer prophylaxis in elderly patients using polyurethane foam or Jay wheelchair cushions, *Int J Rehabil Res* 17:123-137, 1994.

Constantian MB: Etiology: Gross effects of pressure. In Constantian MB, editor: *Pressure ulcers: principles and techniques of management,* Boston, 1980, Little, Brown.

DeLateur BJ et al: Wheelchair cushions designed to prevent pressure sores: an evaluation, *Arch Phys Med Rehabil* 57:129-135, 1976.

Dinsdale SM: Decubitus ulcers: role of pressure and friction in causation, *Arch Phys Med Rehabil* 55:147-152, 1974.

Dunk N, Callaghan J: Gender-based differences in postural responses to seated exposures, *Clin Biomech* 20:1101-1110, 2005.

Ferguson-Pell M, Cardi M: Prototype development and comparative evaluation of wheelchair pressure mapping system, *Assist Tech* 5:78-91, 1993.

Ferguson-Pell MW et al: A knowledge-based program for pressure sore prevention, *Ann N Y Acad Sci,* 463:284-286, 1986.

Fernie G, Letts RM: Seating the elderly. In Letts RM, editor: *Principles of seating the disabled,* Boca Raton, FL, 1991, CRC Press.

Fisher SV et al: Wheelchair cushion effect on skin temperature, *Arch Phys Med Rehabil* 59:68-72, 1978.

Garber SL, Krouskop TA, Carter RE: A system for clinically evaluating wheelchair pressure-relief cushions, *Am J Occup Ther* 32:565-570, 1978.

Geyer MJ et al: Wheelchair seating: a state of the science report, *Assist Tech* 15:120-128, 2003.

Hadcock L et al: Pressure measurement applications for humans, *Proceedings of Association of Canadian Ergonomists Conference,* August 2003, London, Ontario.

Hadders-Algra M, Brogren E, Forssberg H: Development of postural control—differences between ventral and dorsal muscles? *Neurosci Biobehav Rev* 22:501-506, 1998.

Hadders-Algra M et al: Development of postural adjustments during reaching in infants with CP, *Dev Med Child Neurol* 41:766-776, 1999.

Hobson DA: Contributions of posture and deformity to the body-seat interface variables of a person with spinal cord injury, *Proceedings of the Fifth International Seating Symposium,* pp. 153-171, February 1989, Memphis, Tenn.

Hobson DA: Seating and mobility for the severely disabled. In Smith RV, Leslie JH, editors: *Rehabilitation engineering,* Boca Raton, FL, 1990, CRC Press.

Hobson DA, Crane B: State of the science white paper on wheelchair seating comfort, February 2001: www.rerc.pitt.edu/RERC_PDF/Comfort.pdf. Accessed March 16, 2005.

Kangas KM: Creating mobility within mobility systems, *Rehab Manag* 13:58-60, 62, 2000: http://www.rehabpub.com/trehab/672000/3.asp. Accessed October 11, 2006.

Koo TKK, Mak AFT, Lee YL: Posture effect on seating interface biomechanics: comparison between two seating cushions, *Arch Phys Med Rehabil* 77: 40-47, 1996.

Kosiak M: Etiology and pathology of ischemic ulcers, *Arch Phys Med Rehabil* 40:6262-6269, 1959.

Kosiak M: Etiology of decubitus ulcers, *Arch Phys Med Rehabil* 42:19-29, 1961.

Kosiak M et al: Evaluation of pressure as a factor in the production of ischial ulcers, *Arch Phys Med Rehabil* 39:623-629, 1958.

Krause JS et al: An exploratory study of pressure ulcers after SCI: Relationship to protective behaviours and risk factors, *Arch Phys Med Rehabil* 82:107-113, 2001.

Krouskop TA et al: The effectiveness of preventive management in reducing the occurrence of pressure sores, *J Rehabil Res Dev* 20:74-83, 1983.

Lander-Ganz E, Gefen A: Mechanical compression-induced pressure sores in rat hindlimb: muscle stiffness, histology and compression models, *J Appl Physiol* 96:2034-2049, 2004.

Landis EM: Micro-injection studies of capillary blood pressure in human skin, *Heart* 15:209-228, 1930.

Law M et al: *Canadian Occupational Performance Measure,* ed 3, Toronto, 1997, CAOT Publications ACE.

Lemaire et al: Clinical analysis of a CAD/CAM system for custom seating: A comparison of hand-sculpting methods, *J Rehabil Res Dev* 33:311-320, 1996.

Letts RM, editor: *Principles of seating the disabled,* Boca Raton, Fla, 1991, CRC Press.

Low J, Reed D; *Basic biomechanics explained,* Oxford, 1996, Butterworth Heinemann.

Mayall JK, Desharnais G: *Positioning in a wheelchair: a guide for professional caregivers of the disabled adult,* Thorofare, NJ, 1995, SLACK.

McDonald, H: Preventing pressure ulcers, *Rehab Manag* 14:40, 42-46, 2001.

Miller WC, Mortenson B, Garden J: The WhOM: a client specific outcome measure of wheelchair intervention, *Proceedings of the Twenty-Second International Seating Symposium,* p. 65-68, March 2006, Vancouver, British Columbia.

Miller Polgar J et al: Comparison of occupational performance between two methods of pelvic stabilization, *Proceedings of the Tri-Joint Congress,* June 2000, Toronto, Ontario.

Mills T et al: Development and consumer validation of the functional evaluation in a wheelchair (FEW) instrument, *Dis Rehabil* 24:38-46, 2002.

Minkel JL: Seating SCI clients, *Proceedings of the Sixth Northeast RESNA Regional Conference*, 1990, RESNA, Washington, DC.

National Pressure Ulcer Advisory Panel: Statement on pressure ulcer prevention, 1992: www.npuap.org/positn1.htm. Accessed October 10, 2006.

Norton D, McLaren R, Exton-Smith AN: *An investigation of geriatric nursing problems in hospital,* London, 1975, Churchill Livingstone. (Original work published in 1962.)

Pape TL-B, Kim J, Weiner B: The shaping of individual meanings assigned to AT: A review of personal factors, *Disabil Rehabil* 24:5-20, 2002.

Parkinson MB, Chaffin DB, Reed MP: Center of pressure excursion capability in performance of seated lateral-reaching tasks. *Clin Biomechan* 21:26-32, 2006.

Patterson R et al: The physiological response to repeated surface pressure loads in the able bodied and spinal cord injured, *Proceedings of the RESNA International 92 Conference,* pp. 205-206, June 1992, Toronto, Ontario.

Pfeffer J: The cause of pressure sores. In Webster JG, editor: *Prevention of pressure sores,* Bristol, United Kingdom, 1991, IOP Publishing.

Reichel SM: Shearing force as a factor in decubitus ulcers in paraplegics, *JAMA* 762-763, February 15, 1958.

Reswick JB, Rogers JE: Experience at Rancho Los Amigos Hospital with devices and techniques to prevent pressure sores. In Kenedi RM, Cowden JM, Scales JT, editors: *Bedsore biomechanics,* Baltimore, 1976, University Park Press.

Rigby P et al: Effects of a wheelchair-mounted rigid pelvic stabilizer on caregiver assistance for children. *Assist Technol* 13:2-11, 2001.

Savelsbergh GJP, Van der Kamp J: The effect of body orientation to gravity on early infant reaching, *J Exp Child Psychol* 8:510-528, 1994.

Shechtman O et al: Comparing wheelchair cushions for effectiveness of pressure relief: a pilot study, *Occup Ther J Res* 21:29-48, 2001.

Sprigle S: The match game, *Team Rehabil Rep* 3:20-21, 1992.

Sprigle S: Effects of forces and the selection of support surfaces, *Top Geriatr Rehabil* 16:47-62, 2000.

Sprigle S, Press L, Davis K:, Development of uniform terminology and procedures to describe wheelchair cushion characteristics, *J Rehabil Res Dev* 38:449-461, 2001.

Stekelenburg CWJ et al: Compression-induced deep tissue injury examined with magnetic resonance imaging and histology, *J Appl Physiol* 100:1946-1954, 2006.

Stewart SFC, Palmieri BS, Cochran GVB: Wheelchair cushion effect on skin temperature, heat flux, and relative humidity, *Arch Phys Med Rehabil* 61:229-233, 1980.

Stinson M, Porter A, Eakin P: Measuring interface pressure: a laboratory-based investigation into the effects of repositioning on sitting time, *Am J Occup Ther* 56:185-90, 2002.

Swaine J: Seeing the difference, *Rehab Manag:* www.rehabpub/features/112003/4.asp. Accessed October 31, 2006.

Tang S: Seat cushions. In Webster JG, editor: *Prevention of pressure sores,* Bristol, United Kingdom, 1991, IOP Publishing.

Torrance C: Pressure sores: aetiology, treatment and prevention, London, 1983, Croom Helm.

Tredwell S, Roxborough L: Cerebral palsy seating. In Letts RM, editor: *Principles of seating the disabled,* Boca Raton, FL, 1991, CRC Press.

Trefler E, Hobson DA, Taylor SJ: *Seating and mobility for persons with physical disabilities,* Tucson, 1993, Therapy Skill Builders.

Weiss-Lambrou R et al: Wheelchair seating aids: how satisfied are consumers? *Assist Technol* 11:43-52, 1999.

Whimster IW: The trophic effects of nerves on skin. In Kenedi RM, Cowden JM, Scales JT, editors: *Bedsore biomechanics,* Baltimore, 1976, University Park Press.

Zacharkow D: *Wheelchair posture and pressure sores,* Springfield, IL, 1984, Charles C Thomas.

Zacharkow D: Posture, sitting, standing, chair design and exercise, Springfield, IL, 1988, Charles C Thomas.

CHAPTER 7

Human/Assistive Technology Interface

Chapter Outline

DEVELOPMENT OF MOTOR SKILLS FOR USE
OF CONTROL INTERFACES

OUTPUT COMPONENT OF THE HUMAN
TECHNOLOGY INTERFACE
Speech Output

Digital Recording
Speech Synthesis

SUMMARY

Learning Objectives

On completing this chapter, you will be able to do the following:

1. Describe the elements of the human/technology interface and its role within the assistive technology component of the human activity assistive technology model
2. Describe the characteristics of control interfaces
3. Identify and define the basic selection methods
4. Describe the means by which the user's physical control can be enhanced
5. Discuss a framework for control interface decision making
6. Identify technologies for direct selection
7. Identify technologies for indirect selection
8. Discuss the outcomes that can be achieved through implementation of a motor training program and how technology can be used to improve motor response
9. Describe the computer user interface
10. List the major components of a computer system and give the function of each component
11. Describe the major approaches to keyboard and mouse emulation
12. Describe the major approaches to electronic speech generation used in assistive technologies

Key Terms

Abbreviation Expansion
Acceptance Time
Accessibility Options
Activation Characteristics
Automatic Scanning
Circular Scanning
Coded Access
Command Domain
Concept Keyboards
Continuous Input
Control Enhancers
Control Interface
Digital Recording
Direct Selection
Directed Scanning
Discrete Inputs
Distributed Controls

Easy Access
Emulation
General Input Device–Emulating
  Interface
Graphical User Interface
Group-Item Scanning
Indirect Selection
Input Domain
Integrated Control
Inverse Scanning
Linear Scan
Multitasking
On-Screen Keyboard
Parallel Port
Prosodic Features
Rate Enhancement
Rotary Scanning

Row-Column Scanning
Scanning
Selection Methods
Selection Set
Sensory Characteristics
Serial Port
Spatial Characteristics
Speech Synthesis
Step Scanning
Text-To-Speech Programs
Transparent Access
Universal Access
USB Port
Word Completion
Word Prediction

The human/technology interface is a major part of the assistive technology component of the human activity assistive technology model. Bailey (1996, p. 173) defines an interface as "the boundary shared by interacting components in a system" in which "the essence of this interaction is communication or the exchange of information back and forth across the boundary." The human/technology interface is the boundary between the human and the assistive technology across which information is exchanged. This exchange of information is bidirectional and includes both the interface from the person to the device used to control the assistive device and the interface that provides feedback regarding the device's operation from the device to the person.

The exchange of information in the form of input to operate the device takes place by way of a control interface between the user and the device. It may vary from someone who needs an enlarged light switch to turn a light off and on to someone who needs to access a portable communication system with a single switch to someone who needs to control a power wheelchair with a joystick. The exchange of information from the device to the person takes place through a visual or auditory display. These displays, which have an important role in providing feedback to the user, are also considered a component of the human/technology interface. The role of displays in specific assistive technology applications is discussed in subsequent chapters. Alternative displays for people with visual or auditory impairments are discussed in Chapters 8 and 9, respectively.

In this chapter we discuss the various control interfaces, their characteristics, the control methods that provide the link between the person with a disability and the device being controlled, and the use of electronically generated speech as an output for assistive technologies. A framework for matching control interfaces, control methods, and enhancement techniques to the user's needs and skills is also presented.

▧ ELEMENTS OF THE HUMAN/ TECHNOLOGY INTERFACE

The human/technology interface is more than just a piece of hardware with inputs into the device. There are actually *three* elements of the human/technology interface that contribute to the operation of a device: the control interface, the selection set, and the selection method. These three elements are interrelated, and careful attention must be given to each element to have an effective human/technology interface.

Control Interface

The **control interface** (e.g., keyboard, joystick) is the hardware by which the human in the assistive technology system operates or controls a device. It is sometimes also referred to as an *input device*. The control interface generates from one to an infinite number of independent inputs, or signals, defined as the **input domain** (Morasso et al, 1979). The input domain may be either discrete or continuous.

A control interface with **discrete inputs** is one in which each location has a fixed value representing a distinct result with no intermediate steps. For discrete interfaces, the size of the input domain is equal to the total number of targets available to the user. For example, a computer keyboard may have more than 100 keys, each representing a different letter

or symbol, which is the signal that is sent to the processor. Although a single switch has only one signal in its input domain, a dual switch has two signals. With a **continuous input** interface the inputs are continuous, with an infinite number of values. Interfaces that are continuous either vary in quantity along a range, as with a volume control, or maintain an even quantity while providing a continuous input, such as driving straight ahead using a steering wheel to make small adjustments. A proportional joystick and a computer mouse both have a continuous input domain in which there can be an infinite number of possible input signals.

Selection Set

The **selection set** is the items available from which choices are made (Lee and Thomas, 1990). Selection sets can be represented by traditional orthography (e.g., written letters, words, and sentences), symbols used to represent ideas, computer icons, line drawings or pictures, or synthetic speech. The modalities in which the selection set is presented can be visual (e.g., letters on the keyboard), tactile (e.g., Braille), or auditory (e.g., spoken choices in auditory scanning).

The size, modality, and type of selection set chosen are based on the user's needs and the desired *activity output*. Electronic aids to daily living (EADL) or a power wheelchair typically have fewer items in the selection set than an augmentative communication device. The size may also vary according to the user's skills. For example, an individual who spells and has good physical control has the skills to use the selection set of a standard keyboard, which consists of all the letters and function keys. Another individual who is working on developing language and communication skills may have a selection set consisting of only two picture symbol choices displayed on a lap tray. Selection sets are discussed further in Chapter 11.

Selection Methods

There are two basic methods in which the user makes selections by use of the control interface: direct selection and indirect selection. We refer to these as **selection methods.** Currently used indirect selection methods include scanning, directed scanning, and coded access.

Direct Selection.   With **direct selection** the individual is able to use the control interface to randomly choose any of the items in the selection set. The consumer indicates his choice by using voice, finger, hand, eye, or other body movement. In this method of selection the user identifies a target and goes directly to it (Smith, 1991). At any one time, all the elements of the selection set are equally available for selecting; that is, they are not time dependent. Typing on a keyboard or even picking a flower from the garden is considered direct selection. Physically, direct selection requires refined,

Direct Selection

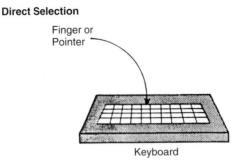

Figure 7-1 Input required to obtain the letter *S* with use of direct selection. (From Smith RO: Technological approaches to performance enhancement. In Christiansen C, Baum C, editors: *Occupational therapy: overcoming human performance deficits,* Thorofare, NJ, 1991, Slack.)

Input	Output
Press S	S

controlled movements and it is the more difficult of the two methods. Cognitively, there is an immediate, direct result from the selection made; therefore, direct selection is more intuitive and easier to use. Figure 7-1 shows the input that is made by using direct selection to obtain the letter *S*. The various types of control interfaces that allow the individual to use direct selection are described in the section on selecting a control interface for a user.

Indirect Selection. With **indirect selection,** intermediate steps are involved in making a selection. The most common indirect selection method is scanning. With **scanning,** the selection set is presented on a display and is sequentially scanned by a cursor or light on the device. When the particular element that the individual wishes to select is presented, a signal is generated by the user. With an assistive device, the control interface used for scanning is a single switch or an array of two or more switches. Depending on the needs of the user, scanning can vary in the format used for the selection set and in the manner in which the control interface is used to make the selection. These various techniques are discussed later in this chapter.

Scanning and direct selection require different physical and cognitive skills. Scanning requires good visual tracking skills, a high degree of attention, and the ability to sequence. The advantage of scanning is that it requires very little motor control to make a selection. Ratcliff (1994) measured speed and accuracy in a four-level direction-following task carried out by children in grades 1 through 5 who were using scanning and direct selection. She found that subjects using direct selection made significantly more errors than those using scanning across all grade and difficulty levels. Overall error rates decreased with increasing grade level. Significant differences were also noted between second and third graders and between fourth and fifth graders at the second difficulty level. No other grade or difficulty level differences were statistically significant. Reasons cited for the differences in selection method error rates include the dependence on visual perceptual skills,

memory, and the vigilance and attention (necessity to wait for the desired selection) in scanning. Scanning is also more complex cognitively than direct selection because there are additional steps imposed between the user's action (e.g., hitting a switch or key) and the resulting input. Ratcliff concludes that scanning is a more difficult task than direct selection even for nondisabled children, which has implications for electronic assistive device application.

Because scanning is inherently slow, there have been a number of approaches used to make it more efficient and faster for the user. Some of these involve the location of letters, word completion and prediction, and other text-based approaches. These are discussed in Chapter 11. However, many of these approaches can actually slow down the scanning because they require a larger amount of concentration by the user. An alternative approach is to automatically adjust the scanning rate (reduce the delay between rows, columns, and entries) and maximize the rate for an individual user (Simpson and Koester, 1999). This approach uses a known text passage in which the user enters that passage at as fast a scan rate as possible. If the number of errors increases, the scan delay is increased (rate decreased) by use of a Bayesian probabilistic model. Simpson and Koseter found that, for non-disabled users, the automatic adaptation of scan rate had the potential to increase rate of text entry without the addition of task complexity that occurs in text-based methods.

Directed scanning is a hybrid approach in which the user activates the control interface to select the direction of the scan, vertical or horizontal. Then the device scans the selection set sequentially. When the desired choice is reached, the user sends a signal to the *processor* to make the selection. This signal is generated either by pausing at the choice, an **acceptance time,** or by activating another control interface to indicate the choice. In directed scanning, both the type of movement made and the point when the movement is made contribute to the selection (Vanderheiden, 1984). A joystick or an array of switches (two to eight switches) are the control interfaces used with directed scanning. Figure 7-2 gives

Directed Scanning

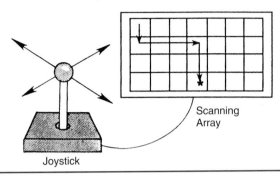

Input	Output
Move Joystick:	S
Down	
Right	
Right	
Right	
Down	

Figure 7-2 Directed scanning showing input required to select the letter *S*. The user selects the direction of the scan, and the items in the selection set are scanned sequentially by the device. When the desired item is reached, the user makes the selection. (From Smith RO: Technological approaches to performance enhancement. In Christiansen C, Baum C, editors: *Occupational therapy: overcoming human performance deficits*, Thorofare, NJ, 1991, Slack.)

an example of the input required to select the letter *S* using directed scanning with a four-position joystick.

Directed scanning requires more steps than direct selection but fewer steps than single-switch scanning. The user needs to be able to activate and hold the control interface and to release it at the appropriate time. If the individual can produce the movements required to use this method, the outcome is faster entry of the desired selections into the device.

Another form of indirect selection is **coded access.** In coded access the individual uses a distinct sequence of movements to input a code for each item in the selection set. Like the other two methods of indirect selection, intermediate steps are required for making a selection. The control interface is a single switch or an array of switches configured to match the code. Morse code is one example of coded access, wherein the selection set is the alphabet but an intermediate step is necessary to obtain a letter. Morse code was developed to be very efficient by assigning the most frequently used letters the shortest codes. This efficiency can be useful in written or conversational communication. In addition, Morse code does not require that a selection set be displayed. The codes are usually memorized, although visual displays, diagrams, or charts can be used to aid in recalling the codes. Morse code and other coded access methods are described in greater detail later in this chapter.

Like scanning, coded access requires less physical skill than direct selection. The advantage of coded access over scanning, however, is that the timing of the input is under the control of the user and is not dependent on the device. The disadvantage is that it takes more cognitive skill, especially memory and sequencing, than direct selection does.

Most current devices can be accessed by more than one type of control interface and selection method. The selection set on most devices can also be varied to match the user's needs. From a manufacturing perspective, versatility of a device allows it to be applicable to a wider population, which

helps to contain the cost of the device and makes it possible to adapt to changing user needs and skills.

The Processor: Connecting the Human/ Technology Interface to the Activity Output

When the user activates the control interface, information is sent via a signal to the *processor.* The processor interprets the information and generates two signals that are converted to (1) feedback to any display that is being used and (2) an activity output, depending on the functions of the assistive technology system. The set of device functions is referred to as the **command domain** (Morasso et al., 1979). For example, the command domain of a joystick on a power wheelchair is typically configured so that the signal for the UP input is transformed into forward movement of the wheelchair, DOWN into reverse movement, LEFT into movement to the left, and RIGHT into movement to the right. That same joystick can be used to control a television set in which the same input domain of UP, DOWN, LEFT, and RIGHT becomes a command domain of television volume up, volume down, channel up, channel down. In an electric feeder the command domain includes lifting up the spoon, rotating the plate, and putting the spoon back down. In a communication device the command domain is the meaning assigned to each input selection, including functions such as print and speak.

For every element in the command domain there must be a corresponding element in the *selection set.* The selection set is presented to the user by the selection method. For example, with direct selection each item in the selection set is labeled on the target itself. In direct selection the size of the input domain (number of independent signals) is equal to the size of the command domain. With indirect selection, the input domain has fewer signals than the number of elements in the command domain. With scanning, each item in the selection set is presented sequentially by the device. Thus we can see how the selection method connects the human/technology interface to the command domain of the processor.

Keyboard- and Mouse-Emulating Interfaces.   Many computer adaptations are mandated by the legislation described in Chapter 1 (e.g., Public Law 508). The best approach to adapting a computer for use by individuals with physical limitations is to begin with the simplest modifications designed for the most minimal of physical limitations on the part of the user. We can then progress to more complex adaptations designed to accommodate even the most severely limited potential user. **Transparent access** is essential for effective access. This term describes two fundamental concepts: (1) 100% of the functions of the computer must be adapted if the user who has a disability is to have full access and (2) all application software that runs on the unmodified computer must also run on the adapted computer. All the keyboard keys, including modifier (e.g., shift, control, alt) and special function keys, and all the mouse functions, such as point, click, and drag, must be available on the adapted input system. If a program (e.g., word processor) works with the standard computer, then it should work with the adaptations. The adaptations also have to be consistent with the operating system of the computer and the hardware configuration (e.g., Windows).

There must be a bridge between the control interface and the computer to use many of the alternatives to keyboard or mouse, such as an expanded keyboard or a single switch, to access a computer. Sometimes this bridge is built into the control interface and other times it is separate. Because the control interface itself is only a switch (or set of switches in a keyboard), pressing a switch or key does not generate any meaningful information for the computer or other assistive device. To make the information meaningful, a *decoder* must be used (Anson, 1997). In the 1980s and 1990s the Trace Center at the University of Wisconsin developed a standard for **general input device–emulating interfaces,** or GIDEIs. The GIDEI standard defines the characteristics of a special-purpose processor that translates (i.e., decodes) the signals from the control interface so they match the command domain requirements of the computer. For example, if the computer application requires the use of ESC or DEL keys, then the input device must provide a way for the control interface to generate these key commands. For older devices, the decoding was accomplished through software in the computer, or an additional hardware component (the GIDEI). With the development of the USB standard, particularly the human interface device (HID) component, nearly all of the functions previously developed requiring a special-purpose GIDEI can now be accomplished through the USB interface (Novak and Olsen, 2001). The decoding previously carried out by the GIDEI is built into the control interface (particularly keyboards) and supplied to the computer through the USB port. An additional advantage of the USB port is that it supplies power to the external device from the computer, which eliminates the necessity for an external power source for USB input devices and is especially valuable for assistive technology applications based on portable computers. Additional software may need to be loaded into the computer to allow customization of the control interface selection setup (discussed later in this chapter). There are, however, challenges involved in using the USB HID standard, and these can result in incompatibilities between assistive technology devices and between the device and the host computer (Vanderheiden and Zimmermann, 2002). The existing USB HID standard provides definitions for common human input devices such as keyboards, mouse pointers, joysticks, and game pads. However, it does not currently have a definition specifically for assistive technology input devices. So, assistive technology products must still emulate one of the defined devices (such as a keyboard or mouse) to provide the specialized input. There are no general standards defined to do this for assistive technology developers to follow, which has resulted in different manufacturers using the USB HID in different ways. This has resulted in incompatibilities between assistive technology products and confusion for the end users. The development of an assistive technology definition for the USB HID standard has been proposed to address the issue of incompatibility. There are no general standards for assistive technology applications, and different manufacturers implement the HID standard in different ways. The development of an assistive technology definition for the USB standard has been proposed to address the issue of incompatibility (Marsden, 2005).

Emulating interfaces have a general set of characteristics that allow the computer to be altered for a given application and for a specific person with a disability. Commercial products may be implemented with features that include some or all of these general characteristics, and specific commercial features can change rapidly. The characteristics of an emulating interface are customized through a *setup,* a concept that originated with the adaptive firmware card (AFC) for the Apple II series of computers (Schwejda and Vanderheiden, 1982). As shown in Box 7-1, a setup consists of three basic elements: (1) an input method, (2) overlays, and (3) a set of options. The features of the setup may be implemented in hardware (electronic circuits) or software (a program) or both. Storage of a setup may be in memory within the emulator hardware or resident in the computer memory. Setups are also usually stored on the computer hard disk drive or in the peripheral device (e.g., an alternative keyboard), which allows them to be loaded into the computer or the emulator as needed. As shown in Box 7-1, the setup is used with an *application* program.

Several examples of setups that may be used with different application programs are shown in Figure 7-3. The setup shown in Figure 7-3, *A,* is intended to be used for text entry

BOX 7-1 Major Features of Commonly Used General Input Device-Emulating Interfaces

A setup consists of the following three parts:

1. Input method
   Keyboard:
   - Assisted
   - Contracted
   - Expanded
   - Virtual
   - Normal

   Morse code:
   - One switch
   - Two switch

   ASCII*:
   - Parallel
   - Serial

   Scanning:
   - Linear or row-column
   - Auto, inverse, or step
   - Single-, dual-, four-, or five switch
   - Switched joystick

   Proportional:
   - Mouse
   - Trackball
   - Joystick

2. Overlay: all three of the following may be the same or they may be different

   User: the selection set arrangement from which the user chooses

   Computer: the character or string of characters sent to the application program when the user chooses

   Speech: synthetic speech used as a prompt to the user or as feedback when a selection is made

3. Options
   Abbreviations: text-based codes
   Autocaps: CAP and 2 spaces after., !, or ?
   Key repeat rate
   Levels: like a shift, can be many levels on one setup; equivalent in scanning is branching
   Macros: codes can include control characters and functions
   Mouse emulation: move, drag, click, and tab
   Multitasking: can interrupt one mode for another
   Predictive entry: previous characters determine user overlay
   Rate: how fast or slow the user can input to the GIDEI
   Screen selection display location: where on the screen the user overlay appears
   Slowdown of programs

   Application program or disk:
   The business, education, or recreational program being used

*Sometimes used with AAC, environmental control units, or powered wheelchair controllers (see text).

	Method	Overlay	Options	Application
A	Virtual keyboard	User: QWERTY Layout Computer: Same Speech: No	Speed of mouse • •	Business, productivity software (word processing, spreadsheet, etc.)
B	Single-switch scanning	User: ETA Array Computer: Same Speech: No	Rate • •	
C	Expanded keyboard	User: [➡] [STOP] Computer: Arrow, Return Speech: "This one," "Next one"	Speech Slowdown • •	Early education matching task with arrow and return
D	Single-switch scanning	User: [--->] [OK] Computer: Arrow, Return Speech: "This one," "Next one"	Rate Speech Slowdown	

Figure 7-3 A GIDEI setup consists of three parts: input method, overlay, and options. **A** to **D**, Four examples of GIDEI setups for different consumers and different applications are shown.

in a business environment. The application software can be a word processor, a spreadsheet, or a database. The major function is the entry of text characters, and the setup includes several options to make this process more efficient. Autocapitalization automatically enters one space and latches the shift function after sentence-ending punctuation (i.e., .?!). Abbreviations allow a few characters to be used as a code for a longer word or phrase. The user of the emulator stores both the sequence of characters and their corresponding abbreviation. When the abbreviation (code) is entered, the emulator automatically expands it into the whole stored word or phrase. For example, typing the two letters *MN* (for "my name") followed by an abbreviation key would result in the user's name and address being entered. Several methods of abbreviation expansion and other types of rate enhancement are discussed in Chapter 11. The setup also includes *macros*, which are codes similar to abbreviations. The macros differ, however, in that they are often used to control application program functions. For example, assume that the word processor requires that the following keys be pressed to set a margin (such as for typing an address on an envelope): SHIFT F8 (shifted function key number 8) 174 ENTER, a total of 6 keystrokes (if SHIFT and F8 are pressed in sequence). A macro for this key sequence could be defined as [ALT]E. This would save four keystrokes (if the ALT key and E were pressed in sequence), and it would also be easier to remember these two keys than the entire key sequence. It is also possible to store mouse functions and "replay" them with one command. Another way to save keystrokes is for the computer to anticipate the words on the basis of previous characters entered. For example, if a *T* is typed, then an *H* is very likely to follow. Likewise, it is possible to predict whole words rather than just letters. This method of input acceleration is called *word prediction* or *word completion*. In some cases the emulator software program keeps track of the words that the user inputs most frequently, and the choices presented is in the order of frequency of use for the specific person using the emulator. We discuss word prediction further later in this chapter. Many of these options are available for both the Windows (see *www.microsoft.com/enable/default.aspx*) and Macintosh (see *http://www.apple.com/accessibility/*) operating systems. Additional information is also available from the manufacturers' Web sites listed here.

This set of options can be used with any of the input methods shown in Box 7-1. The particular input method determines the overlays. The term **on-screen keyboard** refers to those keyboard emulation methods that use a video image of the keyboard on the video screen, together with a cursor. An example is shown in Figure 7-3, *A.* The display of the keyboard layout on the screen can contain key locations for use as macros and it can be arranged to make selections as fast as possible. For a single-switch user, the overlay on the screen may be a scanning array with special characters included, as shown in Figure 7-3, *B.*

A second setup, shown in Figure 7-3, *C* and *D,* is for a young child who is using any of a wide range of software programs that require selection of an answer by matching a cursor (pointer) location with the correct item (Figure 7-4). The task may be to match numbers, letters, shapes, words, or pictures. Often the software requires that one key (e.g., RIGHT ARROW) be used to move the cursor and another key (e.g., RETURN) to select the one that the student believes is correct. Two setups are shown in Figure 7-3 for this application. In this case the user and computer overlays are different, so a speech overlay is also included. Because the user is not likely to have learned to read yet, the speech overlay helps identify the choices to be made. Speech is used as a reinforcer when the choice is made, which is shown as a second speech overlay in Figure 7-3, *C.* This setup is for use with an expanded keyboard. In this case a visual overlay with symbols can be used. An example is shown in Figure 7-5. Another overlay, Figure 7-3, *D,* shows the use of scanning on the screen, which is restricted to text characters. For example, an arrow can be generated with two dashes and the greater than (>) sign. "OK" is used as the label for "this is the one I want" (the student's choice). Both these setups use the speech, scanning rate, and program slow-down options. However, for the second setup (scanning), an option that allows us to place the scanning array on any line of the display monitor is also included. This option is important because the scan line can hide part of the program if it is in a fixed location.

Many USB-based input devices allow other features, such as mouse **emulation** and the use of macro instructions and **multitasking.** Mouse emulation substitutes a set of keys, a scanning array, or Morse code characters for mouse functions (similar to MouseKeys, Table 7-1). Macros can be used to return the mouse cursor to a specific location on the basis of stored information. This feature can save time when

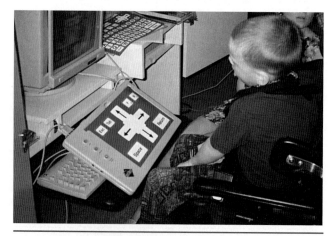

Figure 7-4   A GIDEI overlay for cursor-controlling movement by using arrows. This is being used with an expanded keyboard and an educational software program.

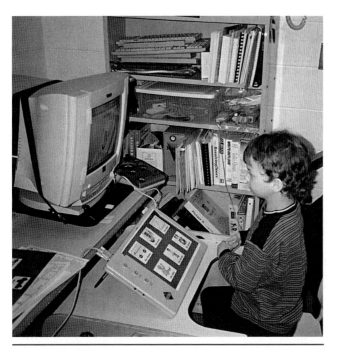

Figure 7-5   A symbol-based GIDEI overlay for use with an expanded keyboard and an educational software program.

TABLE 7-1	Minimal Adaptations to the Standard Keyboard and Mouse*
Need Addressed	Software Approach
Modifier key cannot be used at same time as another key	StickyKeys[†]
User cannot release key before it starts to repeat	FilterKeys[†]
User accidentally hits wrong keys	SlowKeys,[†] BounceKeys,[†] FilterKeys[†]
User cannot manipulate mouse	MouseKeys[†]
User wants to use augmentative communication device as input	SerialKeys[†] in Windows XP or an alternative (like AAC keys)
User cannot access keyboard (Windows Vista)	On-screen keyboard (Windows XP and Vista) Built-in ASR

*Easy Access (part of universal access) in Macintosh operating system, Apple Computer, Cupertino, Calif.; accessibility options in Windows XP, Ease of Access in Windows Vista, Microsoft Corp., Seattle, Wash.
[†]Software modifications developed at the Trace Center, University of Wisconsin, Madison. These are included as before-market modifications to the Macintosh operating system or Windows in some personal computers and are available as after-market versions in others. The function of each program is as follows:
StickyKeys: user can press modifier key, then press second key without holding both down simultaneously.
SlowKeys: a delay can be added before the character selected by hitting a key is entered into the computer; this means that the user can release an incorrect key before it is entered.
BounceKeys: prevents double characters from being entered if the user bounces on the key when pressing and releasing.
FilterKeys: the combination of SlowKeys, BounceKeys, and RepeatKeys in Microsoft Windows.
MouseKeys: substitutes arrow keys for mouse movements.
SerialKeys: allows any serial input to replace mouse and keyboard; this function has largely been replaced by USB standard devices.

scanning is the mode used for mouse emulation. All these features can be incorporated into a setup that can be loaded when it is necessary or desirable to use the mouse. Anson (1997) describes the characteristics of several GIDEIs for both Windows and Macintosh operating systems.

All currently available commercial devices use the USB standard for providing adapted input, and they are designed for either, or both, Windows-based and Macintosh computers. All adapted input devices have a hardware component, and some have software that may be used for operation or customization. All also have provisions for attachment of control interfaces (alternative keyboards, switches, etc.).

Many of the adapted inputs listed in Table 7-2 include keyboard or mouse emulation. Some of these systems may also require a software program to be loaded into the host computer. This software may be used as part of the emulation process, and it also supports specialized setups for the adapted input device to be used with specific software programs (e.g., the educational applications described in Chapter 15).

General-Purpose Emulators. The first general-purpose keyboard emulator to be widely available was the AFC. The original version of this device was intended for use in the Apple II+ computer (Schwejda and Vanderheiden, 1982). The features incorporated in the AFC are still fundamental to most current emulators. In a very real sense, virtually all the basic capabilities have their origins in the AFC. The major advances in emulator design

have been the result of advances in the host computer rather than fundamental insights into the process of keyboard and mouse emulation.

Emulators also use built-in synthetic speech feedback in "talking setups" that allow the user to receive auditory and visual prompting and feedback. This feature is useful for young children who may not be able to read, for visually impaired individuals, and as an added input modality for persons with learning disabilities.

The Kenx was originally designed to provide alternative input to the Macintosh computer and was later ported to the Windows operating system as well. It was originally packaged as a combination of hardware and software that incorporated scanning, Morse code, alternative keyboard, and on-screen keyboard functions. The software became known as "Discover." Today's software, called DiscoverPro (Madentec, Ltd, Edmonton, Alberta, Canada; *www.Madentec.com*), works with a number of alternative input devices, including IntelliKeys (IntelliTools, Petaluma, Calif.; *www.intellitools.com*), IntelliSwitch (Madentec, Ltd), and head pointers such as TrackerPro (Madentec, Ltd), or HeadMouse (Origin Instruments, Grand Prairie, Tex.; *www.orin.com*).

TABLE 7-2	Alternative Keyboards for Direct Selection	
Category	Description	Device Name/Manufacturer
Expanded keyboards	Generally membrane keyboards that have enlarged target areas, often programmable so that key size can be customized; useful for individuals with good range and poor resolution; also useful for individuals with limited cognitive/language skills or visual impairment.	IntelliKeys (IntelliTools); USB King Keyboard (TASH, Inc.); Expanded Keyboard (EKEG Electronics Company, LTD); Big Keys Plus (Inclusive Technologies); Touch and Go and Concept Keyboard (Traxsys Computer Products); Expanded Keyboard (Maltron)
Contracted keyboards	Miniature, full-function keyboards, typically with membrane overlay; useful for individuals with limited range of motion and good resolution.	USB Mini Keyboard (TASH, Inc.); Mini Keyboard (EKEG Electronics Co. Ltd.); The Magic Wand Keyboard (In Touch Systems)
Touch screens/touch tablets	Activated by either breaking a very thin light beam or by a capacitive array that detects the electrical charge on the finger; the electrode array used to detect where the finger or pointer is touching is transparent; touch screen can be placed over the face of a monitor.	Touch Window (RiverDeep); MagicTouch (Laureate Learning Systems, Inc.)
TongueTouch Keypad	Battery-operated, radio frequency–transmitting device with nine pressure-sensitive keys activated by tongue; universal controller processes information sent from keypad to receiver.	UCS 2000 with TongueTouch Keypad (newAbilities, Inc.)
Special-purpose keyboards	Keyboards on special-purpose devices, such as augmentative communication and environmental control devices; available keys may be much more limited in number or may be specific in function compared with standard keyboard.	See Chapter 11

Data from RiverDeep, San Francisco, Calif. (http://rivapprod2.riverdeep.net/); EKEG Electronics, Vancouver, Canada (http://www.ekegelectronics.com/); Laureate Learning Systems, Inc. Winooski, Vt. (www.laureatelearning.com); newAbilities, Inc., Palo Alto, Calif. (www.newabilities.com); IntelliTools, Petaluma, Calif. (www.intellitools.com); Inclusive Technologies (http://www.inclusive.co.uk/catalogue/index.html); In Touch Systems, Spring Valley, N.Y. (www.magicwandkeyboard.com); Maltron-USA (http://www.maltron-usa.com/expanded.htm); Traxsys Computer Products (http://assistive.traxsys.com/staticProductListing.asp); TASH, Ajax, Ontario, Canada, or Richmond, Va. (www.tashinc.com).

Discover can either be enabled at startup (when the power is turned on) or activated by clicking on the Discover icon once the computer has booted. Some of the most useful features of Discover are those that are specifically aimed at the **graphical user interface** (GUI). It is possible with Discover, for example, to set tabs on the screen where the mouse is to point and then store the tab as a code (or macro). When the code is entered (by use of any of the basic selection methods and control interfaces), the mouse carries out the movement stored. By saving a series of mouse movements, it is possible to move to a menu, open it, select a specific entry, and then double-click (to start execution), all with one command. This not only saves many mouse movements, but it also avoids errors during tedious and complex movements. If a particular target software application has keyboard-equivalent commands to perform its functions, those can also be issued directly by Discover. Discover also provides row-column scanning with visually enhanced scanning arrays and audible cues, making it useful for people with multiple disabilities (such as blindness and motor impairments). Other useful features include digitized speech, on-screen keyboards, "invisible" setups (for issuing commands without an on-screen keyboard appearing), and

development and printing of keyboard overlays for use with expanded keyboards.

The DARCI TOO provides for alternative mouse, alternative keyboard, joystick, and switch input to Windows-based and Macintosh computers. Input to the computer is through the serial port and it conforms to the Trace standard for GIDEI design. Both a hardware component for attaching the external device to the computer and software to accept that input are included. Two versions of the DARCI TOO are available. One uses an external hardware box that connects to a serial port on the computer. Five operating modes are available with the DARCI TOO: scanning, Morse code, DARCI code matrix keyboard, and communication device. The DARCI USB supports Morse code alternative input through the USB port. No additional software is required, but the MouseKeys accessibility feature must be activated for use.

The process by which a computer can be adapted by use of a software program is described by Hortsman, Levine, and Jaros (1989). Programs in this category range from those implementing the basic features of Table 7-1 to the use of alternate control interfaces and selection methods (Gorgens, Bergler, and Gorgens, 1990). The programs described by these authors and others provide access to Windows and/or Macintosh operating systems. Anson (1997) describes these and other approaches.

On-Screen Selection Sets.   On-screen selection sets use mouse (point-and-click) approaches or scanning to make selections. The keyboard image, shown in Figure 7-6, *B*, is divided into "keys," each of which is labeled with an alphanumerical character, special character, or function. All the possible keys on the computer keyboard being emulated are included in the on-screen keyboard display. The emulation software places the keyboard or scanning array image on the screen, detects the mouse or scanning cursor position, relates the position to the key label of the on-screen

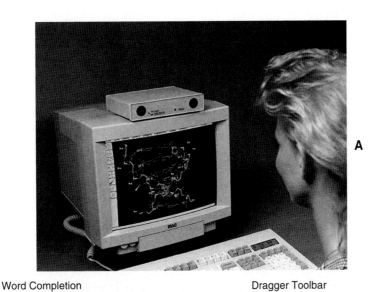

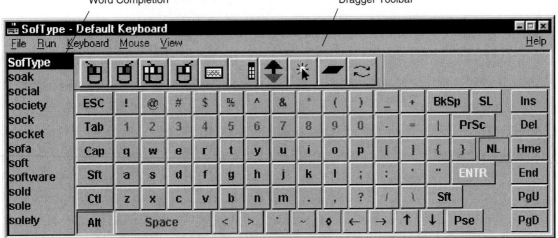

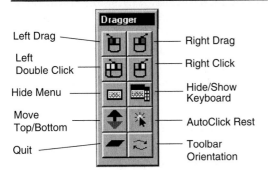

Figure 7-6   **A,** Head-controlled mouse. **B,** An example of an on-screen keyboard screen for Microsoft Windows. (Courtesy Origin Instruments Corporation, www.orin.com.)

keyboard image, and inserts that character into the keyboard routine of the computer so that it is treated as a typed character. Windows also includes a basic on-screen keyboard in its accessibility options. To enter a character or select a function, the user of the on-screen keyboard positions the cursor inside the desired "key" on the screen. Movement of the cursor can be by mouse, trackball, joystick, switch array, or head-controlled mouse. Once the cursor is located inside the targeted key, the user makes the selection either by activating another switch or by holding the cursor on the choice until the device accepts it. Various types of on-screen keyboards allow changes in the keyboard arrangement, size of the on-screen keys, location of the keyboard on the screen, and methods by which this customization can be accomplished. Many of the on-screen keyboard systems also include other characteristics. One of the most common is a word prediction feature that displays frequently used words as the first few characters are typed. Each word may be in a key location or on a list presented in a window. This type of input acceleration is discussed in more detail in Chapter 11. Other features that can be used to optimize performance include horizontal and vertical cursor movement speed, keyboard layouts, and location of the keyboard image on the screen (e.g., top or bottom, depending on the type of application program that is running). Anson (1997) describes several commercial approaches to both hardware and software for on-screen keyboards.

Shein et al (1991) describe the challenges and the approaches that solve some of the problems in the development of emulators for Windows. They indicate that any visual keyboard in a GUI should have several features. First, selecting keys (e.g., with an on-screen keyboard and head pointer) from the visual keyboard should not transfer the internal computer keyboard routines to the new selection but should keep the computer looking for input from the visual keyboard. Typically, the most recently opened window is "on top" of the others. If the keyboard image is in a window, then it must stay on top even if selections from it open another window. Second, the visual keyboard array should send keystroke input information to the application that is active at any given time. Finally, Shein et al state that the visual keyboard should support a range of layouts. These authors have developed one software-based emulator for the Windows and OS/2 GUIs. Several other commercially available products for Windows are available. These products include a variety of input methods (on-screen keyboard with pointing device, scanning in several modes, Morse code), output options (voice synthesis, enlarged screen characters), and optional features (e.g., word prediction, communication device pop-up windows, environmental control interfaces to telephone and appliances).

The use of more than one switch can enable other functions (Shein et al, 2003). In addition to directed scanning described earlier, these additional functions include a cancel function when an incorrect entry is made, a faster scan to get to a region and then scan slowly through the region, reverse and forward scanning, and similar capabilities. Most on-screen keyboard or scanning arrays allow resizing of keys or selection elements, location of the on-screen display anywhere on the screen, word prediction, and abbreviation expansion.

Switch-Controlled Computer Keyboard and Mouse Emulation.   When scanning is used for computer access, the scanning array resembles an on-screen keyboard, and it may occupy up to half of the screen. The result is that the user has two windows open, one for the scanning array and one for the application program. Additional hardware is required to accept from one to five switches as input. The scanning hardware plugs into the computer through a **parallel**, a **serial**, or a **USB port.** One or more of the scanning approaches described earlier may be used. Once a scanning choice is made, the on-screen keyboard software sends the proper code for the element (alphanumerical or special character) to the computer as if it has been typed. There are several general approaches to single-switch scanning for emulation of mouse functions (Blackstein-Alder et al, 2004). With cartesian scanning, a line moves slowly down the screen when the user presses the scanning switch. As it scrolls down the screen, the line intersects various on-screen icons. If the switch is pressed a second time, a pointer or vertical line moves across the screen. When the pointer or vertical line is located over the desired screen icon, a third switch press selects that icon as though the mouse button had been pressed. This function is similar to matrix-type row-column scanning except that the scan is continuous rather than moving discretely between choices.

A second general approach to scanning mouse emulation is cartesian also, but with discrete scanning between screen elements. This method more closely approximates typical row-column scanning. A third approach is rotational scanning that involves two steps, pointing toward a target and then moving the mouse pointer toward the target. When the user activates the switch once, a scan line is drawn from the center to the right-hand side of the computer screen. This scan line rotates about the center at a continuous speed counterclockwise around the screen. When the line intersects an on-screen target, the user activates the switch a second time to stop the rotational scanning. This line remains visible, and a second perpendicular line begins scanning outward from the center. When this line intersects the desired target, the user hits the switch a third time to make the selection.

Commercial programs also allow the user to select what mouse button function (click to select, double-click to open and run the application, or drag to move) is activated with the third switch press. In some cases the selected function is implemented only after an acceptance time. If an additional switch press occurs before the acceptance time (less than a second, typically), the selection is cancelled, which allows for error correction before an entry is made.

Blackstein-Alder et al (2004) carried out a comparative study of mouse emulation scanning. They used the two types of cartesian scanning, rotational scanning, and a hybrid approach that scans quadrants of the screen and then scans within the quadrant (for example, ScanBuddy, Applied Human Factors, Helotes, Tex.; *www.ahf-net.com*). Their subjects were all individuals who had a physical disability with cerebral palsy or a related condition. The subjects were given an opportunity to practice with each of the four techniques before using them in a controlled exercise. The length of practice required varied widely among the subjects. Accuracy (number of correct target selected) was variable. About half the subjects had very similar results for all four methods. For the other half, there was more variability among the methods, with the hybrid approach generating the most errors. Three types of errors occurred: hitting too early (before the cursor reached the desired target), hitting too late, and double switch hits in quick succession (perseveration), which cancelled the entry. Selection times for the two cartesian and hybrid approaches were very similar. Selection times for the rotational approach were more than twice as long as for the other three methods. The majority of users favored the discrete cartesian approach. Cartesian continuous was chosen as the favorite by a second group. None chose rotational scanning as the preferred method. Although not directly applicable to clinical applications because of the use of a simplified scanning program for data collection, these results do point out the value of practice and the difficulties in using a rotational approach. Scan times, scanning line width, dwell time before rest or selection, and other characteristics are adjustable on most commercial products.

Another approach to mouse emulation is the creation of on screen "hot spots" in software applications (for example, ClickIT, Intellitools, Petaluma, Calif.; *www.intellitools.com/*). These are scanned sequentially. This approach optimizes the scan to only those parts of the GUI screen that are active during an application. The hot spot locations are defined by the user (or more typically a supporter of the user) and stored for a particular application. A variety of approaches (e.g., automatic, inverse, and step) can be used to scan the hot spots with one or two switches. Several commercial products provide for mouse functions during scanning (Dragger, Origin Instruments, Grand Prairie, Tex., *www.orin.com*; ScanBuddy, Applied Human Factors, Helotes, Tex., *www.ahf-net.com*). An example is shown in Figure 7-6, *A*. In general, these programs allow the user to select the mouse function after the selection of a target by using any of the scanning or hot spot approaches described here. A more generic approach is one in which all interface objects in Windows are scanned as hot spots until the scan is stopped by switch activation (WIVIK, WiVik; also *http://www.wivik.com/index.html*). This action begins the next sequence (e.g., scanning down a list of choices in an opened menu).

The basic operating system allows the speed of mouse movement, the trail left by the mouse, and other features to be adjusted. For individuals with severe motor impairments, the built-in adjustment of mouse speed, cursor size, and so forth are not sufficient to allow use of the mouse or other pointing device. There are commercial products that extend the range of these adjustments and add other features such as wrapping the cursor around the screen when it reaches one side (i.e., when the cursor hits the right edge of the screen it appears again on the left side; for example, PointSmart, Infogrip, Ventura, Calif., *www.inforgrip.com*).

Single- or dual-switch computer users can also use coded access including Morse code and DARCI (WesTest Engineering, Farmington, Utah; *www.westest.com*) code. Because codes are typically memory based, they do not require a selection display (a set of characters on the screen), as is needed for an on-screen keyboard or scanning array. This method allows the entire screen to be used for the application software being run. When Samuel Morse invented his code in the late 1880s, there were no computers, and therefore basic Morse code does not include ESC or RETURN keys on the computer or characters such as punctuation or \/@#$%. Even more important, Morse saw no need for a SPACE character. He just told his key operators to wait a little longer between dots and dashes (a dot [.] is a short sound and a dash [-] is a longer sound). Unfortunately, the computer requires that a specific ASCII character be sent for SPACE. The absence of standardized codes for anything other than alphanumerical characters (see Figure 7-25) presents a problem with using Morse code for computer access. Examples of codes developed for computer use by several different manufacturers are listed in Table 7-3. Note that in some cases the codes for the same characters are different for the three systems and in other cases they are the same. This variation makes it difficult for the consumer to change from one communication device or adapted input device to another. Once the set of codes is learned and the motor patterns developed, it is very difficult to change to a new set of codes. Computer access with either scanning or Morse code can be accomplished by software programs, hardware adaptations, or combinations of both.

Communication Devices as Alternative Computer Inputs. Many augmentative communication devices (see Chapter 11) can also function as alternative keyboards for computer access. The communication device is connected to the computer through a serial or USB interface. This connection allows the communication device to send characters to the computer as if they were typed from the computer keyboard. Using the communication device has the advantage that the user has access to the same control interface

TABLE 7-3 Nonstandardized Morse Codes Used for Computer Access

Character	Kenx*	Darci Too†
ESC	- - -.	..-...
ENTER	.-.-	.-.-
DELETE	..- -..	-..-.
TAB	-.-..-	-.- -.
.	.-.-.-	.-.-.-
!	.-..-	.-..- -
$	.-.-.	-....-.
SPACE	..- -	..- -
,	- -..- -	- -..- -
"..	-.- -	- -.- -
(	..- -.	....- -.
)	..-.-	-.. - -.
UP ARROW	- -.- -	- ---..
DOWN ARROW	- -..-	------
LEFT ARROW	- - - -	-----.
RIGHT ARROW	..-..-	- -.-.-.
SHIFT	.....-.	..-.-

Note: Standard alphanumerical Morse code characters are shown in Figure 7-25.
*Kenx, Madentec, Edmonton, Alberta, Canada.
†Darci Too for Windows-based computers, WesTest Engineering, Bountiful, Utah.

BOX 7-2 Critical Questions for Evaluating Keyboard Use

1. Can the consumer reach all the keys on the keyboard?
2. Are the size, spacing, and sensory feedback of the keys appropriate?
3. Is the consumer's speed of input adequate for the task?
4. Does the consumer target keys with approximately 75% accuracy?
5. Is the consumer able to simultaneously hold down the modifier key and select another key?
6. Is the consumer able to control the duration for which a key must be pressed before it repeats itself?
7. Does the consumer effectively use the standard keyboard layout?

and selection technique for computer access as he or she uses for communication. This strategy reduces training and skill development time (e.g., no need to learn two keyboard layouts) and allows the user to concentrate on learning how to operate the computer. Another advantage is that any vocabulary (e.g., words or phrases or complete computer commands) stored in the communication device can be sent from the communication device to the computer as a whole by using a serial port. In many currently available communication devices, computer control is a built-in feature. In others it must be added as an option. Accessibility options (Windows) and universal access (Macintosh) provide for input from the communication device with serial keys (see Table 7-1). A standard has been developed to allow all keyboard characters to be sent to the computer, even if the communication device does not have that character. For example, computer keys such as DEL may not be on the communication device, but the user can send a sequence of characters that the computer interprets as the DEL key. Selection of a special-purpose keyboard for a consumer also requires careful consideration of the items presented in Box 7-2.

There are, however, some disadvantages to this approach. One of these is that in many cases the communication device needs to be physically connected to the computer; that is, a cable must be physically plugged in to the computer. An alternative approach is to use wireless links to replace the cable. Most wireless systems use infrared (IR) links, which are similar to the IR environmental control links described in Chapter 14.

A second potential problem is that most communication devices are not able to generate all the possible ASCII codes needed for general-purpose computer access. For this reason, a special standard has been developed for establishing interaction between the computer and the communication device. Table 7-4 lists examples of the character strings used in this standard. All these codes begin with the ESC (escape) code and end with a period (.), and they are intended to be transmitted over a cable to the computer serial port. Unfortunately, not all currently available communication devices support this standard, and it may be necessary for the assistive technology practitioner (ATP) to program the communication device manually to allow use of the computer. For example, one square on a communication device may have the sequence of characters "[ESC]ret." stored; when this square is selected, the computer responds as though the RETURN key has been pressed. These characters must be programmed into the communication device, together with the other sequences in Table 7-4.

CASE STUDY

AUGMENTATIVE AND ALTERNATIVE COMMUNICATION AS A COMPUTER INPUT

You are working with a teenager who has an augmentative and alternative communication (AAC) device that she uses very well (see Chapter 11). She has come to the ATP for development of computer access for writing in school. Which of the accessibility options should the ATP use to interface with her AAC device? What questions should be asked about her AAC device, and what capabilities would it need to have to be functional in this application? What character strings would need to be available in the AAC device for her to be able to input the RETURN, ALT, and SHIFT characters in her word processing program?

TABLE 7-4	Trace Standard for Computer Input by Augmentative Communication Systems and Other GIDEIs

Key Designation	ESC Sequence	Computer
DEL	[ESC]del.	A
DELETE	[ESC]delete.	I, M
CONTROL	[ESC]control.	All
DOWN ARROW	[ESC]down.	All
LEFT ARROW	[ESC]left.	All
ENTER	[ESC]enter.	M, I
RETURN	[ESC]ret.	A, M
TAB	[ESC]tab.	All
BACKSPACE	[ESC]backspace.	I, M
SHIFT	[ESC]shift.	A, I, M*
ALTERNATE	[ESC]alt.	I*
CONTROL	[ESC]ctrl.	A, I,* M*
ESCAPE	[ESC]esc.	All
RESET	[ESC]reset.	A
FUNCTION + #	[ESC]f#	I†
INSERT	[ESC]insert.	I
HOME	[ESC]home.	I
END	[ESC]end.	I
PAGE UP	[ESC]pageup.	I, M
PAGE DOWN	[ESC]pagedown.	I, M
KEYPAD	[ESC]keypad.	I, M‡
SCROLL	[ESC]scroll.	I, M
PRINT SCREEN	[ESC]print.	I
OPTION	[ESC]option.	A, M

A, Apple II series; *M*, Apple Macintosh; *I*, Windows PC.
*Some computers have both left and right shift, control, or alternate keys; use left or right key. For example, LEFT SHIFT = [ESC]lshift., RIGHT ALT = [ESC]ralt., LEFT CONTROL = [ESC]rctrl.
†This sequence is used for each function key, with the key number substituted for the # sign; for example, function key 1 = [ESC]f1.
‡On Macintosh and Windows PCs, the keypad keys are all preceded by kp; for example, 7 on keypad = [ESC]kp7.

According to Table 7-4, to cause a TAB key to be entered, an input device that adheres to the Trace standard looks for the five-character string [ESC]TAB., and when it is received, the program running on the computer reacts as if the TAB key has been pressed by itself from the keyboard. For example, pressing the TAB key in a word processing program moves the cursor five spaces to the right. Another example from Table 7-4 is the entry of a function key. The Trace standard uses the four characters [ESC]F1. as the character string for function key number 1. When this string is sent from the communication device, the computer acts as if the key F1 has been pressed from the keyboard. In many programs, entering this key results in a help menu, and the character string has the same effect as pressing the F1 key.

■ CHARACTERISTICS OF CONTROL INTERFACES

Before the specific types of control interfaces and the selection of a control interface for the user is discussed, it is necessary

to have an understanding of their characteristics. Controls differ according to their spatial, sensory, and activation characteristics (Barker and Cook, 1981). When a control interface is selected for an individual, these characteristics should be taken into consideration. The placement and size of the control interface (spatial characteristics), how it is activated (activation characteristics), and what feedback is obtained as a result of its activation (sensory characteristics) should be considered.

Spatial Characteristics

The **spatial characteristics** of a control interface are (1) its overall physical size (dimensions), shape, and weight, (2) the number of available targets contained within the control interface, (3) the size of each target, and (4) the spacing between targets. Control interfaces can be grouped into broad categories on the basis of their spatial characteristics. For example, a single switch has one target, and the target size is the dimension (height and width) of the switch. Typically, a single switch can accommodate an individual who has limitations in range and only gross resolution for activation. Switch arrays (including joysticks) have two to five switches, each representing a different target. The user's range required to access a switch array needs to be larger than for a single switch but still be relatively small, depending on the spacing between the switches. The user's resolution needs to be more refined than that required for a single switch and less refined than that for a keyboard. A contracted keyboard has keys (targets) of small size in close proximity to each other. Its overall size is also small. The keys on these keyboards range in size from 0.5 to 1.5 cm, and they require relatively fine resolution from the user. The requirement for the user's range is moderate (less than 15 cm in both horizontal and vertical directions). Standard or commonly used keyboards require moderate range and relatively fine resolution of the user. Finally, expanded keyboards have large overall size and enlarged target size, requiring relatively large range and fine resolution. Switch arrays and keyboards can have from two to more than 100 targets.

Activation and Deactivation Characteristics

Many characteristics are related to the activation of the control interface. The **activation characteristics** of a control interface consist of the method of activation, effort, displacement, flexibility, and durability and maintainability. Deactivation, or the release, of a control interface is another characteristic that needs to be considered.

Method of Activation. The *method of activation* is the way in which a signal sent by the user is detected by the control interface and activates the processor. Table 7-5 shows the methods of activation. The first column identifies the

TABLE 7-5   Method of Activation

Signal Sent, User Action (What the Body Does)	Signal Detected	Examples
1. Movement (eye, head, tongue, arms, legs)	1a. Mechanical control interface: activation by the application of a force	1a. Joystick, keyboard, tread switch
	1b. Electromagnetic control interface: activation by the receipt of electromagnetic energy such as light or radio waves	1b. Light pointer, light detector, remote radio transmitter
	1c. Electrical control interface: activation by detection of electrical signals from the surface of the body	1c. EMG, EOG, capacitive, or contact switch
	1d. Proximity control interface: activation by a movement close to the detector but without contact	1d. Heat-sensitive switches
2. Respiration (inhalation-expiration)	2. Pneumatic control interface: activation by detection of respiratory airflow or pressure	2. Puff and sip
3. Phonation	3. Sound or voice control interface: activation by the detection of articulated sounds or speech	3. Sound switch, whistle switch, speech recognition

three ways the user can send a signal to the control interface: movement, respiration, and phonation; the middle column shows how each of these signals is detected by the control interface; and the column on the far right provides examples of each type of control interface.

Movements by the user can be detected by the control interface in three basic ways. The movement may generate a force, external to the body, that is detected by the control interface. These are *mechanical control interfaces,* and they represent the largest category of control interfaces. Most switches, keyboard keys, joysticks, and other controls that require movement or force for activation (e.g., mouse, track-ball) fall into this category. Force is always required to activate a mechanical control interface; however, mechanical displacement may or may not occur. For example, force-controlled joysticks and membrane keyboards have very little displacement when activated. *Electromagnetic control interfaces* do not require contact from the user's body for activation. They detect movement at a distance through either light or radio frequency energy. Examples include head-mounted light sources or detectors and transmitters used with EADLs for remote control (similar to garage door openers). Another example of an electromagnetic control interface is the use of a light beam in a manner similar to the system in many retail stores in which a customer interrupts a light beam when entering or leaving the store. *Electrical control interfaces* are sensitive to electrical currents generated by the body. One type, called a capacitive switch, detects static electricity on the surface of the body. This is similar to the game children play when they attempt to shock someone with static electricity. A common example of this type of interface is seen in some elevator buttons. The switches require no force, and they are therefore useful to individuals who have muscle weakness. Other electrical control interfaces use electrodes attached to the skin to detect underlying muscle electrical activity. The electromyographic (EMG) signal

associated with muscle contraction is the most commonly used signal. Electrodes placed near the eyes can measure eye movements and generate an electro-oculographic (EOG) signal based on eye movements. *Proximity control interfaces,* the last type of interface that detects movement, are also active at a distance, but they detect heat or other signals without coming into contact with the body. Although infrequently used, body heat sensors have been successful as control interfaces when force cannot be generated. In summary, mechanical and electrical switches both require contact with the body, and mechanical types also require the generation of force. Electromagnetic and proximity switches do not require contact with the body.

The second type of body-generated signal shown in Table 7-5 is *respiration.* The signal detected is either air flow or air pressure. The use of this type of control interface, generally called a sip-and-puff switch, requires that the user be able to place and maintain the lips around a tube and produce good control of air flow. When sound or speech is produced by the air flow, we call it *phonation* (see Chapter 3). This is a method of activation that has developed rapidly over the last few years with speech recognition interfaces. Individuals who have physical involvement that makes other means of activating a control interface difficult may be able to produce sounds, letters, or words consistently enough to activate a control interface.

Effort.   The *effort* required by the user to generate the signal from the control interface is the next activation characteristic to consider. Activation effort varies from zero upward to a relatively large amount. For a mechanical interface, this is the force required to cause switch activation. For an electromagnetic interface, the effort is the minimal distance of movement sufficient to cause activation of the sensors. For example, an individual using a light pointer to choose from an array of different items must have sufficient head movement (the effort) to move the light beam from one element (represented by a sensor) to another element (which has a different sensor) and enough stability to hold the light beam on that element. Electrical interfaces require a range of effort from zero (for a capacitive switch) to relatively high for muscle force activation of an EMG. The EMG is measured by electrodes placed on the surface of the skin. The magnitude of the electrical signal is proportional to the amount of force generated by the muscle (the effort). Depending on the muscle and the sensitivity of the measurement system, the effort can vary from a small force to a large force. The level of effort for proximity switches is the distance of movement required for activation. An example is waving a hand close to a heat-sensitive switch. The activation effort of pneumatic control interfaces is the amount of exhalation or inhalation required for activation, which can be either how hard (pressure) or how fast (flow) air is exhaled or inhaled. For example, some power wheelchair processors use a system in which a hard puff (large effort and high pressure generated) is forward, a soft puff (small effort and low pressure generated) is a right turn, a hard sip is reverse, and a soft sip is a left turn. The difference in these control signals is based primarily on effort generated. Phonation signals also have a level of effort related (at the simplest control interface level) to volume or loudness. Noise-activated or sound-activated switches are similar to those found on some toys. For speech recognition control interfaces, the effort also includes proper pronunciation because the detection is based on identification of a particular word (see the section on speech recognition later in this chapter).

Displacement.   Another characteristic that needs to be considered apart from effort is *displacement*. Displacement, which is defined as how far a control interface travels from its original position to its activated position, is unique to mechanical control interfaces. Some mechanical interfaces, such as a force-activated joystick, respond to force and require no displacement (Spaeth and Cooper, 1999). In this case the amount of force that the user exerts determines the output of the joystick. If more force is exerted, the output is greater. Because force is detected, rather than amount of travel or displacement of the joystick, the demands placed on the user change. For individuals who can exert a force over a small distance, this type of joystick is ideal. It also provides more tactile feedback to the user. Many mechanical control interfaces require movement and force for activation. The displacement of these control interfaces provides kinesthetic (movement) feedback as well as tactile and proprioceptive feedback (see Chapter 3). This increased amount of sensory feedback is often of benefit to the user. For example, membrane keyboards have very smaller displacement, and the forces to activate them are often smaller than for switches, which have greater displacement. Without the sensory feedback provided by the displacement, however,

users frequently press harder than necessary, thinking that more force is needed to activate the keys.

Deactivation.   Although we have focused on the activation of control interfaces, we need to keep in mind that there is also a force required to release, or *deactivate,* some control interfaces. Muscle contraction is necessary to remove, or release, the body part from the interface. Weiss (1990) measured both activation and deactivation forces for several mechanical interfaces and found that force was required to release the control interface in all cases but that the deactivation force was approximately one third to one half that required for activation.

Flexibility.   The *flexibility* of the control interface, or the number of ways in which it can be operated by a control site, also needs to be considered. There are many types of keyboards, joysticks, and switches and just as many ways in which the user can activate them. Among individuals with physical disabilities, wide differences in motor performance exist. Depending on the nature of the disability, an individual may or may not have deficits in strength, range of motion, muscle tone, sensation, or coordination. For example, the quality of movement may be smooth or uncoordinated, reflex patterns may dominate movement or be absent, sensory deficits may or may not be present, muscle tone may be normal or increased or decreased, or there may be limitations in range of motion at any joint. Thus one person may push a key with a finger, another may use a thumb, and a third a head pointer. Control interfaces that allow for various ways of activation are considered to be flexible. In general, control interfaces that are activated by movement can typically be activated by several body sites and are considered to be flexible in comparison to control interfaces that are limited to activation by respiration and phonation. Within the category of movement-activated controls, the flexibility varies, for example, from a lever switch, which is most commonly activated by head movement, to a tread switch, which is routinely used for activation by the foot, knee, hand, head, or chin. Some control interfaces, such as the touch switch, have an adjustment for the amount of effort required to activate them. This type of control can be useful for evaluation or for an individual who has fluctuating endurance or a degenerative condition.

The ways in which the control interface can be mounted or positioned for use also contribute to its flexibility. Mounting a control interface at the optimal position in the individual's workspace facilitates activation. Some control interfaces, such as a computer mouse, are not intended for mounting and need to be used on a table or other flat surface, whereas other control interfaces, such as a joystick, can usually be mounted in a variety of locations and can therefore be activated by the chin, hand, or foot. Mounting systems are discussed later in this chapter.

Durability and Maintainability. The *durability* of the control interface is a characteristic that needs consideration as well. Gathering information during the assessment regarding how often the interface is to be used and the amount of force that is to be generated on the interface by the user assists the ATP in making recommendations that correspond to the durability of the control interface. If the control interface is to be used by someone who exerts a great deal of pressure on it because of uncontrolled movements, it must be constructed so it can withstand this type of use. Switches and keyboards made out of plastic, for example, may not hold up well under these circumstances. In the long run it may be cost-effective to buy a more expensive interface made out of metal that will last longer.

A final consideration is the maintainability of the control interface. It is important to consider whether the interface can be easily cleaned and how it should be cleaned so as not to damage any components. Other considerations are whether any of its components need to be replaced periodically and, if so, how difficult a procedure it is. For example, certain switches require a battery to operate, and when the battery dies, it must be replaced. It also helps to know who will be able to repair the control interface if it breaks down and, if it is in need of repair, whether there is a loaner available for the consumer to use in the interim.

Sensory Characteristics

The auditory, somatosensory, and visual feedback produced during the activation of the control interface comprise its **sensory characteristics.** Some control interfaces provide auditory feedback in the form of a click when activated. For example, keyboards that use mechanical switches for each key usually click when pressed, thus providing auditory feedback. Other keyboards have a smooth membrane surface that does not provide any auditory feedback. Somatosensory feedback is the tactile, kinesthetic, or proprioceptive response sensed on activation of the control interface. For example, the texture or "feel" of the activation surface provides tactile data. The position in space of the control site when the user activates the switch provides proprioceptive data. The data generated as a result of movement provide kinesthetic feedback to the user. When the interface is within the consumer's visual field, visual data are obtained through observation of the placement and the movement of the control interface. For some individuals the type of visual data will mean the difference between successful and unsuccessful use of a control interface. For example, someone who has difficulty attending to objects in the environment may be more attentive to a switch that is large and bright red or yellow.

There is usually a direct relationship between the sensory data provided by the control interface and the amount of effort required to activate it. A contact switch that is activated by an electrical charge from the body (i.e., requiring only touch) does not provide the user with any somatosensory feedback. There is no force required and therefore little proprioceptive or visual feedback is provided. The contact switch is also silent, so auditory feedback is absent as well. In some instances we can alter the feedback generated by a control interface. For example, adding a beep to a contact switch provides auditory data or placing a distinguishing texture over the surface of a membrane keyboard provides feedback through the tactile system. Other switches, such as the tread, wobble, and rocker, provide abundant feedback in terms of having a certain feel to them (tactile), an observable movement of the mechanism (visual), and an audible click (auditory).

Generally, interfaces that provide rich sensory feedback facilitate performance. On occasion, sensory feedback may be detrimental to the user's performance. For example, a control interface with an audible click may trigger a startle reflex in the user that interferes with motor movement. The user may eventually adjust to the sound and ignore it, but the ATP may want to consider an alternate control interface. The interrelationship of spatial, sensory, and activation characteristics of control interfaces plays an important role in the design of an assistive technology system. Each of these characteristics must be carefully considered to make effective selections that meet the needs of the consumer.

Rate Enhancement

Rate enhancement refers to all approaches that result in the number of characters generated being greater than the number of selections the individual makes. For example using "ASAP[space]" for "As soon as possible.[space]" saves 16 keystrokes. Because an increased level of efficiency is obtained, the user has to make fewer entries and the overall rate is increased. Rate enhancement goals and approaches differ for direct selection and scanning. In direct selection the goal is to reduce the number of keystrokes while increasing the amount of information selected with each keystroke. In scanning the goal is to optimize the scanning array to reduce the time required to make a desired selection. Specific approaches are discussed later in this section. Rate enhancement is used for many electronic assistive technology applications, including augmentative communication (Chapter 11), computer access (this chapter), cell phone access, and electronic aids to daily living (Chapter 14). Many mainstream software applications use some form of rate enhancement, also called input acceleration. Effective rate enhancement requires that the motor task become automatic (Blackstone, 1990). Motor patterns become more automatic as they are practiced. As the skills improve, motor

TABLE 7-6	Modes (Memory, Chart, Display) of Presentation of Codes to the User		
Type	Memory Based	Chart Based	Display Based
Memory required	Recall	Recognition	Recognition
Advantages	Can be used by those with visual limitations	Can be seen by both user and partner	Can be updated (dynamic display), giving many stored items
Disadvantages	Limited to 200-300 items for most people	Must have chart in visual field; chart can become separated from device	Requires attention to display; can slow down text selection because of split attention

and cognitive tasks become more automatic and the user becomes an "expert." As Blackstone points out, once these motor patterns are established, even small changes in the task may result in dramatic *decreases* in rate.

Direct Selection Rate Enhancement. Rate enhancement techniques for direct selection fall into two broad categories: (1) encoding techniques and (2) prediction techniques. Vanderheiden and Lloyd (1986) distinguish three basic types of codes: memory based, chart based, and display based. These are compared in Table 7-6. A memory-based technique requires that both the user and his or her partner know the codes by memory or that the user has the codes memorized for entry into the device. Chart-based techniques have an index of the codes and their corresponding vocabulary items. This can be a simple paper list attached to an electronic device or a chart on the wall (e.g., two eye blinks equals "call nurse," three eye blinks equals "please turn me," eyes up equals "yes," eyes down equals "no"). Figure 7-7 illustrates both a chart-based and a display-based approach for Morse code (Vanderheiden and Lloyd, 1986). In each device, two switches are used. The right switch produces dots and the left one produces dashes.

Abbreviation expansion is a technique in which a shortened form of a word or phrase (the abbreviation) stands for the entire word or phrase (the expansion). The abbreviations are automatically expanded by the device into the desired word or phrase. Beukelman and Yorkston (1984) evaluated five different coding strategies for abbreviations: (1) random number, (2) alphabetical numerical, (3) numerical groupings with alphabetical codes, (4) alphabetical with alphabetical word groupings, and (5) menu-based (similar to number 4, but provides prompting to the user after the category is entered). The third and fourth approaches included both a category (e.g., food) and an item in that category (e.g., banana). These coding strategies were found to be more effective (measured by accurate selections/minute) than either the numerical (worst performance) or alphabetical codes alone. The menu approach yielded midrange performance.

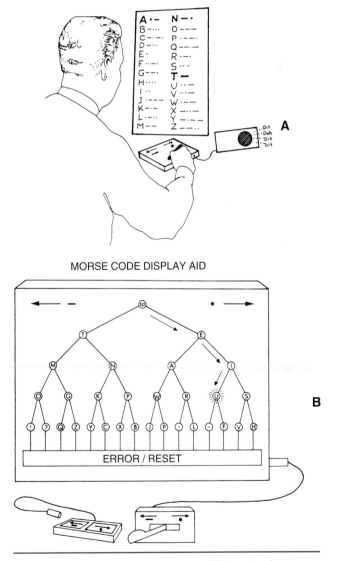

MORSE CODE DISPLAY AID

ERROR / RESET

Figure 7-7   Encoding systems may be either **(A)** chart based or **(B)** display based. (From Blackstone S: *Augmentative communication,* Rockville, MD, 1986, American Speech Language Hearing Association.)

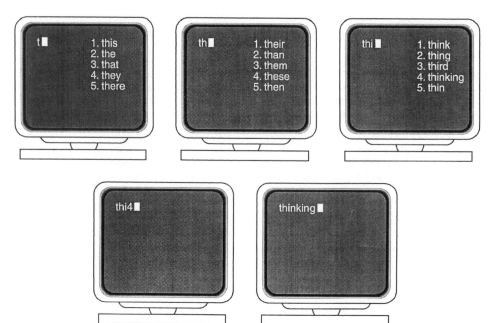

Figure 7-8 Word completion systems present a series of choices based on previous letters entered.

Word prediction or **word completion** approaches use a window on the screen that displays an ordered list of the most likely words on the basis of the letters entered. In word completion, the user selects the desired word, if any, by entering its code (e.g., a number listed next to the word) or continuing to enter letters if the desired word is not displayed (Figure 7-8) (see Case Study: Word Prediction Vocabularies). Word prediction devices offer a menu of words on the basis of previous words entered. (e.g., "*computer*" leads to list of "software," "system," "program," "keyboard"). The most important advantage of this approach is the elimination of the need for memorizing codes. Word prediction (or completion) approaches require that the user redirect the gaze from the input (keyboard keys or scanning array) to a list of words after each entry to check for the presence of the desired word, which can reduce the item selection rate compared with letter-by-letter typing. This reduction in selection rate is due to "cognitive or perceptual load" that can offset the benefits achieved in keystroke savings and result in an overall decrease in text generation rate (Hortsman and Levine, 1996).

If the word lists are placed on the screen at the point in the document where the typed letters appear, then the user does not need to redirect his gaze to check the word list while typing. This approach can result in significantly fewer switch activations in scanning. One application of this approach, called Smart Lists (Applied Human Factors Helotes, Tex, *www.ahf-net.com*), can be used with either keyboard or scanning entry. Smart Keys (Applied Human Factors) is similar to the Minspeak icon prediction. After each entry only the keys that contain a prediction on the basis of that entry are left on the on-screen keyboard, which can make scanning significantly faster because only the relevant keys need to be scanned.

Predictive approaches may be fixed or adaptive. Fixed types have a stored word list that is based on frequency of use that never changes. This method is predictable and consistent for the user and can help in the development of motor and cognitive patterns for retrieval. Adaptive vocabularies change the ordering of words in the dictionary list by keeping track of the words used by the person. The words are always listed in frequency-of-use order. This approach is more directly matched to the user's needs and recent usage.

Current technologies may include combinations of abbreviation expansion and word prediction. Abbreviations are more direct because the user can merely enter the code and immediately get the desired word, and this method allows complete phrases and sentences. Predictions are easier to use because they do not require memorization of codes.

CASE STUDY

WORD PREDICTION VOCABULARIES

Assume that one college student is taking a course in assistive technologies and another student is taking a course in world religions. If both students have word completion/prediction systems, compare the word lists you might expect to be used for writing homework assignments for each course. Would most words be the same or different for the two applications? How would the word lists vary in (1) an adaptive system and (2) a nonadaptive system? What words would you start with as a basic vocabulary in each case?

TABLE 7-7	Comparison of Abbreviation Expansion and Word Completion		
Method	Abbreviation Expansion	Word Completion	Word Prediction
Memory required	Recall	Recognition	Recognition
Language skills	Coding	First letter spelling	Reading
Display type	Memory based (chart for very small lists)	Display based	Display based
Vocabulary	Efficient for content words, greatest rate enhancement for function words	Adaptive or fixed, frequency of occurrence determined	Words
Flexibility	User-determined abbreviations aid recall	Different vocabularies for different contexts	Different vocabularies for different contexts

Word prediction and abbreviation expansion are display- and memory-based versions of the same approach.

These two techniques are actually very similar for fixed predictive systems. For example, in Figure 7-8, the entry for "thinking" is the sequence *thi4*. This could be entered without having to look at the screen, and it would be equivalent to an abbreviation. These two approaches are compared in Table 7-7.

Scanning Rate Enhancement.   Several rate enhancement approaches are possible in scanning (Lesher, Moulton, and Higginbotham, 1998). *Optimization of the row-column matrix* is based on placement of the most frequently used characters near the beginning so that they are scanned first. The matrix layout can also be rearranged by using predictive scanning in which word completion or prediction word lists are presented on the basis of previous scanning input. A computer simulation compared *switch count* (summation of the number of switch hits and the scan times) for seven text samples using each of the 14 techniques relative to a fixed array with the most frequently used characters at the beginning (baseline configuration) (Lesher, Moulton, and Higginbotham, 1998). In a fixed format matrix, placement of symbols (e.g., shift, backspace, and comma) rather than letters is the major factor contributing to switch savings. Changing the matrix with each input using a *dynamic matrix rearrangement* yielded the greatest average switch savings when the prediction was based on the previous four entries rather than fewer (e.g., two or three) previous entries (Lesher, Moulton, and Higginbotham, 1998). The greatest savings when using word and character lists in the scanning matrix was obtained when the list was presented first and then the matrix was scanned. All these results were based on computer modeling, and issues of motor and cognitive skills for persons who rely on AAC can dramatically affect these results (Horstman and Levine, 1996).

■ **SELECTING CONTROL INTERFACES FOR THE USER**

Selecting a control interface for an individual can be a complex process. Understanding the characteristics of control

interfaces as described above and following a systematic process to determine the user's skills and evaluate the effectiveness of control interfaces can make this process easier. Figure 7-9 outlines a framework to guide the ATP through the decision-making process, ultimately leading to the selection of a human/technology interface that matches the user's needs and skills. On the basis of information acquired from

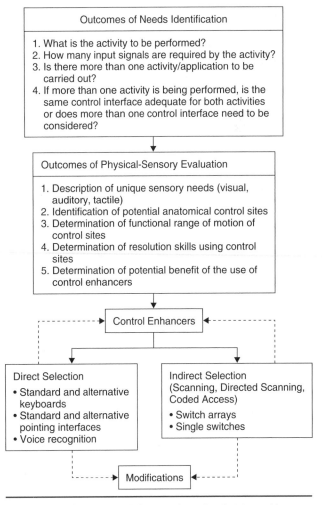

Figure 7-9   Framework for control interface decision making.

the needs identification and physical-sensory components of the evaluation process described in Chapter 4, the ATP makes a decision to pursue further evaluation on one of two paths: (1) interfaces for direct selection or (2) interfaces for indirect selection. In general, control interfaces for direct selection typically have greater numbers of targets and require more refined resolution skills. Control interfaces for indirect selection have eight or fewer targets and are more suitable for individuals with gross motor control. To make an informed decision regarding the most appropriate control interface for a user, the ATP needs to understand the alternatives that are available and evaluate and compare the consumer's ability to operate them. The following sections describe specific control interfaces for both direct and indirect selection and factors that influence the selection of one particular interface over another.

Applying the Outcomes of Needs Identification and Physical-Sensory Evaluations to Control Interface Selection

In Figure 7-9 we list specific information related to human/technology interface selection that is an outcome of the needs identification process. The information gathered reveals particular factors that should be considered during the interface selection process. For example, identifying the activity the consumer wants to perform provides us with information on how large an input domain is required and possible control interfaces to consider. If the consumer is in need of a power wheelchair and is not interested in using a computer, for example, it is not necessary to determine whether he or she can use a keyboard. Alternatively, the consumer may need to perform several functional activities (e.g., communication, mobility, and environmental control), which affects the selection of an interface. In situations such as this, it should be considered whether a different control interface for each function or a single integrated control for all the functions is to be used.

The information gathered during the physical-sensory skills evaluation gives us a profile of the user's skills in these areas, specifically those shown in Figure 7-9. This information can be used to determine the acceptable parameters for potential control interfaces. The *range measurement* determines the consumer's minimal and maximal comfortable reach and defines the geometrical requirements for the individual's workspace. This parameter provides an indication of the possible locations for placement of a control interface (or interfaces) and the maximal distance between the extreme outer edges of the interface (e.g., the overall size of a keyboard or switch array). The *resolution measurement* provides data on the consumer's ability to control his or her movement to select targets.

Given this information on the consumer's skills, potential candidate control interfaces that have similar characteristics

---

CASE STUDY

COMPARATIVE EVALUATION

Max is an 18-year-old man who has cerebral palsy. He lives in a residential facility and attends a work program through United Cerebral Palsy. Max has been referred to ABC Assistive Technology Center for a communication device. He currently communicates with others by using a manual communication board and eye blinks for yes and no.

Through evaluation of Max's range and resolution, it has been determined that his best control sites are his right hand and his head. However, he does not have fine enough control at either site to use direct selection. The ATP decides to perform comparative interface testing by using a tread switch with Max's hand and a lever switch at the side of his head. Data collected during the comparative testing phase of the evaluation show that Max is more accurate and faster activating the switch with his head (versus his hand). However, Max has indicated a preference for using his hand instead of his head.

QUESTIONS

1. Given Max's limited verbal communication, how would the ATP gather information from him regarding his opinion on the hand and the head switches?
2. What type of subjective information would the ATP want to gather from Max regarding his use of and preference for each of these two switches?
3. The data indicate that Max is faster and more accurate using the head switch. However, Max has indicated that he prefers the hand switch. What would the ATP's recommendation be and why?

---

in terms of the number and spacing of the targets and the size of individual switches or keys can be selected. Once candidate interfaces have been selected, comparative testing is conducted. The purpose of comparative testing using the control interfaces is to provide the ATP with information on how fast the consumer can input using the control interface and the accuracy of that input. Methods for carrying out comparative testing are described in Chapter 4. During comparative testing, it is also critical that the ATP gather subjective information from the consumer on each interface that is evaluated. This information includes the ease or difficulty of use.

Control Enhancers: Interface Positioning, Arm Supports, Mouthsticks, Head Pointers, and Hand Pointers

Control enhancers are aids and strategies that enhance or extend the physical control (range and resolution) a person has available to use a control interface. In some cases a person's control may be enhanced to the extent that he or she can select directly. In other cases control enhancers can minimize fatigue. Control enhancers include strategies, such as varying the position or the characteristics of the control interface, and devices, such as mouthsticks, head and hand pointers, and arm supports.

The person and the control interface should both be positioned to maximize function. The importance of proper positioning to maximize an individual's function is discussed in Chapter 6. A person's position should be observed before and during the control interface evaluation. If inadequate positioning appears to be affecting the person's ability to control an interface, it should be addressed before continuing with the evaluation. The position of the control interface can also affect the person's ability to activate it. Changing the height or the angle of the control interface even slightly may enhance the person's ability to control it.

As control interfaces become more sophisticated, control-enhancing features are becoming part of the interface. For example, certain joysticks have a feature called tremor dampening that allows adjustment of the joystick for people who have tremors. Tremor-dampening joysticks are able to distinguish between tremors, which are faster and smaller, and intentional movements, which are slower and larger. The joystick is adjusted so that the tremors are disregarded and only intentional movements are detected. This adjustment enhances the ability of an individual who might otherwise be unable to operate a joystick to control a power wheelchair. A similar feature, called *filter keys,* is used in Windows. When the filter keys feature is activated in Windows, brief keystrokes are ignored and the rate at which keys repeat when being pressed is delayed.

Individuals who have weakness in the arm may not have enough strength to access the full range of a keyboard adequately. A mobile arm support (Figure 7-10, *A*), which props the arm and assists in arm movements by eliminating some of the effects of gravity, may then allow the individual to access a keyboard. For the individual who has the gross motor ability to move his or her arm and hand around a keyboard but has difficulty extending and isolating a finger to depress a key, a pointing aid may help. There are commercially available aids that can be strapped on to the hand to assist in pointing, such as the typing aid shown in Figure 7-10, *B*. In some cases it is necessary to custom fabricate a pointing aid for it to fit the consumer's hand appropriately. These custom-fabricated aids can range from complex hand splints to simple tools such as a pencil with an enlarged eraser.

For individuals who lack functional movement in their arms and hands, a mouthstick or head pointer (Figure 7-11) can be used with head and neck movement to access a keyboard or perform other types of manipulation tasks (e.g., dialing a telephone number or turning pages in a book) (see Chapter 14). For a head pointer, a rod with a rubber tip

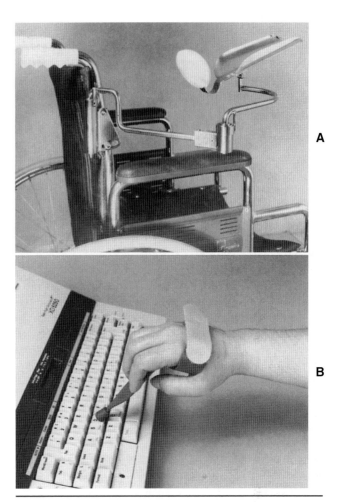

Figure 7-10   Control enhancers. **A,** Mobile arm support used to enhance the control in the upper extremity for accessing a control interface. **B,** Typing aid used to enhance a person's ability to point and access a keyboard. (Courtesy Sammons Preston Co., Bolingbrook, Ill.)

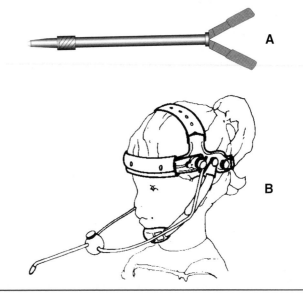

Figure 7-11   Control enhancers. **A,** Mouthstick. **B,** Head pointer.

is attached to a band that is worn around the top of the head. The individual can then use the end of this rod to depress keys. Besides being able to move the head vertically and horizontally, the individual must have the ability to produce a third dimension of movement to depress keys with a head pointer: forward and backward. There are also light pointers that can be worn on the head or held in the hand to control devices. One advantage of head-controlled light pointers is that it is not necessary for the user to move the head forward or backward. Light pointers are described in greater detail in the section on pointing interfaces.

Mouthsticks are often used by individuals who are quadriplegic as a result of a spinal cord injury. A mouthstick consists of a pointer attached to a mouthpiece. The user grips the mouthpiece between the teeth and moves the head to manipulate control interfaces or other objects. The shaft of the mouthstick can be made from a wooden dowel, a piece of plastic, or aluminum. In some cases, interchangeable tips for different functions (e.g., painting, writing, typing) can be inserted into the distal end of the shaft. The mouthpiece can be a standard U shape that is gripped between the teeth or a custom-made insert. Puckett et al (1988) identify a number of criteria for design of a mouthstick. Mouthsticks are also available from several suppliers. Use of a mouthstick requires good oral-motor control; later in this chapter training to develop these skills is discussed.

The consumer's range and resolution with the control enhancer can be determined by using the same methods discussed in Chapter 4. In some cases, particularly if there is a need to extend the consumer's range (e.g., when the head is the likely control site), it is apparent at the beginning of the evaluation that the consumer will benefit from using a control enhancer. When the user has adequate range but resolution is in question, it may not be obvious during the physical-sensory evaluation whether a control enhancer will be beneficial. In these cases it is recommended that comparative testing of candidate interfaces with and without the use of control enhancers be completed. This evaluation provides the ATP with objective data regarding the effectiveness of the control enhancer. Certain control interfaces, however, cannot be activated with a control enhancer. These include displays specially designed to be used with light pointers, eye-controlled systems, or capacitive switches requiring skin contact for activation (Lee and Thomas, 1990).

■ CONTROL INTERFACES FOR DIRECT SELECTION

Because the most rapid selection method is direct selection, it is generally preferable to indirect selection. Control interfaces for direct selection include various types of keyboards, pointing interfaces, speech recognition, eye-gaze, gesture

recognition and cortical signals. Several of these approaches use on-screen keyboards. The critical questions presented in Box 7-2 can assist the ATP in determining the consumer's ability to use any keyboard. As each question is considered, a "yes" answer means that the evaluation is proceeding on the correct pathway and the ATP should continue with the next question. Affirmative responses to all seven questions indicate that the control interface by itself is likely to meet the consumer's needs.

The answer to the first question is determined by asking the consumer to reach the keys at each corner of the keyboard. To obtain an answer to the second question, the consumer should be asked to press several keys located in different areas of the keyboard. The consumer's rate of input can be timed for entering characters. Accuracy can be measured by monitoring errors made during these tasks. In some situations, speed is of primary importance (e.g., in a work setting). In general, speed and accuracy are in opposition; that is, as speed increases, accuracy decreases. In some cases, to be accurate the consumer may make selections so slowly and deliberately that the use of the control interface under investigation becomes impractical. For example, if it takes several seconds to select a key, this rate may be equivalent to the use of scanning to make a selection. Because scanning takes much less physical effort, it should then be considered as an alternative to direct selection. Computer-assisted methods to measure speed and accuracy data are described in Chapter 4. The criterion for accuracy is somewhat subjective and is subject to clinical judgment. We recommend that at least three out of four selections (75%) be correct.

If the answer to any of the questions in Box 7-2 is determined to be "no," then the use of a control enhancer, modifications, or a less-limiting keyboard should be considered. For example, if a standard keyboard cannot be used because of a targeting problem, the following may be considered: (1) an enlarged keyboard with larger targets (less limiting), (2) a keyguard (modification), or (3) a typing aid (a control enhancer). Modifications apply to all types of keyboards and are addressed after the discussion of the different types of keyboards.

Keyboards

For written communication, a keyboard is typically considered the most efficient means of inputting information. The standard keyboard is the first choice for computer access. However, many individuals with disabilities are unable to use a standard keyboard. Fortunately, there are a number of alternatives. Table 7-2 provides examples of some commercially available alternatives to the standard keyboard.

Standard Keyboards.   Some individuals may have difficulty writing because of fatigue or minimally impaired motor control. A standard keyboard on a computer may be all that is needed to allow them to complete writing tasks effectively. Because it is readily available, the standard keyboard is the most desirable interface for direct selection for text entry. The standard keyboard typically has a full alphanumerical array consisting of letters, numbers, punctuation symbols, and special characters such as \/@#$%. Computer keyboards also have special keys. Some of these always have the same effect, such as END, which moves the cursor to the end of a line, or DEL, which erases an entry. Function keys can be assigned to special purposes dictated by a software application. In addition, most computer keyboards contain keys such as SHIFT, CONTROL, and ALT that are referred to as modifier keys because pressing one of these keys while another key is pressed changes the meaning of the second key. Key size, spacing, and amount of distance the keys travel vary depending on the type and manufacturer of the keyboard. To keep the overall size down, laptop computers in particular have smaller keyboards. For this reason, it is wise to have the consumer try the particular type of keyboard he or she will be using.

Built-in Software Adaptations to the Standard Keyboard.
Persons with disabilities often have difficulty in pressing more than one key at a time because they are single-finger typists. They may also have accidental key activation as a result of poor fine motor control. Software adaptations for these and other problems are shown in Table 7-1. These software adaptations are built into Windows and Apple Macintosh operating systems. Collectively these are called **accessibility options** in Windows XP (Microsoft accessibility Web site: *http://www.microsoft.com/enable/products/windowsxp/default.aspx*), Easy Access in Windows Vista (Microsoft accessibility Web site), and **Universal Access** for the Macintosh. They are accessed and adjusted for an individual user through the control panel. Universal access for the Macintosh includes **Easy Access** and CloseView. Easy Access features are those shown in Table 7-1. When StickyKeys is used, the modifier keys are converted to sequential rather than simultaneous use, which allows other effectors (e.g., the head and foot) to also be used to access standard keyboards. In many cases there is also a need for StickyKeys (Windows and Macintosh) and FilterKeys (Windows) or SlowKeys (Macintosh) adaptations. FilterKeys includes the functions of BounceKeys, SlowKeys, and RepeatKeys. In Windows a number of options can be chosen to make the keyboard and mouse faster and easier to use. Options that can be adjusted are described on the Microsoft Web site *(www.microsoft.com/enable/products/windowsxp/default.aspx).*

There is an on-screen keyboard utility in Windows that operates in a manner similar to those described later in this chapter, but it has only basic functionality. Two modes of entry are available when an on-screen key is highlighted by mouse cursor movement: clicking and dwelling. In the latter the user keeps the mouse pointer on an on-screen key for an adjustable, preset time and the key is entered. The on-screen feature also allows entry by scanning with a hot key or switch-input device. Several keyboard configurations are included, and an auditory click may be activated to indicate entry of a character. Windows combines the on-screen keyboard, Narrator, and the magnifier program and a utility manager in its accessibility menu, which is accessed through the start menu. The Accessibility Wizard guides the user through the accessibility options to configure the system specifically for his or her use. Windows Vista also includes a built-in automatic speech recognition system.

Ergonomic Keyboards.
The term *repetitive strain injury* (RSI) encompasses several musculoskeletal disorders that develop as a result of sustained, repetitive movements (Bear-Lehman, 1995). Carpal tunnel syndrome is the most common RSI. It is thought that the use of a standard keyboard with horizontal rows on a flat platform may contribute to RSI in some individuals. Standard keyboards place the hands in an unnatural position with the forearms pronated and the wrists extended and ulnarly deviated. This position causes strain on the tendons and nerves. Numerous alternatives to the standard keyboard have been developed in attempts to reduce this strain on the wrist and hands. These alternatives range from minor rearranging of the keys to major redesign of the keyboard shape and configuration. Here ergonomic keyboards, those keyboards that have been designed with the intent of minimizing the risk of RSI, are discussed. These ergonomic keyboards all use the QWERTY keyboard layout (see Figure 7-12, *A*) with the keys repositioned in some way. Later in this section modifications to the standard QWERTY keyboard layout are discussed.

Ergonomic keyboards attempt to reduce the strain placed on the hands and wrists during the repetitive motion of keying by putting the forearms, wrists, and hands in a neutral position, which is more natural and more comfortable for the typist. There are three basic ways in which the standard keyboard has been redesigned. The first and most common type of ergonomic keyboard is the fixed-split keyboard. In this type of keyboard the layout of the keys is split into two different sections. The center of the keyboard may also be slightly raised with a small slope toward each side. The difference between these keyboards and standard keyboards is that the keys are spaced farther apart and the keyboard is curved so that the hands are placed in a more neutral position. Many of these keyboards have a built-in wrist rest to support the wrists during typing. The Tru-Form Keyboard shown in Figure 7-13, *A*, is one example of this type of keyboard.

The second basic type of ergonomic keyboard is the adjustable-split keyboard. This type also splits the keyboard layout into two parts. A mechanism on the keyboard allows

Standard QWERTY layout

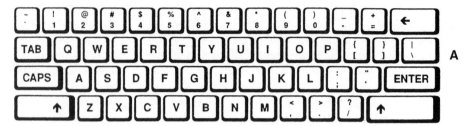

A

Dvorak layout for two hands

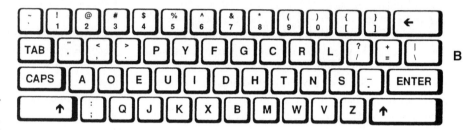

B

Figure 7-12   **A,** Standard QWERTY layout. Dvorak keyboard layouts: **B,** two-hand layout; **C,** one-hand layout, right hand; **D,** Chubon keyboard layout for a typist who uses a single digit or a typing stick.

Dvorak layout for the right hand

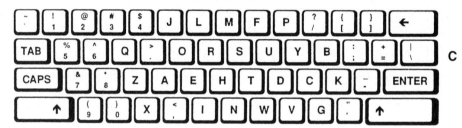

C

Chubon Keyboard Pattern

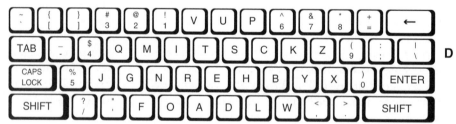

D

one or both sides of the keyboard to be adjusted horizontally and vertically to the position where it is most comfortable. Each section of the split keyboard typically adjusts from 0 to 30 degrees. A user who is a 10-finger typist and does not need to look at the keyboard may be able to take advantage of this range of adjustment. However, for those individuals who need to have the keyboard in the visual field, adjusting the angle too far may make it difficult to see the keys. An example of this type of keyboard is the Maxim Adjustable Keyboard shown in Figure 7-13, *B.*

The third type of ergonomic keyboard uses a concave keywell design. The keyboard layout again is split into two sections, but in this design the keys are arranged in a well such as that shown on the Contoured Keyboard in Figure 7-13, *C.* The principle behind this design is that finger excursion is reduced by having the keys arranged at the same distance from each of the finger joints (Anson, 1997). Other products for all three types of ergonomic keyboards can be found at *www.tifaq.org/keyboards.html.*

Manufacturers of ergonomic keyboards claim that their keyboards reduce the strain placed on the wrist and hands. However, the use of ergonomic keyboards in reducing symptoms of RSI has not been demonstrated in controlled studies. For this reason, it is advised that ergonomic keyboards *not* be

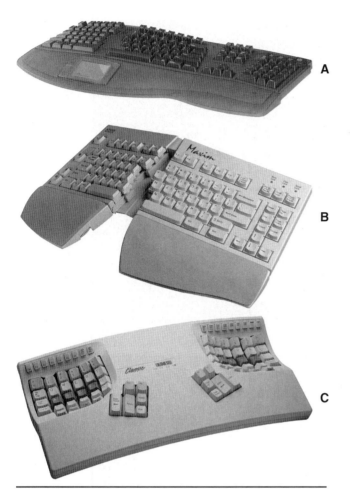

Figure 7-13 Ergonomic keyboards. **A,** The Tru-Form Keyboard. **B,** The Maxim Adjustable Keyboard. **C,** The Contoured Keyboard. (**A,** Courtesy Adesso Inc., www.adessoinc.com; **B** and **C,** courtesy Kinesis Corporation, www.kinesis-ergo.com.)

recommended for the purpose of preventing RSI (Anson, 1997; Tessler, 1993). Situations in which an ergonomic keyboard may be recommended for a consumer include (1) meeting the needs of consumer with physical limitations (e.g., limits in range of motion) and (2) when the consumer finds the ergonomic keyboard more comfortable to use than a standard keyboard. The most critical factor to consider when selecting a keyboard is the user's level of comfort with the different keyboards (Anson, 1997).

Expanded Keyboards. Individuals who do not have sufficient resolution to target the keys on a standard keyboard but still have adequate resolution to select directly may be able to use an expanded keyboard. Expanded keyboards are generally membrane-type keyboards that have enlarged target areas from which the individual can select directly (Figure 7-14, *A*). The minimum size of the target areas on an expanded keyboard is 1 inch square. If the person still has difficulty targeting this size of key, the expanded

keyboard can be customized by grouping keys together to form larger keys. In this way the keyboard can be redesigned to match the skills of the user.

Expanded keyboards vary in overall size and can be chosen depending on the size of the selection set needed by the individual and the key size the individual is able to target accurately. IntelliKeys has a large surface area that can be configured for a variety of key sizes and shapes. It comes with several standard keyboard overlays, such as the one shown in Figure 7-14, *B*. This overlay is an example of a layout that has been configured with different sizes and different shapes of keys on the same keyboard. The IntelliKeys can also be customized to match specific applications by using the companion Overlay Maker software. The keys can be labeled with letters, words, symbols, or pictures. Because they can be customized, expanded keyboards are also useful with individuals who have a cognitive or visual impairment. Examples of expanded keyboards are shown in Table 7-2.

Contracted Keyboards. Some individuals may have sufficient resolution but lack the range of movement to reach all the keys on a standard keyboard. In this situation a contracted, or mini, keyboard may be the solution. These keyboards use either raised keys or a membrane surface. For computer use, contracted keyboards must meet the requirement that all keys of the standard keyboard be represented, which is accomplished by using additional modifier keys. Figure 7-15 shows a consumer being evaluated using a mouthstick with the USB Mini keyboard. This keyboard is approximately 7.25 × 4.2 inches in overall size, with the size of each key approximately one half inch on a side. Several of the keys have multiple functions, depending on which modifier key is pressed first. The functions corresponding to various modifiers can be colored to match the modifier key. The selection set (the alphabet) in Figure 7-15 is not placed in the QWERTY format typical of standard keyboards. The letter placement is based on a "frequency of use" system in which the letters most commonly used in the English language are placed toward the center, with the less commonly used letters placed in the outer edges of the keyboard. This arrangement particularly makes sense to use on a contracted keyboard where the individual's range of motion is restricted. Because of the small key size and closeness of the keys, the user of a contracted keyboard must have good fine motor control. Persons using contracted keyboards type with a single digit, a handheld typing stick, or a mouthstick.

Special-Purpose Keyboards. Keyboards are also used on special-purpose devices, such as augmentative communication and environmental control devices. In these cases the available keys may be much more limited in number or they may be very specific in function compared with the standard keyboard. For example, in portable augmentative

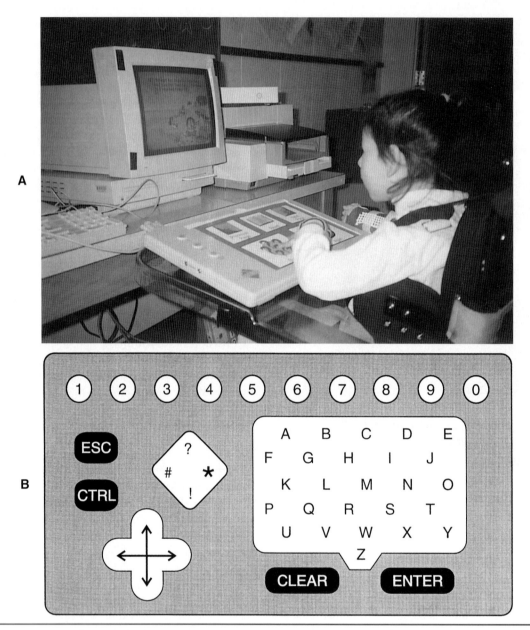

Figure 7-14   **A,** Consumer using an expanded keyboard with thumb. **B,** Expanded keyboard showing configuration with different sizes and shapes of keys on the same keyboard.

communication devices such as the SpringBoard, the keyboards have membrane keys and are restricted to a total of 32 keys (see Chapter 11). These keys are not assigned any specific character or function when manufactured but can be programmed to represent just about anything the user would like. Other devices come with certain keys that have been designated to be specific functions. For example, a key may be designated "SPEAK," and pressing it will cause whatever was entered to be spoken. In all these cases, however, the keyboard provides the same function: direct selection input from the user to the processor.

Dedicated communication devices can also be used as input devices for a general-purpose computer. The communication device is connected to the computer through a serial or USB interface. This connection allows the communication device to send characters to the computer as if they were typed from the computer keyboard. Because the user of the communication device is familiar with the keyboard on the communication device, it is easy for him or her to use it for computer entry and the user does not have to learn another keyboard arrangement. Another advantage is that any words or phrases that are stored in the communication

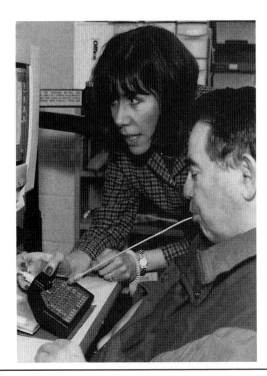

Figure 7-15 Consumer using the WinMini Keyboard and a mouthstick being evaluated.

device can be sent to the computer as words or phrases as well. A standard has been developed to allow all keyboard characters to be sent to the computer, even if the communication device does not have that character. For example, computer keys such as DEL may not be on the communication device, but the user can send a sequence of characters that the computer interprets as the DEL key. Selection of a special-purpose keyboard for a consumer also requires careful consideration of the items presented in Box 7-2.

Automatic Speech Recognition as an Alternative Keyboard

Automatic speech recognition (ASR) technology can be applied to computer access by allowing the user to speak the names of keys or key words and have these spoken utterances interpreted by the computer as if they had been typed. This approach is appealing because human speech is so rapid and voice control is so natural. ASR systems that are extremely reliable, flexible, and easy to use are available for use as full-function keyboard and mouse emulation. For example, if a word processing program is being run, then control functions such as delete, move, and print and the most common vocabulary the person normally uses, a greeting and ending for a business letter, and other similar vocabulary items can be used. If the user changes to a spreadsheet program, he or she can use vocabulary that contains items specific to that application. Microsoft Vista includes ASR as part of the built-in package of accessories.

CASE STUDY

EVALUATION AND SELECTION OF SPEECH RECOGNITION

Marilyn Abraham is a 44-year-old woman who has been diagnosed as having reflex sympathetic dystrophy (RSD) of both wrists. Apparently caused by vasospasm and vasodilation, RSD is a reaction to pain after an injury (Kasch, Poole, and Hedl, 1998). It results in edema; shiny, blotchy skin; and pain. Ms. Abraham is a secretary in a large state office, which she shares with other coworkers. She uses the computer for much of the day. The RSD ensued in her right wrist as a result of the repetitive motion she uses in performing her job. After this injury she received retraining to transfer her hand dominance to her left hand, and the Dvorak one-handed keyboard layout was recommended (see Figure 7-12). Subsequently she broke her left wrist in a motor vehicle accident, which also resulted in RSD. She is able to type or use the mouse for only 10 minutes before her hands and forearms swell. Ms. Abraham has tried different positions and adaptations when typing. For example, she used a pointer held by a cuff in her palm to type so that her forearm remained in a neutral position. This method still resulted in swelling and pain. She also has neck pain when she uses the keyboard.

Ms. Abraham first tried using a trackball with her hand and the on-screen keyboard. After using the trackball for a short time, Ms. Abraham found that it also caused pain. Ms. Abraham next tried using her right foot with an expanded keyboard and then a trackball. There were concerns about the utility of both these approaches because of potential neck strain from looking down and that possibility that the repeated movement of her ankle to input characters using the trackball might lead to repetitive motion problems with her foot.

Next Ms. Abraham tried a head-controlled interface that was worn on a band and attached to her head. She used this interface with an on-screen keyboard and acceptance time to make a selection. She was able to control this interface without difficulty but thought that after a period of use her neck would become tired.

QUESTIONS

1. What other control interfaces could you try with Ms. Abraham?
2. If you evaluate automatic speech recognition for Ms. Abraham, what issues will you need to take into consideration?

Two basic types of ASR systems exist. With a *speaker-dependent system*, the user trains the system to recognize his or her voice by producing several samples of the same element. The method in which the training is handled varies among systems. The system analyzes these samples so that it can recognize variations in the user's speech and generate a computer input (e.g., enter a given letter, a string of letters, or a control key like "return") corresponding to what was spoken. Even after the system has been trained with several speech samples, there likely will be times when the system does not recognize the user's speech and does not produce a response. Recognition accuracy is steadily increasing as advances are made in the computer algorithms used for analysis. Rates can be greater than 90% for general input and nearly 100% for isolated word applications (e.g., command and control, database, spreadsheet). Speaker-dependent systems can be further divided into continuous and discrete categories. Comerford, Makhoul, and Schwartz (1997) describe the development of ASR systems and describe the technical aspects of these systems.

Speaker-independent systems recognize speech patterns of different individuals without training (Gallant, 1989). These systems are developed by using samples of speech from hundreds of people and information provided by phonologists on the various pronunciations of words (Baker, 1981). The tradeoff with this type of total recognition system is that the vocabulary set is small. In assistive technology applications, speaker-independent systems are primarily used for environmental and robotic control (Chapter 14) and power mobility (Chapter 12).

Discrete speech recognition systems require the user to pause between each word for recognition to occur, which is a very unnatural type of speech. There have been reports of voice problems associated with the use of discrete speech recognition systems (Kambeyanda, Singer, and Cronk, 1997). These are due to the abrupt starting and stopping of speech required for these systems, coupled with the monotone quality required for good recognition, both of which are unnatural speech patterns. Continuous ASR systems allow the user to speak in a more normal manner, without major pauses. The rates of input are within the range of normal rates of human speech (150 to 250 words per minute). Although the possibility of damage to the vocal folds is reduced with these systems, it is not totally eliminated. Because the discrete systems are more accurate for single-word recognition, they are sometimes used for commands and control in applications such as spreadsheets and databases. Some manufacturers (e.g., Dragon Systems, Nuance, Inc., Burlington, Mass., *http://www.nuance.com/*) provide both continuous (e.g., Naturally Speaking) and discrete (e.g., Dragon Dictate) ASR, sometimes bundled into the same package. Currently used speech recognition systems are listed in Table 7-8. The majority of these use continuous recognition.

Speech recognition can be used for computer access, wheelchair control, and EADLs. The systems shown in Table 7-8 allow the consumer to use speech to enter text directly into a computer application program. Recognition of control words, such as "save file," used in a word processor is also trained. System vocabulary is also growing rapidly. Early systems had recognition vocabularies (the list of words the system can recognize when spoken) in the 1000 to 5000 range. Current systems have vocabularies of 50,000 words or more. The faster speech rate, larger vocabularies, and continuous recognition all place significant demands on the speed and memory of the host computer. Continuous speech recognition systems require large amounts of memory and high-speed computers. As the cost of this added computer functionality continues to decline, these additional requirements will be less important. However, ASR systems do require more computer resources than other alternative input methods (Anson, 1999).

There are other hardware issues that are important in ASR as well. Foremost of these is the microphone. Anson (1997) discusses considerations in the choice of a microphone for ASR. Although the microphones supplied with ASR systems are satisfactory for use by nondisabled users, they are not adequate when the user has limited breath support, special positioning requirements, or low-volume speech. Most ASR systems use a standard headset microphone. Individuals who have disabilities may not be able to don and doff such microphones independently, and desk-mounted types are often used. Current ASR systems do not require separate hardware to be installed in the computer, and they use commonly available sound cards (Anson, 1999).

EADLs may also use speech recognition to access their functions (see Chapter 14). In such devices the individual can

TABLE 7-8	Speech Recognition Interfaces	
Category	Description	Device Name/Manufacturer
Speaker-dependent systems	Recognition depends on the system's learning the user's speech patterns and building a user vocabulary.	Naturally Speaking and Dragon Dictate (Dragon Systems); Via Voice (IBM); Hear-Say (Voice Pilot Technologies)
Speaker-independent systems	The operation is similar to continuous speech recognition systems, but there is no training required. Generally limited to small, application-specific vocabularies.	Used in special-purpose assistive devices for environmental control or robotic control (see Chapter 14) and wheelchair control (see Chapter 12).

instruct the system to turn lights off and on or perform other functions by voice. The user can train the system to execute these commands with just about any sound, letter, or word.

The questions listed in Box 7-3 can be used to determine the usefulness of speech recognition for a given consumer. The key for success in using speech-activated systems is that the user be able to produce a *consistent* vocalization or verbalization. Differences in speech production are found not only among individual speakers but also within the same speaker. Variability in the user's speech can cause problems with recognition. For this reason, this type of control interface may not be effective for individuals who have dysarthria. Individuals who have had a spinal cord injury and have no functional use of the upper extremities yet have good speech control are potential candidates for a speech recognition system. It is important when considering a speech recognition system to determine whether the user's voice pitch, articulation, and loudness change or fatigue over time. Other noises or voices in the area where the speech-activated system is being used can also confuse the system, resulting in either an incorrect selection or the system having difficulty registering any selection, causing the user to repeat the vocalization several times.

Touch Screens and Touch Tablets

Touch screens are available on augmentative communication devices and laptop, palm, and notebook computers that the user activates by pointing directly to the selection set on the screen. Using a touch screen makes selection cognitively easier for many users, particularly young children, because it is more direct and intuitive. These interfaces are activated by either breaking a very thin light beam or by a capacitive array that detects the electrical charge on the finger. The electrode array used to detect where the finger, or pointer, is touching is transparent, and the touch screen can be placed over the face of a monitor. In either detection method an array of horizontal and vertical sensors is arranged so that an object the size of a finger will be detected. The position in the array determines what the interpretation of the pointing action will be, just as the specific key on a keyboard determines what the

input will be. Separate touch screens can also be attached to the computer monitor or placed over a selection array on a tabletop or other flat surface. The selection set varies with the application program being used.

TongueTouch Keypad

The TongueTouch Keypad, shown in Figure 7-16, consists of nine separate small switches incorporated into a dental mouthpiece that fits in the roof of the mouth. It is a battery-operated, radio frequency–transmitting interface that activates a processor that sends IR signals to the computer. Each of the nine switches corresponds to one choice on a menu presented on a computer screen. The first menu provides choices of environmental control (e.g., television, lights), computer access (keyboard emulation), and wheelchair control. Once one of these categories is chosen, nine more choices pertaining to that category are presented, such as volume and channel control for the television; letters, keyboard array, and mouse movement directions for computer entry; or numerical choices for telephone dialing. This approach is useful for individuals who do not have motor control in their limbs but have good head, neck, and oral-motor control. In particular, the user must have good elevation of the tip of the tongue to activate the individual keys efficiently (Lau and O'Leary, 1993).

Access for Users With Cognitive Limitations

Concept keyboards replace the letters and numbers of the keyboard with pictures, symbols, or words that represent the concepts being used or taught. When the user presses on the picture, the correct character is sent to the computer to create the desired effect. As an example, a child who is having difficulty with basic arithmetic and monetary concepts may be more successful using a concept keyboard in which each key displayed is a coin of a particular denomination, rather than the value (number) or name of the coin (letters). The child can push on the coin and have that number of cents entered into the program. A simple program that asks the child to make change could be used to encourage the child to develop subtraction skills while also learning the value of specific coins. This approach is more motivating for some children and it is easier to press on a key labeled with a quarter than to enter "2" and "5."

Very simple programs may require only two keys. For example, the SPACE key can move a cursor to different matching choices and the RETURN key can select the desired one. This concept can be used to match shapes or numbers or to control any two-choice task. It functions as a keyboard, although only two keys are used.

Another approach to concept keyboards is the use of specially designed software together with special-input keyboards. These systems do not require the use of a special input interface

---

BOX 7-3   Critical Questions for Evaluating Use of Speech Recognition Interface

1. Can the consumer consistently utter all the sounds necessary to access the speech recognition system?
2. Is the recognition vocabulary adequate?
3. Is the consumer's voice articulation, pitch, and loudness consistent enough for accurate selection?
4. Is there likely to be background noise in the consumer's context that will interfere with the speech recognition system?
5. Would an alternative template or vocabulary be beneficial?

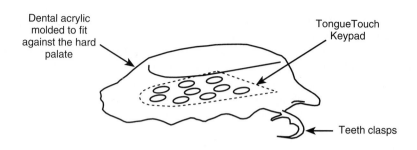

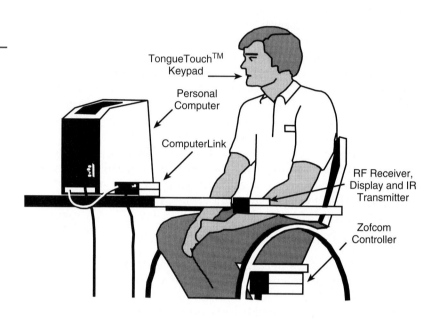

Figure 7-16 Components of the TongueTouch Keypad. (From Lau C, O'Leary S: Comparison of computer interface devices for persons with severe disabilities, *Am J Occup Ther* 47:1022-1029, 1993.)

because they plug directly into a serial, parallel, or USB port. The software also comes with overlays for the keyboard. For example, a program to teach language concepts can be implemented by placing pictures of the concepts on specific keys and having the child generate words by pressing the correct key, causing the concept to be spoken and the picture to be repeated on the screen. When the child plays with the objects described, he or she learns to label his or her actions as well as the objects. Concept keyboards provide a direct relationship between the task and the child's action. For example, by using a picture of the body as the "keyboard" and each body part as a "key," a child can touch the body part when the program instructs him or her to do so. When the child does, the program can repeat the body part name and cause it to be moved on the screen. The Intellikeys (IntelliTools, Petaluma, Calif., *www.intellitools.com*) keyboard is often used as a concept keyboard.

An even more direct concept keyboard is the Touch Window. With this device the user merely touches the screen at the proper place and the touch screen enters the information as though it has been typed. Monitors with built-in touch screens are also available for Macintosh and Windows computers. Moving the finger on the screen can also be used to draw. This device can be placed horizontally on a table or lap tray and used as a concept keyboard with an appropriate overlay. On-screen keyboard arrays can also function as concept keyboards with the choice of on-screen elements.

There are also commercial emulation programs that reduce the complexity of the Windows environment for users who have cognitive disabilities. The Voyager suite of programs from Saltillo (Saltillo, Millersbery, Ohio, *http://saltillo.buyol.com/Item/Voyager_Desktop_Suite.htm*) allows individuals with cognitive disabilities to launch programs, communicate by e-mail, and browse the Web. The entire suite operates with pictures rather than words to present the user with choices removing the necessity for the user to be able to read or write. Receiving e-mail is accomplished by using text to speech to provide an auditory output. The user sends e-mail by selecting a set of pictures that enable the send function, select the recipient by picture or name, and then prompt the user to record a message and send it. Assistive technologies for persons with cognitive limitations are discussed in more detail in Chapter 10.

Eye-Controlled Systems

Often consumers use the direction of eye gaze as the only means of indicating. Manual eye-controlled communication systems have been in use for a long time. In manual systems the user communicates "yes" or "no" though eye blinks or uses the eyes to point to letters on an alphabet board to spell utterances. This manual form of using eye movement as a means of input can be automated by electronically detecting the user's eye movements as a control interface for direct selection.

There are currently two basic types of eye-controlled systems. One type uses an IR video camera mounted adjacent to a computer display. An IR beam from the camera is shined onto the person's eye and then reflected by the retina. The camera picks up this reflection of the individual's eye as he or she looks at the on-screen keyboard appearing on the computer monitor. Special processing software in the computer analyzes the images coming into the camera from the eyes and determines where and for how long the person is looking on the screen. The user makes a selection by looking at it for a specified period, which can be adjusted according to the user's needs. The EyeGaze System, Quick Glance, ERICA (Eye Response Technologies, Charlottesville, Va., *www.eyeresponse.com*), and Tobii (TobiiTechnology, San Francisco, Calif., *www.tobii.com*) are examples of two-eye–controlled systems of this type. The design principles and approach to the ERICA system are described by Lankford (2000). The other type of eye-controlled system uses a head-mounted viewer that tracks the movements of one eye. This viewer is attached to one side of the frame of a standard pair of glasses so that it is in front of one eye. The movements from the eye are viewed and converted into keyboard input by a separate control unit. One example of this type of system is VisionKey. Both types of eye-controlled systems provide the user with computer access for written or verbal communication, Internet access, environmental control, and telephone operation. To operate either type of eye-controlled system, the user must have good vision and control of at least one eye, good head control, including the ability to keep the head fairly stationary, and the cognitive ability to follow instructions.

An eye-controlled system is beneficial for individuals who have little or no movement in their limbs and may also have limited speech, for example, someone who has had a brainstem stroke, has amyotrophic lateral sclerosis, or has high-level quadriplegia. Some disadvantages of eye-controlled systems are that sunlight, bright incandescent lighting, and contact lenses may interfere with system tracking, and the cost of such systems is still rather high in comparison with other input methods. For some individuals, however, it may be the only reliable means of control.

A disadvantage of eye-controlled systems is holding the point of gaze (POG) on a target long enough for selection by a dwell time or separate switch selection. An alternative is to use an EMG control to incrementally move the cursor in small steps by muscle activations. Because the cursor only moves if a muscle is activated, holding on a target is accomplished by

relaxing the muscle, and target acquisition is easier than holding the POG. However, moving large distances on the screen in small steps can be fatiguing. To take advantage of the benefits of POG for moving large distances and the EMG for narrowing down to a precise target and holding, a hybrid POG/EMG system has been developed (Barreto, Al-Masri, and Cremades, 2003). The system calculates the distance from the current cursor location to the POG of an eye tracking system. If this distance is small, then the EMG incremental stepping cursor movement is used. If the distance is large, the POG is used to move to the vicinity of the target. Trials with subjects who are not disabled showed that the hybrid POG/EMG system had faster acquisition times for targets ranging from 8.5 to 22 mm. The variance was higher for the hybrid system, indicating that additional practice and training are required to maximize its effectiveness.

Tracking of Body Features

Another approach to cursor control is the use of a camera to track body features (Betke, Gips, and Fleming, 2002). This system uses a digital camera and image recognition software to track a particular feature. The most easily tracked feature is the tip of the nose, but the eye (gross eye position, not POG), lip, chin, and thumb have also been used. The movement of the feature being tracked is converted into a signal that controls an on-screen mouse cursor. Betke, Gips, and Fleming (2002) describe the technical features of the system software in detail. Trials with nondisabled subjects in an on-screen game in which targets were "captured" by pointing the cursor at them showed that the camera mouse was accurate but slower than a typical hand-controlled mouse. With an on-screen keyboard used for a typing task, the camera mouse was half as fast as a regular mouse, but the accuracy obtained was equivalent on each system. Eleven persons with disabilities ranging in age from 2 to 58 years used the camera mouse. Eight of the 11 were able to control it reliably and continued to use it. With the increasing availability of built-in cameras in computers, the camera mouse requires only a software program to capture the body feature image and interpret its movement as mouse commands, which may make this approach more common.

Brain-Computer Interface

A significant number of people cannot effectively use any of the interfaces described in this chapter. For these individuals, the brain-computer interface (BCI) may offer promise. Although this approach is still primarily in the research stage, there are promising results to date. It is likely that we will see a much greater understanding of the biological/physical interface for the control of computers in the future (Applewhite, 2004). Figure 7-17 is an overview of a typical BCI system (Schalk et al, 2004). Features or signals that

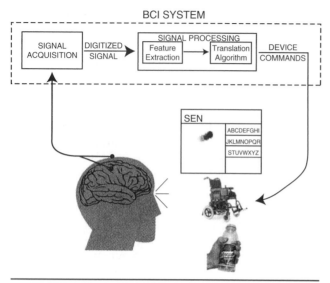

Figure 7-17   An overview of a typical brain control interface system. (From Schalk G et al: BCI2000: a general-purpose brain-computer interface (BCI) system, *IEEE Trans Biomed Eng* 51:1034-1043, 2004).

have been used include slow cortical potentials, P300 evoked potential, sensorimotor rhythms recorded from the cortex, and neuronal action potentials recorded within the cortex. The success of BCI systems depends on the type of brain signal, the methods of signal processing to extract relevant features, the algorithms that translate the features into control signals (most often a mouse-like cursor movement on the screen), user feedback, and user characteristics. BCI systems may be grouped into a set of functional components (Mason and Birch, 2003). The BCI input device provides amplification, feature extraction, feature translation, and user feedback. The control interface converts this signal to those required to control the output device (e.g., power wheelchair, EADL, computer). The device controller provides the actual control signal to the target device (e.g., signals to the motors of a power wheelchair, mouse cursor movement signals to a computer). A typical task for a user is to visualize different movements or sensations or images. An example of differing signals measured on the surface of the cortex for different imagined motor acts is shown in Figure 7-18 (Leuthardt et al, 2004). The unique signal patterns shown in Figure 7-16 can be used to generate control signals. Schalk et al (2004) give technical details of the major approaches to BCI system design. Electrodes located on the surface of the cortex have stronger and more varied signals and less interfering muscle artifact and are more stable than those attached to the scalp (Leuthardt et al, 2004). Some sensorimotor patterns that can be measured from the surface of the cortex under the skull are too weak to be measured outside the skull. The invasiveness of the electrocorticographic signals is the major drawback. In all cases, signals are mathematically analyzed to extract features useful for control (Fabiani et al, 2004).

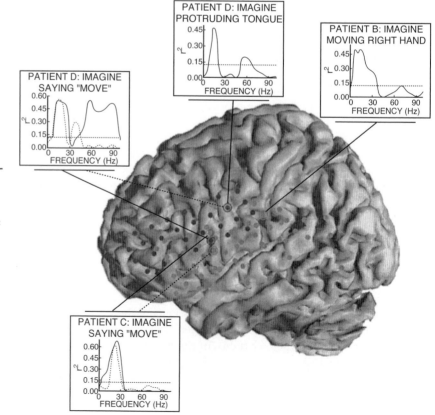

Figure 7-18   An example of differing signals measured on the surface of the cortex for different imagined motor acts. (From Leuthardt EC et al: A brain-computer interface using electrocorticagraphic signals in humans, *J Neural Eng* 1: 63-71, 2004.)

Standard and Alternative Electronic Pointing Interfaces

The other commonly used control interface for direct selection in general-purpose computers is a *mouse*. There are also alternative pointing interfaces that can replace the mouse, such as a trackball, a head sensor, a continuous joystick, and the use of the arrow keys on the keypad (called *MouseKeys*). Box 7-4 identifies the critical questions to consider when assessing an individual for using any type of pointing interface.

It is necessary to determine whether the consumer can use the pointing interface to reach the items in the selection set (targets) and stay fixed on the target while executing the action needed to make a selection. These all imply that the selection targeted is accurate. The person may be able to get to a target area on the screen, but the size of the target may affect his or her ability to maintain that position while selecting it. Any location on the screen can be a target, and these can be of different sizes. Depending on the software program, the size of the target may be fixed or it may be possible to modify the size to meet the user's needs. The user can use one of two techniques to make a selection. With an *acceptance time selection technique,* the user pauses at the selection for a predetermined period (which is adjustable) and that pause signals the selection. With the *manual selection technique,* the user activates another switch to let the device know that the selection has been made. The second approach provides more control for the user, but it also requires additional user motor control.

Pointing interfaces vary in terms of the tactile and proprioceptive feedback that they provide, which may affect the user's performance. Using a pointing interface also requires a significant amount of coordination between the body site executing the movement of the cursor and the eyes following the cursor on the screen and locating the targets. The ATP should determine whether the layout of the items in the selection set is beneficial or detrimental to the user's performance. The selection set and its layout will vary depending on the pointing interface and the software being used.

BOX 7-4   Critical Questions for Evaluating Use of Electronic Pointing Interfaces

1. Can the consumer use the pointing interface to reach all the targets on the screen?
2. Is the size and spacing of the screen targets appropriate?
3. Is the consumer able to complete the action needed to make a selection and perform other mouse functions required by the application software (click, drag, and double click)?
4. Is the sensory feedback provided by the control interface and the user display adequate?
5. Does the consumer use the keyboard layout effectively?

CASE STUDY

EVALUATION AND SELECTION OF A POINTING INTERFACE

David is a 21-year-old man who has muscular dystrophy. He would like to be able to access the family computer for educational and recreational purposes. David would like to play computer-based games and use drawing programs that typically require a mouse. He lacks movement in his four extremities, with the exception of wrist and finger movement. He is able to reach with each hand from within 3 inches of his body to 8 inches out from his body. With his right hand he can reach approximately 5.5 inches to the right of midline and with his left hand he can reach 3 inches to the left of midline. He cannot cross midline with either hand.

David tried a contracted keyboard, and he was able to point to keys in a restricted range near the middle of the keyboard. He was unable to access other areas of the keyboard without assistance for repositioning of his arms. He was able to move a continuous joystick in all four directions and use it with the on-screen keyboard software, but this was difficult for him. A trackball was also used with the on-screen keyboard software to determine whether David could use it. He could easily use the trackball as a pointing device to point to the keys shown on the screen. Using a drawing program and the trackball, he was able to direct the cursor to various parts of the screen with enough precision to draw lines and shapes. However, he was unable to hold the trackball in place with the cursor on the desired selection and simultaneously press the button on the trackball with the same hand to make his selection. The acceptance time selection technique was shown to him, and he was able to easily use this technique.

QUESTIONS

1. From the data given, should the ATP recommend a contracted keyboard for David?
2. From the information given, what would be the optimal control interface for David? What other information is needed regarding David's needs and skills that might influence the recommendation?
3. What other software will David need to operate the recommended control interface?

It is important to know whether the layout of the selection set can be modified for a particular pointing interface and what type of modifications will benefit the user.

Mouse.   The standard computer mouse is a solid box that rides on top of a ball. As the mouse is gripped by the user and moved across a flat surface, the ball rotates, causing the cursor on the screen to move. As the mouse moves, the computer screen shows a pointer that follows the mouse movement. The GUI is used as the selection set. In this type of selection set, the screen contains a list of options, either written words or icons. If the mouse is moved to the option and a button is pressed (usually called *clicking*), then that item is chosen. Two rapid clicks are used to run, or execute, the program related to the icon. If the mouse button is held down while the mouse is pointing to a menu item and then the mouse is moved down the list (called *dragging* the mouse), a new list of choices appears. The GUI reduces the number of keystrokes and provides a prompting display for the user.

The mouse is ideally suited for functions such as drawing, moving around in a document, or moving a block of text. The mouse can be a useful tool for individuals with disabilities who cannot otherwise draw with a pen or pencil. However, mouse use requires a high degree of eye-hand coordination and motor coordination and a certain amount of range of motion. The standard computer mouse is available in many different shapes and sizes. If a consumer is having difficulty using the mouse that came with the computer, the solution may be as simple as finding a mouse that fits his or her hand better. The standard mouse requires a great deal of motor control, however, and many individuals with

disabilities find that the use of a standard computer mouse is difficult or impossible. Another option is to try a different control site for mouse use. If the consumer has better control of his feet than his hands, his foot can be used with a foot-controlled mouse such as the No Hands Mouse. There are also alternatives to mouse use that are easier for many persons with disabilities. Any control interface that can imitate the two-dimensional movement (up/down, left/right) of the mouse can be made to look to the computer like a mouse. Table 7-9 lists the major alternatives to mouse input and sample technologies. Examples of several of these approaches are shown in Figure 7-19.

Keypad Mouse.   For those individuals who are able to use a standard keyboard but have difficulty using a standard mouse, the first alternative to evaluate is the keypad mouse. A numerical keypad is embedded in most standard computer keyboards. *MouseKeys,* included in the accessibility options for Windows and in the Macintosh operating systems, allows use of the keypad to simulate mouse movement. When the NUM LOCK key is engaged, each key on the numerical keypad functions as the number to which it is assigned (1 to 9). When the NUM LOCK key is disengaged

TABLE 7-9   Alternative Electronic Pointing Interfaces

Category	Description	Device Name/Manufacturer
Keypad mouse	Mouse movement is replaced by keys that move the mouse cursor in horizontal, vertical, and diagonal directions. One or more keys perform the functions of the mouse button (click, double click, drag).	R.A.T. (Adaptivation, Inc.)
Trackball	Looks like an inverted mouse; a ball is mounted on a stationary base. Included on the base are one or more buttons that provide the functions of the standard mouse buttons. The base and hand remain stationary and the fingers move the ball. Requires minimal range of motion and less eye-hand coordination.	Big Track, n-Abler (Inclusive Technology); EasiTrax (Inclusive Technology); Trackman Marble Plus (Logitech); EasyBall (Microsoft); Roller Trackball (Traxsys Computer Products)
Continuous input joysticks	Joysticks (continuous input and switched) are used as direct selection interfaces for powered mobility. For computer use, movements are similar to wheelchair control; easy to relate cursor movement (direction, speed, and distance) to joystick movement.	Jouse (Compusult Limited); Roller Joystick II (Traxsys Computer Products); EasiTrax (Inclusive Technology); all manufacturers of power wheelchairs have their own joysticks, which are supplied with wheelchair
Head-controlled mouse	An interface controlled through head movement; the user wears a sensor on the head, which is detected by a unit on the computer. Movement of the head is translated into cursor movement on the screen.	Head Master Plus (Prentke Romich Co.); Head Mouse (Origin Instruments Co.); Tracker (Madentec Ltd. Communications); smartNAV-3 (Inclusive Technology)
Light pointers and light sensors	These devices either emit a light beam that can be used to point to objects or as a control interface, or they receive light and provide an output when the light is reflected from an object or the light beam is interrupted.	Light-operated Ability Switch (Ability Research, Inc.); Lomac (Inclusive Technolgy); Viewpoint Optical Indicator (Prentke Romich); Infrared/sound/touch switch (Words Inc.)

Data from Ability Research, Inc., Minnetoka, Minn. (www.skypoint.com/P5ability/contacts/html); Adaptivation, Sioux Falls, S.D. (www.adaptivation.com); Compusult Limited, Mount Pearl, Newfoundland (http://www.jouse.com/html/about.html); Logitech, Fremont, Calif. (www.logitech.com); Inclusive Technology (http://www.inclusive.co.uk/catalogue/index.html); Madentec Limited, Edmonton, Alberta (www.madentec.com); Microsoft, Redmond, Wash. (www.microsoft.com); Origin Instruments, Grand Prairie, Tex. (www.orin.com); Traxsys Computer Products (http://assistive.traxsys.com/staticProductListing.asp); Prentke Romich Co., Wooster, Ohio (www.prenrom.com); Words+ Inc. (www.words-plus.com).

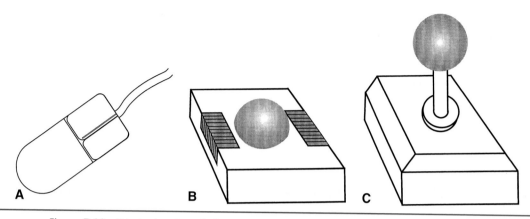

Figure 7-19   Pointing interfaces. **A,** Standard computer mouse. **B,** Trackball. **C,** Proportional joystick.

and *MouseKeys* is running, these keys can perform the same functions as a mouse. The "5" key serves as a mouse click, and the surrounding number keys move the mouse in vertical, horizontal, or diagonal directions. This software interprets the keys as mouse input when MouseKeys is active and interprets them as arrow keys when it is not active. MouseKeys allows adjustment of the mouse speed (distance the cursor moves with each arrow key press) and acceleration (the rate at which the cursor moves).

There are also keypad mice that are external to the standard keyboard, such as the Micro Pad. The advantage of external keypads is that they can be placed in any position in the workspace. The disadvantage is that they take up more space on the work surface. External keypad mice are also available with enlarged keys, such as the Expanded Keypad and the Big Blue Mouse, both of which have 1.5-inch square membrane keys. When a trackball, joystick, or other hardware alternative is substituted for the mouse, it is necessary to accommodate the mouse buttons including clicking (rapid press and release), double clicking, and dragging (holding the button while moving the mouse). Software adaptations replace these mouse button functions by selecting which mouse button function is required and then implementing that function when the user pauses on the selection.

Trackball.   Use of a trackball is one approach that was developed for the able-bodied population but has often been found to be helpful for persons who cannot use the mouse. This device looks like an inverted mouse; a ball is mounted on a stationary base. Included on the base are one or more buttons that provide the functions of the standard mouse buttons. The ball is rotated by moving the hand or finger across it, causing the cursor to move on the screen. Because the base and hand remain stationary and the fingers move the ball, this approach requires less range of motion than the standard mouse and is easier for some disabled users. It is also possible

to use the trackball easily with other body sites such as a chin or foot. On most trackballs the user can latch the mouse button, which allows single-finger or mouthstick users to perform "click and drag" functions without having to hold down a button while simultaneously moving the mouse. Trackballs are available in a variety of sizes, shapes, and configurations. There are trackballs (such as the Trackman Marble Plus) in which the ball is positioned on the side where it can be controlled by the thumb. There are also very small trackballs, such as the Thumbelina Mini Trackball, that fit in the palm of the hand. Having the consumer try the different types of trackballs is important, even if this means taking a trip to a local computer store that has different models available for demonstration.

Continuous Input Joysticks.   A joystick provides four directions of control and is thus ideally suited for use as another alternative to the mouse. There are two types of joysticks: proportional (continuous) and switched (discrete). A proportional joystick has continuous signals, so any movement of the control handle results in an immediate response by the command domain in that direction. By using a proportional joystick, the individual can control not only direction of movement but also the rate of that movement. Proportional joysticks are most commonly used with power wheelchairs. The farther the wheelchair joystick moves away from the starting point, the faster the wheelchair goes. The proportional joystick is also more likely to be used as a mouse substitute because the direction and rate of cursor movement can be controlled by the user. The Jouse is a joystick-operated mouse that is controlled with the chin or mouth. Mouse button activations can be made by using a sip-and-puff switch that is built into the joystick. Just like the proportional joystick used for wheelchair control, the joystick used for a mouse substitute will cause the mouse pointer to move faster the farther away it gets from the center position. A major difference between mouse and trackball use and the use of a joystick is that the joystick is always referenced to a center point, whereas the mouse cursor movement is relative to the current position. This difference in reference point can cause difficulties for the consumer when first using the joystick. The user must spend some time learning how to use this control interface for it to be an effective alternative to the mouse (Anson, 1997).

Head-Controlled Mouse.   For individuals who lack the hand or foot movement to operate a mouse or joystick, there are alternative pointing interfaces that are controlled with head movement (Evans, Drew, and Blenkhorn, 2000). In general, head-controlled mouse systems operate by using a tracking unit that senses and measures head position relative to a fixed reference point. This reference point is the center of the screen for the cursor. As the head moves away from this point in any direction, the cursor is moved on the screen. The technology that is used to sense the head movement differs from one system to another; it may be ultrasound, IR, gyroscopical, or image recognition (video). Each of these relies on transmission of a signal to the sensor on the user's head and detection of a reflected signal that is sent back. An alternative approach is to locate a transmitter on the user's head with a receiver that monitors the change in head position (Evans, Drew, and Blenkhorn, 2000). Different commercial systems implement this reflective measurement in a variety of ways. In early versions of head-controlled interfaces, the headset worn by the user was connected with a wire to the computer, limiting the user's mobility. Most of the systems currently available have a wireless connection, which allows the user to move around more freely. Several devices require only a reflective dot to be placed on the user's face (usually the forehead). This design eliminates the bulky head pointer used in earlier devices.

These systems are intended for individuals who lack upper extremity movement and who can accurately control head movement. For example, persons with high-level spinal cord injuries who cannot use any limb often find these head pointers to be rapid and easy to use. On the other hand, individuals who have random head movement or who do not have trunk alignment with the vertical axis of the video screen often have significantly more trouble using this type of input device.

In one common commercial approach, the user wears a sensor that is attached either to the forehead directly with adhesive, to a pair of glasses, or to a band or headset worn on the head (Figure 7-6, *A*). Through the sensor, a tracking unit on the computer detects head movement and translates it into a signal that the computer interprets as if it were sent by a mouse. By moving the head (with the sensor on it), the person moves the cursor on the screen. For mouse-related tasks (e.g., selecting an icon, opening a window), the head-controlled interface is a direct replacement. Clicking and

double clicking are done by using either an acceptance (or dwell) time (which can be adjusted to meet the user's needs) or a switch. When a switch is used, it is often a puff-and-sip switch that is attached directly to the headset. The person generates a single puff to click and two puffs to double click. To perform the drag function, the user must produce sustained pressure on the puff switch. Some individuals may not have the breath control to perform the drag function. In a later section software programs that can be used to replace the switch for drag-and-click functions are described. For typing, the head-controlled interface must be used with an on-screen keyboard program.

Control of the mouse cursor is either relative (like a joystick) or absolute (like a mouse). With absolute devices the mouse cursor position corresponds to the position of the device (e.g., a trackball, hand-operated mouse, etc.). To operate a relative device, the person moves the cursor by displacing the control. When the cursor reaches the desired location, the control is released. The next movement is then made from that location by displacing the control again. A joystick is an example of a relative pointing device. Because a hand-operated mouse can also be lifted and repositioned, it can act like a relative device. Users with disabilities prefer the relative technique (Evans, Drew, and Blenkhorn, 2000).

Movement times for nondisabled individuals are greater for head-controlled cursor systems than for a conventional mouse (Radwin, Vanderheiden, and Lin, 1990). Movement times are also greater for small versus large targets and for far versus near targets in both healthy individuals and those with cerebral palsy. On the basis of reduction in average movement time as an indicator of relative learning, 15 sets of 48 trials (with one trial defined as mouse cursor movement from center screen to a randomly presented target) were sufficient to attain stable performance using both mouse and head-operated systems in nondisabled individuals. Two participants with cerebral palsy were included in this study. One participant's learning approximated that of the nondisabled control subjects. The other participant's learning was more rapid but also more variable, and both speed and accuracy of head control were dramatically affected by proper trunk stability provided through a seating system.

User operational characteristics, including satisfaction, were evaluated for five currently available mouse alternatives that were based on head tracking by gathering the subjective evaluation of the users (Phillips and Lin, 2003). The users included individuals with high-level spinal cord injuries and those with cerebral palsy. Dependent variables were speed, accuracy, and distance or displacement in target acquisition tasks. Variable performance was reported for participants with cerebral palsy, even when identical interfaces were used. Words per minute and error rate for on-screen keyboards have also been used as dependent variables (Angelo, Deterding, and Weisman, 1991). For individuals with cerebral palsy, direct target acquisition is a faster method than scanning (Angelo, 1992).

Three different technologies (IR with a reflective dot (Tracker 2000, Madentec, Ltd, Edmonton, Canada, *www.Madentec.com*), ultrasound (HeadMaster, Prentke Romich, Wooster, Ohio, *www.prentrom.com*), and gyroscopic (Tracer, Boost Technologies, *www.boosttechnology.com*) were compared in six nondisabled subjects (Anson et al, 2003). Comparisons of speed, accuracy, and user preference were made by using a drawing task with an on-screen cursor. Each of the three approaches was fastest for one third of the subjects and all were equally accurate. The preferred device was the Tracker 2000. This device has only a reflective dot attached to the head, whereas the other two had additional hardware attached. Although results for person with disabilities would likely differ, this study did indicate that all head pointing technologies can yield fast and accurate results.

The impact on performance of repeated trials of the head-controlled mouse (Madentec Tracker One (Madentec, Ltd) system was evaluated in a series of target acquisition tasks for 12 persons with cerebral palsy (Cook et al, 2005). Time to target, time to select, and distance moved to target (i.e., the screen distance traveled over the path between start and finish of a selection movement) were measured. The targets were reduced in size across four once-weekly 1-hour sessions. Nine of the 12 participants were able to achieve a smaller target at the end of the session compared with the initial target size. For the same-size targets, six participants reduced their times to target and seven reduced the distance moved to acquire the target. However, only two participants showed a decrease in their time to select scores, which is an indication of the difficulty of holding a target for a preset dwell time. These results indicate that individuals with cerebral palsy may be able to use head-controlled cursor systems if they are given sufficient practice time with a gradual reduction of target size as skill increases.

Comparison of Key-Pad and Head-Controlled Mouse Alternatives.

When a consumer has difficulty in using the standard mouse, alternatives are considered and it is necessary to make comparisons between different alternatives. Generally, there is little empirical evidence to guide decision making. One study that is useful in this regard compared the use of a head-controlled mouse (Tracker 2000) and an expanded keyboard used as a key-pad mouse (Intellikeys, IntelliTools, Petaluma, Calif., *www.intellitools.com*) (Capilouto et al, 2005). These two devices were chosen because they both require gross motor movements and would likely be considered as alternatives for a specific consumer. The two devices were tested in a target acquisition task by nondisabled university students. Each device was used to acquire a target by moving a cursor from a starting point in the center of the screen. The time to capture a target decreased with practice for both devices, but the head pointer resulted in faster performance. The time to acquire a target was longer for targets spaced further from the starting point, but this effect was less for the head-pointing device. Reaction time was less for the head pointing device as well. All these results are related to the necessity for sequential action in the case of the keyboard (i.e., moving from one key to another to change mouse movement direction compared with continuous movement using the head-pointing system).

Light Pointers and Light Sensors.

A visible light beam may be used as a pointing interface for direct selection. In a simple form the light can be pointed at objects in a room or at letters on a piece of paper. The effectiveness of the light pointer is directly related to how bright and focused it is, and this in turn affects size and weight. Light pointers are most commonly attached to a band worn on the head, but they can also be held in the hand. Highly focused light sources such as laser pens may cause damage if they are shined directly into the eye (Salamo and Jakobs, 1996). The reason for this is the same as the reason for their use: they are a source of highly focused light of high intensity. To illustrate the potential danger of the laser light source, Salamo and Jakobs (1996) compared a 0.001-watt (1 milliwatt) red-light laser with a 100-watt incandescent light bulb. Because the light bulb is not focused and emits light in all directions, the actual light bulb reaching the retina is about 1 milliwatt. Thus, the actual intensity on the retina is the same for both the light bulb and the laser event although the light bulb emits 100,000 times more light than the laser. Despite having the same energy at the retina, the potential danger from the laser is still greater than the light bulb because the size of the image on the eye is 10,000 times smaller (about 1 micrometer in diameter) than the image of the light bulb (about 1 millimeter in diameter), which spreads the heating over a larger area of the retina. This focus of the energy in a small area by the laser is what can lead to burning of the retina and permanent damage to the eye. One other factor that must be considered is the type and duration of exposure. Salamo and Jakobs (1996) recommend an exposure of less that 0.0004 milliwatts (0.4 microwatts) for 1 second as the limit for safe continuous exposure, as might occur in a classroom.

Lasers are grouped into five classes: I (<0.01 milliwatts), II (0.01 to 1 milliwatts), IIIa (1 to 5 milliwatts), IIIB (1 milliwatt to 0.5 watts), and IV (>0.5 watts) (Hyman, Miller, and Neigut, 1992). Only class I lasers meet this criteria; they are so dim that they are not visible in a brightly lit classroom. Laser pointers are at least class II. Because of the continuous use, the possible limitation of protective reflexes that protect nondisabled individuals from exposure to class I laser and the uncontrolled environment the classroom, caution should be exercised when laser pointers are used for choice making and for indicating in the classroom.

IR (invisible) light sources can be used as pointers and computer input devices. A typical computer input system or communication device input consists of three components: (1) the IR transmitter (mounted on eyeglass frames), (2) an IR detector array, and (3) a controller that translates the received IR signals into computer commands corresponding to individual keyboard entries (Chen et al, 1999). Any number of detectors can be used, but typically we use an array of light sensors, one for each element in the selection set. Then the light pointer is used to point to any element. An on-off switch and visible laser light source may also be included to allow greater independence of the user. For example, Chen et al used a tongue-activated switch to turn the system on and off and a visible low-power laser to serve as an indicator of where the user was pointing. They also provide design details on an IR pointing device for computer input. In clinical trials, users who had spinal cord injuries performed as well as users with no disabilities on the basis of speed and accuracy in selecting targets from the sensor array (Chen et al, 2004).

Modifications to Keyboards and Pointing Interfaces

There are several problems that may be experienced by individuals with a physical disability in using any of the control interfaces just described. As mentioned earlier, if a consumer is having difficulty using a particular control interface, there are three paths to pursue. A control enhancer may resolve the difficulty (e.g., when the user has limited range for accessing the interface). Modification of the interface being evaluated is another alternative, and trying a less-limiting interface is the third approach. Before a less-limiting control interface is introduced, modification of the method being evaluated should be considered. Table 7-10 lists the areas of need for which modification of a control interface may be beneficial and approaches that can be used. Each of these difficulties in using a keyboard can be addressed by either hardware or software modifications.

Keyboard Layouts. The QWERTY keyboard layout (Figure 7-12, *A*), the one most familiar to people, was originally designed more than 100 years ago to slow down 10-finger typists using a manual typewriter so the keys would not jam. The QWERTY layout requires much excursion of the fingers and assumes that two hands with 10 fingers will be used. With an increasing number of individuals using computers, there has been a substantial increase in repetitive strain injuries to the hand. Redefining the layout of the characters on the keyboard can reduce the amount of finger movements required by the user to access the keys and may reduce fatigue and the likelihood of an individual's incurring a repetitive strain injury. Furthermore, there are alternative keyboard layout designs that have been developed to accelerate typing speed, such as when the individual is using only one hand or a mouthstick or another alternative access device. With computer keyboards, the definition of the keyboard layout is determined by software in the computer and the keys are labeled with the corresponding characters. The keyboard hardware (other than labeling of the keys) is not modified with any of the alternative keyboard layouts.

Developed in the 1930s by University of Washington Professor August Dvorak, the Dvorak keyboard layout was designed to reduce fatigue and increase speed by placing letters that are most frequently used on the home row of the keyboard. On the left side of the home row are all the vowels, and five of the most used consonants are on the right side of the home row. There are three Dvorak keyboard layouts: one for two-handed typists (Figure 7-12, *B*), one for right hand–only typists (Figure 7-12, *C*), and one for left hand–only typists (similar to that shown for right hand–only typists but flipped). Information on how to redefine the computer keyboard as a Dvorak layout can be found at *web.mit.edu/jcb/www/Dvorak/index.html.*

The Chubon keyboard is a layout pattern that was designed to be used by the single-digit or typing-stick typist (Chubon and Hester, 1988). In this layout (Figure 7-12, *D*) the letters in the English language that are used most frequently are arranged near each other in the center. This layout also places letters that are most frequently used together (e.g., *r* and *e*) in close proximity, which reduces the amount of movement required by the user for entering text and helps to increase the rate of input. For individuals who use a mouthstick or typing stick, an alternative keyboard layout that reduces the amount of travel to keys can significantly increase efficiency.

TABLE 7-10	Modifications to Keyboards and Pointing Interfaces
Need Addressed	**Approach**
User's speed not adequate for task prediction software	Modify keyboard layout, macros, rate enhancement software, word
User has problems making accurate selections	Keyguard, template, shield, delayed acceptance
User has difficulty holding down the modifier key while pressing another key	Mechanical latch, software latch
User cannot release key before it starts to repeat	Keyguard, careful selection of keyboard characteristics; software to disable key repeat function

Another alternative keyboard layout is an alphabetical array. Often individuals who are nonverbal and have been using a manual communication board to spell have learned to use an array in which the letters are placed in alphabetical order. They are very familiar with this arrangement and may be very efficient in selecting characters. For these individuals, it often does not make sense to have them learn a completely new letter arrangement. In this case the keyboard can be redefined, by use of software, to have an alphabetical arrangement.

When a keyboard pattern is selected, several factors need to be considered. The first factor to consider is whether the user is already familiar with one particular keyboard layout. If this is the case, it is important to keep in mind that the time needed for retraining to use a new keyboard pattern is estimated at 90 to 100 hours (Anson, 1997). Another factor to consider is whether the keyboard is shared with other individuals. It is possible to have the computer keyboard defined to use two keyboard patterns (e.g., QWERTY and Dvorak) and to label the keys so that the standard keys are not obscured (e.g., by use of a clear overlay with the new key labels on them, so when placed over the standard keys the original labels are still visible). However, this modification can be confusing to all typists. Finally, there are few data to support the claims that alternative keyboard patterns increase speed or reduce injury. Selecting an alternative keyboard, like other technologies, depends on the needs and skills of the user and which layout he or she feels most comfortable and efficient using.

Keyguards, Shields, and Templates. Some persons may be able to select individual keys directly, but they may occasionally miss the desired key and enter the wrong key. For individuals who have difficulty in accurately targeting and activating keys, a keyguard (Figure 7-20) placed over the keyboard helps by isolating each key and guiding the person's movement. A keyguard is also useful for individuals who produce a lot of extraneous movement each time they bring their hands off the keyboard in an attempt to target a new key. Instead of moving away from the keyboard to make the next selection, the person can rest the hand on top of the keyguard without activating any keys and make relatively isolated, controlled (and thus faster) selections. Although keyguards have been shown to increase the user's accuracy, speed is typically compromised (McCormack, 1990). In nearly all situations a clear keyguard is preferred so that there is minimal obstruction of the labels on the keys. Still, the position of the keyboard with a keyguard needs to be assessed to ensure that the key labels are not being obstructed from the user's view. Keyguards are commercially available for the common computer keyboards. In situations where an individual uses a special terminal in a work setting and would benefit from a keyguard, a custom keyguard can be fabricated from clear plastic.

Similar to the use of a keyguard is the use of a shield on the keyboard to block out certain keys. This modification is typically done with children who are just beginning to use computers and are using software programs that only require the use of a few select keys. To guide the child to the correct keys and increase his or her chances of success with the program, a shield is placed over the keys that are not being used.

A template used on a joystick to guide the individual's movement is akin to the use of a keyguard for a keyboard. The template has four channels that guide the movement of the joystick. The shape of the channel may vary depending on the template and can be a factor in the individual's ability to control the joystick. For example, an individual using the cross-shaped template in Figure 7-21, *A*, may need more precise movement to enter the desired channel but once in one of these channels will be able to stay easily. If the template is like the one in Figure 7-21, *B*, it will be easy for the individual to enter one of the channels but difficult to stay. A compromise solution is to use a template similar to the one shown in Figure 7-21, *C*. In this case, because the entrance to each arm of the cross has been widened, it is easier to move in each direction. Because the end of the slot in

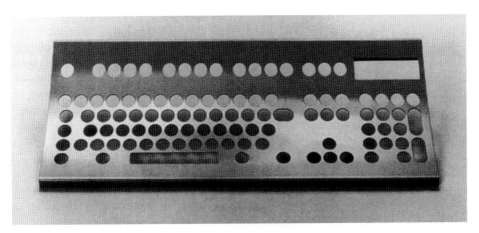

Figure 7-20   Keyguard. (Courtesy TASH, Ajax, Ontario, Canada.)

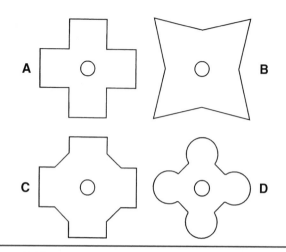

Figure 7-21   **A** to **D,** Four different shapes of joystick templates to maximize user's skills.

each direction retains the cross shape, it is easier to keep the joystick in one direction. We can also improve the performance of the star template (Figure 7-21, *B*) by restricting the travel at the end of the channel once the movement has been made in a direction. This change is shown in Figure 7-21, *D.* For some individuals, the use and type of joystick template means the difference between success or failure in the operation of a power wheelchair.

Technologies for Reducing Accidental Entries. Many keyboards produce multiple entries of characters by prolonged pressing of the key called *key repeat.* Although this feature is useful to nondisabled users (e.g., to obtain multiple spaces or underlines), it can present a problem for persons with disabilities who may not be able to release the key fast enough to prevent double entry. There are a number of ways this can be avoided. Certain types and sensitivities of keyboards that may increase or decrease double entries and auditory feedback (e.g., a beep) when a key is activated may also cue the user to release the key in a timely manner. Both these are sensory characteristics of control interfaces, described earlier in this chapter, that need to be considered as part of the overall assessment. Sometimes the presence of a keyguard helps to diminish the double entries. If the double entries remain a problem, FilterKeys can be used (see Table 7-1).

■ CONTROL INTERFACES FOR INDIRECT SELECTION

When an individual's physical control does not permit him or her to select directly, indirect selection methods are considered. Indirect methods of selection use a single switch or an array of switches and require that the consumer be able to carry out a certain set of skills. Box 7-5 shows the critical

questions to pose during the evaluation to determine whether the consumer has the basic set of skills for switch use.

During the evaluation, it is first necessary to determine whether the user can *activate* the switch, which determines whether there is a match between the sensory, spatial, and activation (e.g., force) requirements of the switch and the physical-sensory skills of the user. If activation is possible, it is necessary to look at other skills related to the way the switch is to be used for indirect selection. The first of these is whether the consumer can *wait* for the desired selection to be presented. This task requires that the consumer have sensory skills for awareness of the selections being presented. Depending on the consumer's sensory abilities, selections can be presented visually or auditorily. An inability to wait can result from problems with central processing or motor control. If the consumer is having difficulty waiting, determining the underlying cause (i.e., sensory, central processing, or motor) may make it possible to modify the task, although the cause is not always easy to determine. The consumer must also be able to *reliably activate the switch at the right time* (i.e., when the desired selection is presented).

Another critical condition is that the consumer be able to *hold* a switch in its closed position for the time it takes the signal from the control interface to register. This time is a variable of the control interface and may differ from switch to switch. In addition, applications such as Morse code input, inverse scanning, and wheelchair mobility require the user to hold the switch closed. Within each of these applications, the length of this hold time varies. For example, for the person using one-switch Morse code, the hold time varies from shorter to longer depending on the input signal (dot or dash). Inverse scanning (see next section) and wheelchair mobility are other applications that require the user to hold down the switch for varying lengths of time. With inverse scanning, the switch is held until the right choice appears; for wheelchair mobility, the switch is held down until the user wants the chair to stop. Frustration, embarrassment, and possibly serious injury in the case of mobility can result if the user cannot carry out precise holding of the switch. If the consumer is having difficulty activating or holding the switch, the switch may require too much force or displacement for activation or the sensory feedback it provides may be inadequate. If this is the case, having the consumer experiment with less limiting switches is recommended. *Releasing* the switch in a timely manner is the next criterion. Inability to release the switch causes inadvertent selections. It is easier for some individuals to activate and hold the switch than to release it. Finally, it should be determined whether the consumer is able to carry out these sets of skills repeatedly.

The ATP can begin evaluating the consumer's skills by using simple technology such as a tape recorder or battery-operated toy as an output when the switch is activated. Once it is determined that the consumer can use the switch on command to control this output, switch activation, holding, and release can be evaluated with software programs designed for that purpose (see Chapter 4). Frequently the use of more than one body control site and candidate interface is considered for a given consumer. Using the critical questions to evaluate each pairing (control site and interface) will help the ATP to make a comparison among them and to develop a recommendation. If the consumer has difficulty with any of these skills, there are certain techniques that can make selection easier.

Selection Techniques for Scanning

The action required by the user to activate the switch to make a selection during scanning and directed scanning usually can be varied to accommodate the user's skills. Table 7-11 lists the three scanning techniques and the level of skill required by the technique for each of the motor acts described earlier. This table is helpful in matching the scanning technique to the user's skills. With **automatic scanning,** the items are presented continuously by the device at a rate that can be set and adjusted according to how fast the user can respond. When the desired selection is presented, the user selects the choice by activating the switch and stopping the scan. Automatic scanning requires a high degree of motor skill by the user to wait for the desired selection and to

activate the switch in the given time frame. It also requires a high degree of sensory and cognitive vigilance for attending to and tracking the cursor on the display. With **step scanning,** the user activates the switch once for each item to move through the choices in the selection set. When the user comes to the desired choice, there are two possibilities for selecting it. Either an additional switch is used to give a signal to select that choice or an acceptance time is used. Step scanning allows the user to control the speed at which the items are presented. The ability to wait is not required for the scan, but it may be for the acceptance of the selection. The ability to activate the switch repeatedly, however, is highly important for step scanning. Motor fatigue can be high because of repeated switch activation.

The last technique is **inverse scanning.** In this type of scanning the scan is initiated by the individual's activating and holding the switch closed. As long as the switch is held down, the items are scanned. When the desired choice appears, the individual releases the switch to make the selection. For accuracy, inverse scanning requires a high level of skill to hold the switch and release it at the proper time. Automatic scanning requires activation of the switch within a specified time frame, so inverse scanning may be easier for individuals who require lots of time to initiate and follow through with movement. Like automatic scanning, motor fatigue is reduced over step scanning because of fewer switch activations; however, sensory and cognitive fatigue is higher because of the vigilance required to attend to the display.

Many devices are capable of providing each of these scanning techniques as options for the user. Angelo (1992) performed a study with six subjects that compared these three scanning techniques. This study found that subjects with spastic cerebral palsy performed poorly with the automatic scanning technique. Step scanning was found to be the most difficult for subjects with athetoid cerebral palsy. It is helpful for the consumer to try each of these selection techniques to experience the subtle differences among them when determining which one is most suitable.

TABLE 7-11	**Selection Techniques for Scanning and Directed Scanning**		
	Automatic Scanning	Step Scanning	Inverse Scanning
Wait	High	Low	Medium
Activate	High	Medium	Low
Hold	Low	Low	High
Release	Low	Medium	High
Motor failure	Low	High	Low
Sensory/cognitive vigilance	High	Low	High

Modified from Beukelman D, Mirenda P: *Augmentative and alternative communication,* ed 3, p. 184., Baltimore, 2005, Paul H. Brookes.

Selection Formats for Scanning

There are a number of formats in which the items in the selection set can be presented to the user for selection in scanning (Box 7-6). In a **linear** format, as shown in Figure 7-22, the items in the selection set are presented in a vertical or horizontal line and scanned one at a time until the desired selection is highlighted and selected by the user. With **circular,** or **rotary, scanning** (Figure 7-23), the items are presented in a circle and scanned one at a time. Because of the slowness inherent in both these types of scanning, Vanderheiden and Lloyd (1986) recommend that the array be limited to 15 choices.

To increase the rate of selection during scanning, **group-item scanning** can replace the single-item scan. In this case

CASE STUDY

EVALUATION AND SELECTION OF SWITCHES

Mrs. Antonelli is a 30-year-old woman who has spastic quadriplegia as a result of meningitis at age 10 years. She lives with her husband and 2-year-old daughter. Mrs. Antonelli was referred for an evaluation for an augmentative communication system for conversation and writing. She has limited functional speech and communicates primarily by finger spelling with her left hand. Her husband interprets the finger spelling, but many others with whom Mrs. Antonelli would like to communicate do not understand her finger spelling. She independently uses a power wheelchair that she controls by a joystick with her left hand.

Mrs. Antonelli showed limited range using either hand, and her resolution seemed fair; therefore, her ability to use keyboards was assessed by use of a contracted keyboard with each hand. She copied words with a great deal of effort and was less than 50% accurate.

Because Mrs. Antonelli uses a switched joystick to control her power wheelchair, a switched joystick was tried with an electronic communication device in a directed scanning mode. Mrs. Antonelli used her left hand with the joystick in approximately the same position as her wheelchair joystick. She was able to move this joystick in all four directions. However, when asked to hold and release the joystick on a specific target, Mrs. Antonelli had difficulty. She was able to do this, but it required significant effort and several attempts to successfully select the desired target.

The pad switch (TASH, Ajax, Ontario, Canada), a pneumatic switch, and a rocker switch (Prentke Romich Co., Wooster, Ohio) were then tried to evaluate the potential for Mrs. Antonelli to use coded access. The switches were positioned one at a time on the right wheelchair armrest to be used with her right hand. Both a single-switch approach, in which a short switch hit produces a dot and a long switch hit produces a dash, and a dual-switch approach (one side produces dots and the other dashes) were tried. Mrs. Antonelli had difficulty with the one-switch mode because she was unable to consistently hold the switch for the appropriate length of time. In the two-switch mode, Mrs. Antonelli was able to move easily between the two parts of the rocker switch to generate dots and dashes. Mrs. Antonelli pressed one side of this switch with her index finger and one side with her middle finger. Mrs. Antonelli felt that the single switches were more difficult to operate than the rocker switch. Mrs. Antonelli also indicated a preference for the dual switch over the joystick for communication. She wanted to continue using her left hand to operate the joystick on her power wheelchair and to use her right hand for Morse code input into her communication device. Mrs. Antonelli acquired the communication system and, with a period of training, quickly memorized the Morse code; her rate of input became rapid.

there are several items in a group and the groups are sequentially scanned. The individual first selects the group that has the desired element. Once the group has been selected, the individual items in that group are scanned until the desired item is reached. When there are a large number of items, a *matrix* scan can be used. In this type of scanning the *group*

BOX 7-6	Scanning Formats

SELECTION SET FORMATS
Linear
Circular
Matrix

ADAPTATIONS TO FORMATS FOR INCREASING
RATE OF SELECTION
Group-item
Row-column
Halving
Quartering
Frequency of use placement

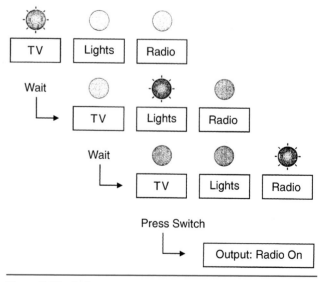

Figure 7-22   In linear scanning, choices are presented vertically or horizontally one at a time.

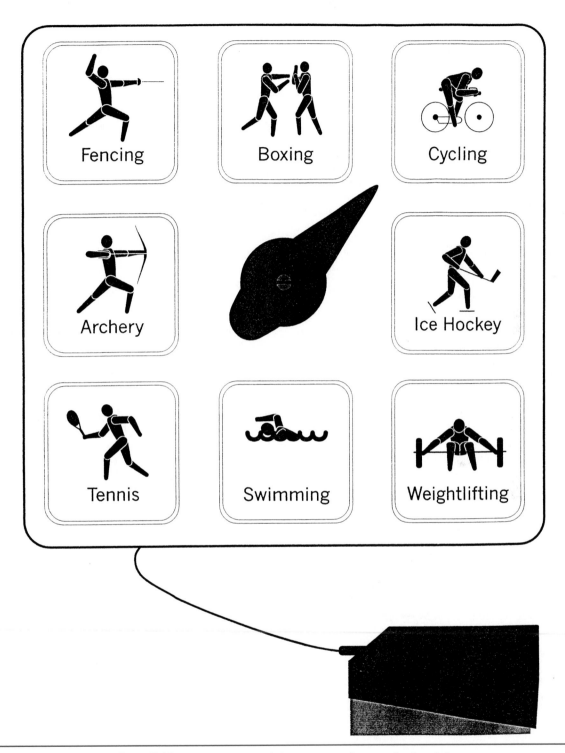

Figure 7-23   In rotary scanning, choices are presented one at a time in a circle.

is a row of items and the *items* are located in columns; thus it is called **row-column scanning.** In row-column scanning there may be several rows of items and each complete row lights up sequentially. The row with the desired item is selected; then each column in that row lights up until the

desired item is selected. Figure 7-24 shows the input required when a single switch is used with row-column scanning to produce the letter *S*.

There are other ways that scanning formats can be adapted to increase the user's rate of selection. *Halving* is

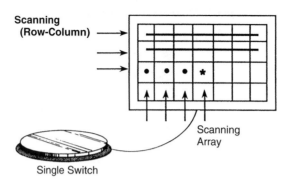

Figure 7-24 Row-column scanning showing the input required for selecting the letter *S*. The rows are first scanned and the user selects the row with the desired item. Then each item in that row is scanned until the desired item is selected. (From Smith RO: Technological approaches to performance enhancement. In Christiansen C, Baum C, editors: *Occupational therapy: overcoming human performance deficits,* Thorofare, NJ, 1991, Slack.)

Input	Output
Press Switch	S
Wait	
Wait	
Press Switch	
Wait	
Wait	
Wait	
Press Switch	

a group-item approach in which the total array is divided in halves. Each half is scanned until the user selects the desired half. The scanning then proceeds in a row-column format as described above until the desired item is reached. This same concept can be used in a *quartering format* in which the array is divided into fourths. Another method used to increase rate of selection is to place the selection set elements in the scanning array according to their frequency of use. For example, if letters are being used as the selection set, placement of *E, T, A, O, N,* and *I* (the most frequently used letters) in the upper left positions of the scanning array results in a significant increase in rate of selection (Vanderheiden and Lloyd, 1986). The application of these principles to augmentative communication is discussed in Chapter 11.

Coded Access

Coded access is another indirect selection input method that requires an intermediate step. As discussed earlier, one of the most common and most efficient methods of coded access is Morse code. Figure 7-25 shows the symbols for international Morse code. The required sequence of movements for obtaining the letter *C* is dash, dot, dash, dot. In two-switch Morse code, one switch is configured to represent a dot and the other switch a dash. Figure 7-26 shows the steps required for obtaining the letter *C* by using two-switch Morse code. In single-switch Morse code the system is configured so that a quick activation and release of the switch results in a dot and holding the switch closed for a longer period before releasing it results in a dash. Letter boundaries

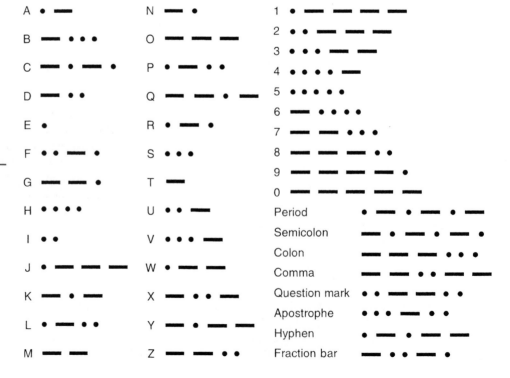

Figure 7-25 International Morse code.

Input	Morse Code	Output
Press Switch 1	▬	
Press Switch 2	●	
Press Switch 1	▬	
Press Switch 2	●	C

Figure 7-26   The input required for selecting the letter *C* by using Morse code.

are distinguished by a slightly longer pause than between dots and dashes within one letter.

Another example of coded access is Darci code. This selection method, used with the DARCI TOO to control a computer, uses an eight-way switch code. An eight-way switch is similar to a four-position switched joystick, with the diagonal positions used as additional switch positions (Figure 7-27, *A*). By use of this code, the letter *C* is generated by moving the switch to position 2, then to position 1, and then to the center (Figure 7-27, *B*). It is this sequence of movements that tells the processor that the desired entry is the letter *C*. With this access method, it is also possible to emulate mouse movements and to access whole words. Other eight-switch (sometimes called *eight-way*) codes have been used in augmentative communication devices (Chapter 11).

Types of Single Switches

Numerous types of single switches are commercially available. It is also possible to custom fabricate switches, but this option is not advised for a number of reasons. Although it may seem less inexpensive to purchase the materials to make a switch, when the time it takes to make the switch is factored in, the cost involved increases significantly. In addition,

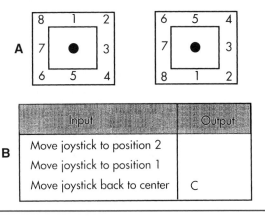

Figure 7-27   **A,** Two alternatives for designating the eight switch locations. **B,** The input required for selecting the letter *C* by using Darci code.

custom-made switches are not as durable as commercially available switches and will not hold up over time.

When a switch is selected for an individual, it is important to consider the spatial, activation-deactivation, and sensory characteristics discussed earlier. Single switches come in many different sizes and shapes and have diverse force and sensory requirements. It is critical that the consumer has the opportunity to try out any switches being considered for a control interface. Table 7-12 summarizes the types of single-switch interfaces and gives a sampling of switches that are commercially available on the basis of the categories shown in Table 7-5.

Mechanical switches are the most commonly used type of single switch, and they can be of various shapes and sizes. Paddle switches (Figure 7-28, *A*) have movement in one direction. On some types of paddle switches the sensitivity can be adjusted according to the user's needs. Wobble (Figure 7-28, *B*) and leaf switches (Figure 7-28, *C*) have a 2- to 4-inch shaft that can be activated by the user in two directions. The wobble switch makes an audible click when activated and the leaf switch does not, making the wobble switch more desirable when the switch is out of the user's visual range, such as during head activation. Lever switches (Figure 7-28, *D*) are similar to wobble switches with the exception that they can only be activated in one direction. This type of switch usually has a round, padded area at the end of a shaft and produces an audible click, which also makes it desirable for activation by the head. There are also various types of button switches that come in different sizes, from a large, round switch such as the Big Red switch, to a small button switch that can be held between the thumb and the index finger, such as the Cap switch. Membrane switches consist of a very thin pad, which also requires some degree of force to activate. These pads are available in various sizes, from as small as 2 inches × 3 inches to as large as 3 inches × 5 inches. The advantages of these membrane pads are that they are flexible, can be paired with an object (by being directly attached to it), and can be used to teach the user to make a direct connection between the object and the switch. The main disadvantage of membrane switches is that they provide poor tactile feedback. This can lead to extra activations or failure to apply enough force to activate the switch. All these switches are activated by body movement that produces a force on the switch. They are considered *passive switches* because they do not require any outside power source. Mercury switches can be used to indicate a change in position such as lifting an arm or finger or tilting the head. This removes the need to activate a mechanical switch.

There are also switches that are activated with body movement but that do not require force or even contact with the switch. These are referred to as *proximity switches*. The switch is activated when it detects an object within its range. The activation range of these types of switches varies from nearly touching the switch to 3 feet away and usually the

TABLE 7-12   **Examples of Single-Switch Interfaces**

Category	Description	Switch Name/Manufacturer
Mechanical switches	Activated by the application of a force; generic names of switches include paddle, plate, button, lever, membrane	Pal Pads, Taction Pads (Adaptivation Corp.); Big Buddy Button, Microlight Switch, Grasp, Trigger Switch (TASH); Big Red and Jelly Bean Switches (AbleNet Inc.); Lever, Leaf, and Tread Switches (ZYGO Industries); Dual-rocking, P and Wobble Switch (Prentke Romich Co.); Access and finger Access (Saltillo); FlexAble, Rocking Action, Plat switch (AMDi)
Electromagnetic switches	Activated by the receipt of electromagnetic energy such as light or radio waves	Fiber Optic Sensor, (ASL); Proximity Switches (AMDi); SCATIR (Tash); Infrared/sound/touch switch (Words+)
Electrical control switches	Activated by detection of electrical signals from the surface of the body	D-Box Standalone EMG Switch (Emerge Medical); Brainfingers 9Cyberlink (Adaptivation Corp.)
Proximity switches	Activated by a movement close to the detector but without actual contact	ASL 204 and 208, Proximity Switch (Adaptive Switch Laboratories, Inc.); Untouchable Buddy (Tash Inc.)
Pneumatic switches	Activated by detection of respiratory air flow or pressure	Pneumatic Switch (Adaptivation); LifeBreath Switch and Sip and Puff Switch (Toys for Special Children); ASL 308 Pneumatic Switch (Adaptive Switch Laboratories); PRC Pneumatic Switch Model PS-2 (Prentke Romich Co.); Pneumatic Switch Model CM-3 (ZYGO Industries); Wireless Integrated Sip/Puff Switch (Madentec)
Phonation switches	Activated by sound or speech	Voice Activated and Sound Activated Switches (Enabling Devices); Infrared/Sound/Touch Switch (Words+)

Data from Ablenet Inc., Minneapolis, Minn. (www.ablenetinc.com); Adaptive Switch Laboratories, Inc., Spicewood, Tex. (www.asl-inc.com); Adaptivation Co Sioux Falls, S.D. (www.adaptivation.com); AMDi, Hicksville, Northwest Territories (http://www.amdi.net/index.htm); Emerge Medical, Atlanta, Ga. (http://www.emergemedical.com/); Madentec Limited, Edmonton, Alberta (www.madentec.com); Prentke Romich, Wooster, Ohio (www.prenrom.com); Saltillo (http://www.saltillo.com/), TASH, Ajax, Ontario, or Richmond, Va. (www.tashinc.com); Enabling Devices—Toys for Special Children, Hastings-on-Hudson, N.Y. (www.enablingdevices.com); Words+ Inc. (www.words-plus.com); ZYGO, Portland, Ore. (www.zygo-usa.com).

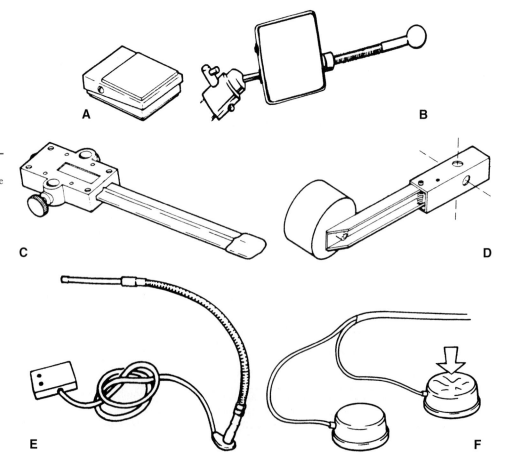

Figure 7-28   Examples of single switches. **A,** Paddle switch. **B,** Wobble switch. **C,** Leaf switch. **D,** Lever switch. **E,** Puff-and-sip switch. **F,** Pillow switch. (**A, C,** and **D,** Courtesy ZYGO Industries, Portland. **B, E,** and **F** from Bergen AF, Presperin J, Tallman T: *Positioning for function: wheelchairs and other assistive technologies,* Valhalla, NY, 1990, Valhalla Rehabilitation Publications.)

activation range is adjustable. Near switches are a series of switches that do not require contact for activation. The switches in this series use different technologies to detect the movement, from photoelectric to fiberoptic. These switches are *active,* meaning they require an outside power source, such as a battery, to operate.

Pneumatic switches are activated by detection of respiratory airflow or pressure and include puff-and-sip and pillow switches. Puff-and-sip switches (Figure 7-28, *E*) are activated by the individual's blowing air into the switch or sucking air out of it. The individual can send varying degrees of air pressure to the switch, which provides different commands to the processor. Pillow switches (Figure 7-28, *F*) respond to air pressure when squeezed (such as with a hand bulb) or when pressure is applied to a cushion.

Switch Arrays, Discrete Joysticks, and Chord Keyboards

Switches are commercially available in preconfigured arrays (two to eight), and any of the single switches we have discussed can be used to design a custom array to meet the needs of the consumer. These offer the advantages of multiple signals while retaining the requirement of low resolution that is typical of single switches.

Paddle switches are often used in switch arrays when two to five input signals are desirable. A type of paddle switch that provides dual input from one control is called a *rocker switch* (Figure 7-29, *A*). A rocker switch is like a seesaw and it does exactly what it says: it rocks from side to side around a fulcrum. This design allows the user to maintain contact with the switch and perform a rotating movement with the control site to activate each side. This type of dual-switch array is often used for Morse code input, with one side signaling dots and the other side dashes. The Slot Switch (Figure 7-29, *B*) is one example of a commercially available paddle switch array that is already configured. The switches in this array are mounted on a base piece that has dividers between the switches. The purpose of the dividers is to help the user isolate the appropriate switch. This array is typically used with the hands or feet by someone who has gross motor skills and a fairly large range of motion. The isolation of each switch helps when the user may not be able to locate the switch visually. There are other switch arrays that are mounted and activated with the head. Switch arrays are often used for power wheelchair control; they are discussed in greater detail in Chapter 12.

At the other extreme, in terms of size, is the Penta switch array. This array consists of five switches, each approximately a fourth inch in diameter. Its overall size is 2 inches in diameter, and it is small enough so that it can be held in the palm of the hand and be activated by the thumb.

A discrete joystick is also considered an array of switches. It consists of four or five switch input signals (UP, DOWN,

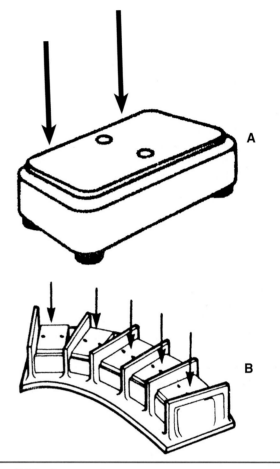

Figure 7-29   Examples of switch arrays. **A,** Dual rocker switch. (Webster JG et al, editors: *Electronic devices for rehabilitation,* New York, 1985, John Wiley and Sons.) **B,** Slot switch. (Courtesy ZYGO Industries, Portland.)

LEFT, RIGHT, and ENTER) that are either open or closed (off or on), with nothing in between. To close the switch, the control handle is moved in the direction of one of the other switches. Switched joysticks require limited range but moderate resolution by the user. They are available with a variety of displacements, forces, and handles to accommodate different grasping abilities of the user. If there is a maximum of five items (e.g., directions of a power wheelchair) in the selection set, the joystick functions as an interface for direct selection. When the selection set is more than five, indirect selection is required by directed scanning. Using the joystick with this method, the individual selects the direction and the device determines the speed of cursor movement.

A chord keyboard is also an array of switches or keys (typically five), each of which is intended to be pushed by one finger. Two-handed versions have 10 or more switches or keys (some have multiple keys for thumb use), and one-handed versions have five or more. The name of these keyboards is derived from the manner in which they are used for text entry. To make an entry, one or more (usually at least two) of the switches are pushed simultaneously, which is analogous to the playing of several notes together on a piano to make a musical chord. The most commonly used chord keyboard is the one used by court stenographers. With this keyboard, a stenographer can transcribe speech as it is spoken, a rate of more than 150 words per minute. For this reason, chord keyboards have often been proposed for rapid text entry by persons with disabilities. However, unless the person has good fine motor control and good coordination of the fingers, this approach is not viable. The degree of finger travel when using a chord keyboard is greatly reduced because generally only the thumb moves from key to key (usually to press a different key to change meaning of the other four keys). It would follow, therefore, that chord keyboards would reduce the incidence of repetitive strain injuries. However, the fingers still need to move to activate the keys. Like the modified keyboard layouts described earlier, there are no studies that demonstrate that chord keyboards reduce the incidence of RSIs.

The chord keyboard is used in a coded access method. Each letter, number, and special symbol is entered by pressing a combination of keys (switches). This combination is interpreted as that character by the processor. For example, to enter the letter *C*, keys 1 and 3 may be pressed together. The codes for each selection must be learned because it is not possible to label the keys with the necessary codes. Therefore the individual using a chord keyboard needs to have good memory skills in addition to good motor skills.

■ INTERNET USE BY PERSONS WITH PHYSICAL DISABILITIES

Persons with physical disabilities who want to use the Internet require only an accessible computer, in contrast to individuals who have visual disabilities and also require carefully designed Web pages (see Chapter 8). The actual use by persons with physical disabilities has not been carefully studied in general, with the exception of people who have sustained a spinal cord injury (Drainoni et al, 2004). A large group (516) of individuals with spinal cord injury from the 16 centers in the Model Spinal Cord Injury System participated in a survey of Internet use. A smaller sample, derived from the larger group, also participated in an assessment of elements of the Health-Related Quality of Life instrument (see Chapter 4). The rate of Internet access was 66% compared with 43% in the general population. There were significant differences in access, however, on the basis of race, employment status, income, education, and marital status. The most significant impact of the Health-Related Quality of Life instrument on Internet use was the pain interference parameter, indicating that significant pain prevented participation in activities of daily living. Frequency of use varied widely from nonuse to rare to frequent use. Most (81%) of

the respondents with spinal cord injuries used the Internet at least weekly. Success in achieving desired outcomes improved markedly from infrequent to rare use, but not from rare to frequent. Primary uses were social (e-mail, chat rooms) and information seeking (health-related information, on-line shopping). A concern regarding Internet access is that it might reduce interpersonal contact and isolate people with disabilities from social interaction. This study indicated that the opposite was true because the use of Internet contact reduced many of the barriers faced by people who have sustained spinal cord injuries (e.g., transportation, telephone use, and need for personal attendants for outside trips).

■ OTHER CONSIDERATIONS IN CONTROL INTERFACE SELECTION

Multiple Versus Integrated Control Interfaces

A long-standing goal of rehabilitation engineers and others is the integration of systems for augmentative and alternative communication (AAC), power mobility, environmental control, and computer access (Barker, 1991; Caves et al, 1991). One of the major reasons for this emphasis is to allow the use of the same control interface for several applications, called **integrated control**. Integration of controls can free the individual from multiple controls and can reduce the jumble of electronic devices surrounding the person.

With recent advances in technology, it is now possible to operate several devices through one processor. The processor is capable of operating only one device at a time, and a method is set up in which the user designates the mode in which he or she would like to function. For example, there are several power wheelchairs with processors that allow the consumer to use one interface, such as a joystick, to control many functions. By selecting the drive mode, the person uses the joystick to propel the wheelchair in all directions. The person can exit the wheelchair drive mode, select the mode designated for environmental control, and turn the lights on and off in the house.

There is an inherent value in the simplification that can result from this type of integration; however, there are also many situations in which separate control interfaces (called **distributed controls**) and devices for each of the functions are warranted. Before deciding whether to use an integrated control or distributed controls, the implications of each method for the consumer should be carefully deliberated. As a guideline, Guerette and Sumi (1994) recommend that integrated controls be used when (1) the person has one single reliable control site, (2) the optimal control interface for each assistive device is the same, (3) speed, accuracy, ease of use, or endurance increases with the use of a single interface, and (4) the person or the family prefers integrated controls for esthetic, performance, or other subjective reasons.

In some cases the consumer may have only one body site that he or she can control, and the person may also have limited range and resolution of this control site. Trying to position more than one control interface for use by this site could be problematic. Using the same control interface for multiple functions would simplify this situation. Next, consider what is the optimal way for the consumer to operate each assistive device. Let's say, for example, that the ATP is evaluating a consumer for control of both a power wheelchair and an AAC device. If the consumer can easily control a joystick, that would be the optimal control interface for the power wheelchair. If this is also the easiest control interface for the consumer to use for controlling an AAC device, it would stand to reason that an integrated control (the joystick) to operate both devices would be beneficial. However, if this person is able to use direct selection with an expanded keyboard for controlling an AAC device, the keyboard would be the optimal control interface for AAC. Integrating the control interfaces by using the joystick for both functions would not make sense in this situation.

Another reason to implement an integrated control interface is the user's preference. The consumer ultimately has the final input into the selection of a control method. The consumer's preference may be based on a sense of having better performance with one method over the other, esthetic reasons, or the importance of independence in going from one function to another. Because integrated controls combine interfaces into one unit, they typically require less hardware and tend to look better than multiple control interfaces. Integrated controls also provide increased independence for the consumer in accessing multiple assistive devices (Guerette, Caves, and Gross, 1992). The consumer does not have to depend on others to set up a different control interface or device. Some consumers place higher value on these issues than other consumers, and what is of importance to the individual consumer must be identified. There is a continuum ranging from wholly discrete systems to fully integrated systems for control interfaces, and there are advantages and disadvantages to different approaches to integration (Nisbet, 1996).

Although there are apparent advantages to using integrated controls, there may be circumstances in which distributed controls are preferred. Guerette and Nakai (1996) identify situations where integrated control may not be appropriate: "(1) when performance on one or more assistive devices is severely compromised by integrating control, (2) when an individual wishes to operate an assistive device from a position other than from a power wheelchair, (3) when physical, cognitive, or visual/perceptual limitations preclude integrating, (4) when it is the individual's preference to use separate controls, and (5) when external factors such as cost or technical limitations preclude the use of integrated controls" (p. 64). In the case example of Mrs. Antonelli, it was easy for her to control her power wheelchair using the joystick with her left hand. However, this method was not the easiest method for her to use to operate the communication device. She had the option, however, of using another body site, and it turned out that the "best" way for her to access the communication device was by using a dual rocker switch with her right hand. If the controls had been integrated and she was to use the joystick for both power mobility and AAC, her activity output for communication would have been significantly compromised. The decision was made to use distributed controls, and her performance in communication was much improved.

In a study that measured consumer satisfaction with integrated controls, Angelo and Trefler (1998) reported that the majority of respondents indicated they were either very satisfied or satisfied with their integrated control device. An increase in independence and the ability to control other equipment such as televisions and computers were reasons the respondents gave for being satisfied with their integrated control devices. Ding et al (2003) reviewed applications of integrated controls in power mobility, augmentative communication, EADLs, and computer access. They also describe the Multiple Master Multiple Slave protocol for interfacing assistive technologies (Linnman, 1996). This protocol is an open network standard for interconnecting electronic rehabilitation devices for power mobility (Chapter 12), EADLs and robotics (Chapter 14), and augmentative communication (Chapter 11). The Multiple Master Multiple Slave standard also includes safety features that allow rapid shutdown of electronic controls (especially wheelchair and robotics) if a failure occurs. It also provides a framework for assistive technology interfaces that makes them more compatible and more easily combined into integrated controls.

Mounting the Control Interface for Use

In all situations it is necessary to address the position and placement of the control interface so that it is optimally accessed by the user. Most keyboards are connected with a cable to the computer, which allows some latitude in positioning them so they are accessible. Keyboards can be placed on stands that raise them (e.g., for mouthstick use) or easels that tilt them (e.g., for easier hand access or foot access). Some keyboards (e.g., contracted keyboards) can be mounted to wheelchairs.

It is also necessary to mount single switches, joysticks, and switch arrays in a convenient location. The most common mounting locations are attachments to a table or desk, to a wheelchair, or to the person's body. There are commercially available mounting systems for table and wheelchair mounting. Some mounting requirements are more challenging than others. For example, it is generally more difficult to position a joystick for foot or chin use than it is to place it for hand use.

There are flexible and fixed mounting systems. Flexible mounting systems (Figure 7-30) can be adjusted and placed in various positions, which is advantageous in settings where more than one person needs a switch mounting. Costs can be controlled by using the same mounting system at different times for several people. This type of mounting system is also advantageous for individuals who require changes in the position of their control interface because of fluctuating skills or needs. The disadvantage of flexible mounting systems is that the position for the control interface must be determined each time it is put in place. Sometimes even a slight fluctuation in the position of the switch can make a significant difference in the individual's ability to access it. Other mounting systems are fixed and are designed for use of a specific control site and switch. The advantage of this approach is that the mounting system is not as likely to move or change position and require adjustment.

Switches are also attached to the individual by straps. Attachment to the body has the major advantage of not being as affected by the person's change in body position. If a switch is mounted to the wheelchair and the person shifts position even slightly, the switch may no longer be reachable or the new position may make it difficult to generate enough force to activate the switch.

The majority of control interfaces have a cable that connects them to the device being used. However, there are wireless keyboards, pointing interfaces, and switches. There are also separate wireless links that can be used with most switches. These links consist of a transmitter that is plugged into the switch and a receiver that plugs into the device. When the switch is pressed, the signal is transmitted to the receiver and the device. Thus the switch is not physically connected to the device. Wireless control interfaces communicate with the processor by IR signals such as those used with television remote controls. Obvious advantages of a remote control interface are that there is one less wire for the user to become tangled in and that it looks better. It can also be advantageous to have a wireless control interface when the interface is mounted on the person's wheelchair. This arrangement allows the person to move to or away from the device being used without having to connect or disconnect the interface. In many situations the person with a disability needs a personal attendant to assist with connecting the cable of the interface to the computer. The use of a remote control interface allows the person to come and go independently, so an attendant is not needed for this task.

■ DEVELOPMENT OF MOTOR SKILLS FOR USE OF CONTROL INTERFACES

In some situations it is necessary to establish a program that develops the individual's motor skills. Three outcomes can be achieved by such a program: (1) the individual can broaden his or her repertoire of motor capabilities and the number and type of inputs that can be accessed, (2) the individual can refine the motor skills he or she has in using an interface to increase speed, endurance, or accuracy, and (3) the individual who lacks the motor skill to use any interface functionally can develop these skills. The amount of training needed will vary in each of these circumstances, depending on the person and the desired outcome. In some cases, such as when the individual has never had the opportunity to control objects physically, this training can be carried out over a period of years. In comparison, a person who needs to develop tolerance for using a mouthstick may require a minimal amount of training. In general, training programs should be interesting, be graded according to the user's skill level, and be age appropriate.

What is initially chosen as the best control site and method for an individual may not necessarily remain constant over time. Kangas (1989) advises that the initial control site and method be considered just that, a starting place for the individual, and that the practitioner remain open to the individual's trying alternative sites and methods for control. Horn and Jones (1996) present a detailed case study in which both direct selection and scanning were used with a child. Although the initial assessment indicated a preference for single-switch scanning on the basis of physical assessment, the child was later able to effectively use direct selection. Horn and Jones discuss this unexpected result in terms of the physical and cognitive skills required for these two selection methods. Their results point out the importance of continuous assessment (see Chapter 4) and the role of training in matching the skills of the user to the control interface.

Kangas (1988) recommends that practitioners encourage users to develop a repertoire of control methods to broaden

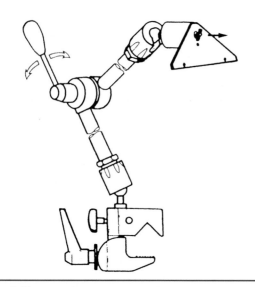

Figure 7-30 Flexible mounting system. (Courtesy ZYGO Industries, Portland, Ore.)

the potential number of devices they can access. For example, if a child who previously used a single switch becomes proficient in the use of a joystick, both these control options can be maintained through different activities. The joystick can be used to play computer games or activate a communication device, and the single switch can still be used to turn on some music. Similar to the concepts presented by Kangas is the *parallel interventions model* (Angelo and Smith, 1989; Smith, 1991). This model proposes that the individual use an initial control interface for accessing a device while simultaneously participating in a motor training program to maximize his or her ability to operate control interfaces. Broadening the person's repertoire allows access to a greater number of devices and may allow the user to lessen reliance on assistive technology. For example, after a period of training, the user may be able to progress from using a single switch to a switch array or from an expanded keyboard to a standard keyboard.

An individual may have the prerequisite motor skills to use a control interface with a device but may require training to refine those skills. Refining these motor skills may result in an increased rate of input, fewer errors, or increased endurance for using the control. For example, a person may be able to select directly but may need training to learn to use a specific keyboard layout to reduce fatigue or to increase speed. There are software programs available that help a person acquire one-handed keyboard skills. Additionally, there are a number of Web sites that provide information on training with different types of keyboard layouts, such as *www.dgp.toronto.edu/people/ematias/papers/ic93*. Refinement of motor skills for mouse use is another example. Again, there are many software programs available that have been developed to gradually improve a person's ability to use a mouse or an alternative to a mouse. These programs include activities for developing targeting skills and mastering point-and-click and click-and-drag skills.

Use of mechanical and electronic pointers worn on the head typically require substantial training to gradually build the consumer's tolerance and effectiveness in using the control enhancer. Similarly, strengthening of the person's existing neck, facial, and oral musculature and a gradual development of tolerance for the mouthstick should take place before he or she performs tasks such as writing or typing. Playing simple board games, painting, or batting a balloon are examples of activities that can be used to develop skills for mouthstick or head pointer use. Many games can also be adapted so that a person using a light pointer practices using the interface through play activities.

Assistive technology provides many individuals who have physical disabilities with their first opportunities to perform a motor act to access communication, mobility, and environmental control. Before this technology became available, those individuals with severe physical disabilities had few or no opportunities to use their existing motor movements.

For this reason, there are many instances in which an individual may have a control site and the ability to activate a single switch, but the ability to activate this control interface is not consistent enough to justify the purchase of an assistive device such as a wheelchair, computer, or augmentative communication system. The intervention then becomes one of improving the individual's motor control.

In these cases a graded approach using technology as one of the modalities for improving the individual's motor skills can and should be implemented. Table 7-13 illustrates some general steps and tools involved in such an approach. The technology then becomes a tool to meet short-term objectives aimed at reaching the long-term goal of participation in an activity by using assistive technology. It is important that this outcome and goal be kept in mind so that the ATP re-evaluates the individual at periodic intervals and allows him or her to move beyond the use of this technology as a tool and into functional device use.

Frequently, an individual engaged in a graded approach is not able to communicate verbally and the question of whether he or she has the cognitive-language skills to access assistive technology also becomes an issue. Therefore this approach (see Table 7-13) starts with evaluating *cause and effect* and providing training at that level as needed. Cause and effect refers to the ability of the individual to understand that he or she can control things in the environment and can make something happen. It encompasses the prerequisite skills of attention and object permanence. The individual must be able to attend to and be aware of the environment and the permanence of objects in that environment. Information can be gathered on the individual's ability to understand cause and effect through the use of a single switch.

TABLE 7-13   Sequential Steps in Motor Training for Switch Use

Goal	Tools Used to Accomplish Goal
1. Time-independent switch use to develop cause and effect	Appliances (fan, blender) Battery-operated toys/radio Software that produces a result whenever the switch is pressed
2. Time-dependent switch use to develop switch use at the right time	Software that requires a response at a specific time to obtain a graphic or sound result
3. Switch within specified window to develop multichoice scanning	Software requiring a response in a "time window"
4. Symbolic choice making	Simple scanning communication device Software allowing time-dependent choice making that has a symbolic label and communicative output

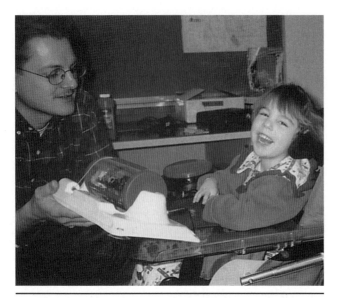

Figure 7-31   Child using a single switch with a battery-operated toy as a reinforcer.

At the first stage, the goal related to assistive technology use is for the individual to be able to activate the switch at any given time and to associate the switch activation with a result. The individual is asked to use a control site to activate a single switch that is connected to some type of reinforcer. Caregivers can provide initial information on what the individual enjoys and finds reinforcing. Objects that can be adapted for switch input and that may be of interest include battery-operated toys, a radio, a blender, or a fan. The child shown in Figure 7-31 is using a switch with a battery-operated toy for the reinforcer. Typically, the individual who is aware that he or she has generated an effect will show some type of response, such as smiling, crying, or looking toward the reinforcer.

If there is success with these activities, computer software programs can be used as an alternative type of reinforcement. These programs provide interesting graphics, animation, and auditory feedback each time the switch is activated. Individuals of all age groups find the programs enjoyable. Data can be collected for each switch activation, including (1) time from prompt to activation, (2) whether the individual activates the switch independently or whether verbal or physical prompting was needed, and (3) the consumer's attention to the result. There are a number of companies that sell software programs to be used at the different stages described in this section.

At the second stage, the goal is for the individual to activate the switch consistently at a specific time. This approach can also be considered one-choice scanning, in which the switch is either hit or not—choice making at its most fundamental level (Cook, 1991). For example, with some computer games the individual needs to activate the switch for

an object to move or to carry out an action such as shooting a basket, hitting a target, and so on. With some programs, as long as the individual successfully activates the switch, the movement of objects on the screen speeds up. Any data provided by the program (e.g., speed, number of correct hits, errors) and data regarding the individual's success in activating the switch at the correct time and whether prompts have been needed are recorded. Burkhart (1987) (see also *www.lburkhart.com*) makes suggestions for computer-based and non-computer-based activities that can be used for motor training. One suggestion for a non-computer-based activity is to use a battery-operated toy fireman that climbs a ladder as long as the switch is activated. To make this a time-dependent activity, a picture of a reinforcer is attached somewhere along the ladder and the individual is asked to release the switch to stop the fireman at the picture and receive the reinforcement.

During the third phase of this training program, the time window becomes more defined as the individual is asked to use the switch to choose from two or more options. Toys, appliances, and computer software programs are also used at this stage. The goal is to increase the number of elements in an array that can be reliably selected by the individual. This progression is important if scanning is to be used for communication or environmental control. One approach is to highlight locations on the screen in sequence. When the switch is hit on a highlighted item, the program provides an interesting result. In some programs the highlighted areas can be limited so that only one is correct, which helps the consumer develop scanning selection skills in the absence of language-based tasks. In addition to the data that have been collected in the previous stages, data on the minimal scan rate the individual can successfully use are recorded.

If the need is for power mobility, then the next step is to use software specifically designed for developing skills in using a joystick. Alternatively, scanning training software aimed at single-switch or dual-switch wheelchair use can be used for training at this stage.

In the final training phase for communication, symbolic representation is added to the choice making. Development of the individual's language skills may have been taking place in conjunction with the motor skills training, and this linguistic step may follow naturally. Selection of symbol systems is discussed in Chapter 11. Through this phase the individual makes the transition from object manipulation (environmental control) to concept manipulation (communication). Greater resources are available at this stage to convey needs, wants, and other information. Simple scanning communication devices or multiple choice computer programs can also be used for further skill development as a precursor to a scanning communication device.

It is assumed that people will improve as a result of repetition of any motor act. It is possible that the quality and speed of their movements may improve, and even the number of movement patterns (e.g., head movement and hand movement) available to them increases. Hussey et al (1992) documented the progress of two young women after the implementation of a motor training program similar to the one described in Table 7-13. Initially, both Janice and Marge lacked the head control to activate even a single switch. The initial control site for both of them was flexion at the elbow, in one case to activate a mercury switch and in the other case a leaf switch. After extensive training with the approach just described, Janice and Marge are now able to select directly from a limited array using a light pointer worn on the head with a portable augmentative communication device. These two cases are representative of the skills that individuals can gain from a systematic motor training program so that use of assistive technology for a functional activity can be achieved.

Skill development varies greatly across different input devices depending on cognitive load, mastery, speed, and user characteristics (Cress and French, 1994). Three groups were included: adults without disabilities who had computer experience, typically developing children between 2.5 and 5.0 years, and children with intellectual disabilities (mental age 2.5 to 5.0 years). Adults without disabilities were able to master all of the devices (touchscreen, trackball, mouse, locking trackball, and keyboard) without training. About 50% of typically developing children were able to master all devices except the locking trackball without training. After training, 80% of these children mastered all devices. The trackball was the easiest to master. Children with intellectual disabilities averaged between 0% and 46% mastery (depending on the device) without training and less than 75% mastery with training. The locking trackball was significantly more difficult to master than the other devices. Adults were able to use the devices faster than the children, and the typically developing children used most devices more slowly than the children with intellectual disabilities. This result is probably related to the greater chronological age of the children with intellectual disabilities. An exception to the general result was the touch screen, which was used faster by the typically developing children. This is probably due to the greater sensory feedback provided by the other interfaces. Performance by typically developing children was related to age and gross motor abilities. In addition to these, performance of children with intellectual disabilities was also related to pattern analysis skills, and the individual input devices showed distinctly different relationships to cognitive and motor development than for the typically developing children. These studies indicate that selection of control interfaces for a given individual depends on cognitive and motor requirements presented by a particular interface and the skills of the individual in these areas, so extrapolation from successful use by adults without disabilities or typically developing children to children with disabilities is not appropriate. The amount of training required for successful use is also generally greater for children who have disabilities than it is for typically developing children or adults.

OUTPUT COMPONENT OF THE HUMAN TECHNOLOGY INTERFACE

Speech Output

Speech is the auditory form of language, and electronic assistive technologies that provide language output rely on artificial speech. The three major applications are screen readers and print-material reading machines for persons who are blind (see Chapter 8), voice output augmentative communication devices (see Chapter 11), and alternative reading formats for persons with cognitive disabilities (see Chapter 10). The two types of speech output are digital recording and speech synthesis. They differ in the manner by which the speech is electronically produced. Table 7-14 lists the features and the typical assistive technology applications for the two approaches.

Digital Recording.   **Digital recording** stores human speech in electronic memory circuits so that it can be retrieved later. The speech to be stored can be entered at any time by just speaking into a built-in microphone. Even a few seconds of speech takes a great deal of memory.

TABLE 7-14	Types of Speech Output Used in Assistive Technologies	
Type of Speech Output	Major Features	Typical Assistive Technology Applications
Digital recording	Uses actual voice and can easily be child, male, female Speech is limited to what is stored Relatively low cost	Augmentative communication
Speech synthesis	Very high quality for single words or complete phrases Intelligibility decreases for unlimited vocabulary with text-to-speech Unlimited vocabulary with text-to-speech Moderate intelligibility with letter-to-sound rules only Highly intelligible with morphemic rules Cost depends on text-to-speech approach	Speech output for EADLs Augmentative communication Screen readers for blind users Speech output for users with learning disabilities Speech output for phone communication by persons who are deaf

For example, 16 seconds of speech may take up to 1 megabyte of memory for storage without signal processing and compression. Current memory technologies are similar to those used for audio music and speech recordings and they can store large amounts of vocabulary. The major advantage of digital recording of speech is that it allows any voice to be easily stored in the device and played back. For example, if the person who is using the AAC system (see Chapter 11) that uses digital recording is a young girl, we can use another young girl's voice to store the required messages.

Speech Synthesis.   **Speech synthesis** generates the speech electronically instead of storing the entire signal. This approach reduces the amount of memory required. Speech output can be created from any electronic text, including that sent to the screen of a computer. A mathematical model of the human vocal system is used to synthesize the speech. One example of a vocal tract model is shown in Figure 7-32. There are two types of sounds in speech, voiced and unvoiced (a hissing sound similar to unvoiced sounds such as *s* or *f*), and both these types of speech must be included in the vocal tract model. These signals are then fed into a model of the vocal tract that is varied to produce the speech in a manner similar to the variation of the tongue, teeth, lips, and throat during human speech. Speech synthesizers can generate any word if the correct codes are sent to them in the correct order.

Prosodic features, which give speech its human quality, are generated by changes in three parameters: (1) amplitude, (2) pitch, and (3) duration of the spoken utterance. As discussed in Chapter 3, human speech consists of both these basic or segmental sounds and prosodic or suprasegmental features. These features allow us to stress a phrase or word, to emphasize a point, or to generate an utterance that portrays a particular mood (e.g., angry or polite or happy). They are also responsible for the inflection changes that distinguish a yes/no question (rising pitch at the end of the sentence) from a statement (falling pitch at the end). For example, the statement, "He is going to dinner" has a falling inflection at the end. However, the inflection in the sentence, "Is he going to dinner?" rises at the end. Murray et al. (1991) developed software, called Hamlet, that used DECTalk (Fonix Corporation, Sandy Utah, *www.fonix.com*) speech synthesizer voice quality to provide vocal emotion effects to the synthetic speech.

Text-To-Speech Programs.   **Text-to-speech programs** convert text characters into the codes required by the speech synthesizer by analyzing a word or sentence. When the speech synthesizer receives these codes, they are combined into the word the user wants to say. There are several approaches that can be taken to generate speech from text input (Allen, 1981). Table 7-15 lists the major approaches and their features. The most common approach is to break words into syntactically significant groups called *morphs* (see Chapter 3), store codes associated with each morph, and match the morph to the letters typed. Approximately 8000 morphs can generate more than 95% of the words in English. To break words down into morphs, and then match the morphs to the speech sounds requires the development of a text-to-speech system. One of the first developments of a morphonemic text-to-speech system was the MITalk-79 system (Allen, 1981).

The commonly used system, DECTalk, uses morphonemic principles of speech synthesis (Bruckert, 1984). This speech synthesizer uses a 6000-entry lexicon that contains basic pronunciation rules similar to those of MITalk-79. The emphasis of this type of system is on maximizing the

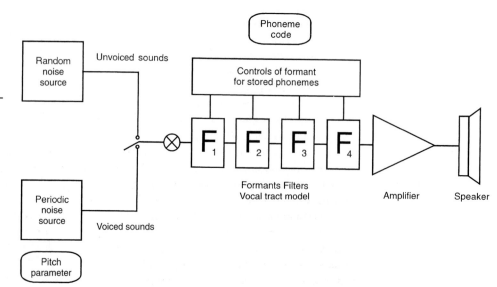

Figure 7-32 Speech synthesis systems are often based on a vocal tract model. Sound sources for both voiced (periodic noise) and unvoiced (random noise), as well as a computational model of the vocal tract characteristics, are included.

TABLE 7-15   **Types of Text-to-Speech Systems Used in Assistive Technologies**

Type of Text-to-Speech System	Major Features	Advantages and Disadvantages
Whole word look-up	Speech pattern for each word stored in memory Look-up of words as they are typed	Requires large memory for even modest vocabulary size Very high intelligibility for words stored Vocabulary limited to words stored
Letter-to-sound conversion	Text is matched to sounds letter by letter according to a set of rules Can use phonemes, allophones, or diphones Limited prosodic features	Unlimited vocabulary with very low memory requirements Relatively low intelligibility Rules have many exceptions and overall quality depends on sophistication of rules
Morphonemic text-to-speech conversion	Relies on combination of stored morphs and letter-to-sound rules Can use phonemes, allophones, or diphones Includes prosodic features	Unlimited vocabulary with moderate memory requirements Relatively high intelligibility Much higher cost than letter-to-sound rules alone

use of prestored pronunciation rules and relying on letter-to-sound rules only for uncommon or user-specific words (e.g., proper names or technical terms). There are seven built-in voices and one user-definable voice. The latter allows the user to pick fundamental frequencies, speech rate, and other parameters to create any voice (e.g., Mickey Mouse or a robot). These built-in voices include children, adult females, and adult males with different features. A small (150-word) user-defined dictionary that can contain words unique to the individual user is also included. Many augmentative communication systems now include this speech output system. The DECTalk has also been used in computer screen readers for individuals who are blind and in automated reading systems (see Chapter 8). Bruckert (1984) describes DECTalk in greater detail. A portable version, Multivoice, is also available. DECTalk and some other commercial speech synthesizers are also available in Spanish, French, and some other European languages (e.g., German, Swedish, and Italian).

Most AAC devices (see Chapter 11) and screen readers for the blind (see Chapter 8) use either DECTalk, Eloquence (Scan Soft, Peabody, Mass., *www.scansoft.com/ speechworks/realspeak/assistive/#eti*), AT&T Natural Voice (AT&T, *www.naturalreaders.com/index.html*), IBM ViaVoice (Austin, Tex., *www.ibm.com/us/*), or a proprietary text-to-speech system (e.g., Dynavox VeriVoice (Pittsburgh, Pa., *www.dynavoxtech.com/*). TMA associates (Tarzana, Calif., *www.tmaa.com/*) provides listings and analysis of text-to-speech and other related products. Aaron, Eide, and Pitrelli (2005) provide an excellent overview and tutorial on speech synthesis.

Audio Considerations.   The intelligibility and sound quality of any speech synthesis system are dramatically affected by the quality of the amplifier and speaker used to provide the final speech output. Many commercial systems use low-power amplifiers and small, low-fidelity speakers. This technology can reduce the quality of the sound and therefore make it more difficult to understand. However, in most AAC applications the speech synthesis system must be portable. Higher-power output amplifiers require larger batteries, and larger speakers that have greater fidelity are heavier than lower-quality speakers. Both these factors affect weight and therefore portability. The most important rule that applies here is that "you don't get something for nothing"; higher quality in speech sound output is obtained only at the cost of increased weight and reduced portability.

Telephone Use.   Telephone lines have a narrower bandwidth (frequency range) and this affects the use of speech synthesis and the intelligibility of speakers with dysarthria (Drager et al, 2004). Adult listeners heard mildly (90% intelligible) dysarthric spoken speech and synthesized speech in both face-to-face and telephone contexts. In the face-to-face situation there are additional cues such as facial expressions, and the acoustic signal is not limited as it is over the telephone. Listeners found the quality of the speech synthesis equivalent to that of the natural speech. Over the telephone, speech quality is degraded more for the natural dysarthric speaker than for the speech synthesis, and the listeners clearly preferred the synthetic speech.

Intelligibility Studies.   The final determination of effectiveness of speech synthesis is how intelligible it is to human listeners. Although personal preference plays a part in this determination, there are objective ways in which to evaluate the intelligibility of various speech synthesizers. The environment in which speech is heard is also a factor in intelligibility. Most intelligibility studies are conducted under very controlled and noise-free conditions. When speech output communication devices are used, it is not in such highly controlled environments. One way to study the degrading of intelligibility in real settings is to add reverberation that simulates more natural conditions (Venkatagiri, 2004). When reverberation is added to simulate a large room and a large lecture hall, the intelligibility of human speech degrades only slightly. Under the same conditions, synthetic speech intelligibility decreased by 28%. These tests were conducted without the benefit of linguistic and communicative context cues that would typically be available to the partners of an AAC user.

■ SUMMARY

In this chapter the elements of the human/technology interface and their relationship to the other components of assistive technology have been defined. The elements of the human/technology interface include the control interface, the selection method, and the selection set. The selection set encompasses the items in the array from which the user can choose. There are two basic methods by which the user makes selections: direct selection or indirect selection. Indirect selection encompasses a subset of selection methods known as scanning, directed scanning, and coded access. Each selection method applies to a different set of consumer skills.

With advances in technology, there is a wide range of control interfaces available for use by persons with disabilities. Control interfaces can be characterized by their sensory, spatial, and activation-deactivation features. Understanding these characteristics can help the ATP sort through the maze of control interfaces. This chapter also described a framework that provides the ATP with a systematic process for matching the interface to the needs and skills of consumers. Critical questions were identified that relate to the user's skills needed to control particular types of interfaces. Addressing these questions during the evaluation can facilitate the selection of an appropriate control interface for the consumer.

Study Questions

1. What is the function of the control interface? Describe the difference between a discrete and a continuous input with examples for each.
2. Define the elements of the human/technology interface and how they are related to the processor and the output.
3. What is a selection set?
4. What are the two basic selection methods used with control interfaces?
5. What are the scanning formats that can be used to accelerate scanning?
6. Why is coded access an indirect selection method? What is the selection set for Morse code?
7. What are the features included in the Macintosh universal access and Windows accessibility options?
8. What is a GIDEI, and what basic functions does it perform?
9. Explain the significance of having a USB HID specific to assistive technologies.
10. What is included in a GIDEI setup?
11. What are the relative disadvantages and advantages of software-based and hardware-based GIDEIs?
12. What does the term *transparent access* mean, and what features are used to implement it?
13. What is an on-screen keyboard?
14. What features are important in matching a specific on-screen keyboard to an individual's needs and skills?
15. List three means of providing input to on-screen keyboards.
16. Examine Table 7-4. Which Morse codes listed in the nonstandard section are the same for both example systems? Why do you think these particular codes happen to be the same, given that there are no standards?

Why do you think that the other codes are different for different systems?
17. What are the somatosensory characteristics of control interfaces that need to be considered in selection of an interface for a consumer?
18. Describe three control interface activation characteristics.
19. How are sensory and activation characteristics of control interfaces related?
20. What two measurements obtained from the consumer during the initial assessment provide information that will assist in identifying spatial characteristics of the control interface?
21. What is a control enhancer? List several examples.
22. Describe tremor dampening.
23. Compare the user profile for a standard, an ergonomic, an expanded, and a contracted keyboard. What user skills would lead the ATP to select one of these over the others?
24. What are the major design goals of ergonomic keyboards?
25. What are the primary considerations that would lead to the choice of speech recognition as an alternative direct selection method?
26. Describe the difference between continuous and discrete speech recognition systems.
27. What is the difference between speaker-independent and speaker-dependent automatic speech recognition systems?
28. What are the most common alternatives to a computer mouse? List at least one advantage and one disadvantage of each.
29. What factors might explain the results in the comparison study of expanded keyboard cursor control of a mouse and head pointing (Capilouto et al, 2005)?

30. What are the two most common approaches to detecting eye position and movement for use as a control interface?
31. What is point of gaze, and why is it a potential limitation in eye-tracking systems?
32. Describe the major components of a brain computer interface.
33. What are the major approaches to BCI development? Which approach do you think offers the most promise? Why?
34. List three types of modifications to keyboards and pointing devices, and give an example of the problems that each solves.
35. Describe the three different selection techniques used with scanning and directed scanning. Which one provides the user with more control and why?

36. What are the relative advantages and disadvantages of the three common scanning methods? Select a client profile that would benefit from each type.
37. Review the description of control interface flexibility in the section on characteristics of control interfaces. Pick three switches from those described in the section on selecting control interfaces, one that is very flexible, one that is moderately flexible, and one that is not flexible. Justify your choices.
38. Describe distributed and integrated control. What are the advantages and disadvantages of each?
39. What outcomes can be achieved through the implementation of training programs for development of motor skills?
40. Describe the steps taken in a training program to develop motor control.

References

Aaron A, Eide E, Pitrelli JF: Conversational computers, *Sci Am* 292:64-69, 2005.

Allen J: Linguistic-based algorithms offer practical text-to-speech systems, *Speech Technol* 1:12-16, 1981.

Angelo J: Comparison of three computer scanning modes as an interface method for persons with cerebral palsy, *Am J Occup Ther* 46:217-222, 1992.

Angelo J, Deterding C, Weisman J: Comparing three head-pointing systems using a single subject design, *Assist Technol* 3:43-49, 1991.

Angelo J, Smith RO: The critical role of occupational therapy in augmentative communication services. In American Occupational Therapy Association, editors: *Technology review '89: perspectives on occupational therapy practice,* Rockville, Md, 1989, American Occupational Therapy Association.

Angelo J, Trefler, E: A survey of persons who use integrated control devices, *Assist Technol* 10:77-83, 1998.

Anson D: Speech recognition technology, *OT Pract* January/February:59-62, 1999.

Anson DK: *Alternative computer access: a guide to selection,* Philadelphia, 1997, FA Davis.

Anson D et al: A comparison of head pointer technologies, *Proc 2003 RESNA Conf:* http://www.resna.org/ProfResources/Publications/Proceedings/2003/Papers/ComputerAccess/Anson_CA_Headpointers.php. Accessed June 28, 2005.

Applewhite A: 40 years: The luminaries, *IEEE Spectrum* 41:37-58, 2004.

Bailey RW: *Human performance engineering,* ed 2, Upper Saddle River, NJ, 1996, Prentice Hall.

Baker JM: How to achieve recognition: A tutorial/status report on automatic speech recognition, *Speech Technol,* Fall:30-31, 36-43, 1981.

Barker MR: *Integrating assistive technology: communication, computers, control and seating and mobility systems.* Presented at Demystifying Technology Workshop, CSUS Assistive Device Center, 1991, Sacramento, Calif.

Barker MR, Cook AM: A systematic approach to evaluating physical ability for control of assistive devices, *Proc 4th Ann Conf Rehabil Eng* June 1981, pp. 287-289.

Barreto A, Al-Masri E, Cremades JG: Eye gaze tracking/electromyogram computer cursor control system for users with motor disabilities, *Proc 2003 RESNA Conf:* http://www.resna.org/ProfResources/Publications/Proceedings/2003/Papers/ComputerAccess/Barreto_CA.php. Accessed June 28, 2005.

Bear-Lehman J: Orthopedic conditions. In Trombly CA, editor: *Occupational therapy for physical dysfunction,* ed 4, Baltimore, Md, 1995, Williams & Wilkins.

Betke M, Gips J, Fleming P: The camera mouse: visual tracking of body features to provide computer access for people with severe disabilities, *IEEE Trans Neualr Syst Rehabil Eng* 10:1-10, 2002.

Beukelman DR, Yorkston KM: Computer enhancement of message formulation and presentation for communication augmentation, *Semin Speech Lang* 5:1-10, 1984.

Blackstein-Alder S et al: Mouse manipulation through single switch scanning, *Assist Technol* 16:28-42, 2004.

Blackstone S: The role of rate in communication, *Augment Commun News* 3:1-3, 1990b.

Bruckert E: A new text-to-speech product produces dynamic human-quality voice, *Speech Technol* 4:114-119, 1984.

Burkhart LJ: *Using computers and speech synthesis to facilitate communicative interaction with young and/or severely handicapped children,* College Park, MD, 1987, Linda J. Burkhart.

Capilouto GJ et al: Performance investigation of a head-operated device and expanded membrane cursor keys in a target acquisition task, *Technol Disabil* 17:173-183, 2005.

Caves K et al: The use of integrated controls for mobility, communication and computer access, *Proc 14th RESNA Conf*, June 1991, pp. 166-167.

Chen D-H et al: Infrared-based communication augmentation system for people with multiple disabilities, *Disabil Rehabil* 26:1105-1109, 2004.

Chen Y-L et al: The new design of an infrared-controlled human-computer interface for the disabled, *IEEE Trans Neural Syst Rehabil Eng* 7:474-481, 1999.

Chubon RA, Hester MR: An enhanced standard computer keyboard system for single-finger and typing-stick typing, *J Rehabil Res Dev* 25:17-24, 1988.

Comerford R, Makhoul J, Schwartz R: The voice of the computer is heard in the land (and it listens too), *IEEE Spectrum* 34:39-47, 1997.

Cook AM: Development of motor skills for switch use by persons with severe disabilities, *Dev Disabil Spec Interest Newsl* 14:3, 1991.

Cook AM et al: Measuring target acquisition utilizing Madentec's tracker system in individuals with cerebral palsy, *Technol Disabil* 17:115-163, 2005.

Cress CJ, French GJ: The relationship between cognitive load measurements and estimates of computer input control skills, *Assist Technol* 6:54-66, 1994.

Ding D et al: Integrated control and related technology of assistive devices, *Assist Technol* 15:89-97, 2003.

Drager KD, Hustad KC, Gable KL: Telephone communication: synthetic and dysarthric speech intelligibility and listener preferences, *Augment Altern Commun* 20:103-112, 2004.

Drainoni M et al: Patterns of internet use by persons with spinal cord injuries and relationship to health-related quality of life, *Arch Phys Med Rehabil* 85:1872-1879, 2004.

Evans DG, Drew R, Blenkhorn P: Controlling muse pointer position using an infrared head-operated joystick, *IEEE Trans Rehabil Eng* 8:107-117, 2000.

Fabiani GE et al: Conversion of EEG activity into cursor movement by a brain-computer interface (BCI), *IEEE Trans Neural Syst Rehabil Eng* 12:331-338, 2004.

Gallant JA: Speech-recognition products, *Electronic Design News* 7:112-122, 1989.

Gorgens RA, Bergler PM, Gorgens DC: HandiWare: Powerful, flexible software solutions for adapted access, augmentative communication and low vision in the DOS environment, *Proc 13th Annu Conf Rehabil Eng*, June 1990, pp. 43-44.

Guerette P, Caves K, Gross K: One switch does it all, *Team Rehabil Rep* March/April:26-29, 1992.

Guerette P, Sumi, E: Integrating control of multiple assistive devices: a retrospective review. *Assist Technol* 6:67-76, 1994.

Guerette PJ, Nakai RJ: Access to assistive technology: a comparison of integrated and distributed control, *Technol Dis* 5:63-73, 1996.

Horn EM, Jones HA: Comparison of two selection techniques used in augmentative and alternative communication, *Augment Altern Commun* 12:23-31, 1996.

Hortsman H, Levine S: Effect of word prediction features on user performance, *Augment Altern Commun* 12:155-168, 1996.

Hortsman HM, Levine SP, Jaros LA: Keyboard emulation for access to IBM-PC–compatible computers by people with motor impairments, *Assist Technol* 1:63-70, 1989.

Hussey SM et al: A conceptual model for developing augmentative communication skills in individuals with severe disabilities, *Proc RESNA Int 92 Conf*, June 1992, pp. 287-289.

Hyman WA, Miller GE, Neigut JS: Laser diodes for head pointing and environmental control, *Proc Int 92 RESNA Conf*, June 1992, pp. 377-379.

Kambeyanda D, Singer L, Cronk S: Potential problems associated with the use of speech recognition products, *Assist Technol* 9:95-101, 1997.

Kangas K: Assessment and training of methods of access and optimal control sites, *Assist Device News* 5, 1988.

Kangas K: The optimal position, *Assist Device News* 5, 1989.

Kasch M, Poole SE, Hedl M: Acute hand injuries. In Early MB, editor: *Physical dysfunction practice skills for the occupational therapy assistant*, St. Louis, 1998, Mosby.

Lankford C: Effective eye-gaze input into Windows™, In *Eye tracking research and applications, Symposium*, pp. 23-27, Palm Beach Gardens, FL, 2000, Association of Computing Machinery.

Lau C, O'Leary S: Comparison of computer interface devices for persons with severe disabilities, *Am J Occup Ther* 47:1022-1029, 1993.

Lee KS, Thomas DJ: *Control of computer-based technology for people with physical disabilities: an assessment manual*, Toronto, 1990, University of Toronto Press.

Lesher GW, Moulton BJ, Higginbotham DJ: Techniques for augmenting scanning, *Augment Altern Commun* 14:81-101, 1998.

Leuthardt EC et al: A brain-computer interface using electrocorticographic signals in humans, *J Neural Eng* 1:63-71, 2004.

Linnman S: M3S: The local network for electric wheelchairs and rehabilitation equipment, *IEEE Trans Rehabil Eng* 4:188-192, 1996.

Marsden R: Personal communication, 2005.

Mason SG, Birch GE: A general framework for brain-computer interface design, *IEEE Trans Neural Syst Rehabil Eng* 11:70-85, 2003.

McCormack DJ: The effects of keyguard use and pelvic positioning on typing speed and accuracy in a boy with cerebral palsy, *Am J Occup Ther* 44:312-315, 1990.

Morasso P et al: Towards standardization of communication and control systems for motor impaired people, *Med Biol Eng Comput* 17:481-488, 1979.

Murray IR et al: Emotional synthetic speech in an integrated communication prosthesis, *Proc 14th Annu Conf Rehabil Eng,* June 1991, pp. 311-313.

Nisbet P: Integrating assistive technologies: current practices and future possibilities. *Med Eng Physics* 18:193-202, 1996.

Novak M, Olsen B: Standards work involving the general input device emulating interface (GIDEI), SerialKeys, and the universal serial bus (USB), *University Wisconsin Trace Enter* (2001): http://trace.wisc.edu/docs/gidei_usb/gidei-usb.html. Accessed August 15, 2005.

Phillips B, Lin A: Head-tracking technology for mouse control: a comparison project, In *Proceedings of the 2003 RESNA Conference,* Washington, DC, 2003, RESNA.

Puckett AD et al: Development of an improved mouthpiece for a mouthstick, *Proc Int Conf Assoc Adv Rehabil Tech,* June 1988, pp. 100-101.

Radwin RR, Vanderheiden GC, Lin ML: A method for evaluating head-controlled computer input devices using Fitts' Law, *Hum Factors* 32: 423-438, 1990.

Ratcliff A: Comparison of relative demands implicated in direct selection and scanning: considerations from normal children, *Augment Altern Commun* 10:67-74, 1994.

Salamo GJ, Jakobs T: Laser pointers: are they safe for use by children? *Augment Altern Commun* 12: 47-51, 1996.

Schalk G et al: BCI2000: A general-purpose brain-computer interface (BCI) system, *IEEE Trans Biomed Eng* 51: 1034-1043, 2004.

Schwejda P, Vanderheiden G: Adaptive-firmware card for the Apple II, *Byte* 7:276-314, 1982.

Shein F et al: WIVIK: a visual keyboard for Windows 3.0, *Proc 14th Annu RESNA Conf,* June 1991, pp. 160-162.

Shein F et al: Beyond single-switch row-column scanning with WIVKI on-screen keyboard, *Proc CSUN Conference* (2003): http://www.csun.edu/cod/conf/2003/proceedings/150.htm.

Simpson RC, Koester HH: Adaptive one-switch row-column scanning, *IEEE Trans Rehabil Eng* 7:464-473, 1999.

Smith RO: Technological approaches to performance enhancement. In Christiansen C, Baum C, editors: *Occupational therapy overcoming human performance deficits,* Thorofare, NJ, 1991, Slack.

Spaeth DM, Cooper RA: Designing a variable compliance joystick for control interface research, *Proc RESNA 99 Conf,* June 1999, pp. 131-133.

Tessler FN: The Apple adjustable keyboard, *MACWORLD,* November 1993.

Vanderheiden G, Zimmermann G: State of the science: access to information technologies. In Winters JM et al, editors: *Emerging and accessible telecommunications, information and healthcare technologies,* pp. 152-184,. Arlington, VA, RESNA Press, 2002: http://trace.wisc.edu/docs/2002SOS-Report-IT/index.htm. Accessed August 20, 2005.

Vanderheiden GC: *A unified quantitative modeling approach for selection-based augmentative communication systems* [dissertation], Madison, 1984, University of Wisconsin.

Vanderheiden GC, Lloyd LL: Communication systems and their components. In Blackstone S, Bruskin D, editors: *Augmentative communication: an introduction,* Rockville, Md, 1986, American Speech Language and Hearing Association.

Venkatagiri HS: Segmental intelligibility of three text-to-speech synthesis methods in reverberant environments, *Augment Altern Commun* 20:150-163, 2004.

Weiss PL: Mechanical characteristics of microswitches adapted for the physically disabled, *J Biomed Eng* 12:398-402, 1990.

CHAPTER 8

Sensory Aids for Persons With Visual Impairments

Learning Objectives

On completing this chapter, you will be able to do the following:

1. Describe the major approaches to sensory substitution, including the advantages and disadvantages of each
2. Describe device use for reading and mobility by persons who have visual impairment
3. Describe how computer outputs are adapted for individuals with visual limitations
4. Describe the major approaches to Internet access for persons with visual impairments

Key Terms

Accessibility
Accessibility Options
Alternative Mobility Device
Alternative Sensory System
Braille
Clear Path Indicator
Closed-Circuit Television
Digital Audio-Based Information
  System
Digital Talking Books

Electronic Travel Aid
Graphical User Interface
Human/Technology Interface
Information Processor
Internet
Magnification Aids
Optical Aids
Optical Character Recognition
Orientation and Mobility
Privacy

Quality
Reading Aid
Refreshable Braille Display
Screen Readers
Spatial Display
Universal Access
User Agent
User Display

When an individual has a sensory impairment, assistive technologies can provide assistance in the input of information. In this chapter, approaches that are used to either aid or replace seeing and hearing are emphasized. This includes sensory aids that are intended for *general use* and assistive technologies that are used specifically for providing visual access to computers. Assessment considerations for sensory function are described in Chapter 4. Patients with low vision were surveyed to determine their major needs for assistive devices (Stelmack et al, 2003). Sixty-three activities in the categories of travel, food and shopping, communications, household tasks, self-care, recreation and socialization, and contrast were included in the survey. The informants were 149 individuals in the age range of 51-96 years (mean 76 years). Two thirds were male. The survey consisted of asking participants whether they could perform the activity independently or if they used a low-vision device or whether they thought it was important to use a device to perform the activity independently. The highest-ranked items involved travel (finding a clear path, identify landmarks, recognize traffic signals, step off a curb), self-care (apply makeup, shave), reading (large print, sign checks, find food in kitchen), and recreation (see television, recognize persons close up); Stelmack et al (2003) provide detailed results. Assistive devices designed to meet the needs identified in the Stelmack survey are discussed in this chapter, beginning with the fundamental principles associated with sensory aids.

■ FUNDAMENTAL APPROACHES TO SENSORY AIDS

Chapters 2 and 3 describe the human component of the human activity assistive technology (HAAT) model in some detail. Two primary intrinsic enablers of the human in this model are sensing and perception. If there are impairments in either of these functions, it is necessary to use sensory aids. When sensory aids are designed or applied, the level of impairment becomes a critical issue. If there is sufficient residual function in the primary sensory system being aided, the input is augmented to make it useful to the person. For example, eyeglasses magnify (augment) the level of visual information. On the other hand, if there is insufficient residual sensory capability, then the sensory aid must use an alternative sensory pathway. For example, braille (tactile pathway) can be used for reading when vision is not functional. We describe both augmentation and replacement for visual information in this section.

Figure 8-1 shows the major components of a sensory aid based on the parts of the assistive technology component of the HAAT model. The *environmental interface* detects the sensory data that the human cannot obtain through his or her own sensory system. This is typically a camera for visual data, a microphone for auditory data, and pressure sensors for tactile data. The environmental interface signal is fed to an **information processor,** the function of which depends on the type of aid. For sensory aids that use the

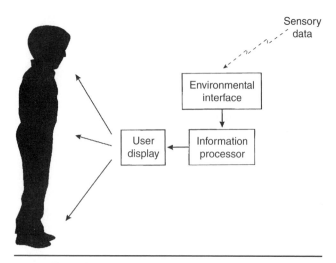

Figure 8-1   The major components of all sensory aids.

same sensory pathway, the information processor primarily amplifies the signal. Examples include **closed-circuit television** (CCTV) for visual input and hearing aids for auditory input. In other cases, the information processor may be more complicated. For example, in an auditory substitution reading device, the information processor may take visual information from the sensor, convert it to speech, and then send it to the user as auditory information. In the case of the sensory aid, the **human/technology interface** is a **user display,** which portrays the sensory information for the human user. The processed information is presented to the user so that the alternative pathway can process it. For the visual pathway this is a visible display (e.g., a video monitor), for the auditory pathway it is an audio display (e.g., a speaker), and for the tactile pathway it is a vibrating pin or electrode array through which pressure or touch data are provided to the user.

Augmentation of an Existing Pathway

For someone who has low vision, the primary pathway (i.e., the one normally used for input) is still available; it is just limited. The limitation may be one of several types. The most common type of limitation is one of *intensity*. For visual information, this limitation means that the size of the input signal is too small to be seen. Eyeglasses are the most common type of aid used for this problem, but other ways can be used to magnify the signal. The second type of impairment is referred to as a *frequency* or *wavelength* limitation. For visual input, this is manifest in inadequacy in discerning colors or the contrast between foreground and background, and this problem can be addressed with filters or by varying contrast (e.g., black on white rather than white on black). Finally, there are *field* limitations. This term is most commonly used in describing visual loss, and the field may be limited in several ways (see Figure 3-4). The most common

approach to problems of this type is to use lenses that are designed to widen the field.

Use of an Alternative Sensory Pathway

When a sensory input modality is so impaired that there can be no useful input of information through that channel, we must substitute an **alternative sensory system.** The use of braille for reading by persons who are blind is an example of tactile substitution for visual input. Tactile and auditory systems replace the visual system, and visual and tactile systems substitute for auditory input of information. Visual and tactile substitutions for auditory information are discussed in Chapter 9. When this type of substitution is made, the assistive technology practitioner (ATP) must be aware of fundamental differences among the tactile, visual, and auditory systems.

Tactile Substitution.   The tactile system has been used as the basis for many visual substitution systems. Visual information is spatially organized (Nye and Bliss, 1970). This means that visual information is represented in the central nervous system by the relationship of objects to each other in space; that is, the left, right, up, down, far, and near features of objects are preserved. In contrast, the auditory system is temporally organized (Kirman, 1973). This means that it is the time relationships in auditory signals that provide information. For example, it is the temporal sequence of sounds in speech that the auditory system uses to form words and derive meaning. Finally, tactile information is both temporally and spatially organized (Kirman, 1973), and sensory input from the tactile system requires both spatial and temporal cues. For example, the fingers are capable of distinguishing fine features such as those found on coins. However, to distinguish one denomination of coin from another, it is necessary to manipulate them in the hand. This movement of the coins provides temporal (time sequence) information that helps clarify the spatial information, and it is very difficult to distinguish two denominations of coins merely by placing a hand on top of them without movement. This combination of movement and texture is referred to as *spatiotemporal information*. The combination of tactile and kinesthetic or proprioceptive information is called the *haptic sensory* system.

Kirman (1973) presents an example that illustrates the differences between visual and tactile information for reading. Print on a page is organized spatially. People read by using saccadic eye movements, which jump from one group of letters to another. With each new point of focus, new information is taken in. This allows the visual system (including the eyes, peripheral pathways, and central nervous system components) to use its spatial feature extraction to recognize shapes as letters, to assemble them into words, and to associate meaning with them. In contrast, a person reading with braille moves his or her hand across the line of raised dots, obtaining both spatial (the organization of the six braille cells) and temporal (the moving pattern under his finger) information. If the sighted person were to use the method used with braille, the text would constantly move before the eyes, and this would result in a blurred image because the spatial information would be constantly changing. Thus we can say that the movement (temporal aspect) interferes with the visual input of information. On the other hand, if the braille user were to use the approach used by the sighted reader, he or she would place a finger on a character, input the information, and then jump to the next character. This would severely limit the input of braille information because the movement required by the tactile system would be absent. Thus the visual and tactile methods of sensory input are very different, which must be taken into account when one system is substituted for the other.

When vision is used for mobility rather than reading, there are some differences. In this case the visual image is constantly changing as the individual walks. The eyes scan the environment, and information is derived from the spatial arrangement of objects and people and from changes in the person's position relative to these objects as he or she moves. The visual system (including oculomotor components) functions to stabilize images on the retina for input of data, even during movement. This maximizes input of changing spatial information. Ways in which persons with visual impairments use other senses and assistive devices for mobility are discussed in the section on mobility later in this chapter.

Auditory Substitution.   The auditory system has been used to substitute for visual information in several ways. Some of these have been more successful than others, and the reasons for success or failure illustrate the challenges of substituting one sense for another. The least successful approaches have been those that converted a visual image of letters into a set of tones. One such device was the Stereotoner (Smith, 1972). The environmental interface for this device was a camera consisting of a set of horizontal slits. As the camera passed over a letter, a black area (i.e., a part of a letter) resulted in a tone being produced and a white area (no letter) resulted in silence. As the camera moved over a letter, a series of tones was heard as changing musical chords. Although some individuals were able to use this information at a reading rate of 40 words per minute, the device was generally unsuccessful. Cook (1982) cites several reasons for this. First, the device required the user to recognize a chord pattern, then to assemble that into a letter, and then to put the letters together into a word that was meaningful in the context of the whole sentence. This is a difficult and unnatural process for the auditory system. Second, the necessity to read letter by letter using this approach resulted in a slow input speed and placed

additional memory requirements on the user. Finally, the Stereotoner was tiring to the user because of the intense concentration required. The major lesson to be learned from this example is that the auditory system is ideally suited to the receipt of language information in certain forms (e.g., speech), but it is poorly suited to complex signals that represent spatial patterns, as in the case of the Stereotoner. This is the primary reason that reading devices using auditory substitution all use speech as the mode of presentation of information.

Devices for visual mobility have used auditory substitution with greater success. This is because mobility depends much more on gross cues than on precise spatial information as in reading. In mobility, the problem becomes one of identifying large objects as potential hazards.

■ PRINCIPLES OF COMPUTER ADAPTATIONS FOR VISUAL IMPAIRMENTS

Computer interaction is bidirectional, and the ATP must understand how computer outputs can be adapted for persons with sensory impairments. User output from a computer is generally provided by a visual display. This type of display is also referred to as *soft copy*. For both general-purpose computers and special-purpose computers built into assistive devices with displays, video display terminals, flat-panel displays, and liquid crystal displays are generally used as output devices. The other type of output from a computer is in a permanent form, or *hard copy*, from a printer. Computers also provide auditory outputs in sound, music, or synthetic speech. These outputs are important to individuals who have visual impairments.

Standard visual computer outputs are not suitable for use by persons who have vision impairments. The term *low vision* indicates that the individual is able to use the visual system for reading but that the standard size, contrast, or spacing are inadequate. The term *blind* refers to individuals for whom the visual system does not provide a useful input channel for computer output displays or printers. For individuals who are blind, alternative sensory pathways of either audition (hearing) or touch (feeling) must be used to provide input. Because low vision and blindness needs are so different from each other, they are discussed separately.

Graphical User Interface

For a human to interact with a computer, there must be an effective communication channel. The most commonly used channel today, the **graphical user interface** (GUI), is established for nondisabled users through the keyboard or mouse for input and a visual display or speakers for output. What makes these peripheral elements into a user interface is the way in which they interact with the internal computer programs. Input of data, storage and processing, and output are all handled by the computer operating system. Some types of user interfaces are more suitable for adaptation of the computer to provide physical or visual access to the computer. The ATP must understand the various types of user interfaces and how they affect access.

The GUI has three distinguishing features: (1) a mouse pointer, which is moved around the screen, (2) a graphical menu bar, which appears on the screen, and (3) one or more windows, which provide a menu of choices (Hayes, 1990). Movement of the mouse or a mouse equivalent (e.g., keystrokes, trackball, head pointer, or joystick) causes the pointer to move around the screen. Two primary characteristics of GUIs are particularly important in assistive technology applications: (1) the use of graphical menus and icons to which the user can point and click for input instead of using the keyboard and (2) multitasking capabilities, which allow more than one program to be loaded and run simultaneously. The creation of a graphical environment can save typing, reduce effort, and increase accuracy, and the use of icons generally helps with recall and ease of use. The GUI allows the use of windows, which partition the screen into smaller screens, each showing a particular application. When an application or function is opened or run by clicking (or sometimes double clicking), a feature (e.g., a calculator) or application (e.g., a word processor) is displayed in a window. Several windows may be open at the same time. Figure 8-2 shows multiple windows open and examples of menus and dialog boxes used for manipulating data and information. Specific implementations of GUIs have slightly different modes of operation, but the basic principles are similar to those described here.

The GUI has both positive and negative implications for persons with disabilities. The positive features are those that apply to nondisabled users. The major limitation of GUI use in assistive technology is that the user may not have the necessary physical (eye-hand coordination) and visual skills. In addition, adaptation for alternative input or output devices is often difficult, and adaptations must be redone when changes are made to the basic operating system. The GUI is the standard user interface because of its ease of operation for novices and its consistency of operation for experts. The latter ensures that every application behaves in basically the same way (e.g., screen icons for the same task look the same, operations such as opening and closing files are always the same). Adaptations of the GUI for persons with disabilities are discussed in following sections.

The GUI presents unique and difficult problems to the blind computer user. Early computer user interfaces used a command line interface (CLI) in which commands were typed and then executed by the computer. There are fundamental differences between the ways in which a text-only CLI and a GUI provide output to the video screen. These differences present access problems related both to the ways in which internal control of the computer display is accomplished and to the ways in which the GUI is used by the computer user (Boyd, Boyd, and Vanderheiden, 1990). CLI-type interfaces used a memory buffer to store text characters for display. Because all the displayed text can be represented by an ASCII code, it is relatively easy to use a software program and to divert text from the screen to

Figure 8-2   An example of a GUI with several windows open for different applications. (From *Microsoft Windows manual,* Microsoft Corp., Redmond, Wash.)

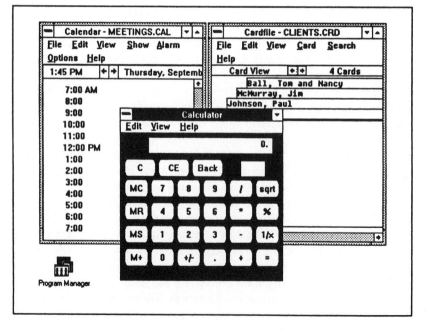

a speech synthesizer. Early screen readers operated on this principle. However, these screen readers were unable to provide access to charts, tables, or plots with graphical features. This type of system is also limited in the features that can be used with text. For example, all text is the same size, shape, and font. Enlarged characters or alternative graphical forms are not possible with a CLI-type of system, and this limits its usefulness to sighted users. The GUI uses a totally different approach to video display control that creates many more options for the portrayal of graphical information. Because each character or other graphical figure is created as a combination of dots, letters may be of any size, shape, or color and many different graphical symbols can be created. This is useful to sighted computer users because they can rely on "visual metaphors" (Boyd, Boyd, and Vanderheiden, 1990) to control a program. *Visual metaphors* use familiar objects to represent computer actions. For example, a trash can may be used for files that are to be deleted, and a file cabinet may represent a disk drive. The graphical labels used to portray these functions are referred to as *icons*.

Another feature of the GUI is that it provides a specific, consistent layout of controls on the screen. This aids the user (especially a novice) in accessing programs because everything is consistent from one application program to another and within an application. Figure 8-2 illustrates a typical GUI with several windows open and an application program running. Note that the icons used are of familiar objects, and each window has a similar look and feel.

GUI Problems and the Blind Computer User

The GUI presents several problems to the blind user. First, the graphical characters are not easily portrayed in alternative modes. Text-to-speech programs and speech synthesizers are designed to convert text to speech output (see Chapter 7). However, they are not well suited to the representation of graphics, including the icons (visual metaphors) used in GUIs. Most icons used in GUIs have text labels with them, and one approach to adaptation is to intercept the label and send it to a text-to-speech voice synthesizer system. The label is then spoken when the icon is selected. Another major problem presented to blind users by GUIs is that screen location is important in using a GUI, which is not easily conveyed by alternative means. Visual information is spatially organized, and auditory information (including speech) is temporal (time based). It is difficult to convey the screen location of a pointer by speech alone. It is difficult to portray two-dimensional spatial attributes with speech. An exception to this is a screen location that never changes. For example, some screen readers use speech to indicate the edges of the screen (e.g., right border, top of screen). A more significant problem is that the mouse pointer location on the screen is relative, rather than referenced to an absolute

standard location. This means that the only information available to the computer is how far the mouse has moved and the direction of the movement. If there is no visual information available to the user, it is difficult to know where the mouse is pointing. Other challenges presented to the visually impaired user of a GUI include the organization of the screen with elements spatially clustered visually; multitasking in which several windows are open simultaneously, with one possibly occluding another (i.e., visually displayed "on top" although both windows are active); spatial semantics (information presented through position in tables, groupings etc.); and graphical semantics (information portrayed through visual elements such as font size, colors, style) (Ratanasit and Moore, 2005). The Microsoft application programming interface for accessibility is a set of technologies that facilitate the development of screen readers and other accessibility utilities for Windows. These technologies provide alternative ways to store and access information about the contents of the computer screen. The accessibility APIs also include software driver interfaces that provide a standard mechanism for accessibility utilities to send information to speech devices or refreshable braille displays.

Ratanasit and Moore (2005) reviewed three primary types of nonspeech sound cues used for representing visual icons used in GUIs: (1) auditory icons, (2) earcons, and (3) hearcons. Auditory icons are everyday sounds used to represent graphical objects. For example, a window might be represented by the sound of tapping on a glass window or a text box by the sound of a typewriter. The Screen Access Model and Windows sound libraries are used in some applications. Earcons are abstract auditory labels that do not necessarily have a semantic relationship to the object they represent. Motives are components of earcons such as rhythm (e.g., the length of a musical note, a Latin beat), pitch (e.g., a musical C vs A), timbre (e.g., sound of a type of instrument), and register (e.g., octaves on the musical scale). An example of an earcon is a musical note or string of notes played when a file, window, or program is opened or closed. Different musical instruments may be used to represent different actions, such as a trumpet representing opening a file and a drum representing closing. In evaluations by blind users, earcons associated with musical characteristics were more effective than those using unstructured sounds (i.e., lacking rhythm, pitch and other cues). Hearcons are either nature sounds or musical works or instruments. Hearcons are completed musical sounds such as those produced by a running river or birds or a musical work, whereas earcons are separate audio components. In an evaluation by visually impaired participants, hearcons did not sufficiently portray semantic relationships to be effective. Font types have been represented by male versus female synthesized voices for normal and hyperlink text or softer and louder sounds for normal versus bold font.

Another obstacle faced by individuals who are visually impaired is the use of graphical information in tables and graphs. Three primary issues are the size of the table (i.e., providing information of the boundaries), overloading with speech information, and knowledge of current location within the table. Various methods have been developed to represent this information auditorally (Ratanasit and Moore, 2005). Nonspeech sounds are used to provide spatial relationships (e.g. a plucked violin string earcon might be used to represent the lines in a table or graph) and the text-based information contained in the table or graph is provided by synthesized speech. Another technique used is to associate higher pitches with larger numbers and lower pitches with smaller numbers in portraying trends and similar graphical data. Evaluation with visually impaired participants indicated greater success in using tables when nonspeech cues were combined with speech-based information. Another graphical approach is to represent numerical values by pitch, as above, but use a different timbre (instrument sound) for each axis.

READING AIDS FOR PERSONS WITH VISUAL IMPAIRMENTS

The major problems faced by persons with visual impairments are (1) access to printed reading material, (2) orientation and mobility (i.e., moving about safely and easily), and (3) access to computers, including the **Internet.** This section first describes reading aids for people with low vision who still obtain information through the visual system. Then tactile and auditory alternatives for people who are blind are discussed. The term *reading* is used here to include access to all print material, including text, mathematics, and graphical representations (e.g., maps, pictures, drawings, and handwriting). As discussed later, some types of reading have very specialized alternatives (e.g., talking compasses in lieu of maps, talking bar code readers for medicines and food cans).

Magnification Aids

There are three factors related to visual system performance for reading: size, spacing, and contrast. This section discusses the principles of low-vision aids for reading print material. These devices are generally referred to as **magnification aids.** Magnification may be vertical (size) or horizontal (spacing) or both. *Magnification* also includes assistive technologies that enhance contrast. There are three categories of magnification aids: (1) optical aids, (2) nonoptical aids, and (3) electronic aids (Servais, 1985). Examples of these are listed in Box 8-1.

Assistive technologies can also be used to enhance visual cues for children who have low vision (Griffin et al, 2002). Color and contrast can be enhanced by using hues (the named color, red, blue, etc.), lightness (perceived intensity), and saturation (perceived differences in color). Deficits in color vision may be difficult to detect in children, and

---

BOX 8-1   Categories and Examples of Low-Vision Aids

OPTICAL AIDS
Hand-held magnifiers
Stand magnifiers
Field expanders
Telescopes

NONOPTICAL AIDS
Enlarged print
High-intensity lamps
Daily living aids
High-contrast objects

ELECTRONIC AIDS
CCTVs
Portable CCTVs
Slide projectors
Opaque projectors
Microfiche readers

Data from Servais SP: Visual aids. In Webster JG et al, editors: *Electronic devices for rehabilitation,* New York, 1985, John Wiley.

Griffin et al provide the following guidelines for use in visual magnifiers, software, or Web site design for children with low vision: use colors that differ as little as possible in lightness, avoid colors from the ends of the spectrum, avoid white or gray with any color of the same lightness, avoid colors adjacent to each other in the color spectrum, and avoid use of pastel colors. Spatial considerations are another consideration in enhancing visual access for children with low vision (Griffin et al, 2002). Space includes size, patterns, outlines, and clarity of text and pictures. Optical magnifiers, software programs, and Web sites can address these features.

Optical Aids.   More than 90% of all individuals who have visual impairments have some usable vision (Doherty, 1993). Thus it is important to carefully choose low-vision devices to meet their needs. The National Institute on Disability and Rehabilitation Research has published a booklet describing clinical assessment methods, equipment, and tools needed for evaluating and matching of consumer's needs to low-vision devices (Doherty, 1993). With the use of **optical aids,** individuals with low vision may be able to see print, do work requiring fine detail, or increase the range of their visual fields.

The simplest of optical aids is the hand-held magnifier. Among the advantages of these devices is that they require little training, they are lightweight and small (can fit in a pocket or purse), and they are inexpensive. Some also have a built-in light to increase contrast, and others have several lenses, which can be used alone or in combination, depending on the application. A selection of optical aids is shown

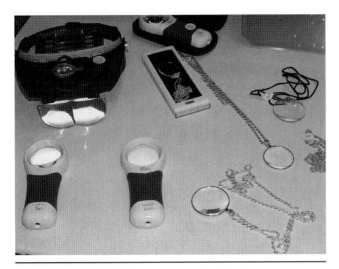

Figure 8-3   A selection of optical aids for low vision.

in Figure 8-3. Sometimes it is difficult to hold a lens and carry out a task (e.g., a two-handed task such as embroidery). In other cases it may be difficult to hold a magnifier steady (e.g., for someone who is elderly or in poor health). In these situations, stand magnifiers, some of which have a built-in light, are useful. Some magnifiers are mounted on eyeglass frames to free both hands.

One approach to limitations of visual field is the use of field expanders. These are generally prisms or special lenses built in to eyeglass frames. When magnifying lenses are used, the expansion of the field reduces the size of the image and a tradeoff occurs. The image is not reduced in size when prism lenses are used to expand the field.

Telescopes assist with distance vision. These may be either worn on the head or held in the hand, and they may be monocular or binocular (Mellor, 1981). They may be used, for example, by students who need to see a chalkboard or an adult who needs to monitor children playing outdoors. Telescopic aids provide an enlarged but narrowed visual field. Head-mounted units may be attached to eyeglass frames or have a separate frame. Head-mounted devices are particularly useful when long periods of wear are necessary, such as when watching television.

Nonoptical Aids.   This approach to magnification is based on changes in the actual material that is to be read (Servais, 1985). Common examples are large-print books or other materials such as menus, programs, and newspapers. High-intensity lamps can significantly increase contrast of reading materials, and high-contrast objects in the environment can aid in localization. For example, brightly colored furniture or dishes can help with visualization. A glass that stands out from a countertop is easier to find and fill with liquid. As Servais (1985) points out, nonoptical aids can be very useful under the right circumstances, but they are limited in application because they are specialized to one or a few tasks.

Electronic Aids.   There are limitations to the amount of magnification and contrast enhancement that can be obtained by optical approaches to magnification. Electronic devices can overcome these limitations. Many electronic low-vision aids are based on CCTV devices. Some manufacturers refer to these devices as *video magnifiers*. There are two primary advantages of CCTV devices. The first of these is that the image size can be increased much more than for optical aids. Equally important is that the image can be manipulated and controlled. For example, contrast can be dramatically affected by the use of color or reversed images (e.g., white type on black background). The overall brightness of an image can also be controlled in CCTV devices, further increasing contrast.

A typical CCTV is shown in Figure 8-4. The major components are a camera (environmental interface), a video display (user display), and a unit that controls the presentation of the image (information processor). The material to be read is placed on a scanning table, which easily moves both left to right and forward and back. There may be mechanical notches that help align the material, and some devices have adjustable margins. When the text is enlarged, the relative position of the material on the page is lost, and a spotlight of high intensity is sometimes used to show the user which part of the page is being imaged. With use of a split video screen, CCTV devices can be operated in conjunction with enlarged computer video displays to allow magnification of both computer data and the CCTV image of standard print material. Other contexts in which CCTV devices are used are to complete job-related tasks, to access educational materials at all levels, and for recreational reading.

All CCTV devices have the major features shown in Figure 8-4. An example of a CCTV device in use is shown in Figure 8-5. There is, however, a relatively wide range of features available in specific devices. The two broad categories of CCTVs are desktop and portable. The first category is by far the largest in terms of commercial products. Size and spacing are controlled primarily by two factors in desktop units: (1) size of the video monitor and (2) amount of enlargement provided by the electronics. Typical video monitors range in size from 12 to 19 inches, and maximal electronic magnification ranges from 45 to more than 60 times. There is a major tradeoff between monitor size and overall space required for the unit. Space requirements are often a significant limitation if a computer terminal, printer, and other office equipment must share space with the CCTV. A split-screen system overcomes this space problem to a large degree. CCTV systems often allow access not only to print material but also to the computer video screen. The technology is virtually the same for print or computer output.

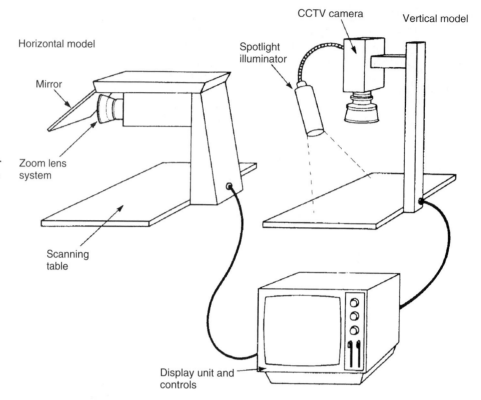

Figure 8-4   CCTV system for low-vision assistance. (From Servais SP: Visual aids. In Webster JG et al, editors: *Electronic devices for rehabilitation*, New York, 1985, John Wiley.)

One such product is Spectrum SVGA, which allows the screen to be split into two. One half is used for CCTV display of printed material and the other is used for enlarged computer output. This system also functions as either a computer screen magnifier only or CCTV only.

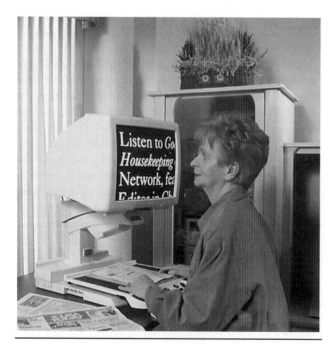

Figure 8-5   A CCTV device in use. (Courtesy NanoPac, Tulsa, Okla.)

A major challenge for people using video magnifiers is navigation around the text because it is often so enlarged that only a portion of a line or two of test is visible. This situation can result in missed words or difficulty in finding the beginning of the next line. One approach is to create a digital image of the page and then let the computer-based magnifier automatically scroll through the text (myReader, Pulse Data Human Ware, Concord, Calif., *www.pulsedata.com*). Automatic reading can be one long row that scrolls across the screen, a column of text whose width is such that it all appears on the screen at once or one word at a time with the user controlling the rate at which each word is displayed. Scrolling rate, magnification, and cursor movement around the text field are all adjustable and controllable by the user.

Contrast enhancement is provided either by gray scale or color. In the former approach the foreground and background contrast is adjustable and may be reversed (e.g., black letters on white or white letters on black). Color adds significant contrast enhancement because the user can choose alternative background and foreground colors. Not all persons with visual impairments have the same color vision, and color vision varies with visual field. Having some control over the foreground-background color combination allows the display to be customized to the needs of an individual user. Another advantage of color displays is that the original color of the print material can be retained. Maps with colored areas can be imaged; a preprinted form that calls for a signature "on the red line" shows the line as red, and so on. The major tradeoff with color monitors is that the image is not as sharp as the black and white image, especially at large magnifications. Color CCTVs are also more expensive than their black and white counterparts.

Most desktop CCTVs are relatively large and heavy primarily because of the video monitor. Liquid crystal displays and flat-panel screens have changed this. Flat-panel displays have different characteristics than cathode ray tubes, and the enlarged images provided by these two technologies are not equivalent or equally useable by all individuals. All desktop units must also be plugged into a wall socket for power. Thus it is difficult to transport them or to use them in contexts such as a classroom (unless a separate workstation is established—a common practice), and desktop units are generally kept in one physical location. Some desktop models have very small cameras (e.g., 1-inch diameter, 3 inches long) that can be connected to any video monitor or television set. This facilitates transportation and use in different locations.

Fully portable CCTVs are designed to be carried with the user. The most significant differences between these portable units and desktop CCTVs are size, weight, and battery power. Portable units weigh as little as 1.2 pounds and measure only about 9 × 3 inches for the display and 4 × 2 inches for the camera (for example, Pico, JBliss Imaging Systems, San Jose, Calif., *www.jbliss.com*; Pocket Viewer, HumanWare, Inc., Concord, Calif., *www.humanware.com*; Carrymate, Clarity, *www.clarityusa.com/*; Magnilink, Vision Cue, *www.visioncue.com/*). Portable units have a hand-held camera that is moved over the page. Maximal magnification varies from 3 to 64 times, and it may be controlled by changing camera lenses or by electronic image enhancement. Some units allow the camera to be connected to a desktop video monitor, standard television set, or portable computer to display the CCTV output. This allows it to be used in a portable or stationary mode, depending on the needs of the user. These cameras are extremely small (e.g., 2 inches × 2 inches × 4 inches, weighing 6 ounces). This flexibility is useful when greater magnification is needed for certain material (e.g., fine print) or at certain times (e.g., at the end of the day, when fatigue is greater) and when the user must travel to different settings during the day.

Access to Visual Computer Displays for Individuals With Low Vision

Screen-magnifying software that enlarges a portion of the screen is the most common adaptation for people who have low vision. The unmagnified screen is referred to as the *physical screen*. There are three basic modes of operation for screen magnifiers: lens magnification, part-screen magnification, and full-screen magnification (Blenkhorn, Gareth, and Baude, 2002). At any one time the user has access to only the portion of the physical screen that appears in this magnified viewing window. Lens magnification is analogous to holding a hand-held magnifying lens over a part of the screen. The screen magnification program takes one section of the physical screen and enlarges it. This means that the magnification window must move to show the portion of the physical screen in which the changes are occurring. Part-screen magnification is similar to lens magnification, except that the magnified portion is displayed in a separate window, usually at the top or bottom of the screen. The magnification program will follow a particular part of the screen referred to as the *focus* of the screen (Blenkhorn, Gareth, and Baude, 2002). Typical foci are the location of the mouse pointer, the location of the text-entry cursor, a highlighted item (e.g., an item in a pull-down menu), or a currently active dialog box. Screen readers automatically track the focus and enlarge the relevant portion of the screen. For example, if a navigation or control box is active, then the viewing window can highlight that box. If mouse movement occurs, then the viewing window can track the mouse cursor movement. If text is being typed in, then the viewing window can follow the text entry cursor and highlight that portion of the physical screen.

Full-screen magnifiers enlarge the entire screen, with the center of the enlarged portion being the cursor location. Thus, at any one time the user has access to only the portion of the physical screen that appears in this magnified viewing window. The size of the text in this window, the *magnification*, varies from 2 to 32 times or more in current magnifier programs. The viewing window must track any changes that occur on the physical screen. The mouse pointer can also be enlarged. Blenkhorn, Gareth, and Baude (2002) describe the design of screen magnification programs, including mouse pointer magnification.

Adaptations that allow persons with low vision to access the computer screen are available in several commercial forms. Lazzaro (1999) describes several potential methods of achieving computer access. The simplest and least costly are built-in screen enlargement software programs provided by the computer manufacturer. One system for the Macintosh, built in to the operating system, is *Zoom*. This program allows for magnification from 2 to 20 times and has fast and easy text handling and graphics capabilities. More information is available on the Apple accessibility Web site *(http://www.apple.com/education/accessibility/technology)*. *Magnifier* (Table 8-1) is a minimal function screen magnification program included in Windows *(http://www.microsoft.com/enable/default.aspx)*. It displays an enlarged portion of the screen (in Windows XP, from 2 to 9 times magnification; in Windows Vista, from 2 to 16 times), uses a part-screen approach and has three focus options: mouse cursor, keyboard entry location, and text editing. Other *Magnifier* options include inverted (e.g., black background, white letters), changing the location of the magnification pane, and high-contrast modes. For individuals who need only the high-contrast option, high contrast provides many color combination options for text, background, windows, and

TABLE 8-1　Simple Adaptations for Visual Impairment

Need Addressed	Software Approach
User cannot see status of CAPS LOCK, NUM LOCK, etc., lights	ToggleKeys
User requires greater contrast between foreground and background or greater size of characters on the screen	Magnifier or high contrast color scheme
User requires speech output rather than visual output	Narrator*

Software modifications developed at the Trace Center, University of Wisconsin, Madison. These are included as before-market modifications to Windows and Macintosh operating systems.

*Windows Vista and XP versions differ. Features of Windows XP Narrator are documented on *http://www.microsoft.com/enable/training/windowsxp/ narratorturnon.aspx*. The out-of-box Windows Vista text-to-speech (TTS) engine speaks U.S. English. This voice is called "Microsoft Anna." In Chinese SKUs of Vista, the TTS engine speaks Mandarin, called "Microsoft Lili." A different voice, perhaps speaking another language, requires the installation of a third-party TTS engine. Narrator will use any Speech Application Programming Interface (SAPI)–compliant TTS engine installed on Windows Vista and configured to be the default TTS engine. Keyboard commands include reading text (a character at a time, word at a time, line, paragraph, document) and navigating text on the basis of font attributes. For example, move cursor to where the font attributes have changed.

other GUI features. This is available in the control panels: **Accessibility Options** for Windows XP, Ease of Access for Windows Vista, and **Universal Access** for Macintosh. None of these built-in options are intended to replace commercially available full-function screen magnifiers. The mouse pointer settings under the Windows "mouse" control panel provide for changing the size, style, and color combination of all the pointers used during GUI interaction.

Screen-magnifying lenses that are placed over the monitor can also enlarge the information, but limited magnification (about two times) and distortion are the major problems. Increased contrast and reduced glare can be achieved with filters placed over the screen. Large monitors can have the effect of increasing text and graphics size, but the magnification is fixed. Adaptations that include both hardware and software provide the greatest compatibility, but they are also the most expensive alternatives.

Many screen magnification programs are available for use with Windows or Macintosh operating systems (for example, Lunar and Lunar Plus from Dolphin, Computer Access, San Mateo, Calif., *www.dolphinusa.com*; MAGic from Freedom Scientific, St. Petersburg, Fla., *www.freedomsci.com*; VIP and ezVIP from JBliss Imaging Systems, San Jose, Calif., *www.jbliss.com*; Zoom Text, Zoom Text Xtra and BigShot from AI Squared, Manchester Center, Vt., *www. aisquared.com*; and Galileo, Baum, Germany, *www.baum.de/*) (see also the Microsoft accessibility Web site, *http://www. microsoft.com/enable/default.aspx*). These software programs offer wider ranges of magnification and have more features

than built-in screen magnifiers. These programs generally offer access to Windows applications, including spreadsheet and word processing, e-mail, and Internet browsers. Many can also run with a screen reader (speech output utility). In some cases the screen reader is bundled with the magnification software, and in other cases the screen magnifier speech output runs in conjunction with a separate screen reader. Magnification of up to 32 times or more is available. The various screen modes described above are available in most screen magnification software. These programs also allow tracking of the mouse pointer, location of keyboard entry, and text editing. The magnification window can be coupled with one or more of these to facilitate navigation for the user. All screen images (including windows, control buttons, and other windows objects) are magnified. Automatic scrolling of the screen (left, right, up, down) is also available to make it easier to read long documents when they are magnified.

CASE STUDY

COMPUTER ACCESS FOR LOW VISION

Cheryl is a college student. Her visual limitations prevent her from using the standard computer display. She has asked the ATP to help her find a way for her to use the computer. The constraints on her situation are that she must use several different computers during the day: her own home computer, a laptop that she carries to class for note taking, and the computers in the student laboratory. What approach would the ATP recommend for her? Would the ATP recommend that she buy special hardware or software to meet her needs, or can she make use of features built into Windows? How would the ATP evaluate the success of your solution for Cheryl?

For individuals who have low vision or blindness, hard copy (printer) output is also a challenge. If the output is to be read by a person with normal vision, the text can be edited on the screen using the methods described earlier and then printed in a standard printer font size. If, however, the user with visual impairment needs to access the hard copy output, then either an enlarged or a braille printout is desirable. For enlarged print, the most common approach is to use a laser printer coupled with a special software program to create larger characters.

Devices That Provide Automatic Reading of Text

Automatic reading of text requires the three components shown in Figure 8-1: an environmental interface, an information processor, and a user display. The environmental interface is a camera that provides an image of the printed page, and the user display can be either tactile (braille) or speech synthesis. A block diagram showing the major components of an automatic reading machine is presented in Figure 8-6. Device operation involves scanning, **optical character recognition** (OCR), and the translation of recognized characters and either text-to-braille or text-to-speech conversion (see Figure 8-6). Most reading machines provide speech output, and some provide braille or both braille and speech. Both software and hardware approaches are used for speech synthesis output in much the same way as those used in screen readers for the blind. Synthetic speech for automatic reading systems is available in a variety of languages. Some automatic reading devices use standard personal computers (PCs) with special software for information processing. The PC is interfaced to a scanner (camera with software) and display (refreshable braille or speech synthesis). Current stand-alone (scanner included in the basic system) automatic reading machines offer simple one-button operation to scan a document and have it read. These units also provide manual access to features such as cursor keys to move around in the text, storing and retrieving files, and transferring the text to a computer or a disk. Automatic reading systems can also be used in conjunction with screen readers and Web browsers.

Camera and Scanner Characteristics for Automatic Reading.

To input the information into the machine, reading devices may use a flatbed scanner, a hand-held scanner, or a combination of the two (Fruchterman, 1991). Flatbed scanners have a glass plate 18 to 24 inches long and 10 to 14 inches wide. Scanners are usually defined as letter or legal size depending on the dimensions of the flat bed. This type of scanner, also called a *desktop scanner*, resembles a photocopy machine; however, the thickness is only about 3 to 4 inches. The material to be read is placed on the surface of the glass, and one advantage of this type of unit is that it can scan almost any kind of document, from a single sheet to a bound magazine or book. An automatic document feeder attachment can also be added to many flatbed scanners. This allows multiple sheets to be loaded and scanned. Scanners are widely used for home or business applications such as scanning photographs for use on Web pages or scanning documents for editing when an electronic copy is not available. For this reason, the technology is improving and the prices are falling as a result of the general market demand (Grotta and Grotta, 1998). This has resulted in advances that benefit blind users of automatic reading systems. Hand-held scanners vary in width from 2½ to 8½ inches (Converso and Hocek, 1990). For scanners narrower than the page, the camera must be moved across a line of text and then moved down to the next line, and so on all the way down the page. This can be difficult for a person who is blind because there is no frame of reference to keep the scanner on one line or to move just one line down. Flatbed scanners overcome this problem. The hand-held scanner can image most types of material, including single sheets and bound documents. An additional advantage is that it can be used with a laptop computer to create a portable reading machine.

All scanners consist of a light source and a camera, and some also contain lenses and mirrors to focus the image on the camera (Converso and Hocek, 1990). Grotta and Grotta (1998) describe both the use of charge-coupled device (CCD) imaging electronics and an emerging technology

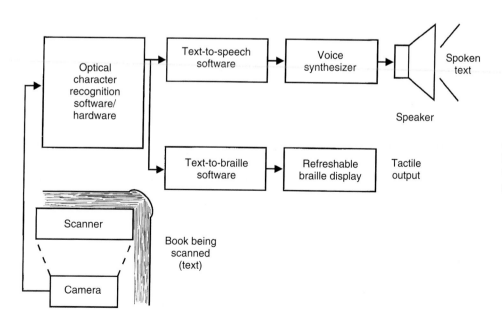

Figure 8-6 The major components of an automatic reading machine for persons with total visual impairment.

called contact image scanners (CIS). CCD cameras use a lens and mirror arrangement that moves across the document with the light source (usually a fluorescent lamp) and that is used to focus the image on the CCD detector. In contrast, CIS systems have a single row of sensors that is positioned just a few millimeters below the document and moves across it, together with an array of light sources, during the scan. The CIS systems draw less power; have a simpler mechanical design, making it possible to have thinner units; and eliminate the delicate optics of CCD devices. The resolution of CIS systems is not as good as that of CCD devices, but it is rapidly improving. The CCD or CIS array serves as a camera that converts the areas of light and dark to an electronic format, and computer software stores it in memory. Hand-held types have only the camera and light source.

The image that the camera stores consists of an array of black and white or color areas called pixels. The density of these pixels in the computer-stored image measures the quality of the scanner image. The units of measure are dots per inch. Scanners have resolutions from 300 to 4800 dots per inch (Grotta and Grotta, 1998). The other major specification that is used is gray-scale levels (for black and white scanning) and color bit depth for color scanning. Typical gray scale values are 256 levels. Color bit depth varies from 24 to 36 bits (Grotta and Grotta, 1998).

Some automatic reading systems have scanners built into them (for example, Ovation, Telesensory, Sunnyvale Calif., *www.telesensory.com*); Sara, Freedom Scientific, St. Petersburg, Fla., *www.freedomsci.com*; Pulse Tech Book Reader, *http://www.plustek.com*; POET-Compact, Baum, *www.baum.de/index-e.php*; ScannaR, HumanWare, Concord, Calif., *www.humanware.com*). These systems include a flatbed scanner, built-in computer, voice output, and hard drive with room for up to 500,000 pages of text. In some cases **Digital Audio-Based Information System** (DAISY) reading capability for digital books (see below) is included. Scanned documents can be saved in MPS, WAV, or plain text format. Many of these systems require only a single button to be pressed to scan and read a document. Some units also provide multiple languages for spoken output. Other reading systems are software products that include optical character recognition and text-to-speech synthesis and are designed to use external commercial scanners and computers (for example, Open Book, Freedom Scientific, St. Petersburg, Fla., *www.freedomsci.com*; Reading Advantage Telesensory, Sunnyvale, Calif., *www.telesensory.com*; Cicero, Dolphin Products, *www.dolphincomputeraccess.com*; An Open Book, Handy Tech Elektronik GmbH, Germany, *www.handytech.de*).

Optical Character Recognition.   The camera and scanner provide an image, consisting of an array of pixels. This image is black and white or color dots, and it is not in a form that can be translated into speech or braille. OCR is used to carry out this conversion. Units, called OCRs, have been developed for scanning print documents into computer-readable form by businesses. They also are used in automatic reading devices for persons who are blind.

The OCR is a software program that runs on a standard PC. The primary function of the OCR is to analyze the raw pixel data and assemble it into letters, spaces (to delineate words), and punctuation. Graphics (pictures or drawings and the elaborate characters sometimes used to begin chapters in books) must be removed from the text before output. There are a number of problems that OCR software must solve. The most significant of these is that letter recognition must occur with different print fonts. OCRs that accomplish this are called *omnifont OCRs*. Most scanners have an OCR product bundled with the scanner. These OCRs provide basic OCR capabilities, but they do not match stand-alone OCR products. Automatic reading systems use the professional stand-alone OCR products to achieve the best possible results. There are several general-purpose commercial omnifont OCR systems commonly used in reading machines for people who are blind. Some companies that provide automatic reading systems have their own proprietary OCR software, and others use professional-quality OCR software developed for business applications. The majority of the commercial software incorporated into automatic reading systems uses either the Xerox or Caere OCR software. Most current scanners use OmniPage LE (Nuance Corp, Burlington, Mass., *www.nuance.com*), the TextBridge (Nuance Corp) Classic, or proprietary OCR software. All OCR software available separately is compatible with the Windows operating system, and several automatic reading systems use standard PCs, OCR software, and an external scanner. Converso and Hocek (1990) present some guidelines for selecting a scanner and OCR for specific applications. They also include a discussion of computer hardware and software (e.g., word processing) factors to consider when scanners and OCRs are obtained.

Braille as a Tactile Reading Substitute

The most widely used tactile substitution device for persons with visual impairments is **braille.** Each braille character consists of a cell of either six or eight dots, as shown in Figure 8-7. The seventh and eighth dots are used to show cursor movement or to provide single-cell presentation of higher-level ASCII codes. This is necessary because the six braille dots can only display 64 different combinations and there are 256 ASCII codes for characters (upper and lower case alphabet, numbers, special symbols, and control characters such as RETURN). Figure 8-7 shows examples of letters and numbers. When text is directly translated into braille letter by letter, it is referred to as *Grade 1*. Also shown in Figure 8-7 are some braille codes for words (called *wordsigns*) and word endings. The use of these contractions

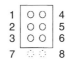

Standard braille cell

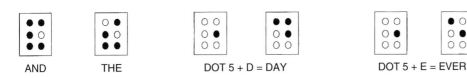

A   B   C   D   E   F   G   H   I   J   K   L

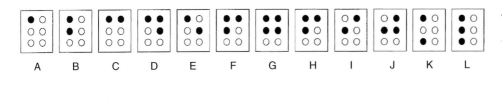

AND   THE   DOT 5 + D = DAY   DOT 5 + E = EVER

Figure 8-7   Examples of braille letters, word signs, and contractions.

significantly speeds up the rate of reading, and this type of braille is called *Grade 2* or *Grade 3*, depending on the number of contractions used. Reading rates with Grade 1 braille are about 40 words per minute. With Grade 3, reading speeds can approach 200 words per minute (Allen, 1971). Traditionally, braille has been produced by embossing on heavy paper, and this method is still widely used. For persons who develop skill with it, braille can be a fast and efficient method for accessing print materials.

Characteristics of Braille.   There are several disadvantages to the use of braille, especially in embossed form. First, the embossed material is heavy and bulky, and each braille page has significantly less information than a printed page of the same size. For example, a braille version of a 400-page print book would fill four books, each the size of an encyclopedia volume (Mann, 1974). A second disadvantage is that the cost of producing braille in an embossed form is high compared with print materials. For this reason, only a fraction of the total print literature is available in braille form. A third limitation is related to the spatial orientation of visual (print) material. When a person scans for a particular piece of information or edits text, this spatial orientation is used to find the particular piece of text needed. This process is difficult when the embossed braille paper format is used. This is partially because of the bulky nature of the material, but it is also a result of the difficulty that braille readers have in scanning text quickly. Finally, braille embossers do not allow corrections to be made. Once the dot pattern is impressed into the paper, it is not possible to remove it.

Braille itself, regardless of format, has limitations as well. The most significant is that very few persons (fewer than 10%) with severe visual impairment learn to use it. This is partially because more than 65% of all persons who become blind do so after age 65 years (Mann, 1974), and many of these cases are the result of diabetes, which also affects the tactile sense, making braille less desirable than other alternatives such as talking books. Despite all these disadvantages, braille is the modality of choice for many persons with severe visual impairment, and the use of a format other than embossed paper significantly enhances the effectiveness of this modality. One of the most widely used of these alternative formats is a refreshable braille cell. Computer output systems use either a refreshable braille display consisting of raised pins or hard copy by use of braille printers.

Refreshable Braille Displays.   Because braille is represented by a series of dots, raised pins can be substituted for the traditional embossed paper format. This approach, called **refreshable braille display,** is shown in Figure 8-8. There are several advantages to this format. The most significant of these is that the refreshable display is controlled by an electronic circuit that can be interfaced to computer displays or braille keyboards. This allows information to be stored electronically and greatly reduces the bulk compared with embossed braille. Second, because the text material is in electronic form, it can be edited, searches can be made, and copies of braille material can be easily produced in electronic form (e.g., on CD removable memory). The refreshable braille cell (or cell array) can also be used as the output mode for an automatic reading machine.

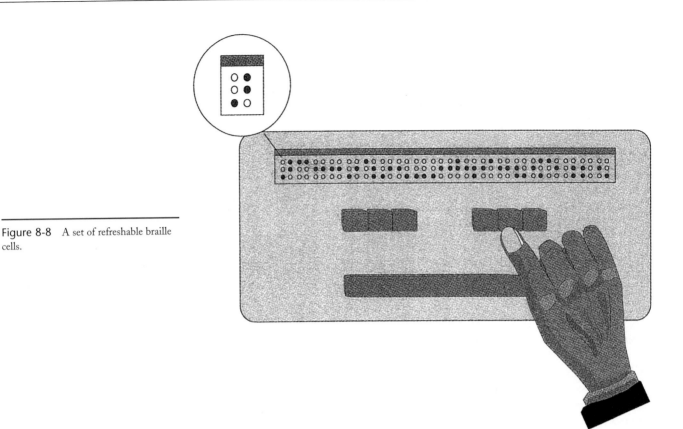

Figure 8-8   A set of refreshable braille cells.

Each refreshable braille cell has a set of small pins arranged in the shape of a standard braille cell. The pins that correspond to the dot pattern for a letter or word sign are raised. Both Grade 1 and Grade 2 braille can be presented on refreshable displays by use of software that converts text from ASCII format to braille. Arrays of from 1 to 80 cells are available.

Stationary refreshable braille displays have arrays with multiple braille cells. Typically the array sizes are 20, 40, or 80 cells (for example, Pulse Data Human Ware, Concord, Calif., *http://www.pulsedata.com*; Freedom Scientific, St. Petersburg, Fla., *www.freedomsci.com*); ALVA Series, Vision Cue, Portland, Ore., *http://www.visioncue.com/*). These arrays, and the hardware and software to control them, typically cost in the range of $3500 to $10,000 depending on the number of cells and the manufacturer. Generally, the standard six-dot format is used for each cell. For an eight-dot cell, the price for a 40-cell array is 20% higher than for the six-dot format. The 80-cell format allows an entire line of a computer screen to be displayed at one time. An eight-dot, 80-cell refreshable display can cost as much as $10,000, a significant increase over the cost of a 40-cell, eight-dot device. Thus price is a major consideration in refreshable braille displays. The refreshable braille arrays we have described generally can be used as an alternative to the screen in desktop computers.

The ALVA (Vision Cue, Portland, Ore., *http://www.visioncue.com/*) braille terminals provide 44-, 70-, and 80-cell refreshable displays for desktop use and 23- and 44-cell displays for portable applications (battery operated). All versions have eight-dot braille cells. All ALVA models also provide extra status cells that display the location of the system cursor, which line of text is displayed in braille, which attributes are active, and the relationship of those attributes to the characters on the screen. This information can be monitored with the left hand while the right hand reads the text on the braille display. USB and serial ports are available for data transfer. Text is provided in both Grade 1 and Grade 2 braille.

Freedom Scientific (Freedom Scientific, St. Petersburg, Fla., *www.freedomsci.com*) makes 40- and 80-cell braille displays. The 40-cell unit includes a Braille keyboard. Both the 40- and 80-cell versions have navigation features accessible through a series of buttons on the display. Combinations of buttons are used to enter commands. Another product, the PAC Mate portable Braille display, is a 20-cell refreshable braille display that is connected to any computer through a USB port. This unit uses a seamless design between braille cells that makes the display feel like paper. It works with most Windows-based software packages. Pulse Data Human Ware (Concord, Calif., *http://www.pulsedata.com*) makes a series of refreshable braille displays, shown in Figure 8-9. The 40-cell and 24-cell Brailliant refreshable braille displays are designed for use with a laptop or desktop computer. The Brailliant 32-, 64-, and 80-cell displays are eight-dot braille displays for desktop computers. All these models are configured for split-window display or as programmable status cells and all include Bluetooth and USB connectivity. The latter are accessed by clicking a sensor located above one of the braille cells to instantly move the mouse pointer or cursor to a new location for editing. Grade 2 braille translation is included on all models.

For computer users who are familiar with braille, this approach can be more effective than screen readers. However, a combination of approaches may be most effective with braille and speech combined. If done thoughtfully and carefully, the hardware and software designed for braille can be used together with that developed for screen reading with speech synthesis. Supernova (Dolphin Computer Systems, San Mateo, Calif., *www.dolphincomputeraccess.com*) provides screen magnification (2 to 32 times) and speech and braille output in one package for Windows applications. There are six different viewing modes: full screen, split screen, window, lens, autolens, and line view (for smooth scrolling). Speech output is available letter by letter during typing or word by word. A variety of languages and speech synthesizers can be used with Voyager. "Hooked access" allows parts of the screen, such as the current line of a word processor, to be permanently displayed. Supernova also supports graphic object labeling and provides speech output and a braille layout mode.

Portable Braille Note Takers and Personal Organizers. Stand-alone data managers or personal organizers vary in size from a compact 4.5 inches square and about 1.5 inches thick to the size of a laptop computer (approximately 9 × 12 inches) (for example, the Braille Lite Series, Freedom Scientific, St. Petersburg, Fla.,

www.freedomsci.com); Braille Desk 2000, Artic Technologies, Troy, Mich., www. artictech.com; Braille Wave, Handy Tech Elektronik GmbH, Germany, *www.handytech.de*; Braille Note and Voice Note, HumanWare, Concord, Calif., *www. humanware.com*); Aria, Sensory Tools, Robotron Proprietary Limited, St. Kilda, Australia, *www.sensorytools.com/products. htm*; MPO 0550, Alva Access Group, Oakland, Calif., *www. alva-bv.nl/*). A typical model is pictured in Figure 8-10.

Some models use a braille keyboard for input and others use a standard QWERTY keyboard. The braille keyboard has one key for each of the six dots in a braille cell. Additional keys are used for eight-dot braille and for control, editing, and data management. Output takes several forms. Synthesized speech is available in all units. Earphone and speaker output for the synthesized speech are also available. Some models include a refreshable Grade 2 braille display (from 8 to 32 braille cells) either alone or paired with synthetic speech. The speech synthesizer and refreshable braille display can also be used as outputs (replacing the output from the video monitor) on the unit or in conjunction with screen reader software on a PC. Additional outputs available on selected models include computer file transfer, Internet, and e-mail access by use of a modem (generally external to the note taker), and print. Some models also dial a telephone automatically from the data in the built-in address book.

Built-in programs vary somewhat among various models. All include some sort of word processing for writing away from a computer (e.g., while sitting by the pool or riding a bus to work), editing documents developed on a PC word processor, and taking notes in class or at meetings. Other programs built into specific models, in various combinations, include a calendar, address book, calculator, timer or watch, e-mail access, Internet browser, and text (ASCII)-to-braille translation. Storage of data is in both random-access memory and flash-read-only memory (ROM). Removable flash memory cards increase both flexibility and growth

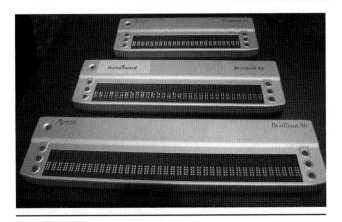

Figure 8-9   Refreshable braille cells are available with a variable number of cells.

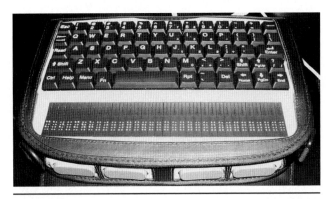

Figure 8-10   A personal organizer with braille display and synthesized speech output.

potential as the capacity is continually being increased. Flash memory card storage through USB ports adds to storage capability and provides an additional means of transferring files between the note taker and a PC. Direct transfer through a USB port is also routinely available. Several portable note takers include productivity software such as word processing and e-mail with full access through speech or braille output. MP3 music players and Web access by Bluetooth or WiFi protocols are also available on many units. Some note takers can also be used as computer keyboards through the built-in USB port or can function as cell phones (e.g., the Alva MPO 0550). Storage and manipulation of information may be in the form of braille or print or both. Control features may be by use of additional keys with specific functions or by use of a speech output menu of choices. The PacMate (Freedom Scientific, St. Petersburg, Fla., *www.freedomsci.com*) is a fully functional pocket PC with voice and Braille options. It includes Microsoft productivity software (e-mail, database, spreadsheet, word processing, scheduling), MP3, Web access, and other features to bring to the blind user the ease of use and functionality that sighted users of portable PCs enjoy.

CASE STUDY

BRAILLE NOTE TAKING IN SCHOOL

Jenny is an eighth-grade student. She uses many pieces of technology to assist her in being successful at school. She has been using a Braille 'n Speak since the fifth grade to take class notes, complete assignments, take tests, keep an assignment notebook, and maintain a personal phone and address book. Review the features of this device *(www.freedomsci.com)* and list those that are likely to benefit Jenny in each of these applications.

Speech as an Auditory Reading Substitute

Because reading is based on visual language, it is logical that auditory substitution for reading also uses language—that is, speech. Audio technology is the primary method for information storage and retrieval used by individuals who are blind (Scadden, 1997). All the approaches discussed in this section have speech as the output mode.

Recorded Audio Material.   The oldest and most prevalent use of auditory substitution for persons with visual impairment is recorded material. Current technology used in recorded audio material is cassette tapes, CDs, and CD-ROMs (for example, Recording for the Blind and Dyslexic, *www.rfbd.org*); National Library Service for the Blind and

Physically Handicapped, Library of Congress, *http://www. loc.gov/nls/index.html*).

The major type of recorded material is cassette tapes. Several models are provided by the National Library Service for the Blind and Physically Handicapped. The major features that are included on some or all of these are $15/16$-inch per second (nonstandard for longer play and copyright protection) and $17/8$-inches per second (standard used for music tapes) playback speeds, variable speed control, portability, automatic reverse or rewind, and frequency compensation to allow increased speed without a "chipmunk" sound. The variable speed allows the listener to review material faster than it was originally spoken. With practice, it is possible to understand speech at rates up to four times normal. Some people also use this type of machine to record lectures and then review the material in lieu of note taking. Cassette tapes can be produced by virtually any local library to make backup copies for distribution.

The use of CD-ROMs allows a great deal of information to be placed on a single disk. One CD-ROM can store a large amount of data. Reproduction costs are low. The major advantages of CD-ROMs for music are greatly increased fidelity resulting from greater frequency response, smaller size of both player and disks than phonograph records, and indexing, which can be used to find a particular track. These features are being exploited in recorded material for individuals who are blind (Scadden, 1997). The use of digitized audio information allows voice recordings to be mixed with headings that allow easier searching of the text. Multimedia presentations are also commonplace with CDs, allowing both visual and auditory presentation of information, thereby increasing the potential market and reducing price. Audio displays are also being used for the presentation of mathematical information by computers and speech synthesizers and as a substitute for data presentation (e.g., tables, charts) (Scadden, 1997). In this form a book can be loaded into a PC word processor (either Windows or Macintosh based) and displayed on the screen. Because the CD-ROM is basically a storage medium for the computer, sophisticated search strategies can be used to find a particular item or place in the text. For persons with low vision or blindness, the availability of CD-ROM–based reading materials opens up many different options for obtaining access to print materials. For example, with an enlarged screen output, reading material on a CD-ROM can be accessed and presented to a person with low vision by use of a computer. More significant, however, is the use of either braille or speech output from the computer to allow individuals who are blind to read from the CD-ROM.

One of the challenges in any electronic format is standardization. Different countries have different recording formats for talking books on tape, and there are many formats for word processors in digital form. For this reason an international group, the DAISY Consortium *(www.daisy.org)*

has developed an international standard for **digital talking books** (Kerscher and Hansson, 1998). This standard includes production, exchange, and use of digital talking books. The goal of the DAISY Consortium is to promote the use of digital books that comply with an international standard. The members of the consortium are associations and organizations across the world that are involved in the provision of reading materials for individuals who are blind. The DAISY standard is hardware platform and operating system independent, and it makes use of the Web accessibility standards developed by the World Wide Web Consortium (W3C). There are several on-line sources for books in the DAISY format (for example, Benetech, *www.bookshare.org;* National Library Service, U.S. Library of Congress, *www.loc.gov/nls;* Recording for the Blind and Dyslexic, *www.rfbd.org;* Dolphin Audio Publishing, *www. dolpjinauiopublishing. com).* These sites have thousands of titles, including books for children and adults, textbooks, and newspapers. Many of the books are available in both DAISY and Braille Reading Foundation (BRF) Grade II braille format for printing books or using refreshable braille displays. Players for DAISY format CDs are available from several manufacturers (for example, Telex, Burnsville, Minn., *www.telex.com;* FSReader, Freedom Scientific, St. Petersburg, Fla., *www.freedomsci.com;* EaseReader, Dolphin Audio Publishing, *www.dolphinaudiopublishing. com;* Victor, Human Ware, Concord, Calif., *www.humanware. com).* A typical DAISY format reader is shown in Figure 8-11.

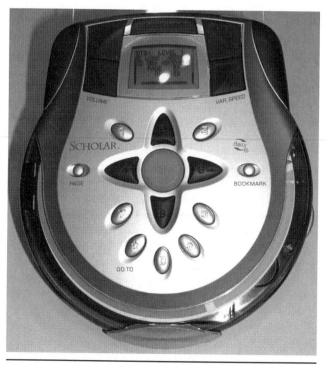

Figure 8-11   Typical DAISY reader.

Synthetic Speech Output Reading Machines.
Auditory output from automatic reading machines is provided by synthetic speech devices. Types of speech synthesis and conversion of ASCII text into speech (called *text-to-speech*) is discussed in Chapter 7. The use of speech synthesis in reading machines for persons with visual impairments or learning disabilities uses the standard types of speech synthesis. There are a variety of both hardware- and software-based speech synthesizers for use with reading programs or aids (see Chapter 7). Because many reading devices are based on PCs, screen readers (programs that provide synthetic speech output from the computer screen, see Chapter 7) can also be used as reading machines.

There are several ways in which information can be converted to ASCII form for use by a screen reading program. The most common is to use a scanner and OCR program as discussed in this section. A second approach is to obtain CD-ROMs that contain computer-readable written material (Dixon and Mandelbaum, 1990). There are services that make books on disk available to persons who are blind. The computer disks have files that can be loaded into a word processor and then read by using a screen reader program. The CD-ROMs provide significantly greater storage than floppy disks, and they are made available to blind readers by publishers. Dictionaries, almanacs, and encyclopedias are among the many publications available in this format. A major advantage of this type of storage is the indexing and searching capability provided by CD-ROM technology. There is now a large and growing amount of literature (especially the classics) available on the Internet in electronic form (called *e-text*). Many newspapers put their whole issues on the Internet, as do on-line news and sports services. Individuals who are blind can read this information by using screen readers and accessible Web browsers.

Access to Visual Computer Displays for Individuals Who Are Blind

For individuals who are blind and need to access a computer, the problem is one of providing input through an alternative sensory pathway, auditory or tactile or both. Auditory output is provided by voice synthesizers (hardware or software based), and tactile output is generally provided by refreshable braille displays and embossed hard copy.

Systems that provide voice synthesis output for blind users are generally referred to as **screen readers.** A computer user who is blind should be able to access all the same graphics and text as a person who is sighted. There are a variety of commercially available speech synthesizers, and many screen readers use their own proprietary speech synthesis software and computer sound cards, as well as compatibility with refreshable braille displays. Windows includes a basic function screen reader utility, *Narrator*, and a *Toggle Keys* in its accessibility options that are accessed through the control panel. These features are described in Table 8-1. The narrator program is a text-to-speech utility for people who are blind or who have low vision; it reads text that is displayed on the screen in an active window or menu options or text that has been typed into a window. The *Toggle Keys* option generates a sound when CAPS LOCK, NUM LOCK, or SCROLL LOCK key is pressed.

A sighted computer user will often scan a screen for a specific piece of information or to obtain a sense of the continuity and flow of the written material, which includes looking for specific screen attributes (such as highlighted or underlined material and features of the GUI). For the user who is blind, duplicating this capability requires that the adapted output system provide reading of text and descriptions of graphics. Finally, screen reader programs provide on-screen messages or prompts for the user input during program operation. Graphic characters should have text labels attached to them. These can be read to the consumer by use of speech synthesis software. Currently available screen reader programs provide navigation assistance by keyboard commands. Examples of typical functions are movement to a particular point in the text, finding the mouse cursor position, providing a spoken description of an on-screen graphic or a special function key, and accessing help information (for example, Screen Reader2 from IBM, Special Needs Systems, Austin, Tex., *www.rs6000.ibm.com/sns;* Jaws for Windows from Freedom Scientific, St. Petersburg, Fla. *www.freedomsci.com;* Zoom Text Xtra Level 2 from AI Squared, Manchester Center, Vt. *www.aisquared.com;* Supernova and Hal from Dolphin Computer Access, San Mateo, Calif. *www.dolphinusa.com;* Magnum and Magnum Deluxe from Artic Technologies, Troy, Mich.; Protalk32 for Windows, Biolink Computer, Vancouver, Canada, *www.biolink.bc.ca;* Window Eyes from GW Microsystems, Fort Wayne, Ind. *www.gwmicro.com/gwie*).

Screen readers also monitor the screen and take action when a particular block of text or a menu appears (Lazzaro, 1999). This feature automatically reads pop-up windows and dialog boxes to the user. Screen readers can typically be set to speak by line, sentence, or paragraph. Other features are also available; for example, Jaws for Windows (Freedom Scientific, St. Petersburg, Fla., *www.freedomsci.com*) allows the user to read the prior, current, or next sentence or paragraph in all applications by using specified keystrokes (e.g., read prior sentence = ALT + UP ARROW; read next sentence = ALT + DOWN ARROW; read current sentence = ALT + NUM PAD). The user may use the standard Windows method of switching between applications (ALT + TAB). There are also special functions for individual programs such as those in Microsoft Office (Microsoft Corporation, Redmond, Wash.), Web browsers, and others. Some screen readers also provide a "window list" in which applications that are running appear in alphabetical order. This allows the user to switch between, close, or see the state

of any active application. This is a faster way to switch between applications when a user has many windows open, rather than moving the cursor to a pull-down menu or "close" box. Hal (Dolphin Computer Access, San Mateo, Calif., *www.dolphinusa.com*) is a screen reader designed to operate with the visible information on the screen. Hal recognizes objects by looking for distinct attributes, shapes, borders, highlights, and so on. This is in contrast to using the standard labels of Windows, and it means that Hal is independent of whether an application has obeyed the rules of Windows programming. Hal recognizes objects by their final shape on the screen, rather than by their Windows attributes. The advantage of this approach is that once set up for one application, all similar-looking applications will talk correctly without any adjustment to the settings. Hal also includes a braille layout mode. These are only examples of product features; as is true for any computer application, rapid advances are common.

Many screen readers have applications for specific types of programs, procedures, or applications. A script is a small computer program that contains sequences of individual steps used to activate and control a wide variety of computer processes. Each script or function contains commands that tell the screen reader how to navigate and what to read under different conditions. Some screen readers allow modification of the scripts (for example, JAWS, Freedom Scientific, St. Petersburg, Fla., *www.freedomsci.com*). Script files can be modified, or entirely new commands can be used to make any application accessible with the screen reader. Scripts can also be created to automate daily tasks or for specific applications (e.g., Web browser, spreadsheet). By analyzing what actions are taking place in a given application, the script can optimize the screen reader for the user.

Window-Eyes (GW Microsystems, Fort Wayne, Ind., *www.gwmicro.com/gwie*) uses the Microsoft Excel DOM (document object model) to communicate directly with Microsoft Word and Microsoft Excel and includes the ability to save specific settings (i.e., headers and totals and monitor cells) for specific documents. VIRGO 4 (Baum, Germany, *www.baum.de/*) uses Microsoft Visual Basic as a scripting language to customize the screen reader for specific applications. Users who have computer programming skills can write their own scripts to automate tasks or to optimize their readers for specific applications.

These applications all require that the special script or application file be developed individually for a particular application. An alternative approach is to develop software that automatically develops a script based on what the user is doing at the time by observing his or her actions (Ma et al, 2004). The software also informs the user when a script exists that is relevant to the application that is being used. Examples of scripts that might be developed are finding a weather forecast or a stock price. The Intelligent Screen Reader (Ma et al, 2004) works with the built-in macro recorder of JAWS and a script generation interface to automatically generate a script with *plan recognition networks* (PRNs). PRNs are probabilistic models of procedures produced by an automated synthesis of plan recognition networks (Huber and Simpson, 2004). The key to this software approach is the ability to identify the user's intentions as the task is being performed. The advantage of this approach is that the user does not need to learn the script programming method and also does not need to depend on the prestored scripts developed by the manufacturer.

Hard copy (printed) output also must be modified for persons who are blind. Typically, braille output is produced by *embossers*. One approach is to design and build a printer specifically for braille embossing from a computer. Embossers are available in both single- and double-sided formats. They include both portable and stationary systems with a variety of printing speeds from 15 to 50 characters per second and with line widths of 32 to 40 characters (single-sided) and 55 characters per second with 56 character line widths (double-sided) (Enabling Technologies, Jenson Beach, Fla., *http://www.brailler.com/index.htm;* Pulse Data Human Ware, Concord, Calif., *http://www.pulsedata.com;* GW Microsystems, Fort Wayne, Ind., *https://www.gwmicro.com/;* View Pluse, Corvallis, Ore., *http://www.viewplus.com*). The Paragon Braille Printer (Pulse Data Human Ware, Concord, Calif., *http://www.pulsedata.com*) is an embosser that prints on tractor-feed paper from 20 to 100 pounds in weight and up to 15 inches in width. The speed of the Paragon is 40 characters per second, which enables it to print more than 120 pages per hour. Vinyl and aluminum sheets can also be embossed to signs with braille markings. The Mountbatten Brailler (Quantum Technology, Sydney, Australia, *http://www.quantech.com.au/index.html*) is a braille writer with a braille keyboard, built-in memory, autocorrection features, and extensive formatting controls. The Mountbatten can be used as an embosser for a computer or as a braille translation device. It can translate from print into braille or braille into print and is available in both electric and battery-operated models. All these embossers include internal software that accepts standard printer output from the host computer and converts it to either six- or eight-cell braille embossed on heavy paper. American Thermoform Corporation (La Verne, Calif., *http://www.americanthermoform.com/index.html*) makes a variety of braille embossers. These cover applications from mass production to systems for individual users.

Braille translation programs are available from Duxbury Systems (Westbury, Mass., *http://www.duxburysystems.com/*). These programs convert ASCII text in many forms (word processor text files, spreadsheets, database files) to Grade 2 braille in hard copy form. Translation of braille cells to text characters and vice versa is not typically on a one-for-one basis. Translation is especially complicated with Grade 2 braille because contractions are used. Formatting of braille

pages also involves issues beyond those affecting print. Duxbury Braille Translation provides translation and formatting capabilities to automate the process of conversion from regular print to braille (and vice versa) and also provides word processing functions for working directly in braille as well as print format. Braille characters can be displayed on the screen for proofreading before printing. Operation of this program has the same features (e.g., menus and screens) for Macintosh and Windows. This software is typically used both by individuals who do not know braille and those who do. The Duxbury Braille Translator allows the user to create braille for schoolbooks and teaching materials, office memos, bus schedules, personal letters, and signs compliant with the Americans With Disabilities Act. The software allows importing of files from popular word processors, including Microsoft Word and WordPerfect, and from HTML sources, as well as others.

Studies of Computer Use by Visually Impaired Adults

It is not surprising that computer use by individuals who are blind or who have low vision is less than by nondisabled individuals. Individuals with visual disabilities have less access to the Internet, are on-line less often, and are more likely to be on-line from work than from home than are individuals without disabilities (Gerber and Kirchner, 2001). Severity of impairment and existence of multiple impairments each reduce the access and use further. Individuals under 65 years of age have greater use and access than do those older than 65 years. This finding is important given the high prevalence of visual impairment in the population more than 65 years old. People who are employed are more likely to use computers and the Internet, regardless of whether they are disabled, and the percentage of people using computes is almost identical for the two groups.

To obtain more detailed information about the computer usage patterns of individuals who have visual impairments, Gerber (2003) conducted a series of focus groups. Four focus groups were used, three at national conferences and one based on subscribers to a technology and visual impairment publication (*Access World: Technology and People With Visual Impairments*, American Foundation for the Blind, New York, *http://www.afb.org/*). Half the participants reported no usable vision, and the other half had variable amounts of vision. Half the respondents had been blind since birth, 85% had some university education, and 73% were employed. This sample represents the group of visually impaired individuals who use computers and the Internet, but it is not representative of the broader visually impaired community. The leading reason why technology was important and helpful was access to employment and the creation of flexibility in finding work. For some individuals computer access allowed telecommuting and access to employment from home.

The computer also allowed employed individuals to create a cultural identity by being successfully employed. The second major benefit of computer use identified was access to information, including newspapers and magazines as well as Web-based sources. This benefit is only recently available because more and more information is available digitally through the Internet. Independence in obtaining this information was a major benefit identified. Respondents talked about how rewarding it was to read for themselves using technology rather than have someone read to them. Improvement in writing skill was identified as a benefit of computer use. A final benefit identified by the focus group participants was the social connections made through the Internet, such as independently sending and receiving e-mail using adapted computers. Participation in on-line discussion groups related to their disability or to other topics of interest helped remove feelings of isolation and loneliness. Lack of training and not having accessible training materials were identified as a major barrier to computer use. Getting help in an accessible form was identified as a major difference between users who had visual impairments and those who did not. Being shut out of advances because of lack of accessibility, especially as computers and software change, was a major fear for many of the participants. For example, if a new version of Windows is developed, it may not be compatible with the accessible screen reader or braille display the person has been using. This issue is discussed further later in this chapter.

As more and more appliances, entertainment products, and productivity tools for work become electronically sophisticated with many new features, people with visual impairments worry that they will be left behind because of lack of access. Universal design (see Chapter 1) principles become very important in this context.

Because training was identified as a major barrier to computer access, Wolfe (2003) conducted a survey of public and private rehabilitation agencies in the United States to determine the availability of training specifically related to individuals with visual impairments. Group technology-related training (general and job related) was provided more frequently than individual training by both public and private agencies. A variety of products including screen readers, screen magnifiers, Web browsers, CCTVs, and electronic note takers were included in the training. These are all described in this chapter. The demand for training was reported to be far greater than the agencies' ability to provide training. The major training challenges reported by Wolfe were changes in technology requiring staff upgrading, lag between new advances in general consumer products and accessible versions, availability of computers and other equipment to use in training, and a shortage of qualified trainers.

To learn more about the need for and value of training, a series of focus groups were held with visually impaired adults who had received training and with trainers (Wolfe, Candela, and Johnson, 2003). The adequacy of training was clustered into positive, neutral, and negative groups. Positive comments focused on the overall quality of the training, greater self-confidence of the trainees after training, and (to a lesser extent) the quality of the trainers. Neutral comments reflected adequacy of the training in general rather than specific areas of training. Negative comments fell into six areas, including (1) training was too short or too infrequent, (2) too few computers were available for hands-on practice, (3) training was not relevant to technology available on the job, (4) the pace of training was too slow or too fast, (5) material was presented at too basic a level, and (6) there was too much variability in trainee experience that limited content that could be covered. The trainers focused on issues of curricular content and trainee preparation for training, but there was no consistency in either of these areas. The need to stay abreast of technology changes was also a challenge listed by this group.

■ VISUAL ACCESS TO THE INTERNET

As the Internet becomes more and more dependent on multimedia representations involving complex graphics, animation, and audible sources of information, the challenges for people who have disabilities increase. The most obvious barriers are for those who are blind. People who have learning disabilities and dyslexia also find it increasingly difficult to access complicated Web sites that may include flashing pictures, complicated charts, and large amounts of audio and video data. It is estimated that as many as 40 million persons in the United States have physical, cognitive, or sensory disabilities (Lazzaro, 1999). Thus, the importance of making the Internet accessible to all is great.

Many of the approaches to computer input and output discussed in this chapter are important to the provision of access to this information for persons who have disabilities. Two useful sources of information are the W3C Web Accessibility Initiative (WAI, *www.w3.org/WAI*) and the Trace Center (*www.trace.wisc.edu/world/web*). Vanderheiden (1998) provides a comprehensive review of the issues related to Internet access by persons with disabilities. He gives both an overview of current approaches and prospects for future developments on the basis of emerging technologies.

User Agents for Access to the Internet

Access to the Internet must be independent of individual devices. This device independence means that users must be able to interact with a *user agent* (and the document it renders) using the input and output devices of their choice on the basis of their specific needs. A **user agent** is defined as software to access Web content (*www.w3.org/wai*).

This includes desktop graphical browsers, text and voice browsers, mobile phones, multimedia players, and software assistive technologies (e.g., screen readers, magnifiers, general input device–emulating interfaces that are used with browsers.

Input devices that are used for Internet access include many of those described earlier in Chapter 7. Mouse and mouse-alternative pointing devices, head wands, keyboards and keyboard alternatives such as on-screen keyboards, braille input keyboards, switches and switch arrays, and microphones can all serve as input devices for user agents. Output devices for Internet access are also those described in this chapter. In addition to the typical computer monitor and audible output, screen readers, screen magnifiers, braille displays, and speech synthesizers are the most commonly used output devices for user agents.

The W3C WAI project is developing guidelines to inform user agent developers of design approaches required to make their products more accessible to people with disabilities. The W3C WAI project also provides practical solutions for the development of accessible user agents on the basis of existing and emerging technologies. These resources will also increase usability for all users. The W3C initiative emphasizes the use of designs that facilitate compatibility between graphical desktop browsers and dependent assistive technologies (e.g., screen readers, screen magnifiers, braille displays, and voice input software). These developments will also benefit those who do not use the standard keyboard and mouse to access the Internet (e.g., those who are mobile and access the Web through palmtop computers, telephones, and auto terminals) (Vanderheiden, 1998).

These guidelines encourage designers of user agents to consider that users access documents in a variety of contexts. Potential users may be unable to see, hear, move, or process some types of information easily or at all. Users may also have difficulty reading or comprehending text, and they may not have or be able to use a keyboard or mouse. They define two classes of user agents. The first are commonly used graphical desktop browsers; their role in obtaining accessibility is discussed later. The second type of user agent is the one who is dependent on other user agents for input or output. These include many of the technologies discussed in this chapter, such as screen magnifiers, screen readers, alternative keyboards, and alternative pointing devices. The guidelines being developed focus on interoperability between these two classes of user agents.

The W3C WAI user agent guidelines are based on several principles that are intended to improve the design of both types of user agents. The first is to ensure that the user interface is accessible. This means that the consumer using an adapted input system must have access to the functionality offered by the user agent through its user interface. Second, the user must have access to document content through the provision of control of the style (e.g., colors, fonts, speech rate, speech volume) and format of a document. Many of the approaches described earlier (e.g., easy scrolling, and viewing windows that follow changes) help ensure access to content. A third principle is that the user agent help orient the user to where he or she is in the document or series of documents. In addition to providing alternative representations of location in a document (e.g., how many links the document contains or the number of the current link), a well-designed navigation system that uses numerical position information allows the user to jump to a specific link. Finally, the guidelines call for the user agent to be designed according to system standards and conventions. These are changing rapidly as development tools are improved. Communication through standard interfaces is particularly important for graphical desktop user agents, which must make information available to assistive technologies. Technologies such as those produced by the W3C include built-in accessibility features that facilitate interoperability. The standards being developed by the W3C WAI provide guidance for the design of user agents that are consistent with these principles. The guidelines are available on the W3C WAI Web page *(www.w3.org/wai)*.

How Web Pages Are Developed

Web pages are a mixture of text, graphics, and sound. These pages are typically developed by using a variety of programming languages. Hypertext markup language (HTML) has become a standard for Web design. HTML is a nonproprietary format that can be created and processed by a range of tools, from simple plain text editors in which the HTML codes are entered from scratch to sophisticated authoring tools. Many word processors convert files from the word processor format to HTML.

The W3C produces recommendations for HTML. These are specifications for developers, and they include guidelines for accessibility and multimedia *(www.w3.org/ MarkUp)*. HTML guidelines also provide access to style sheets. Cascading style sheets allow a Web page to be viewed in any layout chosen by the user (Lazzaro, 1999). Style sheet layouts that are compatible with screen magnifiers, screen readers, and braille are available. The W3C recommends that, wherever possible, developers use a style sheet for formatting their presentation and use HTML purely for structural markup. It is important that developers include options that allow style sheets to be turned off for those people using browsers that do not support style sheets. By using HTML as a standard, problems with file incompatibilities (e.g., from different word processors) can be avoided. One example of an HTML accessibility standard is the alt="text" HTML attribute. This function associates text with each graphic object. By pressing the ALT key on the keyboard, the text associated with the object is displayed. This can also be linked to a screen reader or braille output device.

Because of its capability of allowing a programmer to develop a single version of an application that can be used on a variety of computers and devices, the Java language (Sun Microsystems, *java.sun.com*) is widely used in programming for the Internet. Johnson, Korn, and Walker (1999) describe the Java platform and its accessibility features. The Java Accessibility Utilities provide linkages to help assistive technologies provide access to the GUI by toolkits that implement the Java accessibility application programming interface, a set of packages of software components that provide the basis for building functions such as input and output, data structures, system properties, date and time, internationalization, networking, user interface components, and applets (small application programs that can be run within other applications). Details of these accessibility functions are described by Johnson, Korn, and Walker (1999) and are available at the Java Web site.

Web Browsers

Web browsers for general use incorporate accessibility features to varying degrees. Because most are compatible with Windows, any other accessible products that are also compatible with Windows should work with the browser. That is, however, pure theory, because there are many features of browsers that are independent of the operating system. Thus, the accessibility of browsers varies.

Lynx (hosted by Internet Software Consortium, *http://lynx.isc.org/*) is a text-based browser for the Internet. It is usable by individuals who are blind because it is compatible with braille or screen reading software. Lynx also offers navigational functions.

Microsoft Internet Explorer (Seattle, Wash., *www.microsoft.com/enable/*) contains a range of features for people with disabilities. These include keyboard navigation (among links, frames, and client-side image maps), optional display of text descriptions with images, multiple font sizes and styles, and an optional disabling of style sheets so that the user's font, color, and size settings (the user's personal style sheet) will be used. This allows turning sounds, videos, pictures, and backgrounds off or on. Tool bar button size and icon size, text color, font, and size are all adjustable. Automatic fill-in of user names, passwords, Web addresses, and routine forums is also included. Explorer also uses the high contrast function to increase legibility and incorporates Microsoft Active Accessibility to provide information about the document.

Many of the screen readers described earlier have features that take advantage of Internet Explorer's capabilities. Examples include Hal, JAWS for Windows, and Window Eyes. The features that provide access to the Windows operating system are also used to provide access to Web pages. Many of these screen readers are also compatible with other general-purpose browsers such as Netscape.

Netscape Navigator (Mountain View, Calif., *www.netscape.com*) allows for enlargement, variation in, and colors of fonts. The IBM Home Page Reader speaks Web-based information with a text-to-speech speech synthesizer. Home Page Reader provides audible information from Windows desktop, e-mail and other applications, and Web pages. This information includes tables, frames, forms, and alternate text for images. Home Page Reader speaks information regarding page links or ALT text for objects like images and image maps. The user can navigate and read complex tables, such as television listings, using table navigation mode. In table navigation mode, the user can easily read table rows, columns, and cells, including table cells that span multiple rows or columns. Marcopolo is a plug-in for the Netscape browser that uses a standard PC soundboard to provide access to the Internet by using speech and musical sounds.

Making Web Sites Accessible

The W3C WAI has also developed guidelines for creating accessible Web sites. Their Quick Tips are shown in Box 8-2. These guidelines particularly address the way in which Web sites are laid out and the programming that is done to create the Web site. The guidelines facilitate access to the Web page by people using alternative input or output methods and give designers guidelines for making their content accessible to individuals who have visual, auditory, or manipulation disabilities. The technical terms that appear in the guidelines (e.g., cascading style sheets, HTML, scripts, applets) are defined on the W3C WAI home page.

BOX 8-2 | **Quick Tips to Make Accessible Web Sites**

Images and animations. Use the "ALT" attribute to describe the function of all visuals.

Image maps. Use client-side map and text for hot spots.

Multimedia. Provide captioning and transcripts of audio, and descriptions of video.

Hypertext links. Use text that makes sense when read out of context. For example, avoid "click here."

Page organization. Use headings, lists, and consistent structure. Use cascading style sheets for layout and style where possible.

Graphs and charts. Summarize or use the "longdesc" attribute.

Scripts, applets, and plug-ins. Provide alternative content in case active features are inaccessible or unsupported.

Frames. Use "no frames" element and meaningful titles.

Tables. Make line-by-line reading sensible. Summarize.

Check your work. Validate. Use tools, checklist, and guidelines at *www.w3.org/tr/wai-webcontent*.

For complete guidelines and checklist, see *www.w3.org/wai*.

Vanderheiden and Chisholm (1999) describe the development of authoring guidelines for Web site development. They emphasize the concept of having pages that "transform gracefully" across users, techniques, and situations. By transforming gracefully, they mean that a Web page remains stable regardless of what user, technological, or situational constraints occur. They cite the example of a person with low vision needing to enlarge the entire screen to 36-point text. In this case the author-determined font size will be overridden. They list three guidelines to help authors create documents that transform gracefully. First, authors should ensure that all the information available on the page can be perceived entirely visually and entirely auditorially, as well as being available in text. Second, they recommend that authors separate the content of the site (what is said) and the structure of the content (how it is organized) from the way the content and structure are presented (how the content is accessed by a user). Finally, they advise Web authors to ensure that all pages are operable with a variety of hardware, such as systems without mice, with small or low resolution, or with only speech or text input. They relate these recommendations to the W3C WAI authoring guidelines.

WebXACT is a free on-line service that allows testing of single pages of Web content for **quality, accessibility,** and **privacy** issues *(http://webxact.watchfire.com)*. To analyze a Web site, the URL of the page to be examined is entered into the CAST Web site. Bobby displays a report that indicates any accessibility or browser compatibility errors found on the page. Once the site receives a "Bobby Approved" rating, the Bobby Approved icon can be displayed on the site. The report includes both those things that can be checked automatically and a list of questions regarding checkpoints that must be validated manually. This information must be submitted to CAST before the approval is granted.

Making Mainstream Technologies Accessible

As cellular telephones become more powerful, approaching the power of PCs, there will be significant advantages for people with disabilities, especially those with low vision or blindness. Fruchterman (2003) describes four changes that will occur to make this possible: (1) standard cell phones will have sufficient processing power for almost all the requirements of persons with visual impairments, (2) software will be able to be downloaded into these phones easily, (3) wireless connection to a worldwide network will provide a wide range of information and services in a highly mobile way, and (4) because many of these features will be built into standard cell phones, the cost will be low and reachable by persons with disabilities. A major change in the cell phone industry that will underlie these advances is a move away from proprietary software to an open source approach, much like PCs of today. This will lead to a greater diversity of software for tasks such as text-to-speech output, voice recognition,

and optical character recognition in a variety of languages. Because the operating system will be an open source, many applications for people with disabilities can be downloaded from the Internet. It will be possible for a user to store customized programs on the network and download them as needed from any remote location. Downloading a DAISY reading program into a cell phone can provide access to digital libraries. Outputs in speech or enlarged visual displays can be added as needed by the user. Once the cell phone is accessible and has the capability of adding software for specific functions, a huge range of options will be opened up for the person with a visual impairment. These include calendar/appointments, personal contact database, note taking, multimedia messaging, and Web browsing. With a built-in camera and network access, a blind person could obtain a verbal description of a scene by linking to on-line volunteers who provide descriptions of images.

Although many of these applications are still more in the future than in the present, advances of this type will occur rapidly. One reason for the optimism surrounding these types of advancement is the increasing application of universal design in information technology products (Tobias, 2003). Universal design (see Chapter 1) principles call for mainstream technologies to be accessible to a wide range of individuals with and without disabilities. In the information technology area, there are also government regulations (see Chapter 1 for US legislation) that promote accessibility. Tobias (2003) describes these regulations and the challenges in implementing them. When mainstream technologies use open source operating systems, network-based accommodations can be accessed by users without specially designed equipment. This can reduce cost and thereby increase availability. These applications include automatic teller machines (ATMs), cell phones, vending machines, and other systems that are encountered on a daily basis (Tobias, 2003).

■ MOBILITY AND ORIENTATION AIDS FOR PERSONS WITH VISUAL IMPAIRMENTS

The requirements of devices that aid mobility for persons with visual impairments differ significantly from those for reading. Mobility presents notable problems for persons with visual impairments, and the blind traveler uses many methods to orient himself or herself to the environment and move safely within it (American Foundation for the Blind, 1978). Attention to sensory inputs of smell, sound, air currents, and surface texture alert the blind person to the terrain and environment, and a blind person can learn to pick up cues regarding objects. Sound cues are derived from reflections, sound shadows, and echo location. Temperature changes are also important. For example, passing a window on a cold day or passing under a canopy on a warm day provides information that is used in orientation. Odors from restaurants and crowds and other strong smells also provide information. Input regarding the texture of a sidewalk or grass is provided by the kinesthetic sense. Finally, persons with visual impairments also use travel aids, some of which are discussed in this section.

Reading Versus Mobility

There are several important differences between sensory input for reading and for mobility (Mann, 1974). Inaccuracies in reading result in loss of information, but errors in **orientation and mobility** can result in injury or embarrassment. In a **reading aid** the input is constrained. This means that the information to be sensed is always in a text or graphics form. Although there are differences in text fonts and reading needs, the differences across all reading materials are relatively small. In mobility, however, the range of possible inputs is large. The blind traveler needs to avoid obstacles as varied as a roller skate and a tree. The environment changes frequently (e.g., a chair is moved to a new location), and the blind person must be able to sense these differences. Nye and Bliss (1970) point out that the obstacles of most concern to blind travelers are bicycles, streets, posts, toys, ladders, scaffolding, overhanging branches, and awnings. We define the environmental input required for mobility as being unconstrained because these changes are not predictable and cover a wide range of inputs. To be successful, the design and specification of mobility aids for blind persons must take into account these factors. *Orientation* refers to the "knowledge of one's location in relation to the environment" (Scadden, 1997, p. 141). There are five approaches used to aid blind travel: a sighted guide, dog guides, the long cane, electronic aids, and alternative mobility devices. The last three are discussed in this section.

Canes. The most common mobility aid for persons with visual impairments is the long cane (Farmer, 1978). The standard cane consists of three parts: the grip, the shaft, and the tip. The entire cane is designed to maximize tactile and auditory input from the environment. The grip (which forms the handle) is made of leather, plastic, rubber, or other materials that easily transmit the tactile information to the user's hand. The shaft and tip work together to sense and then relay the tactile information to the grip. The tip (especially a metal tip used on a hard surface such as concrete) is a major source of high-frequency auditory input used by pedestrians who are blind to detect obstacles and landmarks by echolocation. A careful balance is obtained between sufficient rigidity to resist wind and bending and adequate flexibility to transmit the tactile and auditory sense of the surface texture.

Many blind travelers use folding or telescoping canes, which offer the advantage of easy storage when not in use.

Typically these are made of composite materials such as carbon fiber. When collapsed, they can be placed in a pocket or purse.

The primary advantages of canes are the low cost and the simplicity of use. They have significant limitations, however. One of these relates to the range over which sensory information is obtained. In use, the cane is moved in an arc approximately one step in front of the user. Any obstacles outside this range are not detected, and in some cases it is difficult for the blind traveler to adjust and avoid an obstacle within the space of only one step. A second limitation is that the cane only senses obstacles that are below waist level. In many cases, objects above knee level are not sensed until it is too late. For example, if there is a table in the path of the user, the cane may pass between the table legs, under the tabletop. The user will be unaware of the table's existence until he or she runs into it. Obstacles that are above waist height are also not sensed. Those of most concern are head-height obstacles such as tree branches.

Alternative Mobility Devices. The term **alternative mobility device** is used to describe a variety of methods used to aid mobility for individuals who are blind, particularly young children (Skellenger, 1999). Many of these devices are custom made from items such as hula hoops, toy shopping carts, PVC attached to an arm, and similar objects. Skellenger (1999) defines alternative mobility devices as "travel propelled devices other than the long cane that are held relatively statically in front of the traveler and are used primarily to detect obstacles and changes in depth" (p. 517). Skellenger found that these devices are widely used with children under the age of 5 years by orientation and mobility trainers, but they are rarely used with adults. The alternative devices are used primarily for training and are generally replaced by one of the other means of mobility assistance.

Electronic Travel Aids for Orientation and Mobility. **Electronic travel aids** (ETAs) have been developed to overcome some of the limitations of the long cane. These aids supplement rather than replace the long cane and guide dog. They are designed to provide additional environmental information over that sensed with a cane and to detect those obstacles typically missed by the long cane. ETAs also provide information that can assist with orientation for pedestrians who are blind (Scadden, 1997). We discuss both these applications in this section.

ETAs have the three components, as shown in Figure 8-1: an environmental interface, an information processor, and a user display. The environmental interface is typically both an invisible light source and a receiver (usually in the infrared range) or an ultrasonic transmitter and receiver. Both these technologies are similar to those used in television remote controls. The information processor may be a special-purpose electronic circuit or a microcomputer-based device. The user display may be either an auditory tone of varying frequency (e.g., higher as an object gets closer) or a haptic interface. Haptic interfaces are those that provide tactile input by use of vibrating pins or motors. Zelek et al (2003) developed and tested a haptic glove with three separate motors providing vibration to the thumb, middle finger, or little finger, depending on whether an obstacle was to the right, center, or middle of the user. The vibration of the motors was updated two to three times per second. The evaluation of the glove indicated that blind subjects navigated an unknown space efficiently (measured by the length of the path) and accurately (measured by avoidance of obstacles). Zelek et al (2003) also described the concept of visual-tactile mapping. This type of interface could also be used to localize the source of auditory information such as speech descriptions of an object, landmark, or building.

Electronically Augmented Canes.   Over the years several alternatives have been developed to extend the range of the standard cane and add the capability of detecting overhangs. The addition of electronic obstacle sensing also provides better sensing of drop-offs. Figure 8-12, *A,* illustrates the principle of operation of one approach, called the laser cane (Nurion-Raycal, Paoli, Pa., *http://www.nurion.net/*). Three narrow beams of laser light are projected from the cane. One beam is directed upward; it detects obstacles at head height about 2.5 feet in front of the cane tip. If an object is in the path of the beam, the light is reflected to a receiver and a high-pitched tone is emitted. Another beam detects objects directly in front of the traveler at a distance of either 5 or 12 feet (depending on the setting of a switch on the cane handle). If an object is encountered in this beam, the reflected signal causes the vibration of pins. The pins are located in the handle of the cane, where the fingers can comfortably rest on them (Figure 8-12, *B*). The final beam is aimed downward, and it is intended to detect drop-offs deeper than 5 inches (e.g., stairs or curbs) located about 3 feet from the cane tip. If the reflected beam is interrupted (because the drop-off does not reflect light in the same way as with a level surface), then a low-frequency tone is emitted. In some cases the auditory and tactile signals from the laser cane are misleading to the user (Mellor, 1981). For example, the laser beams could travel through a plate-glass door or window without being reflected, and the glass would not be detected. Nonglass portions of the door (e.g., frame or handle) were generally detected, but they had to be recognized as part of a door on the basis of laser cane signals. Highly reflective shiny surfaces also provided confusing reflections to the cane user.

A current ETA based on the cane is the UltraCane (Sound Foresight LTD, Barnsley, United Kingdom, *www.ultracane.com*), which uses ultrasound rather than laser sensing. The UltraCane, shown in Figure 8-13, *A,* provides all the information normally obtained from the long cane and adds two ultrasound beams and sensors. One detects objects directly in front and one detects objects at head height. It comes in seven different lengths from 105 cm (41 inches) to 150 cm (59 inches). The ultrasound beam avoids the problems of transparent glass encountered by the laser cane because the ultrasound beam is reflected from glass or shiny surfaces without distortion. The user display (Figure 8-13, *B*) provides tactile feedback with three vibrating pins located on each side and in the middle to indicate where the detected object is located. The intensity of the vibration indicates how close the object is. In contrast to the earlier laser cane, the UltraCane is collapsible and lightweight. It is used in the same way as the standard long cane. The user sweeps the cane in an arc in front as he or she walks. Although it is not quite as responsive as a standard long cane, primarily because of the added electronics in the handle, the laser cane can also provide conventional tactile and auditory information. One major advantage of the UltraCane is that it is fail safe; if the batteries run down or an electronic failure occurs, the cane can be used like a standard long cane. The laser cane was also used during mobility training, helping the trainee understand how to hold the cane correctly and move it in the correct arc (Mellor, 1981). The UltraCane can be used in a similar fashion. After the training is complete, the trainee can choose either to use the standard cane or to continue with the UltraCane cane. The UltraCane can also provide important information for a congenitally blind child regarding the size of objects and their location in space.

There are several disadvantages to the UltraCane cane. The most significant of these is the cost/benefit ratio. The UltraCane is approximately eight times more expensive than the long cane, and each user must decide how important the additional information received from the UltraCane is to his or her work, lifestyle, or safety.

Another ETA based on the long cane is the EasyGo (Q-tec B.V., The Netherlands, *www.q-tec.nl/uk/easygo.htm*) ultrasound transmitter/sensor that can be attached to a standard long cane. The sensor is aimed forward. When an obstacle is detected by the ultrasound beam, a ring on the handle provides tactile feedback to the user through a ring, which is integrated into the handle. During use, the user's finger rests on the ring, which rotates around the grip when an object is detected. The user can use the cane like a standard long cane while walking. Two ranges are available from the ultrasound sensor by turning the ring to the right (2.5 meters) or left (4 meters).

Ultrasonic Binaural Sensing.   Several devices are intended for use as adjuncts to the long cane. One of these is the Sonic Pathfinder (Perceptual Alternatives, Melbourne, Australia, *www.ariel.ucs.unimelb.edu.au*). This device has five ultrasonic transducers that are mounted on a headband. The two transmitters send out an ultrasound beam that covers the user's pathway. The three receivers (one pointing left,

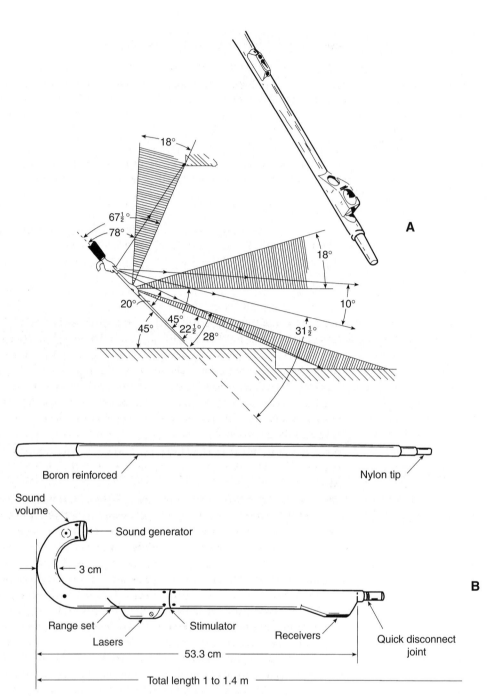

Figure 8-12   The laser cane. **A,** The triangulation method used. **B,** The major components. (From Nye PW, Bliss JC: Sensory aids for the blind: a challenging problem with lessons for the future, *Proc IEEE* 58:1878-1879, 1970.)

Laser Cane Closeup

one right, and one straight ahead) receive echoes when the ultrasound beam is reflected from an object in the user's path. The device is controlled by a microcomputer that processes the echoes and converts them to an audible output. The output is fed to the right, left, or both earpieces, depending on the source of the echo. To simplify the information provided, only the echo of the nearest object is displayed to the user. Priority is also given to objects that are

directly in front of the user. The output of the device can be explained by imagining walking toward a wall. The user hears in both ears the notes of the musical scale descending in order. For every 0.3 meters (1 foot), the pitch drops by one musical note. When the tonic note of the scale is reached, the user is within arm's length of the object. Likewise, if an object is to the right, a tone of constant pitch is played in the right earpiece as long as the user remains at

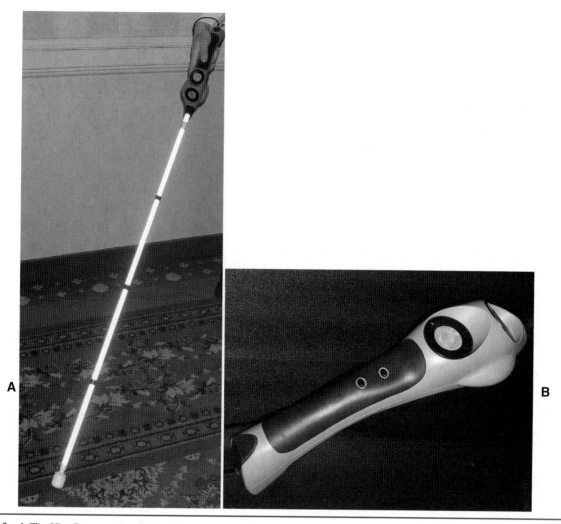

Figure 8-13   **A,** The UltraCane provides all the information normally obtained from the long cane. **B,** Two ultrasound beams and sensors are built into the handle.

the same distance from the object (say a wall). If the user moves closer to the wall, the pitch of the tone drops. The device is silent beyond a distance of 9 meters.

Clear Path Indicators.   Another type of ETA is designed to be a **clear path indicator;** that is, it provides signals to the user only if an object is detected in a field approximately 2 feet in diameter and 6 feet from the user (Farmer, 1978). The Polaron (Nurion-Raycal, Paoli, Pa., *http://www. nurion.net/*) is a device that is either worn on the chest or held in the hand. Ultrasound sensing is used to detect objects within 4, 8, or 16 feet. Feedback to the wearer is by either vibration of the unit or emission of a sound.

The device sends out an ultrasound (i.e., beyond the range of human hearing) beam that creates the clear path cone for detection of signals. This signal is similar to those used in many television remote controls and in electronic aids to daily living. If an object is in the ultrasound beam path, some sound is reflected back to the device, where it

is detected. The length of time it takes the reflected sound to be detected indicates how far away the object is. For objects at a distance of greater than 6 feet, a low-frequency audible sound is emitted from a speaker (the user display). For objects between 3 and 6 feet away, the Polaron emits a series of clicks and a vibration that is felt on the chest. The amplitude (intensity) of the signals increases as the objects get closer. When an object is 3 feet away or less, the tactile vibration is transferred to the neck strap and a higher-pitched beeping sound is heard. In contrast to other ETAs, the Polaron is totally silent when there is no object in its path.

Because both hands are free, the clear path indicators can be used in conjunction with the long cane, and they can be used by a person who requires a wheelchair and needs both hands free for pushing. The combination of auditory and tactile input makes these devices suitable for persons who are both deaf and blind. The simplicity of the feedback provided to the user increases the applicability of these devices, and they can be used by children and adults (Mellor, 1981). However, children may use them more for training and to learn spatial concepts than as travel aids, and the children can use their free hands to reach out and touch objects they have detected. The simplicity of feedback also means that only limited information can be provided to the user, which can restrict the applicability of these devices. Mellor (1981) also points out that heavy clothing may make it difficult to feel the tactile vibration on the chest and to keep these devices aimed in the proper direction.

Miniguide. Although the clear path indicators are intended to supplement the long cane, the Mowat sensor was a popular ETA used alone or with the cane. The Mowat sensor is no longer produced, but its functions have been incorporated into the Miniguide (Hill and Black, 2003). The Miniguide (GDP Research, Adelaide, South Australia, *http://www.gdp-research.com.au/index.html;* available in North America from Sendros, Davis, Calif., *www.senderogroup. com/index.htm*) is 80 mm long, 38 mm wide, and 23 mm thick (3 inches long, 1.4 inches wide, and 0.75 inches thick), about the size of a rectangular flashlight, and weighs less than 50 grams (about 2 ounces). It has an ultrasound transmitter and receiver that emit and receive ultrasound pulses in an elliptical pattern. When an object is detected in the ultrasound beam, the device begins to vibrate gently in the hand. The vibrations become faster for objects that are closer. The device is programmable to meet the needs of individual users. The device has five ranges: 26 feet (8 meters), 13 feet (4 meters), 6.5 feet (2 meters), 3 feet (1 meter), and 1.5 feet (half meter).

The normal use of the Miniguide is to scan the environment to locate specific familiar landmarks (e.g., a bus stop sign) or clear spaces such as doorways. It is small enough to be carried easily in a pocket or purse, and it is generally used to supplement other mobility and orientation devices. If two hands are used, it can detect overhangs with simultaneous use of the long cane. This may, however, be difficult for some persons. Mellor (1981) describes several unique uses of the Mowat sensor that also apply to the Miniguide. For example, it can be used when reaching if touching may be dangerous or undesirable, such as in a machine shop or hospital. It can also be placed on the floor and slowly rotated to find an object that has fallen. Finally, it can be placed on a desk used by a blind receptionist to indicate when someone is standing in front of the desk. The simplicity and relatively low cost of this device make it functional as a supplement to other orientation and mobility devices.

Wheelchair-Mounted Mobility Device for Blind Travelers. The clear path indicator makes it possible for a person to use a wheelchair, but it is not designed specifically for this purpose. For example, it cannot detect walls to the side or drop-offs in front of the wheelchair. Because power wheelchairs can move more rapidly than people normally walk,

the range for detection of objects must be increased to allow adequate time to change direction or to stop to avoid an obstacle. The Wheelchair Pathfinder (Nurion-Raycal, Paoli, Pa., *http://www.nurion.net*) uses a combination of laser and ultrasound beams to sense objects up to 8 feet in front of the user, walls (or other obstacles to the side up to 12 inches), and drop-offs (up to four feet away). Feedback is provided to the user through an audible tone, the frequency of which changes depending on the type of obstacle. There are two components, a master unit and a slave unit. These attach to brackets fastened on each side of the wheelchair. The frequency of the tone emitted by each unit is different, which allows the user to tell the direction of the obstacle.

As Owen (1990) describes, a device such as the Wheelchair Pathfinder can mean the difference between independence and dependence for a blind person who must use a manual wheelchair. Because it mounts on the wheelchair, it frees the hands and allows manual propulsion using the chair's push rims. Because it is optimized to detect obstacles relative to the chair, it provides the most important information to the user and takes into account the ways wheelchairs are used (e.g., how long it takes to stop or turn). Owen provides a description of her transition from being ambulatory and using a long cane with no ETA to using a wheelchair combined with the Wheelchair Pathfinder ETA. When she was ambulatory, she found that the ETAs did not provide her with sufficiently greater information than her long cane, and she felt that most ETAs were merely fancy gadgets. However, when she began to use a wheelchair and she could no longer use her cane because her hands were occupied pushing the wheelchair, she needed the drop-off–sensing aid. This caused her to reassess the value of ETAs in general, and she found that they actually had a greater place in mobility and orientation than she had expected.

Navigation Aids for the Blind

The electronic travel aids for obstacle avoidance do not address orientation that keeps an individual apprised of location and heading. To be effective, a navigation system should (1) keep track of the user's current location and heading as he or she moves through the environment, (2) find the way around and through a variety of environments, (3) successfully find and follow an optimally safe walking path to the destination, and (4) provide information about the salient features of the environment (Walker and Lindsay, 2005). To develop navigation aids, it is necessary to decide what environmental elements are important and then to develop technological approaches to detecting those elements and finally to provide a nonvisual means by which the information can be provided to the user. As described, the most effective auditory method for presenting information is speech, which has been the major approach for descriptive information in navigation aids. Synthetic or recorded speech cues and environmental descriptions are typically used in navigation aids. Other auditory cues are used as well to identify way points along a path (e.g., beacon signals that break down a long path into short segments with an auditory signal toward which the user walks), specific objects (e.g., furniture), locations (e.g., office, laboratory, or shop), or transitions (e.g., carpet to tile, curb cuts). It is important that the presentation of auditory information not interfere with natural environmental cues (e.g., sounds of traffic, water, etc.).

Because of the large number of options for display and sensing and the unconstrained environmental data when developing auditory navigation systems, Walker and Lindsay, (2005) used a virtual environment as a developmental tool. This approach allows the control of environmental obstacles, the evaluation of alternative user display technologies and formats, and alternative environmental sensing methods. They used this virtual environment to develop the System for Wearable Audio Navigation (SWAN) system and evaluated it with both blind and sighted subjects. Three different sound beacon maps were evaluated. A broadband noise beacon provided the best performance because it was easy to localize. Their study also showed that practice significantly improved performance, even over a short number of trials. Walker and Lindsay also concluded that the virtual environment training carried over to natural environmental navigation. They also found few differences in performance by blind and sighted individuals.

A major difficulty in electronic travel aids is the identification of obstacles in a busy or cluttered background. Sonification is the process by which environmental data are transformed into auditory signals to allow interpretation or communication (Nagarajan, Yaacob, and Sainarayanan, 2004). In a natural environment, background objects can dominate the sonification "image." To overcome this problem, Nagarajan, Yaacob, and Sainarayanan used signal processing that mimics the natural human eye. Because the system is used in a real-time mode, the processing time for each signal is short (about 0.7-1 second). Two primary types of processing are used: edge detection and background suppression. Edge detection highlights the boundaries of key objects in the environment, making them stand out. Because some background objects may be important (e.g., a large tree), the background is suppressed, not eliminated. In normal vision, turning the head is used to scan the environment. In the auditory substitution system this technique is also applied, keeping the object of interest in the center of the digital camera used to sense the environment. Stereo signification uses a number of acoustic attributes to add richness to the user display. These attributes include pitch, loudness, timbre (the waveform of the sound that gives a trumpet a different sound than a violin), and location. Localization of objects is aided by the stereo presentation and enhanced by rotating the head and listening to the change in the signals

presented to each ear. Nagarajan, Yaacob, and Sainarayanan (2004) describe the signal processing algorithms used in their system.

When indoor navigation is required, the environment is constrained and the technology can be simplified. Global positioning system (GPS)–based devices (see section later in this chapter) are also not useable indoors. Ross and Henderson (2005) developed an indoor navigation system called "Cyber Crumbs." The concept is to load directions for navigation within a building into a central database. When an individual with a visual disability enters the building, he or she will use an information kiosk to select a desired destination in the building. The kiosk will then compute the most direct route for the person to take and download the route into the person's user's badge in the form of an ordered list of cyber crumb addresses. The stored speech instructions are provided to the user though a bone conduction headset that does not block the input of natural auditory information. As the individual traverses the course toward the destination, the badge detects each strategically located cyber crumb and updates the instructions accordingly. The cyber crumbs are located at key locations such as elevators, hallway intersections, exits, and entrances). The user's badge has a repeat button. Instructions are only repeated when this button is pressed. In a pilot trial of the cyber crumbs system, visually impaired users improved their performance. In baseline trials without the technology, visually impaired individuals took 3.9 times as long to complete a travel path and walked 73% longer distances compared with sighted users. With the cyber crumb technology the time dropped to two times the sighted individuals' time, and the distance traveled to just 8% more than the sighted control subjects.

Global Positioning System–Based Navigation Aids for the Blind. The satellite-based GPS provides precise information regarding features, terrain, vehicles, or buildings. It was initially developed for military applications. The GPS technology is ideally suited to use in navigation systems for persons who are blind. One aspect of wayfinding technology is the concept of "smart environments" (Baldwin, 2003). These environments are conceived as having a series of embedded transmitters (e.g., form signs, intersections, store logos, etc.) that are linked to GPS-based networks and stored maps. The location-based technology has two components: a wireless system for labeling and latitude and longitude geographical databases. These smart environments will be of benefit to the general public (e.g., in navigational aids for traveling) and can be considered part of universal design for the environment (see Chapter 1). If sensors for these networks are built into "wearable computers," the sensing and user display functions will be both unobtrusive and effective in facilitating independent mobility for blind travelers on the basis of existing wayfinding technologies developed for the general public. Baldwin (2003) describes how theses mainstream technologies will benefit blind travelers.

User Preferences for Global Positioning Systems.   Golledge et al (2004) conducted a survey of blind individuals to determine their preferences for the development of GPS-based navigation aids. The most common problems reported were dealing with street crossings, avoiding unknown obstacle hazards, learning new routes, and taking shortcuts. Difficulty in gaining access to navigational information was identified in several areas, including knowing and keeping track of the direction to walk to a destination, knowing which way the person was facing, knowing that they were at a street corner, where to turn, and the location of specific landmarks such as stores and bus stops. The type of needed navigational information identified (in priority order) was information about landmarks, streets, routes, destinations, buildings, and transit. All participants identified automatic speech recognition (see Chapter 7) as the most desirable form of input to the device. Other highly rated input choices were a QWERTY keyboard, braille keyboard, and telephone keyboard. The most acceptable output device for providing navigational information to the user was a collar- or shoulder-mounted speech or sound device. On the basis of the loss of ambient auditory information when headphones were used, this mode was the least acceptable. The Wayfinding Group is collaborating on the development of GPS-based devices (*http://www.senderogroup.com/wayfinding/*).

Global Positioning System Displays.   To determine the most effective user display for a GPS system, Loomis et al (2005) evaluated five spatial displays. A **spatial display** is one that provides direct spatial information about the directions and distances to environmental locations relative to the user. The five displays evaluated were (1) virtual speech, (2) virtual tone, (3) haptic pointer interface (HPI) and tone, (4) HPI and speech, and (5) body pointing. The HPI is like the talking sign technology (see below) that can receive an identifying signal that is produced by an environmental object. Virtual speech and tone provide description information that is localized to the direction from which the signal is received by using a stereophonic user display. The HPI used by Loomis et al. consisted of a hand-held pointer with a compass attached. Their HPI-based displays provided auditory information (tone or speech) that corresponded to the direction in which the pointer was aimed. The body pointing display was identical to the HPI-tone device except that the compass was mounted on the waist rather than held in the hand. Results indicated that the virtual speech was judged to be the best display; body pointing was preferred to the other HPI options and virtual tone displays. One negative feature of the speech was the use of headphones, which limited ambient input. Alternative auditory displays are mandatory.

Commercial Global Positioning Systems.   The simplest devices for assisting with orientation are adapted compasses. The braille compass has the major north, south, east, and west directions labeled in braille and the intercardinal points labeled with raised dots. The face opens, much like a braille watch, so that the direction can be felt. The C2 Talking Compass (Robotron Proprietary Limited, St. Kilda, Australia, *www.robotron.net.au*) uses spoken output to help orient the user. The user points the compass in one direction and presses a button. The compass then speaks the direction as north, east, south, west, or intermediate directions (e.g., northwest). The compass can be purchased with two languages installed, and 20 languages are currently available.

Atlas Speaks (Sendros, Davis, Calif., *www.senderogroup.com/index.htm*) is a talking map on a personal computer (Scadden, 1997). A digital map is generated by software, and the user can navigate through the map by moving the cursor. Street names and other points of interest are spoken as they are encountered by the cursor. Personal points of interest may also be noted. These might include bus stops, favorite restaurants, frequently visited shops, friends' houses, public buildings, landmarks, and museums. Pedestrians who are blind can use Atlas Speaks to plan trips. The user can also create points of interest by entering them into the computer. Several directional formats are available (compass, clock face, or degrees). Once a route is created, it can be saved on a tape recorder, copied to portable note taker, or printed on a braille printer.

Another aid for travelers who are blind is Talking Signs (Talking Signs, Inc., Baton Rouge, La., *www.talkingsigns.com*). Street signs and building signs provide a significant amount of orientation for sighted travelers. Individuals who are blind or who have trouble reading require that same information to maintain their orientation as they travel. Developed at Smith-Kettlewell Eye Research Institute, Talking Signs voice message originates at the sign and is transmitted by infrared light to a hand-held receiver at a distance. Because of the nature of infrared transmission, the transmission is directionally selective. As the user aims the receiver directly at the sign, the intensity and clarity of the message increases. This allows the user to focus the Talking Signs system and orient himself or herself to her actual location. Talking Signs transmitters must be installed as adjuncts to all signs. This is a large task, but many signs have been installed. Talking Sign can also be used to label objects such as building entrances, drinking fountains, phone booths, or rest rooms (Scadden, 1997).

The Trekker (Humanware, Concord, Calif., *http://www.humanware.ca/*) is a system that uses GPS and digital maps to help blind persons find their way in urban and rural areas. The palm-sized device helps guide the visually impaired through the environment as an adjunct to other travel aids (e.g., white canes and guide dogs). Trekker provides information by speech and allows users to record both vocal and written notes. A wide variety of maps from Navteq are available, covering most Western countries. Maps can be downloaded from the Internet or obtained on CD or Compact Flash cards. Navteq *(http://www.navteq.com/)* creates and maintains a database containing all street names and ranges of addresses for urban areas and for more than 1,500,000 points of interest both in North America and Europe. Trekker can be combined with the functions of a personal digital assistant: agenda, text notes, voice notes, address book, DAISY reader (Victor Reader Pocket), media player, e-mail manager, Web browser, calculator, clock, and alarms in the Maestro system.

The BrailleNote GPS (Humanware, Concord, Calif., *http://www.humanware.ca/)* is a cell-phone-size GPS receiver that is an accessory to portable braille or voice note takers. It relays information from GPS satellites that can be used by the portable note taker to calculate where the user is and to plot a route to a destination of choice. The user can calculate the distance and direction to a street address or intersection, find out the relative location of points of interest, and automatically create routes for either walking or riding in a vehicle; it also provides detailed information about speed, direction of travel, and altitude.

■ SPECIAL-PURPOSE VISUAL AIDS

In developing the HAAT model in Chapter 2, three performance areas were defined as part of the activity: self-care, work and school, and play and leisure. Persons with blindness or low vision may have needs in each of these areas, and there are special-purpose devices that can provide assistance. These devices are in addition to those serving needs for reading and orientation/mobility, which are used in all three performance areas. This section describes some of the special-purpose devices that serve these needs. Publications and devices are available; the American Foundation for the Blind (New York City, for example, Bradesco, Brazil, *www.bradesco.com.br*), Sensory Access Foundation (Palo Alto, Calif.),Smith-Kettlewell Eye Research Institute, Rehabilitation Engineering Center (San Francisco, Calif.), and the New York Lighthouse, Inc. (New York, *www.lighthouse.org*) are good sources of information regarding specific needs. There are companies that sell large numbers of products for all three performance areas (LS&S Group, Northbrook, Ill., *www.Lssgroup.com;* Maxi Aids, Farmingdale, N.Y., *www.maxiaids.com;* Independent Living Aids, Inc, Plainview, N.Y., *www.independentliving.com).*

Devices for Self-Care

Auditory or tactile substitutes can be used for many household tasks. For example, braille tape (similar to the tape used for labeling with raised letters) can be used to label canned foods and appliance controls. Another approach to identification of household objects is the use of bar codes and recorded speech (Crabb, 1998). Bar codes are typically used in supermarkets for checkout scanning. However, the codes used are stored in the grocery store computer, so they cannot be read at home. Crabb developed a device, called the I.D. Mate (En-Vision America, Normal, Ill., *www.envisionamerica.com*) that allows a sighted individual to sweep a reader over the bar code and then record a short spoken message describing the contents (e.g., "Campbell's tomato soup"). This information is then played back to the blind user when he or she scans a similar can at the grocery store. Other household items can also be scanned. Approximately 90% of the items sold in the United States have bar codes on them. This includes playing cards, cassette tapes, CDs, and many other items. There are two commercial products that read bar codes. ScanTalker is a bar code reading accessory for the PAC Mate portable note taker. It has a built-in database that matches the bar code with a wide variety of food and personal care products. The product information is provided to the user by speech. The ScanTalker also provides other information, such as nutritional information and preparation instructions, from product labels. The id mate II (Sendros, Davis, Calif., *www.senderogroup.com/index.htm)* is a self-contained device that has a unidirectional bar code reader and hand-held user display that provides product identification and extended information in speech form. More than one million items are contained in the id mate II database. The id mate can also be personalized by entering a bar code and recording a corresponding message. This can be useful for labeling household objects, clothing, and similar personal items.

Voice output is also available on some appliances, such as microwave ovens. Kitchen timers, thermometers, and alarm clocks are available in both enlarged and auditory or tactile forms. Talking wristwatches are used by individuals who are blind. Electrical appliances often have controls marked with tactile labels to allow a blind person to adjust the control. Raised or enlarged print telephone dials can also be obtained from local telephone companies. There are also devices that read paper money and speak the denomination of the bill. These are similar to change machines or those used for automatic purchase of public transportation tickets in many cities. A portable paper money reader is shown in Figure 8-14 (Note Teller, Brytech, Ottawa, Canada, *www.brytech.com/)*. When a paper monetary note of $1 to $100 value is inserted into the device, it automatically turns on and speaks the denomination of the note. Both English and Spanish voice outputs are available, and a headphone may be used for privacy. When the note is removed, the unit automatically turns itself off. Versions specifically for U.S. and Canadian currencies and a universal model are available.

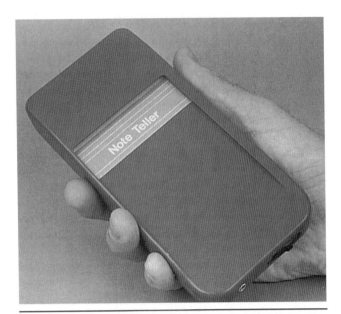

Figure 8-14 The Note Teller paper money reading device. (Courtesy Brytech, Nepean, Canada.)

ATMs usable by both sighted persons and persons with visual impairments are available. These will eventually replace all ATMs in the United States and Canada. Worldwide usage of this technology is likely to occur in the future. Banking over the Internet is also available for persons who are blind or who have low vision. Regulations concerning ATMs are contained in the Americans with Disabilities Act Access Guidelines (*http://www.access-board.gov/ada-aba/adaag/about/guide.htm#Automated*). These guidelines provide performance standards for people with vision impairments. Braille instructions and control labels are used to provide nonvisual information from ATMs. For user feedback during use, audible devices and handsets are recommended to provide access while maintaining privacy. Braille output is not required. Touchscreens with appropriate software and hardware can also be made accessible to persons who are blind. The major provisions of the standards are (Trace Center, University of Wisconsin, *trace.wisc.edu*) differentiation of each control or operating mechanism by sound or touch, provision of opportunity for input and output privacy, marking of function keys with tactile characters, provision of both visual and audible instructions for operation, dispensing of paper currency (if available) in descending order with the lowest denomination on top, and options to receive a receipt in printed or audible form or both.

A leading cause of blindness is diabetes, and there are insulin injection devices that provide independence for blind users. Specially adapted syringes and holders for bottles are available. The holder guides the syringe into the bottle, and the syringe can be set to allow only the amount necessary for one dose to be drawn out of the bottle. Other home health care devices include thermometers with speech output and sphygmomanometers (for blood pressure measurement) that use either raised dots on the pressure meter face or synthesized speech output.

Devices for Work and School

The major needs within vocational and educational applications are for access to reading, mobility, and computers. The approaches and devices in the sections on reading and mobility in this chapter and computer access in Chapter 7 often meet these needs. To be operated as they were designed, many tools require the use of vision. It is possible to use either tactile or auditory adaptations to make these tools available to individuals who have visual impairments. A carpenter's level with a large steel ball and center tab has an adjustment screw on one end. The screw is calibrated with half a degree of tilt corresponding to one turn. To level the device, the carpenter adjusts the screw until the ball is at the center. The user then knows how many degrees of tilt there are and can correct for the tilt. There is also a tactile tape measure with one raised dot at each quarter-inch mark, two at half-inch increments, and one large dot at each inch mark. Calipers, protractors, and micrometers use a similar labeling scheme. An audible device is used by machinists to determine depth of cut when using a lathe. There are also talking tape measures, calculators, scales, and thermometers. Many of these also have tactile versions.

Many electronic test instruments use digital (numerical) displays, which are easily interfaced to speech synthesizers. The output of the meter (e.g., a voltage measurement by a technician) is heard instead of read. Oscilloscopes are also available in both auditory and tactile forms. Electronic calculators that have speech output provide an alternative to visual display–based devices. It is possible for a person with total visual impairment to perform virtually all the tasks required for electronic or mechanical design, fabrication, and testing by using adapted tools and instruments. The Color Teller (Brytech, Ottawa, Canada, *www.brytech.com/*) is a hand-held device that detects colors, tints, and shades like pink, pale blue-green, dark brown, and vivid yellow. The color is spoken in English, French, or Spanish with adjustable volume. It can also be used to determine whether the lights in a room are on or off.

Devices for Play and Leisure

Almost any common board game can be obtained in enlarged form. There are also enlarged and tactually labeled playing cards, and braille or other versions exist for common board games and dice. Computer games that emphasize text rather than graphics can be used with computer screen reading software.

More active games include "beeper ball," in which auditory signals replace visual cues. In this softball-like game, the ball contains an electronic oscillator that emits a beeping sound. The batter can aim for the sound. Bases are also labeled with sounds. Similar approaches are available for playing Frisbee, soccer, and football. In each case the object to be thrown or kicked emits a beep and goals are labeled with auditory markers. Individuals who are blind can snow ski with the assistance of both sighted guides and auditory signals from barriers such as slalom poles and fences.

CASE STUDY

CHANGING NEEDS FOR VISUAL AIDS

Ken has enrolled this fall semester as a student at the state college. He has retinitis pigmentosa. Retinitis pigmentosa is a midperipheral ring scotoma that gradually widens with time so that central vision is frequently reduced by middle age. Night blindness occurs much earlier, and total blindness may eventually ensue. Ken has recently noticed that his vision seems to have deteriorated significantly. He would like to study to become a journalist. Ken lives alone in an apartment close to campus so he can walk to school or, when it is raining, take the bus. As Ken's retinitis pigmentosa advances, what types of assistive technology for sensory impairments might be useful to enable him to continue with his activities in the following areas: (1) school, (2) home/self-care, and (3) recreation/leisure?

■ SUMMARY

For persons who have low vision, it is possible to improve performance by increasing size, contrast, and spacing of the text material. Low-cost magnification aids and filters can help in this regard, but electronic aids provide much greater flexibility. Reading aids for persons who are blind rely on either tactile or auditory substitution. The most effective of these are language based (e.g., speech or braille). Fully automated reading devices are capable of imaging print documents and converting them to speech by use of voice synthesis.

ETAs for persons who are blind serve a useful but limited purpose in aiding mobility and orientation for blind travelers. Just as reading aids use alternative sensory pathways of auditory and tactile input, so do ETAs. The basic structure of a sensory aid shown in Figure 8-1 applies to ETAs as well as to reading aids. The environmental interface is either a light (laser or infrared emitter and sensor) or sound (ultrasound), and the user display is either an auditory tone or series of tones of varying frequency and amplitude or tactile vibration. The information processor converts the reflected light or ultrasound information to the audible or tactile display information presented to the user. Current technology provides only limited substitution or augmentation for the long cane. Future developments will most likely be in the extraction of useful features from the visual image for display to the blind traveler (see Adjouadi, 1992, for example). By concentrating on achieving input that is more informative regarding obstacles and the orientation and location of objects in the environment, the utility of these devices will be greatly enhanced. Electronic aids that assist blind travelers with orientation are also available; some make use of GPS information.

Study Questions

1. What are the two basic approaches to sensory aids in terms of the sensory pathway used?
2. List the three basic parts of a sensory aid and describe the function of each part. Pick one example from visual aids, one from auditory aids, and one from tactile aids and describe the three parts that make up each aid.
3. Compare the visual, auditory, and tactile systems in terms of their basic function and as substitutes for each other.
4. What are the three types of scanners used in reading machines, and how do they differ?
5. What is an OCR, and what function does it perform in a reading machine for the blind?
6. List three output modes available for reading machines.
7. Computer disks or CD-ROMs with text stored on them can be used to provide access to reading material for persons who are blind. What components (e.g., adapted output devices) must be included in such devices, and what role does the computer play?
8. What is a GUI? What advantages does it provide for persons with disabilities?
9. What special problems does the GUI present for persons who are blind?
10. What are the features included in Universal Access and Windows Accessibility options that assist individuals who have low vision or blindness?
11. List three limitations of current voice-only screen reading programs developed for visual access.
12. What are the three factors that must be considered when accommodating for low vision? How are they normally dealt with in access software?
13. Describe the relative advantages and disadvantages of software and hardware approaches to obtaining enlarged displays for persons with visual impairments.

14. How is *magnification* defined for a screen-enlarging program?
15. What are the three modes used in screen magnification software?
16. What is meant by *focus* in a screen magnification program?
17. What is the primary tactile method used for computer output?
18. What are the three approaches to using nonspeech sound for representing GUIs?
19. What is an auditory icon?
20. What are the attributes of an earcon, and how are they used to portray graphical information?
21. What are the two major types of hearcons? How are they used to represent visual components of the GUI?
22. What is the difference between an earcon and a hearcon?
23. What special adaptations are made to braille specifically for computer output use?
24. What adaptations are made to provide hard copy for users with low vision?
25. What adaptations are made to provide hard copy for users who are blind?
26. Define *scrolling* as applied to screen reader programs.
27. What does the term *navigation* mean in describing a screen magnification or screen-reading program?
28. Describe the major benefits of computer use reported by individuals who are blind or who have low vision.
29. What are the major barriers to computer use reported by individuals who are blind or who have low vision?
30. What are the primary challenges in obtaining Web access for persons who have disabilities?
31. What is the WAI?
32. What is a user agent? What are typical user agents for persons with disabilities? What guidelines are used to ensure that a user agent is accessible?
33. How are Web pages developed, and what steps are necessary to ensure that they are usable by persons with disabilities?
34. What is a Web browser? What features are necessary in a Web browser to ensure that people who have disabilities can use it?
35. List the major features of accessible Web sites. What tools are typically used to test accessibility of Web sites?
36. What are the major differences in the effects of errors in reading and in mobility devices?
37. What are the major limitations of the long cane for use as a mobility aid by persons who are blind?
38. What is an electronic travel aid?
39. List three advantages and three disadvantages of the laser cane.
40. What is a clear path indicator, and how is it used in mobility for people who are blind?
41. What are the major assistive technologies applied to orientation for people who are blind?
42. Pick a tool or measurement instrument and figure out how to adapt it for both a person with low vision and one who is blind.

References

Adjouadi M: A man-machine vision interface for sensing the environment, *J Rehabil Res Dev* 29:57-76, 1992.

Allen J: Reading aids for the severely visually handicapped, *CRC Crit Rev Bioeng* 12:139-166, 1971.

American Foundation for the Blind: *How does a blind person get around?* New York, 1978, The Foundation.

Baldwin D: Wayfinding technology: a roadmap to the future, *J Vis Impair Blindness* 97:612-620, 2003.

Blenkhorn P, Gareth D, Baude A: Full-screen magnification for Windows using directx overlays, *IEEE Trans Neural Syst Rehabil Eng* 10:225-231, 2002.

Boyd LH, Boyd WL, Vanderheiden GC: The graphical user interface: crisis, danger, and opportunity, *J Vis Impair Blindness* 84:496-502, 1990.

Converso L, Hocek S: Optical character recognition, *J Vis Impair Blindness* 84:507-509, 1990.

Cook AM: Sensory and communication aids. In Cook AM, Webster JG, editors: *Therapeutic medical devices*, Englewood Cliffs, NJ, 1982, Prentice-Hall.

Crabb N: Mastering the code to independence, *Braille Forum* June:24-27, 1998.

Dixon JM, Mandelbaum JB: Reading through technology: evolving methods and opportunities for print-handicapped individuals, *J Vis Impair Blindness* 84:493-496, 1990.

Doherty JE: *Protocols for choosing low vision devices*, Washington, DC, 1993, National Institute on Disability and Rehabilitation Research.

Farmer LW: Mobility devices, *Bull Prosthet Res* 30:41-118, 1978.

Fruchterman JR: Reading systems for the visually and reading impaired, *Proc 1991 CSUN Conference*, Northridge, CA, California State University, Northridge, 1991.

Fruchterman JR: In the palm of your hand: a vision of the future of technology for people with visual impairments, *J Vis Impair Blindness* 97:585-591, 2003.

Gerber E: The benefits of and barriers to computer use for individuals who are visually impaired, *J Vis Impair Blindness* 97:536-550, 2003.

Gerber E, Kirchner C: Who's surfing? Internet access and computer use by visually impaired youth and adults, *J Vis Impair Blindness* 95:176-181, 2001.

Golledge RG et al: Stated preference for components of a personal guidance system for nonvisual navigations, *J Vis Impair Blindness* 98:135-147, 2004.

Griffin HG et al: Using technology to enhance cues for children with low vision, *Teaching Except Child* 35:36-42, 2002.

Grotta D, Grotta SW: Desktop scanners: what's now...what's next, *PC Mag* 17:147-188, 1998.

Hayes F: From TTY to VDT, *Byte* 15:205-211, 1990.

Hill J, Black J: The Miniguide: a new electronic travel device, *J Vis Impair Blindness* 97: 655-658, 2003.

Huber MJ, Simpson R: Recognizing the plans of screen reader users: Proceedings of the AAMAS 2004 workshop on modeling and other agents from observation (MOO 2004), New York NY: www.marcush.net/irs_papers.html. Accessed March 8, 2006.

Johnson E, Korn P, Walker W: A primer on the Java platform and Java accessibility: Proceedings of the CSUN conference (1999): (http://www.dinf.org/csun_99/session0193.html).

Kerscher G, Hansson K: Consortium—Developing the next generation of digital talking books (DTB): Proceedings of the CSUN conference (1998): (http://www.dinf.org/csun_98_065.htm).

Kirman JH: Tactile communication of speech: a review and analysis, *Psychol Bull* 80:54-74, 1973.

Lazzaro JL: Helping the web help the disabled, *IEEE Spectrum* 36:54-59, 1999.

Loomis JM et al: Personal guidance system for peoples with visual impairment: a comparison of spatial displays for route guidance, *J Vis Impair Blindness* 99: 219-232, 2005.

Ma L et al: Effective computer access using an intelligent screen reader, *Proc 26th RESNA Conf*, Atlanta, Rehabilitation Engineering and Assistive Technology Society of North America, 2004.

Mann RW: Technology and human rehabilitation: prostheses for sensory rehabilitation and/or substitution. In Brown JHU, Dickson JF, editors: *Advances in biomedical engineering*, New York, 1974, Academic Press.

Mellor CM: *Aids for the '80s*, New York, 1981, American Foundation for the Blind.

Nagarajan R, Yaacob S, Sainarayanan G: Computer aided vision assistance for human blind, *Integrated Computer-sided Eng*, 11:15-24, 2004.

Nye PW, Bliss JC: Sensory aids for the blind: a challenging problem with lessons for the future, *Proc IEEE* 58: 1878-1879, 1970.

Owen MJ: Close encounters of a technological kind: a personal transformation, *J Vis Impair Blindness* 84:491-492, 1990.

Ratanasit D, Moore M: Representing graphical user interfaces with sound: a review of approaches, *J Vis Impair Blindness* 99:69-93, 2005.

Ross DA, Henderson VL: Cyber crumbs: an indoor orientation and wayfinding infrastructure: Proceedings of the 28th annual RESNA conference (June 2005): http://www.resna.org/ProfResources/Publications/Proceedings/2005/Research/TCS/Ross.php. Accessed November 26, 2005.

Scadden LA: Technology for people with visual impairments: a 1997 update, *Technol Dis* 6:137-145, 1997.

Servais SP: Visual aids. In Webster JG et al, editors: *Electronic devices for rehabilitation*, New York, 1985, John Wiley.

Skellenger A: Trends in the use of alternative mobility devices, *J Vis Impair Blindness* 93:516-521, 1999.

Smith GC: The Stereotoner—a new sensory aid for the blind, *Proc Annu Conf Eng Med Biol* 14:147, 1972.

Stelmack JA et al: Patient's perceptions of the need for low vision devices, *J Vis Impair Blindness* 97:521-535, 2003.

Tobias J: Information technology and universal design: an agenda for accessible technology, *J Vis Impair Blindness* 97:592-601, 2003.

Vanderheiden GC: Cross-modal access to current and next-generation Internet—fundamental and advanced topics in Internet accessibility, *Technol Disabil* 8:115-126, 1998.

Vanderheiden GC, Chisholm W: The ongoing evolution of the WAI authoring guidelines: Proceedings of the 1999 CSUN conference (http://www.dinf.org/csun_99/session0094.html).

Walker BN, Lindsay J: Using virtual environments to prototype auditory navigation displays, *Assist Technol* 17:72-81, 2005.

Wolfe KE: Wired to work: an analysis of access technology training for people with visual impairments, *J Vis Impair Blindness* 97:633-645, 2003.

Wolfe KE, Candela T, Johnson G: Wired to work: a qualitative analysis of assistive technology training for people with visual impairments, *J Vis Impair Blindness* 97:677-694, 2003.

Zelek JS et al: A haptic glove as a tactile-vision sensory substitution for wayfinding, *J Vis Impair Blindness* 97: 621-632, 2003.

CHAPTER 9

Sensory Aids for Persons With Auditory Impairments

Chapter Outline

FUNDAMENTAL APPROACHES TO AUDITORY
 SENSORY AIDS
Augmentation of an Existing Pathway
Use of an Alternative Sensory Pathway
Tactile Substitution
Visual Substitution

AIDS FOR PERSONS WITH AUDITORY IMPAIRMENTS
Hearing Aids
Electroacoustical Parameters of Hearing Aids
Types of Hearing Aids
Basic Structure of Hearing Aids
Types of Hearing Aid Signal Processing
Cochlear Implants
Electrodes
Transmission of Power and Data
Speech Processing
User Evaluation Results
Telephone Access for Persons Who Are Deaf
Telephone Devices for the Deaf
Visual Telephones for the Deaf
Voice Over Internet Protocol
Technology for Face-to-Face Communication Between
 Hearing and Deaf Individuals

Alerting Devices for Persons With Auditory Impairments
Assistive Listening Devices
Small-Group Devices
Large-Group Devices
Captioning as an Auditory Substitute
Closed-Captioned Television and Movies
*Real-Time Captioning for Education and Business
 Applications*
Captioning by Automatic Speech Recognition
Basic Principles of Computer Adaptations for Auditory
 Impairments
*Built-in Options to Increase Usability by Persons
 Who Are Deaf*
*Access to the Internet When Auditory Information Is Difficult
 for the User*
Aids for Persons With Both Visual and Auditory
 Impairments
*Devices for Face-to-Face Communication With Individuals
 Who Are Deaf and Blind*
Automated Hand for Finger Spelling

SUMMARY

Learning Objectives

On completing this chapter, you will be able to do the following:

1. Describe the major approaches to sensory substitution, including the advantages and disadvantages of each
2. Describe the design and specification of hearing aids
3. Describe adaptations of common devices for use by a person who is hard of hearing or deaf
4. Discuss the major approaches used to provide input for individuals who have both visual and auditory impairments
5. Describe how computer outputs are adapted for individuals with auditory limitations

When an individual has a sensory impairment, assistive technologies can provide assistance in the input of information. This chapter emphasizes approaches that are used to either aid or replace seeing and hearing. This chapter is restricted to sensory aids that are intended for *general use*. Chapter 8 discusses assistive technologies that are designed to assist people who have visual limitations. This chapter focuses on assistive technologies designed to meet the needs of persons with auditory limitations.

▪ FUNDAMENTAL APPROACHES TO AUDITORY SENSORY AIDS

Chapter 8 describes the fundamental approaches to sensory aids. Figure 8-1 applies to auditory as well as visual sensory aids. Augmentation of an existing pathway and use of an alternative pathway are the two basic approaches to sensory assistive technologies. When applied to the auditory system, the alternative pathways are tactile and visual. Each of these approaches is discussed in this chapter.

Augmentation of an Existing Pathway

When someone is hard of hearing, the primary pathway (i.e., the one normally used for input) is still available; it is just limited. Insufficient intensity means that the signals are too weak to be heard, and an amplifier is required. Certain frequencies may be more limited than others for people who are hard of hearing, and the hearing aid must be designed or specified to take this into account. For example, in aging there is usually a greater hearing loss in high rather than low frequencies. Augmentation of the auditory pathway is by use of hearing aids, cochlear implants, or assistive listening devices.

Use of an Alternative Sensory Pathway

There are two alternate sensory pathways available to someone who is deaf. The most common example is the use of manual sign language (visual substitution for auditory). Chapter 8 discusses the fundamental differences among the tactile, visual, and auditory systems.

Tactile Substitution.   Substitution of tactile input for auditory information differs from the substitution of tactile input for visual information (i.e., braille). One major difference is that the rate at which the auditory information changes is relatively high compared with the time required for the tactile system to input information. Engineers refer to this as the relative *bandwidths* of the two systems. The auditory system has a broader bandwidth (more information can be handled in a given amount of time) than the tactile system. Because auditory information is a sequence of sounds, these must be translated into tactile information for presentation to the user. These tactile signals are then detected and assembled into meaningful units by the central nervous system. Because the tactile system requires spatial and temporal information, its rate of input is slower than for the auditory system. Another major limitation of the tactile system for auditory input is that it lacks a means of converting sound (mechanical vibrations) into neural signals. This is the function normally carried out by the cochlea.

The only tactile method for input of auditory information that has been successful is the *Tadoma method* used by individuals who are both deaf and blind. In this method, which was used by Helen Keller, the person receives information by placing his or her hands on the speaker's face, with the thumbs on the lips, index fingers on the sides of the nose, little fingers on the throat, and other fingers on the cheeks. During speech, the fingers detect movements of the lips, nose, and cheeks and feel the vibration of the larynx in the throat. Through practice, kinesthetic input obtained from these sources is interpreted as speech patterns. One reason for the success of this method is that there is a fundamental relationship between the articulators (reflected in the movements of the lips, nose, and cheeks) and the perceived speech signal, and this relationship is at least as important as the acoustic information (pitch and loudness) in the speech signal for individuals using the Tadoma method (Lieberman, 1967).

Visual Substitution.   Visual displays of auditory information can take several forms. One example, sometimes used in speech therapy or as an aid to deaf individuals who are learning to speak, is to display a picture of the speech signal on an oscilloscope-like screen. Often a model pattern portraying the ideal is placed on the top half of the screen, and the pattern from the person learning to speak is placed on the bottom half of the screen. The learner attempts to match the model through practice. Some current devices also use computer graphics to make the process more interesting and motivating. This type of sensory substitution of visual for auditory information is a rehabilitative technology that is not practical for assistive technologies. The reasons for this parallel those presented for the Stereotoner in relation to auditory substitution for vision (see Chapter 8).

Visual substitution for auditory information has been successful in several areas. These include visual alarms (e.g., flashing lights when a telephone or doorbell rings) and the use of text labels for computer-generated synthetic speech. Speech is the most natural auditory form of language. Likewise, written text is the most natural way of presenting visual language. Thus, a major design goal for assistive devices that use visual substitution for auditory communication is to provide speech-to-text conversion. In this type of device, speech is received and converted by computer to text and displayed so that the person with an auditory impairment can read it.

■ AIDS FOR PERSONS WITH AUDITORY IMPAIRMENTS

Helen Keller, who was both deaf and blind, is reported to have been asked whether she would prefer to have her vision or her hearing if she could have one or the other. She responded that she would prefer to have her hearing because she felt that people who are blind are cut off from things, whereas those who are deaf are cut off from people. It is important to keep this concept in mind in the following discussion of aids for persons who are deaf or hard of hearing. Auditory impairment is often not as obvious as visual impairment, and society does not view it as having the same degree of significance as visual impairment. It is natural for a person to wear glasses as a part of the inherent process of aging. However, many people are embarrassed to admit hearing loss sufficient to require a hearing aid. Despite these considerations, hearing loss is significant, and it can be socially isolating. Assistive technologies can provide great improvement in the lives of persons who have either partial or total auditory impairments.

Hearing Aids

Hearing aids are often conceived of as simple devices that amplify sound, primarily speech. Although hearing aids do contain amplifiers, hearing loss is rarely consistent across the entire speech frequency range. As discussed in Chapter 3, hearing loss is generally greater at some frequencies than at others. This presents a problem in the design of hearing aids. If all frequencies are amplified the same amount, the

sound will be unnatural to the user. An additional difficulty encountered in providing hearing aids of high fidelity is that the components are small, and this miniaturization can limit the frequency response of the microphone and speaker, further reducing the quality of the aided speech.

Approximately 60% of the *acoustic energy* of the speech signal is contained in frequencies below 500 Hz (Berger, Hagberg, and Rane, 1977). However, the speech signal contains not only specific frequencies of sound but also the organization of these sounds into meaningful units of auditory language (e.g., phonemes), and more than 95% of the *intelligibility* of the speech signal is associated with frequencies above 500 Hz. For this reason, speech intelligibility rather than sound level is often used as the criterion for successful application of hearing aids.

Electroacoustical Parameters of Hearing Aids. Hearing aid output is typically specified in decibels (dB) referred to a standard of 20 micropascals (see the discussion of sensory function in Chapter 3). Sound pressure level (SPL) is used to designate this parameter. Standards for hearing aid specification have been developed by the American National Standards Institute (S3.46, 1997; *http://web.ansi.org/*) and the *International Electrotechnical Commission* (60 118-0-10; *http://www.iec.ch/*). These standards allow for the comparison of hearing aids from different manufacturers, and they specify parameters that are used in this comparison.

When hearing aids are fitted, it is important to know the output levels from the hearing aid that are delivered to the listener. Average conversational speech can range from 40 to 80 dB SPL depending on both how far away the talker is from the listener and the talker's vocal effort (Olsen, 1988). Therefore, the hearing aid output is assessed in response to a variety of input types and levels (e.g., pure tones and speech or speech-like signals). Powerful hearing aids are capable of producing output SPLs of 130 to 140 dB. These levels can damage the hearing mechanism even if the duration of the input is short. Therefore, the maximum power output of a hearing aid also needs to be specified to ensure that the level of the hearing aid output will not cause further hearing loss. Readers interested in the electroacoustical performance and measurement of hearing aids are referred to Dillon (2001) for a thorough review.

Types of Hearing Aids. Conventional hearing aids can be divided into two types: air conduction and bone conduction. All air conduction hearing aids deliver the hearing aid output into the listener's ear canal. However, some people are unable to wear air conduction hearing aids as a result of chronic ear infections or malformed ear canals. For these individuals, a bone conduction hearing aid is most appropriate. The most common type of bone conduction hearing aid is a BAHA (bone-anchored hearing aid) (Figure 9-1). Inputs to this type of hearing aid are converted to mechanical

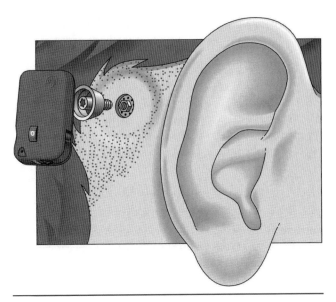

Figure 9-1   Bone-anchored hearing aid. (Courtesy Cochlear Corporation–Bone Anchored Solutions.)

vibrations that shake the skull. BAHAs take advantage of the fact that, at a sensory level, it does not matter whether sounds come from an air-conducted hearing aid or a bone-conducted hearing aid. An air-conducted and a bone-conducted 1000-Hz tone will sound the same provided they are both at the same level of audibility. Snik et al (2005) provide a review of consensus statements regarding BAHAs.

Air conduction hearing aids are available in several different configurations (Stach, 1998). Figure 9-2 illustrates several commonly used types of aids. The major types of ear level aids are behind-the-ear (BTE), in-the-ear (ITE), in-the-canal (ITC), and completely-in-the-canal (CIC) aids. Body-level aids are used in cases of profound hearing loss. The processor is larger to accommodate more signal processing options and greater amplification and is mounted at belt level. The body-level aid is usually used only when other types of aids cannot be used

BTE hearing aids, which fit behind the ear, contain all the components shown in Figure 9-3. The amplified acoustical

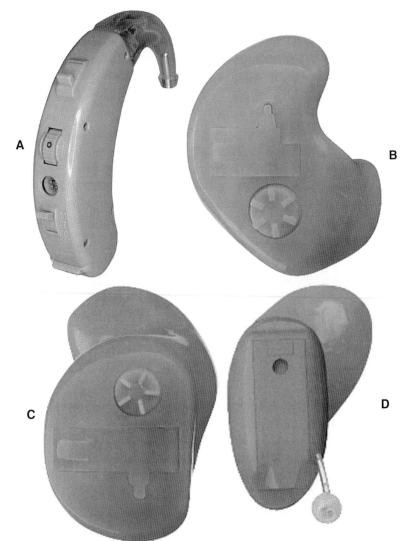

Figure 9-2   Types of hearing aids. **A,** Behind the ear (BTE). **B,** In-the-ear (ITE). **C,** In-the-canal (ITC). **D,** Completely in-the-canal (CIC). (Courtesy Siemans Hearing Instruments, Inc.)

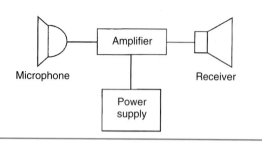

Figure 9-3   The major components of a hearing aid.

signal is fed into the ear canal through a small ear hook that extends over the top of the auricle and holds the hearing aid in place. A small tube directs the sound into the ear through an ear mold that serves as an acoustical coupler. This ear mold is made from an impression of the individual's ear to ensure comfort to the user, maximize the amount of acoustical energy coupled into the ear, and prevent squealing caused by acoustic feedback. When the mold is made, a 2-ml space is included between the coupler and the eardrum. A vent hole can also be added to an ear mold, which can add to acoustical feedback and distortion and preventing the ear from being blocked. The vent hole allows sound to travel to the tympanic membrane directly. An external switch allows selection of the microphone (M), a telecoil (T) for direct telephone reception, or off (O). The MTO switch and a volume control are located on the back of the case for BTE aids.

The ITE aid makes use of electronic miniaturization to place the amplifier and speaker in a small casing that fits into the ear canal. The faceplate of the ITE aid is located in the opening to the ear canal. The microphone is located in the faceplate. This provides a more "natural" location for the microphone because it receives sound that would normally be directed into the ear (Stach, 1998). External controls on the ITE include an MTO switch and volume control. The ITC is a smaller version of the ITE. The CIC type of hearing aid is the smallest, and it is inserted 1 to 2 mm into the canal with the speaker close to the tympanic membrane. Because this type does not protrude outside the ear canal, it is barely visible. Any controls for the aid are fit onto the faceplate of the ITE, ITC, and CIC types of aids.

Basic Structure of Hearing Aids. Figure 9-4 illustrates the basic components of analog and digital hearing aids. The microphone is the **environmental sensor;** it is the component that receives the speech signal. Overall fidelity of the hearing aid is directly related to the quality of this component. Several types of microphones are used in hearing aids (see Stach, 1998). The function of the microphone is to convert the acoustical speech waveform

Figure 9-4   Three approaches to the electronic design of hearing aids. **A,** An analog hearing aid. **B,** A digitally controlled analog hearing aid. **C,** A digital signal processing hearing aid. (Modified from Stach BA: *Clinical audiology,* San Diego, 1998, Singular Publishing Group.)

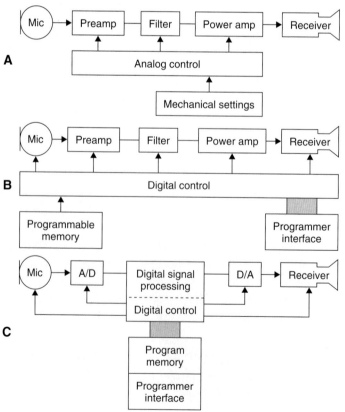

into an electrical signal, which is sent to the amplifier. Microphones may be omnidirectional (amplify sound from any direction) or directional. They also include noise reduction properties to obtain the best input signal possible.

The information processor (see Figure 2-5, *B*) in a hearing aid is the amplifier. It performs several functions. The first and most basic of these is amplification of the input signal with a frequency response (amplifier gain between the input and output, which is different at different frequencies) that is matched to speech signals. Amplifiers may be linear or nonlinear (sometimes called *curvilinear*) (Stach, 1998). Linear amplifiers increase the gain in signal from input to output by the same amount for all intensities of input. This means that a small speech signal and a large noise signal are both amplified the same amount. Linear amplifiers restrict the output to a level that is not harmful to the ear by clipping the signals that are large enough to cause damage. This approach is called *peak clipping* (see below). In a nonlinear or curvilinear amplifier, the output signal does not have the same proportional relationship to the input as in a linear amplifier. The nonlinear approach provides for compensation for louder signals and greater amplification of speech signals through a variety of approaches. Nonlinear amplification is also more versatile in the processing options it allows. Second, the information processor limits loud input signals to prevent distortion and protect the user from damage to the peripheral auditory system. Finally, signal processing is provided to minimize noise and maximize the speech signal.

In an ideal amplifier, all signals are amplified in such a way as to preserve the shape of the input curve at the output of the device. Because the input shape (SPL versus gain plot) is determined by the speech signals picked up by the microphone, maintenance of this shape is important to the signal's intelligibility. Any difference in the shape of the input and output signals is called *distortion*. Distortion can arise from several factors and can appear in several ways (Stach, 1998). Two of the most important types of distortion are frequency distortion and noise distortion. Frequency distortion results when certain frequencies are amplified more than others and when there are shifts in the relationship between different frequency bands in the input and output signals. Noise distortion is the result of nonspeech signals being introduced into the amplified output of the hearing aid, which results in decreased intelligibility. Noise may originate within the components of the hearing aid or outside the aid. Examples of external distortion are skin or other materials rubbing against the microphone. Obviously, the lower this noise level, the greater the fidelity and intelligibility of the output speech signal.

With the increase in capability and decrease in size of digital signal processing (including miniaturized computers), there have been significant advances in hearing aid design. The major advantage of using this type of signal processing is that it can be more exactly matched to the acoustic properties of the auditory system than can the less-sophisticated analog signal processing approach of Figure 9-4, *A*. Preves (1988) describes several of the digital signal processing approaches used in hearing aids (Figure 9-4, *B* and *C*). Among the advantages are lower distortion, less acoustical feedback, more precise compression of loud signals, and greater fidelity and intelligibility in the speech signal supplied to the ear.

As stated earlier, the maximal allowable acoustic input at the ear is 130 to 140 dB. One way of limiting this signal is to set a maximal value for the output and cut off any signals that exceed this value. This is referred to as *peak clipping*. The net result is that loud signals have the peaks of the waveform cut off, or "clipped." Peak clipping often results in distortion and a decrease in intelligibility of the speech signal (Dillon, 1988). To reduce the negative effects of peak clipping, a concept known as *automatic gain control* is used in analog hearing aids to automatically decrease the amplifier gain whenever a loud signal is provided at the input. Figure 9-5 shows how this type of compression works. As the input signal is increased in amplitude, the amplifier senses this and reduces the gain. The amount of time that it takes for the amplifier to respond is referred to as the *attack time* of the circuit. When the input signal is reduced, the amplifier again responds as shown in Figure 9-5. The time it takes the amplifier to recover and increase its gain back to normal is called the *response time*. These two times are often part of a hearing aid specification. This type of hearing aid compression does not decrease intelligibility of the speech signal for large acoustic inputs (Dillon, 1988).

Nonlinear circuits allow more complex compression methods to be used (Stach, 1998). Nonlinear compression not only limits the effect of loud sounds as described above for analog compression, but it also provides nonlinear gain with various input levels within the user's dynamic range. Dynamic range is the difference between the softest detectable signal and the loudness of input that causes discomfort. This varies from individual to individual. For individuals who have normal hearing, the dynamic range is up to 100 dB. An individual with significant hearing loss of 50 dB would have a dynamic range of only 50 dB. This might be further reduced if recruitment occurs in the cochlea and auditory nerve, resulting in an increase in the loudness of the signal. Recruitment is common in sensorineural hearing loss (see Chapter 3). One goal of nonlinear speech compression techniques is to fit the input speech into the user's dynamic range. Low-intensity signals are amplified to be in the user's range, and high-intensity signals above the user's comfort range are reduced. Because low- and high-intensity signals require different levels of amplification, a nonlinear approach is needed. This type of nonlinear processing is called *dynamic range compression* (Stach, 1998). Compression may be applied at the input or output of the hearing aid circuitry. With input compression, the microphone and preamplifier trigger the compression when a signal above a preset threshold

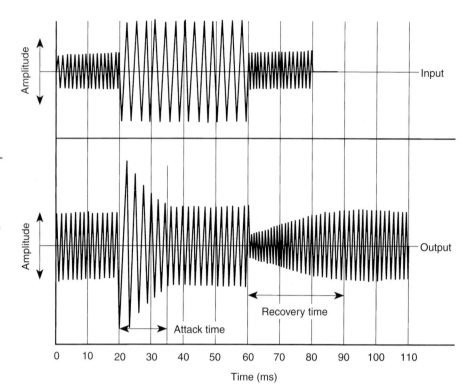

Figure 9-5 The compensation response of a hearing aid to sudden changes in input (top waveform); sound intensity is shown in the bottom trace. (Data from Staab WJ: *Hearing aid handbook*, Blue Ridge Summit, PA, 1978, TAB Books.)

is detected. Alternatively, a high output level may be used to activate the compression. This is termed *output compression*. It is possible to adjust several of the compression parameters, which makes it easier to match the characteristics of the hearing aid to the needs of the user.

The user display (see Figure 2-5, *B*) for a hearing aid is the *speaker*. This component is often referred to as the *receiver*, and it converts the electrically amplified signal to an acoustical waveform that is coupled to the ear. The small size of these devices severely limits the frequency response of the hearing aid for signals above the range of speech. As mentioned previously, most receivers are air-conduction types, which acoustically couple the speech signal to the ear canal. However, when the middle or outer ear precludes the use of an ear mold (e.g., chronic draining ears, atresia, absence of the pinna), bone conduction receivers may be required.

Types of Hearing Aid Signal Processing. Current hearing aids use one of the three design approaches shown in Figure 9-4 (Stach, 1998). Figure 9-4, *A*, illustrates the classical analog approach to hearing aid design. The majority of hearing aids made have been of the analog type. Analog hearing aids operate directly on the acoustical signal detected by the microphone; this signal is continuous. In an analog hearing aid, the time-varying input acoustical signal is amplified and filtered and compression is applied if necessary. The signal is then fed directly to the speaker.

The second type of hearing aid circuitry is referred to as *digitally controlled analog* or *hybrid* (Levitt, 1997; Stach, 1998).

As shown in Figure 9-4, *B*, the signal path (amplification, filtering, and compression) is still analog, but the control of these circuits is set by digital parameters. Because the digital parameters control the device and can be stored in memory, this device is very flexible. Digitally controlled analog devices can be customized to meet the needs of the user with the parameters stored in the digital memory. Parameters that can be digitally controlled include gain, frequency response, compression parameters, and electroacoustical parameters. The primary reason for the development of the hybrid type of hearing aid was that early pure digital hearing aids were bulky and consumed larger amounts of power than did corresponding analog aids. The hybrid approach gave increased flexibility without the larger size and greater power requirements.

With the development of low-power, small digital signal processing circuits, digital hearing aids (see Figure 9-4, *C*) are possible. This type of hearing aid uses stored control parameters like the hybrid type; the signal is converted to digital form and then processed. Even these hearing aids have analog preamplifiers to boost the signal to a level sufficient for analog-to-digital conversion. One of the advantages provided by digital circuitry is the capability of shaping the frequency response of the hearing aid. This provides the possibility of canceling acoustical feedback and increasing the signal-to-noise ratio of the hearing aid (Levitt, 1997). Digital aids also can use adaptive filtering to shape the frequency response on the basis of the spectral characteristics of the incoming signal. Currently available digital hearing aids have the computational capability of a small computer. The major limitation at this time is not signal processing capability but rather our limited understanding of the most effective way to process speech signals for people who have hearing aids (Levitt, 1997). As in many areas of assistive technology application, we are limited by our understanding of the clinical and biological aspects of the problem, not by the available technologies.

Cochlear Implants

If there is damage to the cochlea of the inner ear, an auditory prosthesis can provide some sound perception. The first reported use of electrical stimulation of the inner ear was made by the Italian physicist Alessandro Volta (for whom the volt is named) more than 200 years ago. He inserted wires into his ear and connected them to a 50-volt battery, and he experienced an "auditory sensation" when the voltage was applied. More recently, engineers and physiologists have developed sophisticated aids that accommodate lost cochlear function.

These devices, termed **cochlear implants,** have the components shown in Figure 9-6 (Feigenbaum, 1987). As long as the eighth cranial nerve is intact, it is possible to provide stimulation by use of implanted electrodes. Cochlear implants have been shown to be of benefit to adults and young persons who have adventitious hearing loss (i.e., hearing loss after acquiring speech and language) (Stach, 1998). Significant benefits have also been reported for cochlear implants in young prelingual children (Balkany et al, 2002; Waltzman et al, 2002). Children as young as 18 months old are developing speech largely through auditory input. In recent years, younger and younger children have received cochlear implants to take advantage of their neural plasticity (Ramsden, 2002). There are two major parts of most cochlear

implants (Ramsden, 2002). External to the body are a microphone (environmental interface), electronic processing circuits that extract key parameters from the speech signal, and a transmitter that couples the information to the skull. The implanted portion consists of an electrode array (1 to 22 electrodes), a receiver that couples the external data and power to the skull, and electronic circuits that provide proper synchronization and stimulation parameters for the electrode array. Ten-year failure rates are reported to be less than 3% for the internal and external elements combined (Ramsden, 2002).

Candidates for cochlear implants must meet certain audiological and age criteria. Severe or profound (>90 dB) bilateral pure tone hearing loss, sentence recognition scores of less than 30%, and age 2 years or more with >90 dB loss in children are the primary criteria for cochlea implants (Loizou, 1998). Age at implant for children and duration of deafness for adults are important factors in obtaining success (Ramsden, 2002). Better results occur for children at younger implant ages and for adults who have had shorter periods of deafness.

Surgical procedures consist of insertion of the electrode array into the cochlea and implantation of the internal components and linking antenna for transcranial transmission of data and power. Ramsden (2002) describes the surgical procedures and possible surgical complications. After the implant is inserted, a period of 1 month or so is allowed for healing, and then a process of "switch-on and tuning" is carried out. Two thresholds are measured: minimal perception of sound and the level at which the sound just ceases to be comfortable. Then the electrode array is tested and signal processing is applied.

The operation of a four-channel cochlear implant system is shown schematically in Figure 9-7 (Loizou, 1998). Sound received by an external microphone is sent to a speech processor. The processed signal is coupled through the skin by a radio frequency transmitter-receiver pair. The internal signal is then fed to the electrode array implanted

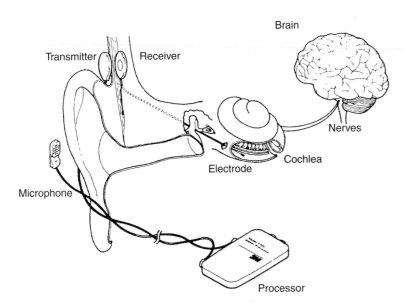

Figure 9-6   The components of a cochlear implant. (From Radcliffe D: How cochlear implants work, *Hearing J* November:53, 1984.)

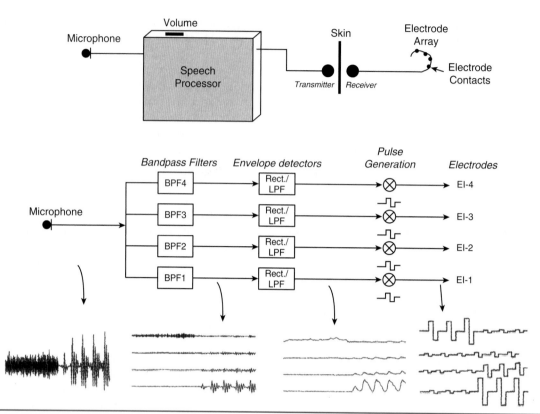

Figure 9-7   Diagram showing the operation of a four-channel cochlear implant. Sound is picked up by a microphone and sent to a speech processor box worn by the patient. The sound is then processed, and electrical stimuli are delivered to the electrodes through a radiofrequency link. Bottom figure shows a simplified implementation of the CIS signal processing strategy using the syllable *sa* as an input signal. The signal first goes through a set of four bandpass filters that divide the acoustic waveform into four channels. The envelopes of the band-passed waveforms are then detected by rectification and low-pass filtering. Current pulses are generated with amplitudes proportional to the envelopes of each channel and transmitted to the four electrodes through a radiofrequency link. Note that in the actual implementation the envelopes are compressed to fit the patient's electrical dynamic range. (From Loizou P: Mimicking the human ear, *IEEE Signal Process Mag* 15:101-130, 1998.)

in the cochlea. One type of process is also illustrated in Figure 9-7: a bank of filters processes the speech information and then converts it into pulses that are sent to the electrodes. Signal processing is discussed in more detail later in this section. The resulting electrical signals at each point in the system are illustrated at the bottom of Figure 9-7. Current approaches to cochlear implants differ in several important respects. The main distinguishing characteristics, shown in Box 9-1, are discussed in depth by Loizou (1998) and summarized in this section.

Electrodes.   The three major considerations in design of electrodes are (1) biocompatibility of materials, (2) placement of electrodes, and (3) the number of electrodes in the array (Shallop and Mecklenberg, 1988). The stimulating portion of most electrodes in current devices is made of platinum-iridium because it is electrically stable and does not react with biological tissue. The "leads," wires that connect the stimulator to the platinum-tipped electrode, need to be flexible enough to curve around the cochlea, but they also must be rigid enough not to bend as they are inserted. The electrode array and the lead wires are coated

with polytetrafluoroethylene (Teflon) or silicone to insulate them from each other and from the tissue. If there are small holes or breaks in the insulation, the tissue near the break will be exposed to electrical current. This can damage both the wire and the tissue. The insulation material must also be impervious to leakage of ionic fluids in the body.

Electrode placement is intracochlear (inside the cochlea), and the size of the electrode is dictated by the microanatomy of the cochlea. The average cochlea is about 32 mm long,

---

BOX 9-1   **Varying Characteristics of Cochlear Implant Systems**

Electrode design: Number of electrodes, electrode configuration
Type of stimulation: Analog or pulsatile
Transmission link: Transcutaneous or percutaneous
Signal processing: Waveform representation or feature extraction

From Loizou P: Mimicking the human ear, *IEEE Signal Process Mag* 15:101-130, 1998.

and electrode arrays can be up to 25 mm long for insertion into this cavity (usually the scala tympani). Stimulation is either monopolar or bipolar. Monopolar stimulation places one reference electrode outside the cochlea and an array of single electrodes inside the cochlea along the basilar membrane. This arrangement requires less power for stimulation but results in less specific and less focused stimulation in the cochlea. Bipolar stimulation places electrode pairs along the membrane. This results in much more localized and specific stimulation, but it requires more power. Greater power means larger size, and this dictates the type of external packaging. The external package may be in either a BTE or body-level type. The majority of cochlear implants to date have been body-level types. As miniaturized technologies have been enhanced, BTE types have become more prevalent. The minimal spacing between electrode tips, on the basis of electrical stimulation parameters, is 0.5 to 4 mm (Loizou, 1998; White, 1987). This sets a practical limit of 22 electrodes in an array. Several different numbers of electrodes have been used in cochlear implants. Initially all devices used only one electrode. Currently available types of cochlear implants (Clarion, Advanced Bionics Corp., Sylmar, Calif., *www.cochlearimplant.com/*; Nucleus 24, Cochlear Inc., Lane Cove, Australia, *www.cochlear.com/*; PUL SARCI, Med El, *www.medel.com/*) have 12, 16, or 22 electrodes (Loizou, 2006).

Transmission of Power and Data.   Because the microphone and speech processing components of cochlear implants need to be adjusted and because of their size and weight, they are placed outside the skull. The electrode array must be inside the cochlea, and there must be a connection through the skull. Initially this was done with wires that passed through the skull and a percutaneous plug that was used when the wires were removed. This type of percutaneous connection is subject to infection, and it has been replaced by a transmitter-receiver approach (Ramsden, 2002). A small induction coil on the external skin surface is connected to the transmitter. This coil transmits through the skin to the receiving coil located directly opposite, under the skin. The receiving coil is connected to the internal electronics and the electrode array. Power for the internal electronics is also coupled through the skin. In some cases the internal circuitry is totally passive and merely passes the stimulation signal to the electrodes. In other cases (such as that shown in Figure 9-6), the internal circuitry processes the incoming signal and distributes it to the different electrodes in the array. This consumes power, which is normally coupled through the skin just as the data are.

Speech Processing.   The purpose of the cochlear implant is to provide an electrically triggered physiological signal that can be related to speech and environmental sounds. The process by which the cochlea, auditory nerve, and higher centers process speech is complex, and it is difficult to design an electronic speech processor that provides physiologically meaningful data to the electrode array.

The area of speech processing or coding of the signals to be sent to the electrode is one in which differences exist among different cochlear implants. Digital processing of the speech signal is aimed at extracting the relevant speech data from the microphone and converting it to a form that provides the most possible information to the user by stimulation of the auditory nerve. To recognize speech, it is necessary to encode frequency, intensity, and temporal patterns (Loizou, 1998, 2006). One approach, shown in Figure 9-7, uses a "vocoder" approach in which the incoming signal is broken down into a set of signals of different frequency through a filter bank. Frequency is encoded in the normal cochlea by location along the basilar membrane (referred to as *tonotopic organization*). A multiple electrode array can provide different frequencies at different locations along the basilar membrane, but the normal cochlea uses other, more sophisticated methods to further encode frequency (Loizou, 1998). Intensity or amplitude (what we subjectively perceive as loudness) can be encoded by the magnitude of the stimulus at any electrode location. However, the normal cochlea also uses "recruitment" of adjacent hair cells to reflect increased intensity. Recruitment or interaction between the electrode channels can also happen with electrical stimulation of neural tissue as the intensity of the stimulus increases.

Continuous interleaved sampling (CIS) signal processing was developed to avoid some of the problems of channel interactions by delivering temporally offset trains of pulses to each electrode (Loizou, 1998; Wilson et al, 1993). CIS is based on the use of nonsimultaneous interleaved stimulation. In interleaved stimulation, electrodes at different parts of the cochlea are stimulated in sequence rather than those adjacent to each other being stimulated in sequence, and only one electrode is stimulated at one time, helping to eliminate interaction between channels. A key feature is a relatively high rate (greater than 800 pulses per second) of stimulation on each channel, which provides the basis for tracking rapid variations in speech by use of pulse amplitude variations presented to the electrodes. The tradeoff for use of high stimulation rates is more cross-channel interaction. The amplitude of the incoming speech signal must be compressed to avoid damage resulting from overstimulation. As in hearing aids, this process is called compression. Because of the nature of the auditory system, a nonlinear (logarithmic) compression is typically used in cochlear implants (Loizou, 1998, 2006). Intensity of the electrical signal in microamps is analogous to the intensity of the acoustical stimulus in dB. A refinement on the CIS processing approach detects the peaks of the speech signal in several bands. The number of frequency bands is greater than the number of electrodes, and the signals sent to the electrodes are based on the bands with the highest output at any given time. This approach is called ACE (previously called SPEAK) and is implanted on the Nucelus-24 devices (Cochlear Inc., Lane Cove, Australia, *www.cochlear.com/*). Sentence recognition tests with the CIS, SPEAK, and ACE signal processing approaches demonstrated that significantly higher scores were obtained with the ACE than with the SPEAK or CIS strategies (Loizou, 2006). Loizou (1998, 2006) discusses speech processing for cochlear implants in depth and describes current commercial approaches.

Major cochlear implant manufacturers also provide software that is used to program the signal-processing characteristics of the implant to match the needs of the user. These are used after the surgery has been completed and healing has taken place. Signals are supplied to the implant and psychophysical measurements are made to determine the optimal type of signal (pulse or analog) and electrode combinations. This uses pure tone responses. Then speech input is evaluated and adjustments are made to maximize speech intelligibility.

User Evaluation Results. Almost all postlingually deaf individuals can obtain some degree of open set (the test words or sentences are not known) speech perception without lip reading by use of cochlear implants (Ramsden, 2002). Some users can also communicate over the telephone. The degree of improvement depends on many factors, including the characteristics of the cochlear implant technology used. In general, more channels or electrodes result in greater speech perception (Loizou, 1998). Increasing the number of electrodes or channels will not be effective if there is a smaller number of surviving auditory neurons. The type of signal processing also affects cochlear implant outcomes. For example, the spectral processing method yields greater than 90% correct speech recognition even with a small number of channels, whereas the CIS processing method required up to eight channels to achieve similar results (Loizou, 2006). An area of continued research is aimed at increasing music perception and enjoyment.

In the case of prelingual children, the need for effective auditory perception is critical in the development of spoken language. For deaf children, the cochlear implant has been shown to facilitate development of language at a rate comparable to that of typical hearing children (Balkany et al, 2002). These results are dependent on a number of factors, including age at implantation, length of deafness, and length of use (habituation to the cochlear implant) (Waltzman et al, 2002). Children who receive an implant at an age younger than 5 years perform much better on speech perception tests than do children who are older at the time of implantation. Children who receive an implant before the age of 2 years perform equally well with children who are between 2 and 5 years old when they receive their implant. The minimum age is now 12 months (Balkany et al, 2002). Children who use the cochlear implant full time perform significantly better than those who do not. In general, as the duration of use increases, the performance improves (Balkany et al, 2002; Waltzman et al, 2002). In one study, word recognition scores increased from less than 1% before implantation to 8.9% at

1 year, to 30% at 3 years, and eventually reached 65%, and sentence recognition scores increased from 18% (1 year) to 42% (3 years) to 80% (Waltzman et al, 2002). These average scores were affected by age at implantation (higher scores for those implanted at younger ages).

Waltzman et al (2002) describe the recommended criteria for selecting candidates for implantation and for choosing the ear to be used. Cochlear implants are typically implanted in only one ear. This makes auditory localization more difficult and can result in uneven auditory input. Although there is work on bilateral cochlear implants (Loizou, 2006), the technical problems of stimulation, signal processing, and synchronization are formidable. An alternative approach when there is some residual hearing in one ear is to use a hearing aid in one ear and a cochlear implant in the other (Ching et al, 2001). Clear benefits have been demonstrated from having the combination of hearing aid and cochlear implant, but there are several factors that are important to consider. The use of the cochlear implant may lessen the desire for using the hearing aid because the hearing aid is less attractive or is perceived to interfere with the speech perception from the cochlear implant. If the child is used to the hearing aid, the cochlear implant may not be used as often as is necessary for habituation. Ching et al (2001) present four case studies of children fitted with both a hearing aid and a cochlear implant; they describe success factors and strategies for optimizing effectiveness of this combination of devices.

Telephone Access for Persons Who Are Deaf

The isolation imposed on deaf persons by the telephone is ironic given that Alexander Graham Bell was working on an aid for the deaf when he invented it. For some individuals, additional amplification is sufficient to make the telephone accessible. This may be built into the person's telephone or it may be an add-on unit that can be placed over the earpiece of any telephone. Both types of devices are available from local telephone companies. As discussed in the previous section, many hearing aids have a magnetic induction feature (telecoil) that allows the output of the telephone to be coupled to the hearing aid electromagnetically.

For many individuals with severe hearing loss, even increased amplification does not make the telephone signal audible. For these persons to obtain access to telephone conversations, a device that can visually send and receive telephone information is used. These individuals also often use master ring indicators, which either amplify the ringing of the telephone or connect the ringer to a table lamp that flashes when the telephone rings. These adaptations are also available from local telephone companies.

Telephone Devices for the Deaf. Originally, deaf individuals used teletype (TTY) devices designed for sending weather and news information over telephone lines to provide a "visual telephone." Many of these TTYs were donated by IBM and other companies to help deaf people talk to each other. The original TTY, now obsolete, consisted of a typewriter and electronic circuitry for converting the typed letters to pulses that could be sent over the telephone line to another TTY. The second TTY converted the pulses back into text that was typed on paper on the remote TTY. Because of their low cost, especially for surplus units, TTYs were very popular with deaf individuals, and some are still in use. A good source of information is the Gallaudet University Technology Assessment Program *(http://tap. gallaudet.edu)*.

Electronic versions of earlier TTYs are still referred to as TTYs (for example, Ameriphone, by Clarity, Chattanooga, Tenn., *http://www.clarityproducts.com/products/categories/ category345.asp;* Krown Mfg., Inc., Fort Worth, Tex., *www. krowntty.com;* Ultratec, Inc., Madison, Wis., *www.ultratec. com*). They use a keypad, a visual display, and a modulator-demodulator (modem) to convert the electronic signal to pulses. Connection to the telephone service is by one of three methods: (1) an acoustical coupler that couples the pulses directly to the telephone handset, (2) direct connection to the telephone line by a cable, and (3) cable connection to a cell phone. Some TTYs also function as telephones with additional amplification for users who are hard of hearing. Several models of current TTYs are lightweight, battery-powered devices for portable use. Some of these units are compatible with cell phones, further increasing access for users who are deaf. Additional features include built-in printers or connections for external printers, automatic answering messages, storage of phone numbers, answering machine capability, storage of conversations, and identification to the person being calling that a TTY is being used. TTYs should be thought of more as a phone than a data modem. An example of a TTY is shown in Figure 9-8. An acoustic coupler is required when calling from a pay telephone. In computer-to-computer telephone line communication, each computer can send and receive at the same time. Thus, if one device is sending, the other unit can interrupt it. This type of operation is called *full-duplex.* Because of their design, TTYs are only able to send (originate) or to receive at one time, not both; this is called *half-duplex* mode. After each transmission, the user must type *GA* (go ahead) to indicate that he is finished and then wait for a response. Half-duplex is also useful when voice communication is occurring because line discontinuities at switching stations or over long distance lines can result in a reflected signal that is heard as an echo by the speaker. Half-duplex switches the direction of transmission based on voice-activated sensors. Full-duplex operation requires that the sending and receiving computers solve the problem of echoes, but it is more rapid and it allows interruption of a long transmission if an error occurs. TTYs are extremely

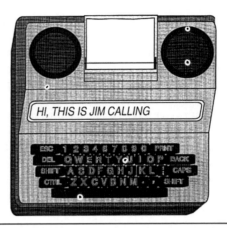

Figure 9-8   A typical TTY has an electronic display and a keyboard for typing messages.

easy to set up and use in the basic configuration. Advanced TTY features include use with an answering machine, remote retrieval of messages, message notification via paging, and a printer. The printer function gives both a permanent record of the conversation and a chance to review messages before responding to them. Some TTYs plug directly into cellular and cordless telephones to allow mobile use.

The TTYs also use a unique coding approach based on five bits of data, rather than the customary eight used in computer ASCII transmission. This code, called Baudot, is widely used by the deaf community, and it is still used in modern TTYs although it does not match the standard for all other computer communication, which is based on the ASCII code. When data are in ASCII form, they can be displayed on a computer screen, enlarged, combined with time or date information, and stored in files for later use. In contrast to ASCII, Baudot does not require a carrier signal, it uses only two frequencies (1800 and 1400 Hz), and it does not require "handshaking" protocols. As discussed in Chapter 7, communication between a computer and a peripheral or another computer is either parallel or serial. In serial transmission a rate of transmission, called the baud setting, must be the same for the receiving and the transmitting devices. TTYs typically use a rate of 110 to 300 baud. Computer modems typically use rates of 2400 baud or higher. The slower TTY speed offers an advantage when single-line displays are used because it is slow enough to be read during the transmission. Three hundred baud is the maximum that can be used easily with an acoustic coupler.

There are two primary ways to use the TTY with the telephone. If both parties have a TTY, then each simply types a message, sends a "go ahead" (the letters *GA*) command to indicate that he or she is finished, and then waits for an answer. If the deaf person needs to talk to someone who does not have a TTY, then the telephone company provides a relay operator. The operator, who has a TTY, reads the message sent by the deaf person to the hearing person. The response is then spoken to the operator, who types the message to the deaf person's TTY. Under the provisions of Title IV (telecommunications) of the Americans With Disabilities Act (ADA), all telephone services offered to the general public must include both interstate and intrastate relay services for persons who use TTYs. The Federal Communications Commission (FCC) issued the rules for Title IV, and this agency monitors compliance. These rules also require that both ASCII and Baudot capabilities be provided by the relay services. Approximately 95% of the calls through a relay operator use Baudot data format. Title IV regulations also specify the conduct of relay operators. The most important features of these rules are complete confidentiality and verbatim transmission of messages.

AT&T uses an interesting combination of the technologies described in this chapter in its relay services (Halliday, 1993). A blind operator serves as a relay communications assistant. Incoming voice messages are relayed by typing on a computer terminal that sends the message to the deaf person's TTY. Incoming TTY messages are converted to braille by use of a refreshable braille display and are then relayed by voice to the hearing person. This is a unique combination of technologies for persons who are deaf and who are blind, and it takes advantage of the skills of each individual.

There are a large number of deaf persons who have and use TTYs (Baudot protocol), and there are also many individuals who have personal computers with modems that use the ASCII protocol. Therefore, current TTYs often include both ASCII and Baudot protocols, and some computer programs that convert from one code to another are available. To use a computer for TTY communication, the user must have both TTY software and a modem that can emulate a TTY (Baudot at 300 baud) (for example, Next TalNXi Communications, Inc., Salt Lake City, Utah; Phone-TTY, Inc., Parsippany, NJ, *www.phone-tty.com;* Ultratec, Inc., Madison, Wis., *www.ultratec.com;* Soft TTY (Macintosh only), *www.softtty.com/*). The TTY software generates the Baudot codes and sends information to the TTY modem (hardware plugged into the computer). The modem then communicates with a stand-alone TTY at 300 baud. The modem must meet all the transmission protocols (e.g., frequency, five-bit code, half-duplex communication) of the Baudot TTY for the communication to be successful. These protocols are not available on standard computer modems, and that is the reason that a special TTY modem (with a setting of 300 baud to communicate in Baudot code with other TTYs) is required for successful communication with a TTY. A typical screen shot of a software-based TTY

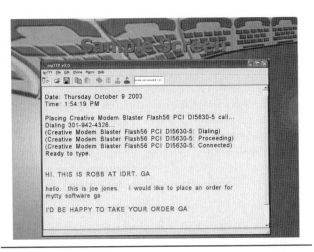

Figure 9-9 A screen shot of a software-based TTY system. (Courtesy SoftTTY, Inc.)

program in use is shown in Figure 9-9. Several windows are used, including incoming and outgoing messages, a phone book, and a log of past messages.

One of the major advantages of the Baudot-based TTYs is simplicity because all have the same transmission protocol. Use of ASCII offers a variety of protocols that differ in significant ways, and a successful transmission depends on both the transmitting and the receiving parties having the same setup. This requires that the sender know the protocol of the receiver. A hearing person can obtain this information by voice, an option not available to the deaf caller.

Williams, Jensema, and Harkins (1991) compared the features of 11 ASCII-based TTY products to determine their compatibility with Baudot devices. To determine compatibility of ASCII-based TTYs with each other, Williams, Jensema, and Harkins used each of the 11 devices in their sample to call each of the others. This resulted in 110 calls. The purpose of this study was to determine the degree to which deaf people could place a phone call successfully to other TTY products. To parallel the use of Baudot-based TTYs, in which the user can turn on the unit and immediately begin sending and receiving, no adjustment was made in the ASCII protocol other than to set it at the default settings.

Of the 110 outgoing calls, 77 (70%) were unsuccessful (e.g., receiving unit automatically switched to Baudot, garbled, or failed transmission). For incoming calls, 81 (74%) were unsuccessful. Combining incoming and outgoing results, only 12% of the total calls were successful on both ends. Many of the calls resulted in both ends being automatically switched to Baudot, eliminating all the advantages of using ASCII. Also, not all units had automatic switching (three for outgoing, seven for incoming).

CASE STUDY

SELECTING A TTY PROGRAM

The educational audiologist at a local school approached the assistive technology practitioner (ATP) for advice regarding a young child who is profoundly deaf. The family does not have a stand-alone TTY, but they do have a computer. They are interested in using it as a TTY. The computer has the advantage of being a full-screen, full-keyboard computer that may be easier for the child to use and to read than one-line, cramped-keyboard traditional models. However, the computer is not as portable. Also, if the phone rings with a TTY call while the computer is off, the call will be missed. The price of each approach is about the same. What approach should the ATP take to help the family make this choice? Special attention should be paid to helping them (1) decide whether their computer and modem will work with TTY software and (2) determine the tradeoffs between the stand-alone TTY and a computer-based TTY with TTY software.

Visual Telephones for the Deaf. Because it requires typing of each utterance, TTY telephone transmission is slow, typically one third to one fourth the rate of human speech (Galuska and Foulds, 1990). Visual sign language, on the other hand, results in communication rates comparable to human speech, and it is the primary form of communication used by individuals who are deaf. It does, of course, require that both the speaker and the listener understand sign language or that an interpreter be available. There are many situations in which this option is unavailable or impractical. For example, in a work setting it is not always practical to have an interpreter available for casual or unscheduled conversations. If standard telephone lines could be used to send visual images of manual signs, it would significantly increase communication rates over those obtained with use of TTYs.

There are several difficulties with sending video information over standard telephone lines. The most significant of these is that video signals contain much more information than audio signals. The way in which this larger amount of information is accommodated is to allow a wider bandwidth for the signals. The bandwidth is a measure of how much information can be accommodated. Because the telephone is intended to serve only voice communication, its bandwidth is very narrow (as low as 3000 Hz). In contrast, television channel bandwidths are measured in megahertz. Thus we have two choices: (1) increase the bandwidth of the telephone or (2) decrease the bandwidth of the video signal. If video telephones come into widespread usage in homes, then the first option will be realized. However, to allow use over any existing telephone line, the second approach is most practical. Narrowing the bandwidth of the video signal is accomplished by data compression (Galuska and Foulds, 1990). In this process the video signal is sent with lower bandwidth, and the intelligibility of the visual signing is used as a criterion for acceptability. Using a test instrument designed to simulate different bandwidths, Harkins, Wolff, and Korres (1991) tested four rates of transmission (slower rates are analogous to lower bandwidths). They found that intelligibility decreased with decreasing bandwidth and that a bandwidth about one third of the normal television signal provided was optimal. Decreases below this level resulted in significantly poorer intelligibility, but bandwidths greater than one third of the normal yielded only marginal improvement. Harkins, Wolff, and Korres (1991) also found that finger spelling at normal rates was less intelligible than whole words at normal rates or reduced-speed finger spelling.

In a work environment there is an alternative to the visual telephone that can provide many of the same benefits: the use of personal computers (PCs) and local area networks (LANs). LANs are typically used to transfer data and messages (e.g., electronic mail) from one PC to another within an office or over a wider network. When PCs and LANs are used in conjunction with a simple video camera and software, visual images can be sent from one computer to another (Galuska, Grove, and Gray, 1992). This allows two individuals with hearing impairments to communicate by sign language. Another, more far-reaching application is to use a LAN to provide interpretive services to a deaf employee or customer. The interpreter can be connected by video on the network to the employee. A speakerphone provides audio connection from the meeting to the interpreter and from the hearing impaired person (by the interpreter) to others at the meeting. The network video provides signed interpretation to the individual with a hearing impairment from the interpreter and from the hearing impaired individual to the interpreter for voice relay to the meeting.

SignWorks *(www.deafstudiestrust.demon.co.uk/text/Projects/sworksum)* is a project of the Deaf Studies Trust at the University of Bristol in the United Kingdom. The goal is to support deaf business within the United Kingdom. Because there is very little business activity in the United Kingdom by people who are deaf, SignWorks also helps new businesses get started and works with deaf entrepreneurs, managers, and professionals. A key element in this project is the use of multimedia information services. SignWorks uses on-line information services and visual telecommunications to create a system of advice for deaf people in business. SignWorks provides a range of services (e.g., job counseling and training support) and facilitates the development and application of telecommunications equipment. A key element of this project is the use of sign language on the telephone, allowing people who are deaf to conduct daily business on an equal standing with hearing people. The video telephone being used in the project is the mm220 by Motion Media Technology (Bristol, U.K., *www.mmtech.co.uk*). The videophone will be installed at libraries, schools, support organizations for the deaf, and companies that have deaf employees. The mm220 videophone is about the size of a traditional business telephone. It is one of the first videophones whose picture quality and speed can successfully transmit and receive sign language. It includes a built-in camera, microphone, and video screen. It can also be connected to a PC for two-way data sharing for documents, files, and interaction with Internet-based meetings software.

Another approach is to take advantage of the Internet and to use an interpreter located at a remote location who hears the conversation and then signs it over video for the individual who is deaf (Sorensen Communications, Inc. Salt Lake City, Utah, *www.sorenson.com/*). This approach is enabled by a broadband videophone appliance specifically designed for deaf and hard-of-hearing individuals (Sorenson VP-100). Sorenson Video Relay Service is a free service to conduct video relay calls with family, friends, and business associates through a certified sign language interpreter, Sorenson videophone, television, and a high-speed Internet connection. The deaf user sees an interpreter on their television and signs to the interpreter, who then contacts the hearing user by a standard phone line and relays the conversation between the two parties.

The use of an intermediary relay operator has been extended by one company to include a person who listens to the call as it comes in and captions the auditory information onto a small display built into the telephone (CapTel, Ultratec Madison, Wis., *www.captionedtelephone.com/*). Figure 9-10 shows how the system works. With this system, the user dials a call as on any other telephone. As the call is dialed, it is also connected to a captioning service. When the call is completed, the other party is connected to the caller in the normal way. In addition, the user captioning service transcribes everything the other party says into written text by use of voice-recognition technology. The written text appears almost simultaneously with the spoken word on a visual display on the captioning phone. The cost of the captioning service is covered by Telecommunications Relay Service funds as part of Title IV of the ADA. This approach requires both a special phone and the availability of the CapTel captioning service as part of the relay service provided by the state. This system also works with external voice answering machine messages.

Voice Over Internet Protocol.   Most telephone calls are made over the public switched telephone network, or PSTN. Increasingly, hearing users are moving to Internet-based telephone service, referred to as voice over Internet protocol (VoIP). There are many advantages to this change, including lower cost, inclusion of multimedia, and the features commonly available with cell phones or land-based networks, such as voicemail, caller ID, three-way calling, and other features included in the basic price of VoIP software or a VoIP service subscription. Originally Internet phone calls stayed within the Internet (PC to PC), but VoIP now bridges to the PSTN.

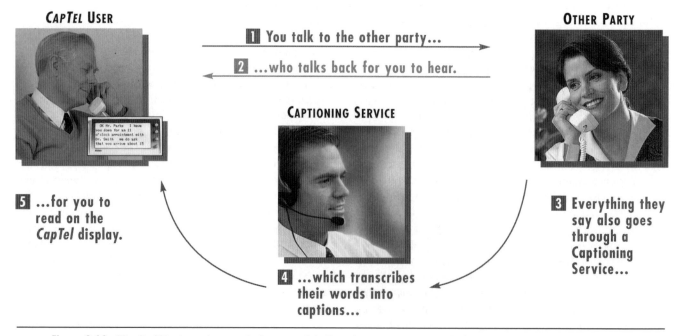

Figure 9-10   The CapTel private phone captioning system is built on the same concept as a telephone relay operator. (Courtesy CapTel.)

Although there are many reasons that both hearing and deaf users are attracted to VoIP, there are some issues of accessibility for VoIP (Harkins, 2004). One disadvantage is relay operator service, which is mandated by the PSTN regulator (FCC) under the ADA and into which PSTN companies pay a fee from each user. VoIP companies do not participate in this program and do not typically provide relay service. A second accessibility issue is that VoIP will often garble TTY messages, especially with heavy traffic on the network. TTY messages can also be garbled if lower-quality speech coding is used for the call to save bandwidth. Many TTYs cannot connect to VoIP phones and some VoIP phones cannot connect to any TTY except by acoustical coupling. This reduces access below that of the hearing user. There is technology (NexTalk VM, NXI, *www.nxicom.com/products-biz/nextalk_vm.html*) that allows Internet protocol (IP)-to-IP text inside an organization's IP network and allows outside communication with TTYs that are on the public switched telephone network. This is a limited solution relevant only to the organizations that have this technology, not the entire network. Voice quality can also vary over VoIP, which can affect individuals who are hard of hearing. The multimedia aspect of VoIP can lead to more effective use of video and its application to the use of sign language interpreters or lip reading. Advances will undoubtedly be made rapidly in VoIP as it becomes more popular, and this will include TTY compatibility.

Technology for Face-to-Face Communication Between Hearing and Deaf Individuals

The Sorenson method can be effective for face-to face conversations, but it requires time for setup and must be planned in advance for work meetings or casual conversations. For these purposes, assistive technologies that allow communication without speech or sign language interpretation can be very effective. One product, the Interpretype (ITY, Interpretype, Rochester, N.Y., *www.interpretype.com/index.php*) is designed specifically for this application. This system consists of a preprogrammed laptop-style computer that is able to send typed messages to other ITY units or a computer (Gan, 2005). A built-in display shows the text that is received from the communication partner and displays messages typed into its keyboard. The major advantage of this approach is its simplicity; however, these stand-alone devices are expensive relative to TTYs. For this reason some companies have developed simple modifications to TTYs to allow them to be used a face-to-face communication devices (Modern Deaf Communication, Inc, Danbury, Conn., *www.danbury.org/moderndeafcommunication/about_comm_equip.htm*) In this case the TTYs are interconnected, rather that being connected to a telephone line. Once connected, they function like the ITY device: one person types and the text show up on the other person's screen. The primary advantage of using simple technology for face-to-face communication is that it is simple to set up, lightweight to carry, and intuitive to use. Because many deaf individuals have portable TTYs, the modification for face-to-face use is more cost-effective. They still need to buy a second unit, but the total cost for both units can be less than $600 and the total weight can be less than 3 pounds (1.5 kg) (Modern Deaf Communication, Inc).

Alerting Devices for Persons With Auditory Impairments

There are many environmental sounds other than speech about which a person who is deaf needs to know. Examples are telephones, doorbells, smoke alarms, and a child's cry. There are **alerting devices** available that detect these sounds and then cause a vibration, a flashing light signal, or both to call attention to the sound. Some devices are very specific. For example, one device is tuned to the frequency of a smoke alarm and it responds only to that sound. When the smoke alarm auditory signal is detected, the visible smoke detector transmits a flasher, which can be connected to a standard lamp. The lamp flashes as long as the smoke detector is active.

Telephone alerting devices include amplified ringers that plug into a standard telephone jack and provide up to 95 dB of ringing sound (McFadden, 1996). Another approach is to use a flashing light that is connected to the telephone line. This can alert the person who is deaf that there is an incoming TTY call. Some systems have a strobe light connected to them; others use a table lamp plugged into the alerting device. The only modification required for these adaptations is a two-plug telephone adapter to allow plugging in of both the adapted alerting device and the telephone.

Doorbells can be both directly wired into a flashing light or detected by a microphone and then converted into a visible (typically a flashing light) or tactile (vibration) signal. For more general sound detection, there are silent alarms that can detect any signal and then transmit to a wrist-worn receiver. This both vibrates and flashes a light to indicate that the sound has occurred. Some devices can accommodate 16 or more channels, and different lights flash for each sound. A microphone and transmitter can be placed in each of the locations where an important sound may occur. For example, one can be near the front door, another near the telephone, another in the baby's room, and a final one near the back door. When a sound is detected at any of these locations, the wrist unit vibrates and one light is illuminated to indicate which sound has been detected.

Alarm clocks for persons who are deaf generally are either visible (flashing light on a bedside table) or tactile (vibration under the pillow). They may either be built in to an alarm clock (e.g., the entire face of the clock flashes) or they may detect the clock's alarm and then cause the vibration or flashing light (or both).

One of the major difficulties faced by persons who are deaf is the lack of awareness of sounds associated with traffic. Sirens, horns, and ambient traffic noise all contribute to our ability to drive. Miyazaki and Ishida (1987) developed a device that detects specific sounds and displays a visible alarm to the driver. Traffic horns of different types (air horn on a truck versus a car horn), sirens, railroad crossings, and motorcycles are typical of the sounds detected and displayed.

Assistive Listening Devices

All the devices discussed in this chapter have been designed for use by hearing-impaired individuals. There is also a class of assistive devices that are intended to be used in group settings, such as lecture halls, churches, business meetings, courtrooms, and broadcast television. These are called **assistive listening devices.**

Small-Group Devices. For many individuals who have auditory impairments, hearing aids are only effective for one-on-one conversations at close range (and possibly for telephone use). When these individuals are in a group, even a small group of five or fewer persons, it is very difficult for them to understand what is being said; *small-group* or *personal listening devices* are helpful in this situation (Williams and Snope, 1985). These devices consist of a microphone and a battery-powered radio transmitter that are worn by the speaker and a receiver that is carried by the person with an auditory impairment. The output of the receiver can either be fed into earphones (personal FM system) or coupled directly to the hearing aid (similar to the telephone aids described earlier). If the person does not normally use a hearing aid or the hearing aids used do not accommodate direct coupling of the signal, the earphones are used. The speaker uses a microphone and whatever he or she says is then transmitted to the listener with a high signal-to-noise ratio. For small-group meetings with several participants, the speaker and microphone can be placed in the middle of the conference table to pick up all the voices. Small-group devices can have multiple receivers for one transmitter if there is more than one person requiring amplification.

Several acoustical parameters affect speech perception in a classroom environment (Crandell and Smaldino, 2000). These are signal-to-noise ratio (SNR), reverberation time (RT), and distance from the speaker.

Classroom noise can be external to the classroom (outside the building such as street noise or inside the building such as other classes, hallway noise, etc.) or inside the classroom (other students talking, heating and air conditioning, moving of furniture). The SNR is the relationship between the speech amplitude from the teacher and the background noise. As the noise level increases, the perception of speech by children with and without hearing impairment falls. The decrement in speech perception is greater for children with sensorineural hearing loss. The greatest effect is on consonant perception. Because noise tends to mask frequencies above it in frequency, the effect is greater with low-frequency noise. Crandell and Smaldino (2000) recommend a SNR of at least +15dB.

RT is the prolongation or persistence of sound as it reflects off hard surfaces, specified as a time delay. Shorter RTs are better for speech perception. RT is longer with lower frequencies because sound is absorbed more readily at high frequencies. Like SNR, RT has a greater effect on children with hearing loss than for typically hearing children. Recommended RT values for classrooms are lower than 0.6 seconds (Crandell and Smaldino, 2000).

The final factor is distance from the speaker. As this distance increases, the sound level decreases up to a critical value determined by the volume of the room, directionality of the speech signal relative to the listener, and the RT. Beyond the critical distance reverberated signals arrive from sources closer than the speaker (e.g., walls, ceiling) and mask the original signal to a greater extent. Positioning a child in the front of the room near the teacher does not solve the problem because reverberated signals and other speech (e.g., a child participating in a discussion) come from throughout the room. These factors indicate that a room that is acoustically well designed (low noise sources, short RT) and have a uniform speaker-to-listener distance will be most effective for children with and without hearing limitations. Classrooms designed within these guidelines have been shown to positively affect academic performance in reading, spelling, concentration, and attention (Crandell and Smaldino, 2000).

One approach to achieving uniform sound throughout the room and avoiding the problems of distance from the speaker is the use of sound field systems (Ross and Levitt, 2002). As shown in Figure 9-11, the teacher's voice is transmitted to speakers located around the room, so the teacher's voice is presented uniformly throughout the classroom. The original systems used FM radio transmission. Recently, infrared (IR) transmission systems have come into use. The primary advantage of the IR systems is that the signal is contained within the classroom and there is no interference between classrooms or from outside radio sources. Research shows that sound from a teacher typically is at a level only about 6 dB above background noise in a typical classroom. Sound field systems can boost this to 8 to 10 dB which is a much more suitable SNR (Ross and Levitt, 2002). The effectiveness of these systems depends on sound acoustical room design to maximize SNR and minimize RT. The maximum benefit of sound field systems is to children with mild hearing loss and those with attention deficit and learning disabilities. For children with more profound hearing loss, sound field systems also allow direct transmission to

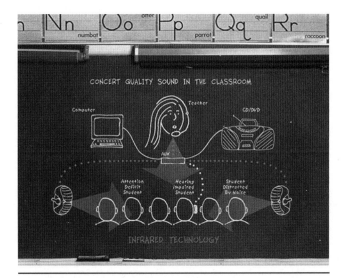

Figure 9-11   A typical sound field system setup. (Courtesy Telex.)

an individual student through earphones by coupling to a personal FM system. Sound field systems have been shown to increase speech perception, improve academic skills (reading, spelling), and address learning disabilities (e.g., attention). Typically hearing students have also been shown to benefit from sound field systems and teachers benefit from greater student attention and less vocal strain. One additional benefit of some sound field systems is the use of ambient noise compensation (ANC) (Ross and Levitt, 2002). ANC uses digital signal processing to automatically increase amplification if the noise level rises temporarily because of factors such as a transient noise (e.g., air conditioning starting up) or a decrease in the teacher's speaking volume. Adjustment for these changes in the ANC allows the sound field system to maintain a constant SNR for the student.

Several manufacturers produce devices that combine a conventional BTE hearing aid with an FM system (for example, the Extend Ear, AVR Communication Limited, Eden Prairie, Minn., *www.avrsono.com;* Microlink, Phonak Staeta, Switzerland, *www.phonak.com*). Some manufacturers use a "boot" that fits over the bottom of the BTE device and directly couples the amplified sound to the hearing aid. Other manufacturers have built the FM receiver directly into the case of the BTE. In either case, a transmitter sends the radio signal from the person who is speaking to the wireless receiver attached to or built in to the BTE device. The hearing aid user can switch between hearing aid only, hearing aid plus FM, and FM-only modes. In the FM-only mode, the user would hear only the speech of the person wearing the transmitter. However, if the user wanted to monitor his or her own voice or hear another child's answer to a question in class, the hearing aid plus FM mode might be more appropriate.

Large-Group Devices.   The problems addressed by small-group devices also exist in large meeting rooms such as concert halls, lecture auditoriums, and churches. Under the provisions of the ADA, these areas must be equipped with assistive listening devices. There are several approaches possible, all of which are directly coupled to the public address system of the facility being equipped. These are (1) hard-wired jacks for plugging in earphones, (2) FM transmitter-receiver setups similar to small-group devices, and (3) audio induction loops for transmission to hearing aids equipped with telecoils (Williams and Snope, 1985). Hard-wired systems have the advantage of privacy (there is no transmission over the air) and simplicity of technology. There are two primary limitations of this approach, however. First, rewiring a facility has a high cost and, unless the wiring is done during construction, it is usually not feasible. Second, persons requiring the use of the assisted listening device are forced to sit in a few predetermined locations (where there are earphone jacks).

The audio induction loop devices have their roots in Europe. They require that the user's hearing aid have an induction coil (*telecoil*). The major limitations of the induction coil approach are the large amount of power required to drive the induction coil transmitter and susceptibility to interference. FM transmission has a lower level of interference, a large transmission range, and a transmission band specifically for use by persons with hearing impairment (72 to 76 MHz). However, recently the 72- to 76-MHz transmission band has been inundated with interference from cellular telephones, pagers, and other devices. The FCC has put out a notice of proposed rulemaking to secure the band from 215 to 217 MHz for FM system use. FM systems have the advantage that the listener can sit anywhere within range, and they can easily be wired into the normal public address system. Limitations of this approach include varying degrees of strength in the signals being received by the receivers in different hearing aids and a nonuniform transmission pattern resulting in unequal signal strength.

Other assistive listening devices have been developed for television viewing and for use as personal amplifiers (Stach, 1998). Personal amplifiers are hard-wired microphones connected to an amplifier and to earphones worn by the person who is hard of hearing. They are used in hospitals and similar situations for temporary amplification when hearing aids are not available or not worn. Television listeners are assistive listening devices that connect directly to the audio of the television set and transmit the signal to a receiver by FM or ultrasound. The user has earphones connected to the receiver.

Captioning as an Auditory Substitute

Captioning is a process whereby the audio portion of a television program is converted to written words, which appear in a window on the screen. Captioning substitutes visual (text) information for auditory (voice) information. The most common application is in commercial television and films. Captioning is also used as an alternative to sign language interpreters in classrooms, meetings, and for face-to-face conversations.

Closed-Captioned Television and Movies. When captioning is used in public media (television, movie theaters), it is **closed captioning.** It is called closed because the words are not visible unless the viewer has a closed-caption decoder. In the United States the Telecommunications Act of 1996 (see Chapter 1) resulted in FCC regulations requiring television broadcasters to provide closed captioning. New programming released after January 1, 1998, must be "fully accessible." *Fully accessible* means that 95% of the nonexempt programming must be closed captioned. A tele-caption decoder can be connected to a television set, video-cassette recorder, or cable television receiver to decode the captioning signal and display the words on the screen. All television sets currently being produced have a built-in closed caption converter. It takes between 20 and 30 hours to close caption a 1-hour television program. The individual broadcasters make decisions regarding which programs are captioned consistent with the regulations described above. Some programs, such as live newscasts, are captioned on the fly, whereas others are captioned in postproduction. With approximately 20 million new televisions sold in the United States each year, every household was expected to have at least one caption-capable set by the year 2000.

More than 3000 titles of home videos and nearly 500 hours of network, cable, and independent programming a week are now available in closed-caption form. Closed captioning includes movies, network news, comedies, sporting events, dramas, and educational, religious, and children's programming. In excess of 550 national advertisers have closed captioned more than 13,000 commercials. The National Captioning Institute (NCI) can also caption live programs such as news broadcasts, presidential speeches, and coverage of the Olympics. Captions can aid those learning English as a second language and provide assistance in efforts to eradicate illiteracy.

People who are deaf or blind can enjoy first-run movies in theaters. A project carried out by the CPB/WGBH National Center for Accessible Media (*www.wgbh.org/ wgbh/pages/ncam/*) in Boston has developed systems that enable these populations to access movies through closed captions (for deaf patrons) and descriptive narration (for blind patrons). Both these adaptations have been developed to avoid altering of the movie-going experience for the general audience. Reversed captions are displayed by the Rear Window Captioning System on a light-emitting diode text display that is mounted in the rear of a theater. Deaf and hard-of-hearing persons use transparent acrylic panels

attached to their seats to reflect the captions so that they appear to be superimposed on the movie screen. The caption users can sit anywhere in the theater because the reflective panels are both portable and adjustable. Blind and visually impaired moviegoers can hear the descriptive narration on headsets using the DVS Theatrical system. The narration is delivered by IR or FM listening systems. These descriptions provide information about key visual elements such as actions, settings, and scene changes. This makes the movies more meaningful to people with vision loss. Initially only available in specialty theaters, these technologies are being introduced into conventional movie theaters. The captioning and descriptive narration systems are integrated into the movie projection sound system by use of CD-ROM technology. A reader attached to the film projector reads a time code printed on the film. The caption and descriptive narration tracks are recorded on a separate CD-ROM, which plays alongside the other disks in the movie sound player. The information on the movie time code signals the CD sound player to play the audio descriptions synchronously with the film soundtrack. The CD player also sends the captions to the light-emitting diode display and the descriptive narration to the IR or FM emitter. WGBH is working with all the major studios and exhibitors to encourage them to adopt these technologies and make closed captions and descriptive narration available for movies on a continuing basis.

Real-Time Captioning for Education and Business Applications. Computer-assisted realtime (or remote) transcription (CART) has been applied in several different ways (Figure 9-12). For lectures or meetings where there is one deaf participant, CART can be provided one-on-one where a stenographer translates speech into text in real time and it is displayed on a monitor for the individual who is deaf. For meetings in which there is more than one deaf participant, the text output is projected on a screen, generally from a computer. The Internet can also be used to assist deaf individuals with spoken language interpretation. The stenographer has voice connection through the Internet to the meeting or classroom and enters text with a stenotype machine. The text is translated through computer software to text, transmitted over the Internet back to the classroom or meeting, and then read by the deaf individual. Several vendors provide CART services (for example, Hear Ink, *www.hearink.com/*; Caption First, *www.captionfirst.com/*).

Another example is computer-assisted notetaking (CAN) (Youdelman and Messerly, 1996). A fast typist enters text with a standard computer keyboard and with use of abbreviations (see Chapter 7) to maximize speed of data entry. As in the CART method, text is displayed on a screen. The rate of entry is too slow for the speech to be converted directly to text, so a summary is used. The accuracy of the summary is estimated to be in the 90% to 95% range. In an evaluation study, Youdelman and Messerly (1996) found

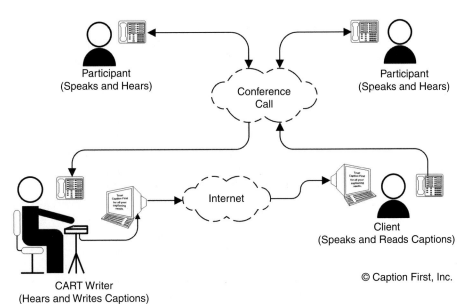

Figure 9-12   Schematic representation of a computer-assisted realtime (or remote) transcription (CART). (Courtesy Caption First, http://www.captionfirst.com/.)

that notetakers found this approach to be superior to pencil and paper methods because speed could be increased without sacrificing legibility, text could be easily edited, printed copies could be made available to students immediately, and emphasis of important points could be enhanced by bold, italic, or underline formats. The teachers felt that the CAN approach helped students obtain more information than they had with previous methods and that the printed method improved spelling skills. Because CAN was applied to uncaptioned videotapes and other media, it had an additional benefit. The teachers also noted a positive impact on the entire class, not just on the hearing-impaired students, because it helped the entire class focus on the material covered and helped them develop good note-taking skills. The hearing-impaired students stated that CAN helped them understand the material and keep up with the teacher. The children without hearing impairments observed that it was helpful to glance at the display as the teacher was talking to gain information missed orally. They also benefited from the printed notes.

Captioning by Automatic Speech Recognition.
Students who are deaf depend on oral lectures for information in the classroom in elementary, secondary, and postsecondary education, and there is an increase in auditory information on the Web. Given the cost of interpreters ($50 per hour or more) and stenographers for real-time captioning ($100-200 per hour), the cost of making an educational experience accessible for a deaf student is high for universities (Bain et al, 2005). All these factors add to the problems. One possible solution to access to information for people who are deaf is the use of automatic speech recognition (ASR) (see Chapter 7) in captioning systems

(Bain et al, 2005). In an ideal system the auditory information would be translated into text and displayed for the deaf user. Current ASR systems are speaker dependent, requiring training of the software to recognize the speech patterns of the speaker. Thus, a general-purpose ASR captioning device that would recognize any speaker's voice is not currently feasible.

As an intermediary step, IBM in conjunction with a number of universities has developed what they call the Liberated Learning Project (Bain et al, 2005). In this system the ASR system is trained by a professor at the beginning of a course, creating a personalized voice profile. The IBM software, called ViaScribe *(www-306.ibm.com/able/ solution_offerings/ViaScribe.html)*, is an ASR application that produces real-time closed-captioning of spontaneous speech. Because the final text is also printed, the system serves as a note-taking application as well. A proof of concept project using VisScribe was conducted in conjunction with St Mary's University in Nova Scotia, Canada (Bain et al, 2005). This project successfully implanted the basic concept of real-time automatic closed-captioning with significant overall cost savings to the universities involved. ViaScribe allows the instructor to speak naturally without interjecting punctuation (e.g., saying "period" at the end of a sentence), as is required by most ASR systems. When the speaker pauses, the text display skips to the next line. If the ASR makes an error, ViaScribe presents errors written phonetically rather than presenting an incorrect word. The program automatically synchronizes captions with slides or videos. The instructor says commands such as "next slide" or "start presentation" and the captioning appears with the visual information. ViaScribe uses the synchronized multimedia integration language (see Chapter 8) to create a file that synchronizes various media with the text transcript used for captioning. Options include multiple screens or single screens with multiple windows and editing before printing. After a presentation, the multimedia lecture and presentation notes are made available by webcast over the Internet. The Liberated Learning Project evaluation substantiated the promise and feasibility of the concept of ASR to captioning as a viable technology for classroom use in universities (Bain et al, 2005). There needs to be continual improvements in the accuracy and reductions in the time for editing to ensure that this approach is both feasible and cost-effective in the long run.

Basic Principles of Computer Adaptations for Auditory Impairments

The basic characteristics of the graphical user interface are described in Chapter 8. Increasingly, there is auditory information that is included with programs or Web pages. For persons who are deaf, this information may be inaccessible. If an individual is hard of hearing, the system volume can generally be increased. It is also possible to use headphones and link more directly to the user's auditory system. Computer interaction is bidirectional, and the ATP must understand how computer outputs can be adapted for persons with sensory impairments. Persons who are deaf or hard of hearing also may have difficulties in recognizing auditory computer outputs, such as sounds or speech.

Built-in Options to Increase Usability by Persons Who Are Deaf.
Adaptations that facilitate some of these functions and that are included in the **accessibility options** in Windows and Macintosh are shown in Table 9-1. ToggleKeys (Windows XP) generates a sound when the

TABLE 9-1	Simple Adaptations for Auditory Impairment
Need Addressed	Software Approach
User cannot hear speech and sounds produced by programs or Web pages	ShowSounds, Flash Screen, Visual Notifications*
User cannot hear sounds used to signal change of operation or error during program operation	SoundSentry

Software modifications developed at the Trace Center, University of Wisconsin, Madison. These are included as before-market modifications in most personal computers.
*ShowSounds: Windows XP, Microsoft, Redmond, Wash. (*www.microsoft.com/enable/*); Flash Screen: Macintosh, Apple Computer, Cupertino, Calif. (*www.apple.com/education/accessibility/technology/*); Visual Notifications: Windows Vista, Microsoft, Redmond, Wash.

CAPS LOCK, NUM LOCK, or SCROLL LOCK keys are pressed. ShowSounds (Windows XP) displays captions for speech and sounds. SoundSentry (Windows XP) generates a visual warning when the system generates a sound. The Flash Screen feature (Mac OS X) provides a visual indication of alert sounds. When a sound is emitted, Flash Screen will also flash the screen once. In addition to the benefit to hearing-impaired students, non-hearing-impaired students my also appreciate the option of having visual rather than auditory alerts. A variety of screen flash options are available. Windows Vista uses Visual Notifications to replace system sounds with visual cues, such as a flash on the screen, so system alerts are announced with visual notifications instead of sounds. The way in which the warning from Sound Notifications is presented is also variable. Vista also allows the user to display text captions for spoken dialog in multimedia programs. By using this option, the user can also cause Windows to display text captions in place of sounds to indicate that an activity is happening (for example, when a document starts or finishes printing).

Access to the Internet When Auditory Information Is Difficult for the User.
Because Web pages are a mixture of text, graphics, and sound, they can present challenges to individuals who are deaf or hard of hearing. As the amount of auditory Web content increases, people who are deaf are also prevented from accessing information. Chapter 8 describes general issues of access and how Web pages are developed, including the use of programming languages such as hypertext markup language. The World Wide Web Consortium (W3C) (see Chapter 8) recommendations include accessibility for deaf and hard of hearing users. By using the Microsoft Synchronized Accessible Media Interchange, authors of Web pages and multimedia software can add closed captioning for users who are deaf or hard of hearing. This standard simplifies captioning for developers, educators, and multimedia producers and designers and is available to the public as an open (no licensing fees) standard. This approach is similar to the use of closed captioning for television viewers. The W3C Web Accessibility Initiative synchronized multimedia integration language is designed to facilitate multimedia presentations in which an author can describe the behavior of a multimedia presentation, associate hyperlinks with media objects, and describe the layout of the presentation on a screen. These features allow integration of timing of multimedia presentations into hypertext markup language programs. The W3C Quick Tips shown in Box 8-2 include auditory adaptations.

Aids for Persons With Both Visual and Auditory Impairments

Individuals who are both deaf and blind must use tactile input to obtain information about the environment and to communicate. There are two basic methods used by this group of people. The Tadoma method (described earlier in this chapter) is used to understand speech; finger spelling, with the deaf-blind individual sensing the signs in his hand, is used when both persons in the conversation know signing or one person acts as an interpreter.

Devices for Face-to-Face Communication With Individuals Who Are Deaf and Blind.

A common approach to communication between a nondisabled person and individual who is both deaf and blind is to use a standard keyboard and visual display for the nondisabled person and a braille keyboard and display for the person who deaf/blind (for example, ITY, Intertype, Rochester, N.Y., *www.interpretype.com/index.php;* FSTTY and FSCommunicator, Freedom Scientific, St Petersburg, Fla., *www.freedomscientific.com/fs_products/FlyerPDFs/FSTTYFlyer.pdf;* Braille-TTY telephone, Krown, Ft Worth, Tex., *www.krownmfg.com/html/products/vtouch_tty.html;* Telle-touch, Perkins, Watertown, Mass., *https://support.perkins.org/store_product.asp?key={F4F388C9-3A81-4157-A660-841A8B2E2232};* Braillephone, *http://www.av-mart.com/Braillephone.htm*). This configuration enables direct face-to-face communication with individuals who have no knowledge of sign language or braille to communicate with a person who is both deaf and blind. One approach uses a portable note-taking device (PACMate, Freedom Scientific) with built-in Braille keyboard and refreshable display (see Chapter 8) with PC-based TTY software. An early method (Telle-touch, *https://support.perkins.org/store_product.asp?key={F4F388C9-3A81-4157-A660-841A8B2E2232}*) uses a regular QWERTY keyboard and a single braille cell. As the hearing user types, the deaf-blind user feels the text one letter at a time. An expansion of that concept has a braille display, TTY, QWERTY keyboard and visible display all built into the same case (Braillephone; Braille-TTY telephone). The TTY function provides the capability for the deaf-blind person to talk to other people who have a TTY or, through a relay operator, anyone with a telephone. The keyboards (braille and QWERTY) and displays (braille and visual) allow face-to face communication. Finally, another approach uses two separate devices connected by cable or wireless transmission (ITY, Intertype). Both the hearing and deaf-blind user have a keyboard and display, which may be QWERTY or braille keyboard and visual or braille display. The advantage of this approach is that the two people communicating can have a more comfortable physical spacing as they communicate because they each have their own devices. The device can either be a stand-alone system designed for this purpose or a computer running special software.

Automated Hand for Finger Spelling.

One of the difficulties for deaf-blind individuals who depend on finger spelling is that the speaker must be able to finger spell or

there must be an interpreter present. A further limitation is that the deaf-blind person gives up privacy when an interpreter is used. One approach, still under development, is the use of a mechanical hand connected to a keyboard (Gilden and Jaffe, 1987). The hand is fully articulated; that is, all joints of each finger are independently adjustable. The finger positions for each letter are stored in the computer and are generated when a letter is typed from the keyboard. The mechanical hand can also be connected to a TTY for telephone conversations and to a remote computer by a modem for bulletin boards. Because it is programmed to accept computer input from a keyboard, it can also accept alphabetical characters from a computer. This allows it to be connected to a text-scanning computer in place of the normal voice synthesizer. An evaluation of the second generation of this hand by a group of deaf-blind individuals showed that some could easily interpret the finger patterns, whereas others had great difficulty (Jaffe, Harwin, and Harkins, 1993). On the basis of these results, as well as advances in mechanical design, a third generation of this hand was developed (Jaffe, Harwin, and Harkins, 1993). This version is faster, smaller, and more portable. Finger positions are also more accurately portrayed. Because many deaf-blind individuals are born deaf and blindness develops over the course of the late teenage years, they learn to finger spell early but do not learn braille. Therefore, by the time they become blind they desire a system they can use easily, and the mechanical finger meets this need.

◾ SUMMARY

Hearing aids provide assistance for persons whose hearing is inadequate for conversation. Recent trends in hearing aid design have focused on improved fidelity and digital speech processing. An individual who has damage to the cochlea may benefit from the use of cochlear implants. Emphasis on speech processing algorithms will continue to provide better understanding of how stimulation by cochlear implants can aid speech recognition.

Aids for persons who are deaf use either visual or tactile systems as alternatives. Speech-to-text (sound-to-visual display) devices are not as well developed as text-to-speech aids, and visual information is most commonly used for alarms rather than for communication. Exceptions to this are telephone communication using telephone devices for the deaf (TTYs).

Aids for persons who are both deaf and blind must use tactile substitution. The major approach is braille output with a text-based keyboard for communication between a sighted and a deaf-blind individual. A mechanical device that emulates finger spelling (commonly used by deaf-blind persons) and is driven by a computer with keyboard entry provides communication between a sighted person who does not know finger spelling and a deaf-blind person who does.

Study Questions

1. What are the two basic approaches to auditory sensory aids in terms of the sensory pathway used?
2. List the three basic parts of an auditory sensory aid and describe the function of each part.
3. Discuss the major differences between blindness and deafness in terms of the effect on the individual's social, work or school, and private lives.
4. What are the major parts of a hearing aid, and what is the function of each?
5. What are the four types of hearing aids?
6. What is acoustic coupling, and how does it affect hearing aid performance?
7. How does a bone-anchored hearing aid function, and when is it used?
8. List the major functions that a cochlear implant must accomplish.
9. What are the major differences among analog, digitally controlled analog, and digital hearing aids?
10. What is meant by *compression* in hearing aids?
11. What is the difference between linear and curvilinear amplification in hearing aids?
12. How are data and power coupled to cochlear implants?
13. What is the relationship between the number of electrodes and the functional performance for a cochlear implant?
14. What are the major differences between a channel and an electrode in cochlear implants?
15. Describe the major approaches to signal processing used in cochlear implants. What are the advantages and disadvantages of each?
16. What is a TTY, and why is the Baudot code used?
17. What is CapTel and how does it work?
18. Compare a stand-alone TTY with a computer TTY modem using Baudot coding. What advantages does each offer to a deaf user?
19. Why can't a standard computer modem be used to communicate with a TTY without special software?
20. What are the major limitations to the use of standard telephone lines for visual information transmission (such as for manual signing)?
21. What is computer-assisted realtime transmission and how does it apply to education, business, and personal use?
22. Explain how ViaScribe makes automatic speech recognition a viable captioning option. What are the constraints on this application?
23. What are "alerting devices"? For what purposes are they normally used?
24. What are FM transmission systems for group listening, and how are they typically used?
25. What are the three major assistive technology approaches used for deaf-blind individuals to obtain communication input? What are the relative advantages of each approach?
26. Discuss the major differences between blindness and deafness in terms of the effect on the individual's social, work or school, and private lives?

References

Bain K et al: Accessibility, transcription, and access everywhere, *IBM Syst J* 44:589-603, 2005.

Balkany TJ et al: Cochlear implants in children—a review, *Acta Otolaryngol* 122:356-362, 2002.

Berger KW, Hagberg EN, Rane RL: *Prescription of hearing aids: rationale, procedures and results*, Kent, Ohio, 1977, Herald.

Ching TYC et al: Management of children using cochlear implants and hearing aids, *Volta Rev* 103:39-57, 2001.

Crandell CC, Smaldino JJ: Classroom acoustics for children with normal hearing and with hearing impairment, *Lang Speech Hearing Serv Schools* 31:362-370, 2000.

Dillon H: Compression in hearing aids. In Sandlin RE, editor: *Handbook of hearing aid amplification*, vol 1, Boston, 1988, Little, Brown.

Dillon H: *Hearing aids*, New York, 2001, Thieme.

Feigenbaum E: Cochlear implant devices for the profoundly hearing impaired, *IEEE Eng Med Biol Mag* 6:10-21, 1987.

Galuska S, Foulds R: A real-time visual telephone for the deaf In *Proceedings of the 13th Annual RESNA Conference*, pp 267-268, Washington, DC, 1990, RESNA.

Galuska S, Grove T, Gray J: A visual "talk" utility: Using sign language over a local area computer network. In *Proceedings of the 15th Annual RESNA Conference*, pp 134-135, Washington, DC, 1992, RESNA.

Gan K: Interpretype—assistive technology for face-to-face communication, Proceedings of the CSUN Conference (2005): http://www.csun.edu/cod/conf/2005/proceedings/2168.htm. Accessed April 2007.

Gilden D, Jaffe DL: Speaking in hands, *SOMA* October:6-13, 1987.

Halliday J: How can braille help people who are deaf, *Hum Awareness Newsl* Autumn, 1993.

Harkins J: Voice over IP: Some accessibility issues. In *The Blue Book: 2005 TDI national directory and resource guide*, pp. 21-23, Silver Spring, Md, 2004, TDI.

Harkins JE, Wolff AB, Korres E: Intelligibility experiments with a feature extraction system designed to simulate a low-bandwidth video telephone for deaf people. In *Proceedings of the 14th Annual RESNA Conference*, pp 38-40, Washington, DC, 1991, RESNA.

Jaffe DL, Harwin WS, Harkins JE: The development of a third generation finger spelling aid. In *Proceedings of the 16th Annual RESNA Conference*, pp 161-163, Washington, DC, 1993, RESNA.

Levitt H: Digital hearing aids: Past, present and future. In *Practical hearing aid selection and fitting*, pp. xi-xxiii, Washington, DC, 1997, Department of Veterans Affairs.

Lieberman P: *Intonation, perception and language*, Cambridge, Mass, 1967, MIT Press.

Loizou P: Mimicking the human ear, *IEEE Signal Processing Mag* 15:101-130, 1998.

Loizou P: Speech processing in vocoder-centric cochlear implants, *Adv Otorhinolaryngol* 64:109-143, 2006.

McFadden GM: Aids for hearing impairments and deafness. In Galvin JC, Scherer MJ, editors: *Evaluating, selecting and using appropriate assistive technology*, Rockville, MD, 1996, Aspen Publishers.

Miyazaki S, Ishida A: Traffic-alarm sound monitor for aurally handicapped drivers, *Med Biol Eng Comput* 25:68-74, 1987.

Olsen W: Average speech levels and spectra in various speaking/listening conditions: a summary of the Pearson, Bennett and Fidell (1977) report, *Am J Audiol* 7:21-25, 1988.

Preves DA: Principles of signal processing. In Sandlin RE, editor: *Handbook of hearing aid amplification*, vol 1, Boston, 1988, Little, Brown.

Ramsden RT: Cochlear implants and brain stem implants, *Br Med Bull* 63:183-193, 2002.

Ross M, Levitt H: Classroom sound-field systems, *Volta Voices* 9-2:7-8, 2002

Shallop JK, Mecklenberg DJ: Technical aspects of cochlear implants. In Sandlin RE, editor: *Handbook of hearing aid amplification*, vol 1, Boston, 1988, Little, Brown.

Snik AFM et al. Consensus statements on the BAHA system: where do we stand at present? *Ann Otol Rhinol Laryngol* 114(Suppl 195):1-12, 2005.

Stach BA: *Clinical audiology*, San Diego, 1998, Singular Publishing Group.

Waltzman S et al: Long-term effects of cochlear implants in children, *Otolaryngol Head Neck Surg* 126:505-511, 2002.

White RL: System design of a cochlear implant, *IEEE Eng Med Biol Mag* 6:10-21, 1987.

Williams NS, Jensema CJ, Harkins JE: ASCII-based TDD products: Features and compatibility. In *Proceedings of the 14th Annual RESNA Conference*, pp 41-43, Washington, DC, 1991, RESNA.

Williams PS, Snope T: *Assistive listening devices: professional practices*, Washington, DC, 1985, American Speech-Language and Hearing Association.

Wilson BS et al: Design and evaluation of a continuous interleaved sampling (CIS) processing strategy for multichannel cochlear implants, *J Rehabil Res* 30:110-116, 1993.

Youdelman K, Messerly C: Computer-assisted note taking for mainstreamed hearing-impaired students, *Volta Rev* 98:191-200, 1996.

PART 4

The Activities: Performance Areas

CHAPTER 10

Assistive Technologies for Cognitive Augmentation

Kim Adams, Roger Calixto, Al Cook, Lui Shi Gan, Andrew Ganton,

J. Andrew Rees, Tyler Simpson, Rebecca Watchorn

Chapter Outline

Learning Objectives

On completing this chapter, you will be able to do the following:

1. Apply the human activity assistive technology model to help identify appropriate assistive technologies for individuals with cognitive disabilities
2. Identify cognitive skills that underlie functional performance for persons with cognitive disabilities
3. Understand what cognitive faculties are commonly compromised in specific disorders
4. Understand the role of assistive technologies in aiding cognitive function
5. Identify and describe some of the assistive technologies that are currently available to assist individuals with cognitive impairments

Key Terms

Alternative Input	Developmental Disabilities	Mild Cognitive Disabilities
Alternative Output	Encoding	Problem Solving
Attention	Generalization	Prompting
Attention Deficit Hyperactivity	Information Processing	Smart House
Disorder	Intellectual Disability	Stimuli Control
Autism Spectrum Disorder	Knowledge Representation	Tracking and Identification
Cerebral Vascular Accident	Learning Disabilities	Traumatic Brain Injury
Cognitive Prosthesis	Media Presentation	Vigilance
Dementia	Memory	

The majority of currently available assistive technologies are designed to meet the needs of individuals who have motor or sensory limitations. Those assistive devices are the subject of most of this book. Recently, designers of assistive technologies have turned their attention to the needs of individuals whose limitations are primarily cognitive. An example of this type of technology is shown in Figure 10-1. This chapter explores cognitive applications of assistive technologies beginning with a description of the primary cognitive disorders that lead to assistive technology needs. After the description of disorders, several cognitive skills, the major characteristics of cognitive assistive technologies, and applications that aid or replace specific cognitive abilities are described.

Recall that the human activity assistive technology (HAAT) model (see Chapter 2) consists of four elements: human, activity, context, and assistive technology (see Figure 2-2). This chapter focuses on the human skills in the area of cognition. To apply the HAAT model, a desired activity would be identified. For example, the activity might be carrying out a sequence of steps such as for making a bed. The context would also be identified, and in this example it is the home. Given the activity and the context, the required set of skills to accomplish the activity can be determined. If there is a gap between the skills required to complete the task and the skills that the individual brings to the task, the use of assistive technologies to aid or replace the required skill should be considered. In this case, if the person has an **intellectual disability** that affects his or her ability to remember the required sequence of steps to make the bed, then a prompting device might be helpful. For any particular disability a skill set and possible limitations can be identified. Note that the expected skills and limitations presented in this chapter are general and that every individual is unique. The process of identifying and applying assistive technologies for cognitive assistance is illustrated in the case studies of William and Darrell.

CASE STUDY

INTELLECTUAL DISABILITY AND TASKS OF DAILY LIVING

William is a 38-year-old man with an intellectual disability. He lives in a group home with five other men. He is expected to carry out duties to contribute to the program at the home. His task is to set the table for dinner. Currently he is only successful in completing this task if he has continuous prompting from a member of the staff. This is limiting both to William, because he is not independent, and to the home because the staff is occupied making dinner during the time William is to carry out this task. Fortunately, there are assistive technologies available to assist William in this task. List the characteristics you think such a technology should have and then look at the descriptions later in this chapter of approaches that have been taken. Did you come up with better ideas than what is available?

■ COGNITIVE SKILLS

The basic mechanisms of human thought are important in understanding human behavior in many different circumstances. Understanding the underlying thought processes that are involved in various tasks can help us understand why an individual may find a seemingly simple task to be very difficult, whereas a seemingly difficult task may be carried out virtually effortlessly. The field of cognitive psychology attempts to discover mental representations and the processes that operate on them (Willingham, 2001). Unfortunately, cognitive psychology is still a relatively new field, and therefore many possible representations and processes are waiting to be discovered. Thus, a complete atlas detailing all

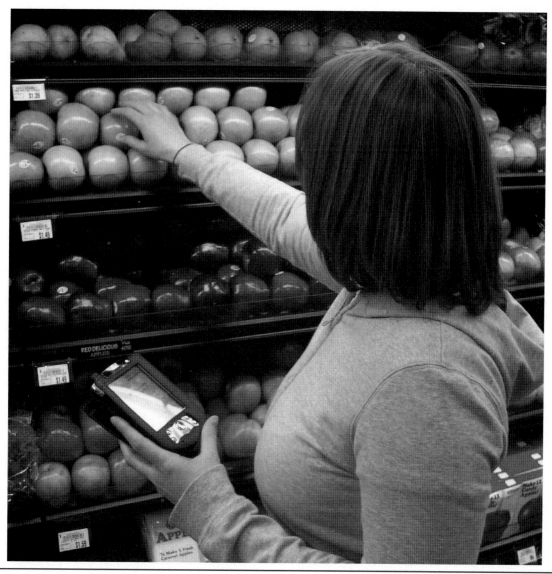

Figure 10-1   A specially programmed PDA can help an individual with a cognitive disability to achieve a greater level of independence. (Courtesy AbleLink Technologies, http://www.ablelinktech.com/.)

mental processes is impossible to provide at this time. There is a solid research-based foundation in key areas such as **memory, attention, information processing,** and **problem solving** (Sternberg, 2003). Box 10-1 highlights some of the cognitive skills for which assistive technologies may serve as a compensatory device. This list of cognitive skills is not meant to be exhaustive, nor is it the only way in which cognition might be depicted as being partitioned, but it serves the purpose here of categorizing the needs to be met by assistive technologies. Each skill listed will be described briefly in this section; for more detailed descriptions, refer to a cognitive psychology textbook (e.g., Sternberg, 2003).

Perception

Perhaps one of the most fundamental questions in cognitive psychology involves how our sensory systems identify what is in the outside world and how we then make sense of that information. Sensation refers to the signal that arrives at the body, such as those to the eyes, ears, and skin; technologies that meet sensory needs are discussed in Chapters 8 and 9. Perception involves interpretation of the sensory information (Anderson, 2000). There are assistive technologies designed to aid people in the area of perception. For example, if someone with an intellectual disability has a weakness in visual perception, then enlarged letters and auditory feedback may

BOX 10-1　Definitions of Cognitive Skills

PERCEPTION

Interpretation of the sensations received from environmental stimuli (through the sense organs)

ATTENTION

Link between the limited amount of information that is actually manipulated mentally and the enormous amount of information available through the senses, stored memories, and other cognitive processes

Signal detection: Detecting the appearance of a particular stimulus

Vigilance: Paying close and continuous attention

Search: Active scanning of the environment for particular stimuli or features

Selective: Tracking one stimulus or one type of stimulus and ignoring another

Divided: Allocating available resources to coordinate performance of more than one task at a time

MEMORY

Drawing on past knowledge to use it in the present

Encoding: Physical and sensory input is transformed into a representation that can be stored in memory

Storage: The movement of encoded information into memory and the maintenance of information in storage

Sensory: The smallest capacity for storing information (i.e., for only a fleeting sensory image) and the shortest duration for memory storage (i.e., for only fractions of a second)

Short-term: A modest capacity (i.e., for about seven items) and a duration of a number of seconds unless strategies (e.g., rehearsal) are used for keeping the information in the short-term store for longer periods of time

Long-term: A greater capacity than both the sensory store and the short-term store, and it can store information for very long periods of time, even indefinitely

Retrieval: Recovery of stored information from memory, by moving the information into consciousness for use in active cognitive processing

Implicit: Enhanced performance on a task, as a result of prior experience, despite having no conscious awareness of recollecting the prior experience

Explicit: Consciously recalling or recognizing particular information

Recall: Retrieving memories with no hints

Recognition: Retrieving memories with hints

ORIENTATION

Knowing and ascertaining one's relation to self, to others, to time, and to one's surroundings

Place: Awareness of one's location, such as one's immediate surroundings, one's town or country

Time: Awareness of day, date, month and year. Also, *time management*: ordering events in chronological sequence, allocating amounts of time to events and activities

Person: Awareness of one's own identity and of individuals in the immediate environment

Quantity: Activity involving numbers (counting) and other incremental problems

KNOWLEDGE REPRESENTATION

The mental representation of facts, objects, and skills

Mental Representation

Declarative: Recognition and understanding of factual information about objects, ideas, and events in the environment ("knowing that")

Procedural: Understanding and awareness of how to perform particular tasks or procedures ("knowing how")

Grouping

Categorization: The characterization of the relationship among objects, concepts, or thoughts

Sorting: Organizing objects, concepts, and thoughts into defined categories

Sequencing: Ordering objects or activities according to a set of rules

PROBLEM SOLVING

A process for which the goal is to overcome obstacles obstructing a path to a solution.

Problem identification: Awareness of and definition of the problem

Judgment: Ability to make sound decisions, recognizing the consequences of decisions taken or actions performed

Decision making: Selecting a course of action from defined alternatives

Reasoning

Deductive: To draw a specific conclusion from a set of general propositions

Inductive: To reach a probable general conclusion on the basis of specific facts or observations

Planning: Anticipating events so as to formulate a course of action to achieve a desired outcome

Evaluation and iteration: Monitoring the status of the problem, evaluating if the goal has been achieved, and if not, making another iteration of the problem-solving cycle

Transfer: The carryover of knowledge or skills from one context to another

LANGUAGE

A system of communicating objects, concepts, emotions, and thoughts through the systematic use of sounds, graphics, gestures or other symbols

Data from Sternberg RJ: *Cognitive psychology*, ed 3, Belmont, CA, 2003, Wadsworth.

aid the person when using a computer for word processing. As technologies gain sophistication, especially in interpretation of input data according to more and more complex algorithms, there will be an increasing ability to aid individuals whose primary needs are perceptual.

Attention

Attention can be understood to mean the mechanism for continued cognitive processing (Willingham, 2001). It can also be thought of as the ability to focus on a particular stimulus and incorporates several different levels. At the lowest level, attention is the ability to detect and respond to a stimulus. At higher levels it refers to the shifting attention between competing tasks (also called divided attention), sustaining attention and selectively attending to a stimulus while ignoring another (Golisz and Toglia, 2003). Many different models of attention have been proposed, which can broadly be classified as bottleneck theories, which explain how information selection occurs when a certain information processing stage becomes overloaded, or capacity theories, which explain our limitations as a function of a limited amount of mental effort that we can distribute across tasks (Reed, 2000). The characterization of different types of attention provides insight into different areas in which people may have strengths and weaknesses and for which assistive technologies may be able to help.

Three main types of attention are signal detection, selective attention, and divided attention. Signal detection is a process by which an individual must detect the appearance of a particular stimulus. Signal detection occurs in two ways, one requiring **vigilance,** or paying close and continuous attention over a prolonged period, and the other requiring *search*, the active scanning of the environment, in pursuit of particular stimuli or particular features. Although vigilance requires the person to wait for the signal to appear, search requires the person to actively, and sometimes skillfully, seek out a target. For example, after an earthquake a person might be vigilant in watching for smoke, and if smoke were detected, he or she might then actively search for the source of the smoke (Sternberg, 2003).

Selective attention is the process by which we filter out distractions and focus on the event we have chosen (Ashcraft, 1998). How a person can attend to what one person is saying while ignoring what other people are saying is referred to as the "cocktail party problem" (Cherry, 1953). Cherry found it was relatively easy for most people to accurately repeat a message they were attending to, but not surprisingly, they were not able to recall much from a second message they were intentionally ignoring. However, Cherry was surprised to find that very few people picked up even seemingly obvious changes to the distracter message, such as reversing the speech or changing it to another language. In their day-to-day lives many people probably experience variability in their selective attention skills and it is easy to imagine that some people may struggle with selectively attending more than others. For example, children with attention deficit disorder have difficulty focusing on the teacher in class. Assistive listening devices (see Chapter 9) in which the child wears headphones hooked up to a microphone that the teacher wears can help to better focus attention and minimize distractions.

In contrast to selecting only one stimulus to attend to, at some times it is necessary to allocate attention to multiple stimuli at one time. This is referred to as *divided attention,* such as listening to a lecture and taking notes. Research in this area has shown there are serious limits to the number of things people can do at one time. Often, rather than attending to multiple stimuli simultaneously, people actually switch their attention back and forth between tasks so rapidly that they are unaware of the switching. As the individual tasks become more and more cognitively demanding, it becomes harder to do and they are less likely to be able to truly perform the tasks concurrently (Galotti, 2004).

Memory

Many people are aware of a certain amount of variability from task to task within their own memory abilities and how their memory abilities differ from others around them. Many models of memory, such as the modal model, account for this variability, in part by distinguishing between kinds of memory on the basis of the length of time the information is stored. The modal model assumes that information is received, processed, and stored differently for each kind of memory (Atkinson & Shiffrin, 1968). When information is first presented, it is held in the *sensory store*, but only for a very brief moment. *Short-term memory* is where information that is attended to is stored for up to about 20 seconds. Various strategies, such as rehearing the information to be remembered, can be used to maintain information in the short-term store. To remember something for a longer period of time it is necessary for it to be transferred to *long-term memory*.

Distinctions have been made between the **encoding** of a memory, which is how a physical or sensory input is transformed into a representation that can be stored in memory, and the actual *storage* of a memory, which refers to the movement of encoded information into memory and the maintenance of information in storage. Although one person might experience memory problems as a result of difficulty in the storage or maintenance of the memory, another person's memory problem may result from a difficulty encoding the information into a representation that had the possibility of being stored. Stored memory is accessed through a *retrieval* process, by which stored information is moved into consciousness for use in active cognitive processing. Often people are aware of their memory retrieval and are able to accurately report that they are using information they have previously stored. This is referred to as *explicit* memory. A second type of memory, *implicit* memory, is demonstrated when an individual shows enhanced performance on a task as a result of prior experience, despite having no conscious awareness of the prior experience. Many devices make use of implicit memories in one form or another. Implicit memory can be demonstrated through word-stem completion tasks where a person is given the first few letters of a word and asked to fill in the rest of the letters to complete the word, where at least two possibilities would work.

This type of memory plays a key role in word completion and word prediction used in some assistive devices for cognitive function described later in this chapter and augmentative communication (Chapter 11) and computer access for motor disabilities (Chapter 7). People are more likely to complete the word stem to form a word they recently saw, or were primed to think of, even if they have no conscious recollection of this word. People who have amnesia have difficulty with explicit memory but perform as well as nonamnesic participants on implicit memory tasks (Shimura, 1986). Thus, it seems that amnesia may selectively impair explicit memory while sparing implicit memory. Another example of implicit memory is *procedural* memory, for example, knowing how to ride a bicycle. Although people are quite capable of performing the action, most people are unable to consciously say what it is they have learned (Anderson, 2000). Amnesia also tends to leave procedural memories intact.

There are two common ways of probing memory. In a *recall* task the participant is asked to state what he or she remembers. Free recall tasks provide virtually no hints at all, whereas cued recall tasks add in a small amount of information about the material the participant is supposed to recall (Willingham, 2001). *Recognition* tasks, on the other hand, provide the target (material to be remembered) along with other material meant to distract the person. Free recall is generally the most challenging, followed by cued recall, and then recognition. In everyday life, distracters may mislead someone's memory, although not intentionally. An awareness of how these different types of probing aid memory and how distractors hinder it is important in certain assistive technology tasks. For example, symbols on an augmentative communication display serve as recognition probes for vocabulary content, but too many choices could deteriorate performance.

Further distinctions in memory were made by Tulving (1972, 1983), who claimed that there are separate and distinct, yet interacting, systems for memories for events and memories for general knowledge. Memories for events are termed *episodic* memories and include personal experiences of events or episodes, such as memories from the last birthday party or a first date. *Semantic* memories are a person's general knowledge, or "mental dictionary and encyclopedia combined" (Ashcraft, 1998, p. 132). For example, knowledge of the fact that the capital of Canada is Ottawa is a semantic memory. Semantic memories also include language and the conceptual knowledge that relates concepts and ideas to one another (Ashcraft, 1998). An example of semantic memory is the effective use of pictures that trigger memories and lead to increased vocabulary use in storytelling by individuals with aphasia (McKelvey et al, in press). Placing a familiar picture (e.g., a family photograph of a trip to Hawaii) in the center of an augmentative communication display triggers the use of vocabulary that was unavailable to be retrieved by the person without the prompt of the picture.

Orientation

The human mind constantly receives information related to its surroundings. A simple walk down the street during lunch hour provides an abundance of information about the noisy construction site, the smell of the flowers, or the number of cars waiting at a stoplight. These things, as well as all the other information that the mind attends to on a constant basis, require the series of skills defined so far. We need perception to notice the sights and sounds; attention also plays a role as the person focuses on different stimuli, and memory helps to recognize and relate things. This information processing happens continuously throughout the day.

In this little walk down the street, or while driving to work, the person must constantly be aware of where he or she is and where he or she is going. Usually a person finds the way on the basis of a series of clues such as streets and landmarks or by knowing that home lies east, but, more important, people have the ability to guide themselves from point A to point B. This ability, called orientation to *place*, is what people rely on to orient themselves, and other objects or people, in their surroundings (World Health Organization [WHO], 2001). Assistive technology can aid people who have limitations in this ability, for instance, with the use of way-finding devices.

A similar concept, but applied to the abstract notion of time instead of physical space, is orientation to *time*, the *temporal* processing awareness of time and date (WHO, 2001). It is what permits us to know it is lunch time and that we can go on our daily walk. Assistive technology developers have created devices to aid people with time scheduling without the user having to know how to read a clock. Recognition of self, or the awareness of our own identity and that of others in the environment, brings us to the last of the orientation skills: orientation to *person* (WHO, 2001). This particular mental facet is most commonly affected in disorders such as dementia and traumatic brain injury (TBI), where people forget not only who others are, but also who they are. An example of low-tech assistive technology for people who become lost and cannot tell others how to help them find their way home is a card listing the person's address and phone number, which they can present to a passerby if they become lost.

If we are looking at the number of cars at an intersection, we may consciously decide there are too many to allow a safe crossing of the street or we might notice the number of people on the sidewalk around which we have to navigate. This numerical processing is what we call *quantitative* orientation and constitutes the mental activities involving numbers (counting) and other incremental problems.

Knowledge Representation

An individual's acquired knowledge is all the information and skills that have been learned, including the alphabet, how to wash the hands, that gravity makes things fall, and the colors of the rainbow. These are all **knowledge representations,** which help us relate to things, ideas, and events. The mental representation of facts, objects, and skills is also related to memory and can further be divided by the type of memory used. For example, declarative *memory* is used when recollecting what something is (e.g., a ball). *Procedural memory* is the mental capacity to correctly remember a sequence of operations necessary for performance of a task or procedure (e.g., tying a shoe or washing hands) and does not necessarily require conscious recollection. Declarative memory is related to knowing *what* something is, whereas procedural memory is knowing *how* to do something. Both of these can be important in the application of assistive devices to aid cognitive function.

The cognitive processes involved in *grouping* play a role in the design and application of assistive devices. As an example of grouping, a bag with red blocks and yellow balls is given to a boy. If he is told to group them, he will go through a process of evaluation of the characteristics of these objects and how they relate to each other. This cognitive process, called *categorization*, is the basis for ordering and organizing objects, concepts, or thoughts. In this case the child would most probably group the blocks and the balls, exercising the second step of grouping, called *sorting*. Sorting is the cognitive process of organizing objects, concepts, or thoughts into defined categories. There are numerous alternative categories that could be used. The child may sort them into the blocks and balls he likes and those he doesn't like, which is still a valid sorting even if it may appear to be random to an observer. If these objects had numbers on them, the child could be asked to put them in order. In this case the order is much more rigid as the task of *sequencing* requires items to be placed in the correct numerical order. Sequencing requires the ordering of objects or activities according to a set of rules, rather than to a user-defined category. People who have intellectual disabilities may benefit from assistive technology that aids these skills. For instance, many workshop activities require sorting of items into boxes, and a slot which only allows items of a particular shape to pass through into a box could be helpful.

Problem Solving

There are several ways of looking at problem solving from the cognitive psychology point of view. One of these ways focuses on how people think about the relationships between elements of a problem. "Gestalt" is a German word that translates very loosely to the concept of a whole pattern or configuration. Thus, *the Gestalt approach* focuses on the

reorganization of the elements of the problem. One aspect of intelligence in the Gestalt approach may be seeing the relationships among stimuli that prove to be useful rather than focusing on individual elements, or meaningless relationships (Ashcraft, 1998). In contrast, *the information-processing approach* deconstructs problem solving (for example, examining successful problem-solving computer programs) in an attempt to discover processes that contribute to problem solving (Hunt and Ellis, 1999). From the systems perspective, information processing has three components: input (sensory input), throughput (the processing component), and output (the motor action or verbalization). The processes are influenced by both feedback and feed-forward loops.

Newell and Simon (1972) identified three general characteristics of problem solving. The first is the *task environment*, which refers to how the problem is presented to the person and includes not only the context in which the problem is presented, but also the information, assumptions, and constraints presented (Hunt and Ellis, 1999). These factors may influence the cognitive processes a person goes through in solving a problem and must be taken into account. In assistive technology design this implies that steps required for operation of a device must be logical and intuitive from the user's point of view, not just from the designer's point of view. For example, a navigational aid designed for someone with intellectual disabilities needs to present information by voice in simple direct commands (e.g., "go to the white building") rather than in more abstract general terms (e.g., turn right 45 degrees and walk 20 meters, then turn right 30 degrees).

Newell and Simon (1972) identify the person's mental representation of the problem and the various solutions that may be attempted as the *problem space*. This construct includes the hypotheses and ideas the person develops about how the problem might be solved and the various mental representations of the problem the person holds as progress is made toward a solution. In the hierarchy of Box 10-1, it is suggested that the person must first *identify the problem*. Various mental skills are required for a person to accurately carry out this important first step in problem solving. If a person has difficulty identifying problems, various devices such as ones that prompt or cue may help (e.g., The Independent Living Suite, Ablelink Technologies, Colorado Springs, Col., *www.ablelinktech.com*). Both accurate and inaccurate mental representations of what the problem is are included in the problem space. The last characteristic of problem solving that Newell and Simon identify is selection of an appropriate *operator*, or sequence of operations, to move from one problem state to another, ultimately to the final goal state.

Box 10-1 lists possible skills a problem solver might need in selecting the appropriate operations. *Judgment* is the ability to make sound decisions, recognizing the consequences of decisions taken or actions performed. *Decision making* is the cognitive process of selecting a course of action from defined alternatives. *Planning* is the process of anticipating future events so as to formulate a course of action to achieve a desired outcome. The frontal lobes of the brain are involved in all three of these processes as well as impulse control and controlling and executing behavior. A person's ability to perform these tasks may be affected in the presence of specific types of injuries or conditions that result from damaged or not yet fully developed frontal lobes. For these individuals, the best approach may be to reduce the number of alternative solutions, make the options clear, and reduce the reliance on anticipation of future consequences of decisions.

Another skill used in problem solving is *reasoning*. Two types of reasoning include deductive reasoning and inductive reasoning. *Deductive* reasoning is a process by which an individual tries to draw a logically certain and specific conclusion from a set of general propositions. For example, when using an assistive device that requires touching a screen location (a button) to create an action, the statements, "All buttons make something happen when you push them" and "This is a button" leads to the conclusion, "Something will happen if this button is pushed." *Inductive* reasoning is a process by which an individual tries to reach a probable general conclusion on the basis of a set of specific facts or observations. This conclusion is likely to be true on the basis of past experience, but there is no guarantee that it will absolutely be true (Hunt and Ellis, 1999).

Another type of reasoning is analogical reasoning, which is using a solution to a related problem to help in solving the current problem (Reed, 2000). Although one might think analogical reasoning would be a sophisticated skill only developing in mature thinking, there is evidence that even very young children use analogies to solve problems. After watching their parents perform a similar task, 10- to 12-month-old children were able to move an obstacle and pull an appropriate string to obtain a toy, even when the superficial features of the problem presented to the children differed in all aspects from those in the problem they saw a parent solve (Chen, Sanchez, and Campbell, 1997). The problem is illustrated in Figure 10-2. The child was required to remove a barrier by pulling on a cloth, which brought a string attached to a toy close enough for the child to reach. The child then pulled on the string to bring the toy within reach. A second cloth had a string that was not attached to the toy. The three situations in Figure 10-2 differ in all aspect of the superficial features (color and texture of the cloth, the type of barrier [transparent or opaque], and the type of toy). Parents demonstrated the solution to the problem on the first trial, and the babies obtained the toy more readily on each subsequent trial, suggesting that they had

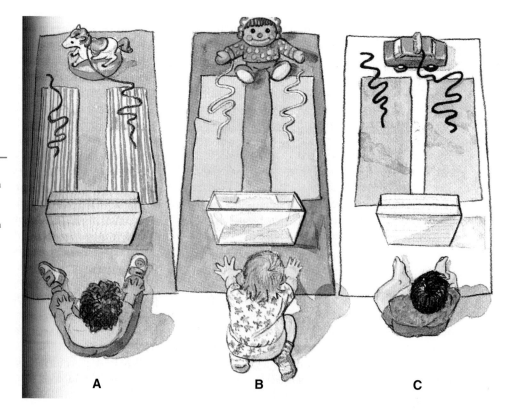

Figure 10-2   An example of analogical reasoning. (Adapted from Chen Z, Sanchez RP, Campbell T: From beyond to within their grasp: the rudiments of analogical problem solving in 10- to 13-month-olds, *Dev Psychol* 33:792, 1997.)

A   B   C

a mental representation of behaviors to access out-of-reach objects.

One of the best predictors of whether people will use an analogy to solve a problem is whether there is *surface similarity* between the problem seen before and the new problem. Surface similarity is how similar the elements in the problem are to the elements in the analog. Although it encourages analogy use, surface similarity can also interfere with performance when the similarities are only superficial, which often occurs with electronic assistive devices whose generic characteristics may be similar but whose function has significant differences. As illustration of this concept, there are many assistive technology applications that use personal digital assistants (PDAs). For example, PDAs have been programmed to function as augmentative communication devices (see Chapter 11) and as cognitive assists (see Figure 10-1). Both applications use an input method of a touch screen or small keyboards, and they both have an output of either speech or visual characters and text. As these two diverse applications illustrate, these are superficial features that may be operated in many different ways. These surface features of the two applications may appear to be identical, and indeed the same device could be used for both applications with a change in software. However, the function will be very different because of the characteristics of the software loaded into the device. If the user attends only to the existence of the input and output features and the size, color, and shape of the PDA, then some of the operational parameters of the device may not be understood. If he or she has previous experiences with one type of device that uses a PDA, then he or she may assume, on the basis of this superficial characteristic, that a new device operates the same as the previous one just because it also uses a PDA.

Structural similarity, on the other hand, is how similar the content or structure of the two problems are to each other (Willingham, 2001). It is important to establish parallels between the structures of the problems to help the person map elements from the source of the analogy to the target (Ashcraft, 1998). Analogical reasoning is one method of **generalization**, the carryover of knowledge or skills from one kind of task or one particular context to another kind of task or another context. Knowledge is most likely to be generalized when the conditions under which the knowledge is to be used are very similar to those under which the knowledge was acquired (Hunt and Ellis, 1999). As with many cognitive skills, it would be inaccurate to describe people as "possessing" or "not possessing" reasoning abilities or generalization skills, but we might imagine how certain technologies could aid a person with disabilities in these areas. Examples of these devices are described in a later section of this chapter.

The last step in problem solving involves *confirming the successful conclusion of the task*. The problem solver must evaluate the outcome of his or her actions and determine whether the task has ended successfully or whether it requires continuation or repetition. In the example of analogical reasoning used above, if the baby did not receive the toy after pulling the string, he might try again after evaluating the outcome of his actions.

Language and Learning

Language is fundamental to cognitive task representation. Through language, the process of exchanging information, we can express our thoughts, needs, and ideas. *Language* is a method of communication that is composed of rules (grammar) and symbols, expressed by gestures, sounds, or writing. When a skill or task is taught, language is used to portray the desired outcome. *Learning* is the process by which knowledge, skills, or attitudes are acquired; it can be attained through study, experience, or teaching. In Box 10-1 learning is placed at the end of the hierarchy because it builds on the previously mentioned skills, like building blocks. *General learning* refers to the basic ability to acquire knowledge, skills, or attitudes, used as a necessity for the more specific types of learning: *mathematics, reading*, and *writing*. The ability of someone to learn and comprehend in each of these categories helps define both the features the technology must have and the skills the person needs to use it.

■ DISORDERS THAT MAY BENEFIT FROM COGNITIVE ASSISTIVE TECHNOLOGIES

This section describes disorders in which a person's cognitive skills may be compromised. The disorders are broken into two groups: congenital, those that occur at birth, and acquired, those that are acquired after birth. Intellectual or **developmental disabilities (DD), learning disabilities (LD), attention deficit hyperactivity disorder (ADHD),** and **autism spectrum disorder (ASD)** are congenital disorders, whereas **dementia, traumatic brain injury (TBI),** and **cerebral vascular accidents (CVA)** are acquired disorders. This group of disorders, summarized in Table 10-1, is a representative subset of those for which assistive technology has been found useful to address cognitive limitations.

There are physical disorders that may have some cognitive involvement. Aging is a physical process that limits motor function and also affects cognitive skills such as memory. Individuals with cerebral palsy (CP) may have a concurrent intellectual disability. People who have multiple sclerosis (MS) may have cognitive involvement, including behavior changes as the disease progresses. Longitudinal studies have evaluated cognitive impairment in relation to the clinical course of the disease. Results of one such study found impairment of specific cognitive functions, most commonly

TABLE 10-1 Disorders That May Benefit From Cognitive Assistive Technologies

Disorder	Incidence	Characteristics
Intellectual disability	8 individuals per 1000 (http://www.cdc.gov/mmwr/preview/ mmwrhtml/00040023.htm)	Limitations in functional skills, impairments in memory, language use, and communication, abstract conceptualization, generalization and problem identification/problem solving (Wehmeyer, Smith, and Davies, 2005)
Learning disability	2% of children	Significant difficulties in understanding or in using either spoken or written language; evident in problems with reading, writing, mathematical manipulation, listening, spelling, or speaking (Edyburn, 2005)
ADHD	4% (Daley, 2006) and 5%-7% (www.adhd.com)	Typical capacity to learn and to use their skills confounded by factors that make it difficult to fully realize that potential; easily frustrated, have trouble paying attention, prone to daydreaming and moodiness; fidgety, disorganized, impulsive, disruptive, or aggressive (Schuck and Crinella, 2005) (www.adhdcanada.com)
ASD	1 child per 165, 25% exhibit intellectual disability, 4 times more prevalent in boys than girls (Chakrabarti and Fombonne, 2001)	Varying degrees of impairment in communication and social interaction skills or presence of restricted, repetitive, and stereotyped patterns of behavior
Dementia	0.5%-1% (<65 years), 7%-10% (65-75years), 18%-20% (75-85 years), 35%-40% (85+ years)	(1) Decline of cognitive capacity with some effect on day-to-day functioning, (2) impairment in multiple areas of cognition (global), and (3) normal level of consciousness (Rabins, Lyketsos, and Steele, 2006)
TBI	Mild: 131 per 100,000 Moderate: 15 per 100,000 Severe: 14 per 100,000 people (21 per 100,000 if prehospital deaths included) (Dawodu, 2006)	See Table 10-6
CVA	160/100,000 (overall), 1000/100,000 (age 50-65 years), 3000/100,000 (>80 years) (Demaerschalk and Hachinski, 2006)	Visual neglect, apraxia, aphasia; dysphagia; perceptual deficits, impaired alertness, attention disorders, memory disorders, impaired executive function, impaired judgment, impaired activities of daily living (O'Sullivan and Schmitz, 1994)

long-term verbal memory, but did not find a global cognitive impairment (Piras et al, 2002).

Congenital Disabilities

Intellectual Disabilities. Intellectual disability is typically defined as a disability where the person has a below average score on an intelligence or mental ability test and a limitation in functional skills (Wehmeyer, Smith, and Davies, 2005). These functional skills include but are not limited to communication, self-care, and social interaction *(http://www.cdc.gov/ncbddd/dd/ddmr.htm)*. The terms *developmental disability, cognitive disability,* or *mental retardation* are often used to describe individuals with intellectual disabilities. Intellectual disability can range in severity from mild to severe.

Learning Disabilities. LDs are disorders in which the person has near-normal mental abilities in general but a deficit in the comprehension or use of spoken or

written language. These disabilities may be manifested as a significant difficulty with reading, writing, reasoning, or mathematical ability. Because students with LDs tend to perform poorly on standardized tests, it was long thought that LDs were a mild form of intellectual disability. This assumption is untrue; LDs can be thought of as a deficit in the processing and integration of information in an area (e.g., reading) as opposed to limitations in the basic ability in that specific area of learning. People with LDs have typical age-related capacity in all areas. Table 10-2 lists abilities associated with learning disabilities. However, processing deficits lead to the hallmark difficulties that are commonly experienced (Johnson et al, 2005).

Attention Deficit Hyperactivity Disorder. ADHD is defined as a pattern of inattention, hyperactivity, or impulsivity that is more frequent or severe than for typical people of a given age *(www.nimh.nih.gov/publicat/adhd.cfm)*. The delay aversion hypothesis of ADHD posits that the child with ADHD distracts himself or herself from the passing of

TABLE 10-2	**Categorization of Abilities Associated With Learning Disabilities**
Explicit Abilities	Implicit Abilities
Reading skills (dyslexia)	Visual or auditory discrimination
Mathematical skills (dyscalculia)	Visual or auditory closure
Writing skills (dyslexia, dysgraphia)	Visual or auditory figure-ground discrimination
Language skills (dysphasia)	Visual or auditory memory
Motor-learning skills (dyspraxia)	Visual or auditory sequencing
Social skills	Auditory association and comprehension
	Spatial perception
	Temporal perception

time when he or she is not in control by daydreaming, inattention, and fidgeting (Daley, 2006). Children (and adults) with ADHD have a normal capacity to learn and to use their skills but have confounding factors that make it difficult to fully realize that potential (Schuck and Crinella, 2005). Particularly, those with ADHD can be easily frustrated, have trouble paying attention, are prone to daydreaming and moodiness, and are fidgety, disorganized, impulsive, disruptive, or aggressive.

Autism Spectrum Disorder.   ASD is a developmental disorder that is characterized by varying degrees of impairment in communication and social interaction skills or the presence of restricted, repetitive, and stereotyped patterns of behavior. A commonly used definition for autism is that of the *Diagnostic and Statistical Manual of Mental Disorders– Fourth Edition* (DSM-IV) (American Psychiatric Association [APA], 2000), which classifies autism as a *pervasive development disorder (PDD)*. As the term implies, this disorder covers a wide spectrum of conditions, with individual differences in number and kinds of symptoms, levels of severity, age of onset, and limitations with social interaction. Major subtypes of ASD include *autistic disorder, Asperger's syndrome, Rett syndrome, childhood disintegrative disorders,* and *PDD not otherwise specified (NOS)*. Individuals with ASD typically demonstrate deficits in communication skills including delay in, or total lack of, spoken language and *spontaneous speech*; unusual speaking patterns (e.g., *echolalia* or idiosyncratic language); and underdeveloped social interaction skills (including problems interpreting facial expressions, gestures, and intonation while interacting with other people). They might also seem evasive, avoid eye contact, and appear to lack initiation and desire to share joy or interest. Children with ASD also have inflexible adherence to specific routines and demonstrate unusual persistence and intense focus on a specific subject or activity. Many children with ASD have unusual (hypersensitive or hyposensitive) responses to

sensory information, which could lead to the lack of or aversive response to sensory input.

Individuals with ASD also have strengths and unique abilities. For example, some individuals with ASD have unusually good spatial perception and visual recall or accurate and detailed memory for information and facts, are able to concentrate for long periods of time on particular tasks or subjects, and are more attentive to details then most people. These abilities may allow them to excel in areas of music, science, math, physics, and other specialized areas.

Acquired Disabilities

Dementia.   The word dementia comes from the Latin *de mens*, which means "from the mind." Dementia is best defined as a syndrome, or a pattern of clinical symptoms and signs, that can be defined by the following three points: (1) decline of cognitive capacity with some effect on day-to-day functioning, (2) impairment in multiple areas of cognition (global), and (3) normal level of consciousness (Rabins, Lyketsos, and Steele, 2006). Dementia is distinguished from congenital cognitive disorders (such as intellectual disability, LDs, etc.) by its age of onset and its degenerative component. It is also important to note that, although it must affect multiple areas of cognition, not all areas are affected. Rabins, Lyketsos, and Steele (2006) define the "*three pillars of dementia care.*" First is to treat the disease, which helps identify current needs and future necessities as the disorder progresses. Second is treatment of the symptoms. By treating the symptoms, the quality of life of the client will improve in the cognitive, functional, and behavioral domains. Medications and technology are the two main ways to accomplish this task. Third, client support is important and leads to ensuring that the client's needs are met and quality of life is improved as much as possible.

Traumatic Brain Injury.   People who have a TBI often lose significant cognitive function. A TBI may occur when the head or brain is struck by an external force, such as from a fall, gunshot wound, or motor vehicle accident. The causes of TBI are described in Table 10-3. The extent of the trauma to the brain is the determining factor in diagnosing TBI, not the injury itself. For instance, it is possible to incur TBI as the result of both open-head injuries (the brain is exposed to air) and closed-head injuries (no brain exposure). The effect of a TBI on an individual's cognitive ability varies from case to case, in terms of both severity and the set of skills affected. Not all head injuries give rise to TBI, and there is an accepted method for diagnosing such an injury. One tool available to assist with diagnosis is the Glasgow Coma Scale (GCS), a rating system used for describing the severity of a coma (Dawodu, 2006). The GCS ranks comas on a scale of 3 (most severe) to 15 (mildest) according to eye response, verbal response, and motor response categories. A score on the

TABLE 10-3	Data on Causes of Traumatic Brain Injury (Injury Control Research Center)
Cause	Percentage of Total
Motor vehicle crashes	64%
Gunshot wounds	13%
Falls	11%
Assault	8%
Pedestrian	3%
Sports	1%

Data from *TBI Inform*, June, 2000. Published by the UAB-TBIMS, Birmingham, AL. © 2000 Board of Trustees, University of Alabama, http://main.uab.edu/tbi/show.asp?durki=27492&site=2988&return=57898#cause.

TABLE 10-5	Return to Driving		
	Percent Return to Driving		
	No	Partially	Yes
6 months	69%	13%	19%
12 months	60%	10%	30%

Data from ICRC Study, 1999, http://www.neuroskills.com/whattoexpect.shtml.

GCS of 12 or lower is a mild brain injury and below 8 is considered a severe injury.

If the GCS does not indicate TBI, one of the following two criteria must be satisfied for a TBI diagnosis: either the client has amnesia for the traumatic event or the individual has a documented loss of consciousness. It is common to have a *recovery period* after the injury. This recovery usually plateaus within 12 months after injury, and the extent of recovery is both variable and unpredictable (Cicerone et al, 2005). A good measure of the extent of an individual's recovery from a TBI is his or her return to preinjury activities of daily living. Two main recovery indicators are the return to work and the return to driving, both important tasks for independent living. Data on the return to work are summarized in Table 10-4, and similar data for the return to driving are shown in Table 10-5 (Novack, 1999). In both cases, very little improvement was observed beyond 12 months after injury. Typical cognitive and behavioral difficulties that a person with TBI may encounter are listed in Table 10-6 (Novack, 1999; Rehabilitation Engineering Society of North America, [RESNA], 1998). Two areas of importance are memory and language skills because these may benefit from intervention with assistive technology.

Stroke. A *stroke*, or CVA, is an incidence of irregular blood flow within the brain causing an interruption in

brain function. A stroke may arise from a lack of blood flow to the brain (known as an *ischemic stroke*) or from ruptured blood vessels in the brain (a *hemorrhagic stroke*). The neurological damage incurred as the result of a stroke produces symptoms that directly correspond to the injured area within the brain (O'Sullivan and Schmitz, 1994). A CVA causes acute damage to the brain; there are no degenerative effects after the onset of injury. As with TBI, persons who have sustained a stroke often have a recovery period where portions of the brain learn to compensate for damaged areas. Typical cognitive and behavioral difficulties associated with stroke are shown in Table 10-7. Most recovery (as observed by the return to activities of daily living) occurs within 6 months after onset (Bruno, 2004). The majority of persons with CVA are able to return home after the initial hospitalization period. A summary of discharge locations after hospitalization for stroke is shown in Table 10-8. These data suggest that the number of people returning home after a CVA is increasing, which might be attributed to improvements to hospital care at the onset of stroke. Children may have a more pronounced recovery than adults because their brains have a greater degree of plasticity. Also, women may display greater recovery of lost language skill than men because the language centers of the brain are larger in women than in men.

COGNITIVE SKILLS RELATED TO SPECIFIC DISORDERS

Figure 10-3 identifies the skills that are most often affected by different disorders. Cognitive skills are listed along the

TABLE 10-4	Return to Work				
	Student	Employed	Home	Retired	Unemployed
Onset	11%	57%	1%	11%	21%
6 months	7%	17%	None	10%	67%
12 months	7%	26%	None	8%	57%

Data from IRCR Study, 1999, http://www.neuroskills.com/whattoexpect.shtml.

TABLE 10-6   List of Typical Cognitive and Behavioral Difficulties After TBI

Type of Difficulty	Examples
Cognitive	Processing of visual or auditory information
	Disrupted attention and concentration
	Language problems (i.e., aphasia)
	Difficulty storing and retrieving new memories
	Poor reasoning, judgment, and problem solving skills
	Difficulty learning new information
Behavioral	Restlessness and agitation
	Emotional lability and irritability
	Confabulation
	Diminished insight
	Socially inappropriate behavior
	Poor initiation
	Lack of emotional response
	Projecting blame on others
	Depression
	Anxiety

TABLE 10-7   List of Typical Cognitive and Behavioral Difficulties After Stroke

Type of Difficulty	Examples
Cognitive	Visual neglect, hemianopsia
	Apraxia
	Language problems (i.e. aphasia, dysarthria)
	Perceptual deficits (i.e., figure-ground impairment, disorientation)
	Impaired alertness, attention disorders
	Memory problems, both short-term and long-term
	Perseveration
	Decreased executive function
Behavioral	Impaired judgment
	Impulsiveness
	Emotional lability
	Confabulation
	Poor initiation
	Mood alterations
	Depression

TABLE 10-8   Discharge Data for Stroke From the Canadian Heart and Stroke Foundation

Discharge Destination	1993	1999
Home	33%	56%
Inpatient rehabilitation	41%	32%
Nursing home or long-term care	26%	11%

Data from Heart and Stroke Foundation of Canada. Stroke statistics: http://ww2.heartandstroke.ca/Page.asp?PageID=33&ArticleID=428&Src=stroke&From=SubCategory/ Accessed April 16, 2005.

top row and disabilities and disorders along the vertical axis. The cognitive skills in Figure 10-3 are the same ones covered in the first section of this chapter and are summarized in Box 10-1. The cognitive skills are roughly arranged so that, moving from left to right, the skills build on each other and are higher order. The disabilities listed are those that manifest primarily with cognitive limitations.

This table illustrates *possible* skills that may be affected for a person with a specific disorder. The inclusion of skills and the definition of categories were based on the applicability of the table to assistive technology applications, and all listed cognitive skills are judged to be those that could be aided or replaced with the help of assistive technologies. Most of the disorders and disabilities that have cognitive implications are quite variable from individual to individual. Thus, not all of the possible limitations included in Figure 10-3 will exist in all cases. In Figure 10-3, items marked with an X are the skills that may be limited or absent in the corresponding disorder. For each entry in this table, the frame of reference is the person with a disability (i.e., the skill is restricted or absent in the person). Figure 10-3 could be used during an assessment as a checklist to ensure that the assistive technology practitioner (ATP) assesses skills that may be affected and to reduce the chance of missing a crucial skill or deficiency. If there is a gap between the skills required to complete a task and the skills that the individual brings to the task, the use of assistive technologies to aid or replace the required skill should be considered. The possible substitution or augmentation for these skills with assistive technologies is discussed in the next section and displayed in Figure 10-3.

■ CHARACTERISTICS OF ASSISTIVE TECHNOLOGIES THAT ADDRESS COGNITIVE NEEDS

General Concepts

Considerations for Individuals With Mild Cognitive Disabilities. On one hand, the application of assistive technologies to meet the needs of individuals with **mild cognitive disabilities** is easier than for more severe disabilities simply because the human skills are greater than for some other disabilities. On the other hand, the needs that these individuals have are more subtle and harder to define than in the case of physical disabilities or more severe cognitive disabilities. For example, learning disabilities typically involve significant difficulties in understanding or in using either spoken or written language, and these difficulties may be evident in problems with reading, writing, mathematical manipulation, listening, spelling, or speaking (Edyburn, 2005). Although there are assistive technologies that are specifically designed to address these areas (discussed later in

Category	Skill	Subskill	ID	LD	ADHD	ASD	DEMENTA	TBI	CVA
Perception				X		X		X	X
Attention	Signal Detection	Vigilance			X			X	X
Attention	Signal Detection	Search			X	X		X	X
Attention	Selective				X		X	X	X
Attention	Divided				X	X	X	X	X
Memory	Encoding						X	X	X
Memory	Storage	Short Term			X	X	X	X	X
Memory	Storage	Long Term					X	X	X
Memory	Retrieval	Recognition					X	X	X
Memory	Retrieval	Recall					X	X	X
Orientation	Place				X		X	X	X
Orientation	Time				X		X	X	X
Orientation	Person				X		X	X	X
Orientation	Quantitative				X		X	X	X
Knowledge Representation and Organization	Mental Representations	Declarative/know what				X	X	X	X
Knowledge Representation and Organization	Mental Representations	Procedural/know how				X	X	X	X
Knowledge Representation and Organization	Grouping	Categorization				X		X	X
Knowledge Representation and Organization	Grouping	Sorting				X		X	X
Knowledge Representation and Organization	Grouping	Sequencing				X		X	X
Problem Solving	Identify Problem					X		X	X
Problem Solving	Judgment			X	X	X	X	X	X
Problem Solving	Decision Making			X	X	X		X	X
Problem Solving	Reasoning	Deductive				X	X	X	X
Problem Solving	Reasoning	Inductive				X	X	X	X
Problem Solving	Planning					X		X	X
Problem Solving	Evaluation and Iteration					X	X	X	X
Problem Solving	Transfer/Generalization					X		X	X
Language						X		X	X
Learning	General					X	X	X	X
Learning	Mathematics					X	X	X	X
Learning	Reading					X	X	X	X
Learning	Writing					X	X	X	X

Figure 10-3 Skills versus disorder matrix. *ID*, Intellectual disability; *LD*, learning disability; *ADHD*, attention deficit hyperactivity disorder; *ASD*, autism spectrum disorder; *TBI*, traumatic brain injury; *CVA*, cardiovascular accident (stroke).

this chapter), many of the technological tools are useful for all students and are part of instructional technology (Ashton, 2005). Even the so-called assistive technologies have features (e.g., multimedia, synthetic speech output, voice recognition input) that are useful to all learners. Chapter 1 distinguishes between educational technologies (or instructional technologies) and assistive technologies. This distinction works well for sensory and motor assistive technologies. The distinction is much more blurred for cognitive assistive technologies (Ashton, 2005; Edyburn, 2005). For example, some spell checkers, word prediction, and talking word processors have been specifically designed for individuals with learning disabilities (e.g., Co-Writer and Write-Outloud, Don Johnston, Inc, Volo, Ill., *www.donjohnston.com*). These programs are discussed later in this chapter. As Ashton (2005) points out, each of these technologies is potentially useful to all students, not just those with learning disabilities. In that sense they are educational or instructional technologies. Edyburn has suggested that the term technology-enhanced performance be used instead of assistive technology. The advantage of this conceptual shift is that emphasis is placed on performance and outcomes, not on assessment and selection of the technology. The emphasis on human performance is important and reflected in the HAAT model. However, the move away from assistive technology to technology-enhanced performance does not recognize the unique features of assistive technologies that are described in Chapter 1 (see Box 1-1), particularly that of being an individualized system that meets unique needs for an individual.

Edyburn (2005) carries the concept of technology to enhance performance further by pointing out that many other productivity tools can function as "assistive technologies" for individuals with mild disabilities. He cites the example of the *Ask Jeeves* Web search engine *(www.askjeeves.com)*, which could provide assistance to a child who has difficulty retrieving information. Edyburn poses the following question: if the student knows that he or she can find the names of all the U.S. presidents using this or another search engine, then isn't that as useful an educational outcome as having memorized the names for a test? The question of information retrieval using the Web is part of the larger issue of compensation versus remediation in cognitive assistive technologies (Edyburn, 2002). Throughout this text a four-part approach to assistive technology applications has been emphasized: human, activity, assistive technology device, and context (the HAAT model of Chapter 2). When the ATP is dealing with motor disabilities, the starting point is a careful description of the activity to be performed. An evaluation of the individual's skills relevant to the activity leads to a clear picture of what assistive technology needs he has. The context (physical, social, and cultural milieu and institutional environment) then moderates the choices of assistive technologies. The assistive technology includes

both soft technologies (training, strategies) and hard technologies (devices) or, in Edyburn's (2002, 2005) terminology, remediation (soft technology) and compensation (hard technology).

For sensory or motor disabilities, we don't much care how the function is accomplished as long as the activity can be satisfactorily completed. Other issues, such as how much energy it takes to walk versus to use a power wheelchair for someone with severe cerebral palsy, are matters of personal choice. The situation changes dramatically, however, in dealing with cognitive assistive technologies. Should the child in our example be required to learn the presidents' names (remediation) or be allowed to use an assistive technology (Ask Jeeves) as a compensatory tool, and why is its use considered "cheating" by some educators and parents (Edyburn, 2005)?

A related concern is the concept of time in educational contexts. Time is fixed and accomplishment varies (Edyburn, 2005). This is not true in the case of sensory or motor disabilities where additional time (e.g., for an individual who is blind to cross the street using a long cane) is an accepted part of human performance. In vocational settings, completion time for a task also varies from individual to individual and is acceptable within wide limits. Why, then, is this not the case in an educational context? As Edyburn (2005) points out, restricting time, learning activities, instructional approaches, and other classroom variables to a "one-size-fits-all" constraint in educational settings means that high standards of performance cannot be achieved. Although many students with special needs are given extra time to complete an examination, the level of competence they achieve is still variable and time (even expanded time) is fixed. If achievement were to be fixed then each student would be allowed as much time as necessary to complete the task. If uniformly high performance and preparation for later vocational success are the goals, then compensation, using both hard and soft assistive technologies, must be an alternative for individuals with mild cognitive disabilities as it is for their counterparts with motor and sensory disabilities.

Considerations for Individuals With Moderate to Severe Intellectual Disabilities.

Several ways of characterizing cognitive needs have been used in consideration of assistive technology applications for individuals who have intellectual disabilities. One method considers the cognitive impairment exhibited, such as impairments in memory, language use and communication, abstract conceptualization, generalization, and problem identification/problem solving (Wehmeyer, Smith, and Davies, 2005). Assistive technology characteristics that address these impairments include simplicity of operation, capacity of the technology to support repetition, consistency in presentation, use, and inclusion of multiple modalities (e.g., speech, sounds, and graphical representations). Wehmeyer, Smith and Davies (2005) discuss assistive technology characteristics and approaches for each of these impairments. Many of these technologies are covered in the subsequent sections of this chapter.

Granlund et al (1995) take a different approach and define five content areas for technological assistance to individuals who have moderate to severe intellectual disabilities. The content areas, on the basis of cognitive structures, are the following:

- Quality (What is this?)
- Causal patterns (Why? And if so?)
- Space (Where?)
- Quantity (How much? How big?)
- Time (When? Duration?)

Within these content areas, individuals with intellectual disabilities typically have difficulties in organization and reorganization, performing operations with cognitive structures, and symbolic representation. Within these content areas, adults with cognitive disabilities may encounter problems in activities such as choosing a leisure activity, using public transportation, being on time for work, and preparing meals. Typical assessment questions and assistive technology examples for each content area are listed in Table 10-9.

Wehmeyer et al (2004) described eight primary factors of cognitive ability: (1) language, (2) reasoning, (3) memory and learning, (4) visual perception, (5) auditory perception, (6) idea production, (7) cognitive speed, and (8) knowledge and achievement. They argue that the promise of technology for aiding individuals with intellectual disabilities lies in enhancing human capacity in these areas rather than compensating for deficits. An important element in this approach is the application of the principles of universal design (see Chapter 1) to ensure that mainstream technologies are designed in such a way that individuals with a range of intellectual abilities can access them. The design of the human

technology interface (see Chapter 2) in the HAAT model is an example of the difference between a compensation approach and the concept of enhancement of the technology characteristics to make it more accessible. If an individual with an intellectual disability has difficulty accessing a screen because of language problems (e.g., reading), one approach is to use a compensatory approach and provide auditory output instead of text, avoiding the necessity for reading. If the problem is too much clutter on the display, then the best approach may be to simplify the display (i.e., enhance it) so that the information is more accessible. The following sections of this chapter describe technology approaches that use both enhancement and compensation strategies. For individuals with intellectual disabilities, Wehmeyer et al (2004) present a thorough literature review of approaches that have been taken to enhance performance in each of the eight cognitive factors.

Considerations for Individuals With Acquired Disabilities. Individuals with acquired cognitive disabilities resulting from injury (e.g., TBI) or disease (e.g., CVA or dementia) retain a wide variety of remaining cognitive skills. The majority of assistive technologies and strategies that have been used to aid persons with acquired cognitive disabilities are designed to compensate for deficits by building on remaining strengths (LoPresti, Mihailidis, and Kirsch, 2004). Collective technologies and strategies that help a person with cognitive deficits function more independently in certain tasks have been called assistive technology for cognition (ATC) (LoPresti, Mihailidis, and Kirsch, 2004) or **cognitive prosthesis** (Cole and Mathews, 1999). An ATC or a cognitive prosthesis is an entire system of hardware, software, and personal assistance that is individualized to meet specific needs. A more accurate descriptor would be *cognitive orthosis* because the intent is to augment cognitive function rather than to replace it. However, Bower (2003) uses "prosthesis" in his description, which states that a "cognitive

TABLE 10-9	Assessment Questions and Assistive Technology Examples	
Content Area	Typical Assessment Questions	Examples of Applicable Assistive Technology
Quality	How does person classify objects? Are one, two, or more dimensions used?	Sorting jigs, graphic symbol labels for categories
Causal patterns	How many steps in a process or chain can be understood? Can outcomes of accomplishing a task in different ways be compared?	Sequencing jigs, PDA-based prompting and cuing
Space	Can the person find his or her way with a map? Does he or she use shortcuts? Can he or she ask directions?	Paper maps, dynamic display an GPS on PDA with speech output
Quantity	How is money handled? Is conservation of volume present?	Money-sorting jigs, matching task rather than counting, parts-counting jigs
Time	Can a watch be used? Is the duration of an activity or waiting period understood?	Quarter hour watch, electronic pocket calendars with reminders, PDA with reminder and voice output

From Granlund M et al: Assistive technology for cognitive disability, *Technol Disabil* 4:205-214, 1995.

prosthesis is a computational tool that amplifies or extends a person's thought and perception, much as eyeglasses are prostheses that improve vision…a cognitive prosthesis magnifies strengths in human intellect rather than corrects presumed deficiencies in it. Cognitive prostheses, therefore, are more like binoculars than eyeglasses." As the HAAT model (see Chapter 2) implies, a cognitive prosthesis includes a custom-designed computer-based compensatory strategy that directly assists in performing daily activities (Institute for Cognitive Prosthetics, *http://www.brain-rehab.com/definecp.htm*). It may also include additional technologies such as a cell phone, pager, digital camera, or low-tech approaches.

Cognitive Skills Assisted by Technology

Figure 10-4 relates cognitive skills to categories of assistive technologies. This characterization is similar to that used by others (e.g., Cole and Mathews, 1999; Edyburn, 2005; Granlund et al, 1995; LoPresti, Mihailidis and Kirsch, 2004; Wehmeyer et al, 2004; Wehmeyer, Smith, and Davies, 2005). Cognitive skills are listed along the top row and assistive technology categories on the vertical axis. This table can be used to identify assistive technologies (rows) that aid or replace skills (columns) to enable a person to carry out functional tasks. It can be used to identify both compensatory and enhancement approaches to the use of assistive technologies for individuals who have cognitive disabilities. Entries in Figure 10-4 are marked with X, A, or R, where X indicates that the skill is required by the technology, A indicates that the technology aids that skill, and R indicates that the technology replaces that skill. Figure 10-4 is based on clinical experience and published literature regarding assistive technologies frequently used by people with cognitive limitations. Similar devices are grouped and category names have been assigned.

Memory. Memory aids are those devices or software packages that augment or replace memory by providing a means to store commonly used information or aiding in the retrieval of information. These devices can be subdivided into three categories on the basis of their primary tasks: recording, word completion/prediction, and information retrieval. Recorders are devices that store information that can be replayed at a later time to aid in the recall of facts or appointments. The most common devices in this category are those that record voice information as short memos. This feature is often built into PDAs, cell phones, and small dictaphones. Word completion and prediction solutions are software packages that aid memory during a written communication task by giving a user a series of contextually significant words/phrases that he or she may wish to use. This technology is also discussed in Chapter 7, where its use was to speed up time to input text or to reduce the number of required keystrokes.

Information retrieval systems are devices or software packages that categorize and organize words/phrases so that they may be retrieved through associations. A number of information retrieval aids have been designed that use palm top computers (often called personal digital assistants or PDAs). Features of these devices that are particularly useful include small size for portability, flexibility in programming for customization, large storage capacity, a variety of input and output modalities, and interfacing to other technologies (e.g., desktop or notebook computers, cell phones) (Szymkowiak et al, 2005). When PDAs are used with individuals who have disabilities, two usability issues arise: changes in sensory processing and the small size of the keyboards and screens. Individuals with cognitive limitations from aging, injury (TBI or CVA), or dementia often have accompanying visual problems (declining acuity and contrast sensitivity, including color discrimination). The interconnectivity of PDAs provides the opportunity for interfacing with the Internet to retrieve a much wider range of information. However, small screen and keyboard features are particularly limiting in long sessions of data retrieval (Szymkowiak et al, 2005).

PDA daily schedulers and reminder alarm devices (both of which are produced in a wide variety of formats) (Figure 10-5) are technologies that tend to provide the most immediate benefit to people with TBI (Kim et al, 1999; Van Hulle and Hux, 2005), CVA, and aging (Szymkowiak et al, 2005). Software packages for these devices have also been designed to include prompting cues to aid memory (Bergman, 2002). These specially designed systems can be customized to meet the needs of a specific user and they have user-friendly interfaces and are easy to carry (Gorman et al, 2003). The PDA-based information retrieval aids require the user to display some degree of sensory perception, language use, memory, or learning skill to be of practical benefit. Because the software can be customized, the complexity of these functions can be adjusted to fit the skills of a wide variety of users. The following case study illustrates the application of a PDA as a memory and organization aid.

Memory Message (Saltillo, *www.saltillo.com/*) (Figure 10-6) is a commercially available memory aid designed to assist individuals by reminding them of activities and tasks throughout the day. The small size (6.3 inches × 4 inches × 1.1 inches, 12.5 ounces) makes the device easy to carry. A standard clock face is built into the front of the device that shows the current day and time, and a button is available to provide audible time information. Up to 280 alarms can be set with 40 separate recorded instruction messages. When an alarm occurs, the user can either acknowledge the alarm (by pressing "OK") or have it repeated by pressing (:?"). A caregiver programs alarms and messages through a keyboard. Alarms can be set for a single event or for a recurring activity. The WatchMinder2: Training and Reminder System, which is described in the time management section, can also serve as a memory aid.

	Attention – Signal Detection – Vigilance	Attention – Signal Detection – Search	Attention – Selective	Attention – Divided	Perception	Memory – Storage – Short Term	Memory – Storage – Long Term	Memory – Encoding	Memory – Retrieval – Recognition	Memory – Retrieval – Recall	Info Proc. – Quantitative	Info Proc. – Visuospatial	Info Proc. – Temporal	Info Proc. – Personal	Knowledge – Categorization	Knowledge – Sorting	Knowledge – Sequencing	Knowledge – Mental Rep. – Declarative/know what	Knowledge – Mental Rep. – Procedural/know how	Problem – Identify Problem	Problem – Judgment	Problem – Decision Making	Problem – Reasoning – Deductive	Problem – Reasoning – Inductive	Problem – Planning	Problem – Evaluation and Iteration	Problem – Generalization	Language	Learning – General	Learning – Mathematics	Learning – Reading	Learning – Writing
Memory Aids – Recorders	X	X		X	X	R	R			R			A					R	X									X	X			
Word completion/prediction	X	X		X	X	R	R		X	A									X									X	A		X	A
Information retrieval		X	X		X		X		X	A								A	A			X						A	A			A
Time Management	A	X		X	X	R	R		X	R			R				X	A	X			X		X		X		X	X			
Prompting / Cueing					X	R	R		X	R			R					X	X			X				X		X				
Stimuli Control – Auditory (noise reduction)	A	A	A	A	A	R			R	R	A				X			R	R	R	R	R	R	R	R	R			R	R	R	R
Visual field		A	A	R	R							A								A	R	R	R	R	R	R	A		A	R	R	
Media presentation	A	A	A	A	A																											
Concept organization		A	A	A	X	A	A	A	A	X	A	A			A	A	A	X	X			A	A	X	A	X	A	X	A		A	
Language Tools	X	X		X	X	X	X		X	R	R				X		X	A	X			X	X	X		X		X	A		X	X
Alternative Input		X		X	X						A								X							X		A	X		A	A
Alternative Output	X		X		R						A	R		R														A	A	A	A	A
Tracking	X					R	R		R	R								R		R						R						
ID						R	R		R	R				R				R	X	R											A	R

Figure 10-4   Skills versus assistive technology matrix. An "X" indicates means that the cognitive skill is required to use that type of assistive technology. An "A" means that type of assistive technology might aid the cognitive skill in an activity. An "R" means that type of assistive technology might replace the requirement for that cognitive skill in an activity. Note that these entries are with respect to the assistive technology.

CASE STUDY

MEMORY CHALLENGES AFTER TRAUMATIC BRAIN INJURY

Darrell is a 30-year-old man who sustained a TBI 3 years ago. His ability to read and write was severely affected, but he is able to communicate well through speech. Darrell also has trouble with time management and often forgets to complete daily tasks. He acknowledges his weaknesses and has been actively seeking out technologies that could help him to live more independently. One of Darrell's main concerns is addressing his forgetfulness. Ever since returning to work, he has had to rely on constant reminders from his supervisor to complete tasks. He has found that his inability to read or write was not affecting his job performance, but it was limiting his ability to use written reminders to help with his memory difficulties. In addition to seeking help completing his work duties more independently, Darrell was also hoping to find something that would help him remember to take his medication at the right times throughout the day.

Essentially, what Darrell requires is both a "things-to-do" checklist and an alarm capable of signaling reminders at preset times throughout the day. One major restriction is that he must be able to interact with the device in some way that does not require reading or writing. Aside from that, Darrell has said he would prefer that the device be portable, and that it should have at least enough battery life to last an entire 8-hour work shift.

A PDA device with voice recognition software was recommended for Darrell. After a brief training period, he was able to dictate a list of things he needed to do, store them in the PDA's memory, and then play them back for future reference by use of the device's text-to-voice synthesizer. In this manner, Darrell was able to set up a schedule in the mornings and complete his work duties without constant reminders from his supervisor. He was also able to program a spoken reminder that indicated when it was time to take his medication. Darrell enjoyed the flexibility of this system because, after some training with the device, he was able to program new checklists and alarms as needed. Overall, he was very satisfied with the independence he gained from using the device.

What other alternatives to voice input/output would be appropriate for Darrell's needs? If Darrell was able to read and write, would this affect the choice of technology? Could the same functionality be obtained with a less costly device or combination of devices? Is there a "low-tech" solution?

Time Management. Time management technologies are those devices that aid in the planning, prioritizing, and execution of daily and time-dependent tasks. One class of devices uses an alternative format for representing time to make it more accessible to individuals with intellectual disabilities.

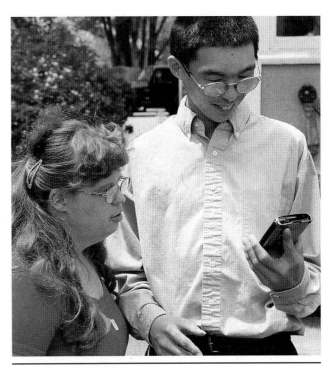

Figure 10-5   PDAs can be used by persons with intellectual disabilities for a variety of tasks. (Courtesy AbleLink Technologies, http://www.ablelinktech.com/.)

Examples of such devices are the Quarter Hour Watch (made by Handitek AB, Sweden, available from ZYGO Industries, Portland, Ore., *www.zygo-usa.com*) (Figure 10-7), a device that offers an alternative and potentially more intuitive representation of the passage of time (Granlund et al, 1995). The Quarter Hour Watch uses an entirely different concept of time by presenting a 2-hour time frame in 8 one-quarter-hour steps. Rather than clock hands or numbers, the watch display has eight circles, one for each quarter hour.

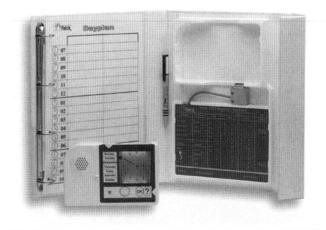

Figure 10-6   The Memory Message system provides reminders of activities throughout the day. (Courtesy Saltillo, www.saltillo.com.)

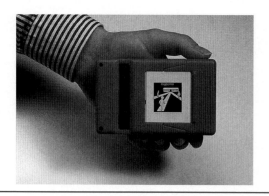

Figure 10-7   The Quarter Hour Watch. (Courtesy ZYGO Industries © GEWA, AB, Portland, Ore., www.zygo-usa.com.)

The user of the watch must understand elapsed time rather than absolute time based on standard clocks. Events are represented by pictures on plastic chips (about the size of 35 mm slides) that are placed into the Quarter Hour Watch. A care provider sets the time of the event on the back of the plastic chip, which is read by the watch. When the chip is inserted into the watch, the display indicates how much time remains until the event should occur. If the time to the event is greater than 2 hours, then all eight circles are dark. After each quarter hour, a circle turns from dark to light until they are all light. At that time a signal sounds and the circles flash. The individual using the watch chooses the chip (e.g., time for favorite TV program, time to go to work) and then is able to tell when that time has arrived.

The WatchMinder (Irvine, Calif., *www.watchminder.com*) (Figure 10-8) is a device that reminds a user when a given, preprogrammed task or event is scheduled to occur. This device was designed for people with attention deficit disorder, ADHD, LD, chronic diseases, stroke, or brain injury. A silent vibrating reminder system or beeping alert, with 30 programmable alarms, is included with both a training and reminder mode. The reminder mode is for remembering

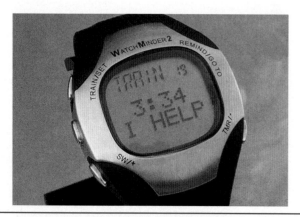

Figure 10-8   WatchMinder. (Courtesy WatchMinder, Irvine, CA, Watchminder.com.)

BOX 10-2	Examples of WatchMinder2 Preset Messages

BATHRM (bathroom)
BE POS (be positive)
BREATH (breathe)
COUGH
FOLDIR (follow directions)
FOLRUL (follow rules)
GIVPOS (give positive reinforcement)
GOODJB (good job)
HANDUP (raise hand)
IGNORE
POSIMG (positive image)
POSTUR (posture)
PRAY
PYATTN (pay attention)
RELAX
REST
SIT
STOP
STRTCH (stretch)

specific tasks such as taking medication and doing homework or chores. The training mode is for behavior change and self-monitoring. Box 10-2 shows preset messages for the WatchMinder2. This device can also be programmed with three personalized messages. The WatchMinder2 has two possible schedule modes: *fixed* (every 2, 3, 5, 10, 15, 20, 30, 45, or 60 minutes) or random (central processing unit randomly chooses from 2, 3, 5, 10, 15, 30, and 60 minutes). The person programming the device chooses one of these modes and the daily start (S) time and end (E) time.

The 24-hour Electronic Time Panel (Saltillo, *www.saltillo.com/*) (Figure 10-9) is a planning board or day planner that facilitates the sequencing and organization of an individual's tasks and events for a given period of time. This panel helps teach concepts such as understanding units of time (e.g., "How long is an hour?") and elapsed time (e.g., "Why can't I have lunch now?"). This device also helps individuals to independently answer daily life questions (e.g., "Do I have time to eat before the bus comes?" or "How long until we go swimming?"). Like the Quarter Hour Watch, the 24-hour Electronic Time Panel uses a lighted display on the one side with increments of 15 minutes from 7 AM to 11 PM. A similar column of lights on the other side shows the times from 11 PM until 7 AM. The time slot adjacent to each light can be labeled with an activity by using text, pictures, or other symbols. The current time is represented either by a column of lights starting with the current time and proceeding in 15-minute intervals or by a single dot of light. The time until a desired activity is indicated by the length of the column of lights from the present time to the start time of the event. Alarms can be set for

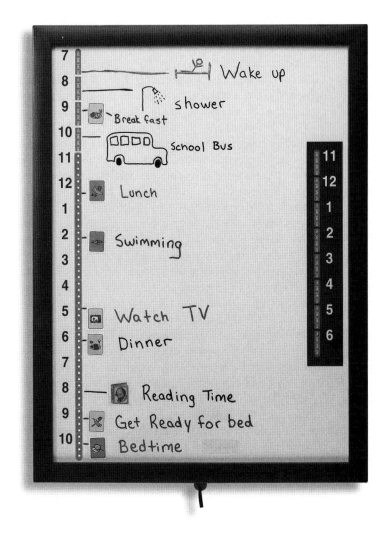

Figure 10-9   The 24-hour Electronic Time Panel. (Courtesy Saltillo, www.saltillo.com.)

each 15-minute increment. The Electronic Time Panel can be used in an individual living arrangement, group living setting, or a classroom.

Davies, Stock, and Wehmeyer (2002) evaluated a palmtop-based time management and scheduling system (Schedule Assistant, AbleLink technologies, Colorado Springs, Col., *www.ablelinktech.com*) designed for individuals who have intellectual disabilities. The Schedule Assistant was evaluated in a pilot study with 12 participants who had intellectual disabilities. Each participant was asked to complete an eight-item schedule using the Schedule Assistant and using a traditional written schedule. A care provider entered a schedule of daily events into the Schedule Assistant and the device provided visual and auditory (speaker or earphone) prompts that correspond to those events at the appropriate time. A typical use of this type of device is shown in Figure 10-5. The reminders can be replayed automatically until acknowledged or by a request from the user. Results showed that participants required significantly less assistance when using the Schedule Assistant than with the written instructions, leading to the conclusion that

electronic scheduling and prompting systems have value for individuals who have intellectual disabilities.

Prompting/Cueing/Coaching.   Prompting systems are those devices or software packages that inform a user that an action should be taken and provide visual, verbal, or auditory cues as to how to accomplish a task. In most cases the systems allow a care provider to enter the relevant information regarding events, times, and frequency. Some devices also allow collection of data regarding ease of use, and others feature communication with a central station for data logging, emergency assistance requests, or tracking of an individual's actions and location.

Prompting people to take their medication is one of the main uses of prompting systems. Low-tech medication reminders, boxes with seven or more compartments labeled by the day or type of medication, have been in widespread use for many years. However, these devices do not alert the person that it is time for the medication. If an alert is needed, then electronic medication reminders are required (Mann, 2005). A watch-based medication reminder (e.g., Cadex Medication Reminder Watch, *http://www.cadexproduct.com/?source=overture&OVRAW=http%2F%2F%3Acadexproducts.com)%5C&OVKEY=http%20cadexproducts.com&OVMTC=standard)* provides up to 12 daily reminders that have an audible alarm and a display of the required medication. Although this format is convenient because of its small size, it has a small display and limited memory. Pagers and cell phones are also used as medication reminders (e.g., MedPrompt Medical Paging System, *www.medprompt.com*) with dosage, type of medication, and instruction provided by text messaging from a central service. Software for PDAs (e.g., On-Time-Rx of Palm OS, *www.ontimerx.com*) provides medication alerts with detailed information regarding pill type and dosage, a medication log, refill reminder, and emergency information (Mann, 2005).

The ISAAC Cognitive Prosthesis System is a wearable and highly customizable device that provides procedural information and personal information storage (Cole and Dehdashti, 1998). This system is a fully individualized cognitive prosthetic system that assists the user to live and work more independently through the organization and delivery of individualized prompts and procedural and personal information. A care provider enters the content with use of an authoring system. The content is then delivered to the individual with a cognitive disability in English or Spanish as synthesized speech, audio, text, checklists, or graphics. Prompts can be delivered on the basis of specified conditions, such as the time of day, to prompt for an action by the user. User input is through a pressure-sensitive touch screen.

Mihailidis, Fernie, and Barbenel (2001) developed a prompting system for handwashing to assist individuals who have dementia. The system, called COACH, uses a video camera, personal computer, and artificial intelligence software. The system monitors progress of the person and provides auditory prompts when steps are skipped or mistakes are made. The system also learns the patterns of the individual users and adapts its settings and cues to match them. In a single subject design study with 10 elder participants, the COACH system led to significant improvement in completion of hand washing tasks without caregiver assistance (Mihailidis, 2004).

Individuals with Alzheimer's disease often have periods of forgetfulness and disorientation. The disorientation can lead to wandering behavior that is unsafe to the person and very worrisome to the caregivers and family. Global positioning systems (GPS) have been used to assist these individuals by providing their location to the caregiver (Mann, 2005). The GPS Locator Watch (Wherify, *www.childlocator.com/*) is designed to track children, but its features apply well to persons with dementia. The watch has a wireless transmitter/receiver that transmits the location of the person and allows transmission of information to the watch. To prevent individuals whose disability makes it difficult to understand the purpose of the watch and who try to remove it, the watch has an electronically activated

lock to keep it in place. The lock can be remotely released for removal. The device also has a built-in pager, clock, and emergency call function. A navigational device based on a GPS cell phone, called Opportunity Knocks, was designed specifically for people with cognitive limitations (Kautz et al, 2004). This device learns the patterns of the user, and uses that pattern to help the user find the most familiar (not necessarily the shortest) route, recover from mistakes, and receive prompts when needed. If an error occurs (e.g., a user misses a bus stop that is routinely taken), the device verbally prompts the user with prompts such as "I think you made a mistake" or "May I guide you to [location]?" The user can indicate which location by touching a picture of it on the display of the cell phone. Then a mode of transportation (e.g., walk or bus) is chosen in the same way. Using the stored patterns, the system then directs the user to that location. Using stored information, the system can also determine whether the user is on the wrong bus and direct him to get off at the next stop. Instruction can then be provided to get the person back on track to his or her destination.

The concept of a **smart house** (Figure 10-10) has been used to denote living environments in which automation is used to provide automatic functions including monitoring, communication, household functions (lights, air conditioning/heating, door locks), physiological measurements, and medication alerts (Mann, 2005). Smart houses have the potential to allow individuals with cognitive limitations greater independence, and in the case of elderly individuals, a chance to stay in their homes rather than move to group living facilities. Mann (2005) describes levels of smart house from basic communications (Internet, phone) through complex monitoring and tracking of the resident's health, behavior, and needs. The core of the smart house is a processing and communication system linked to a sensory array. One example of a monitoring application is described in the following case study. The system aids a user in performing common tasks of daily living by assessing the person's current physiological state and the state of various utilities throughout the home and providing the user with feedback should they become disoriented or confused on a given task (Haigh, Kiff, and Ho, 2006). Mann (2005) describes several smart house projects.

CASE STUDY

DEMENTIA: ASSISTIVE TECHNOLOGY TO ALLOW STAYING AT HOME

Eighty-six-year old Emily has lived in her own home for many years. She and her husband (deceased) raised their family in this home, and her daughter still lives nearby. Emily now lives alone in the home. She has had difficulty remembering things and occasionally gets confused since she sustained a series of ministrokes a few years ago. Although her daughter helps out as much as she can, her own family and full-time job limit her availability. Emily's confusion and memory loss have resulted in her leaving the gas cooker in her house turned on but not lit. Several possible solutions were proposed by the local assistive technology clinic. Because Emily still enjoyed cooking her own meals, turning off the gas permanently was ruled out. An electric cooker was suggested, but Emily had spent her life cooking on a gas stove and didn't want to "learn how to cook all over again." A microwave oven was ruled out for the same reason. The solution that was implemented involved using a gas sensor connected to a shut-off valve. The sensor was originally connected to an audible alarm, and its use to control the shut-off valve required modification. The system was also set up to notify a central home monitoring system that a gas leak had been detected. The home monitoring center then notified Emily's daughter, who was able to go to the home and turn the gas back on. This approach allowed Emily to remain at home and to continue preparing her own meals. In the past year or so, her daughter has only had to reconnect the gas about four times in total.

Adapted from the Safe Home Project,
www.tunstall.co.uk/6_3casestudies.htm.

The COACH and the smart house are examples of *context-aware cognitive orthoses* (LoPresti, Mihailidis, and Kirsch, 2004). Each of these systems provides cueing and prompting on the basis of a combination of prestored information and data obtained from sensors in the environment. The use of context-based information can relieve anxiety, reduce the cognitive load, and overcome a lack of initiation by the individual using the device. In terms of the HAAT model, this functionality provides important information about one of the four elements of the model: the context. LoPresti, Mihailidis, and Kirsch (2004) describe other examples of context-aware cognitive orthoses.

Low-tech devices can also aid a user in performing a task by providing concrete feedback as to the proper course of action to undertake. For example, a microwave button shield only lets a user see/use those buttons that are needed for a specific task or raised lines on paper give a user an idea of where symbols should be placed to enhance readability. Task-specific jigs enable people to perform tasks that they may not otherwise be able to perform. For example, weighing and counting tasks in manufacturing and assembly can be difficult for workers who have cognitive disabilities. One approach to modifying weighing and counting is to use a talking scale connected to a controller that provides prompting and feedback as necessary

(Erlandson and Stant, 1998). For counting tasks, a bin with a specified number of locations is weighed. If the bin is properly filled, the weight is correct and the user is prompted to proceed with the next step. If the weight is too low, the user is told to check all the bins, and if it is too high the user is prompted to be sure only one element is in each bin. For weighing, objects placed on the scale are compared with stored weight limit values, and the user is prompted if the weight is above or below the weight range. Visual and auditory prompts are included. Erlandson and Stant (1998) describe the successful use of this system in a nail counting task for a construction supply company by a woman with mild intellectual disability.

Prompting systems have been used with autistic individuals for initiation, maintenance, or termination of an activity (Goldsmith and LeBlanc, 2004). Coyle and Cole (2004) reported a decrease of off-task behavior in three autistic students when an auditory timer was used to prompt self-monitoring of on-task behavior in classroom settings. Taber et al (1999) similarly reported a decrease in teacher-delivered prompts and in off-task and inappropriate behavior in a 12-year-old student when a self-operated auditory prompting system was used. Tactile systems were investigated in a few studies to increase verbal initiation (Shabani et al, 2002; Taylor and Levin, 1998) and to seek assistance when lost (Taylor et al, 2004).

Although most of the studies report a positive outcome of a prompting system, these reports consist of mainly preliminary or anecdotal results, with small, if not single numbers of case studies. More systematic studies should be conducted to demonstrate the efficacy of prompting systems in assisting social initiation in individuals with ASD. With the increasing popularity and advancement in small electronic devices (e.g., cell phones, PDAs, MP3 players, etc.), these systems could provide a more cost effective and socially valid assistive technology for ASD.

Stimuli Control.   The family of **stimuli control** devices includes technologies that address attention or perception problems by limiting or manipulating the information presented to the user. They can be subdivided into three categories that best capture their intended application: noise reduction techniques, visual field manipulation, and media presentation techniques. Auditory (noise reduction) devices are those devices that filter out extraneous noise so the user may focus on one specific source. An example of such a system is a transmitter/headphone receiver link between a student and teacher in a classroom setting similar to those used for students who are hard of hearing (see FM systems in Chapter 9). Visual stimuli can be altered in a similar fashion, through the use of prism glasses or special lenses that correct for double vision or neglect (e.g., in TBI).

Media presentation is an important design consideration for many visual display applications. Web sites, computer monitors, and other visual displays need to be carefully

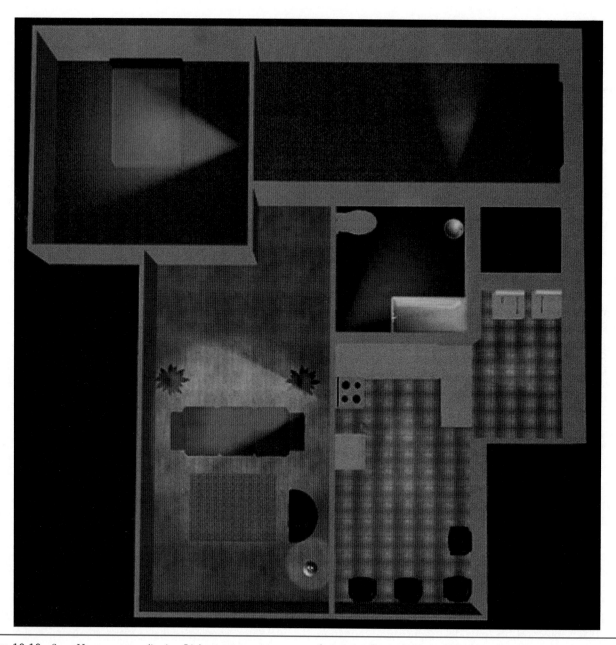

Figure 10-10   SmartHouse conceptualization. Light areas represent sensor field for detecting movement by room. (Courtesy Medical Automation Research Center, University of Virginia, https://smarthouse. med.virginia.edu/index.php.)

designed to avoid extraneous information that might be distracting to a person with an attention disorder. By reducing clutter, increasing clarity, and simplifying visual displays, information can be presented in a way that is best perceived and understood by a broad target audience. Key concepts in Web design for individuals with cognitive disabilities are shown in Table 10-10. The WebAim project (Center for Persons with Disabilities, Utah State University, *www.webaim.org*) has many useful resources for making Web sites accessible to individuals who have cognitive disabilities. These include evaluation packages to check Web sites for accessibility, guidelines

for developing accessible Web sites, and tools for making Web sites more accessible to this population.

Internet access for individuals with intellectual disabilities can provide benefits in self-esteem and self-confidence, independence in vocational and living contexts, opportunities for training, self-directed activities, and use of their time for pursuits that are stimulating and informative (Davies, Stock, and Wehmeyer, 2001). Unfortunately, access to the Internet for this population is often limited by standard Web browsers that require high-level cognitive skills, particularly in reading and writing. A pilot project

TABLE 10-10   Key Concepts in Web Design for Individuals With Cognitive Disabilities

Challenges	Solutions
Users may become confused at complex layouts or inconsistent navigational schemes.	Simplify the layout as much as possible. Keep the navigational schemes as consistent as possible.
Users may have difficulty focusing on or comprehending lengthy sections of text.	Where appropriate, group textual information under logical headings. Organize information in manageable "chunks."
One method of input may not be sufficient.	Where appropriate, supplement text with illustrations or other media, and vice versa.

Data from WebAIM, http://www.webaim.org/techniques/cognitive/.

was designed to compare a specially designed Web browser (Web Trek, AbleLink Technologies, Colorado Springs, Col., *www.ablelinktech.com/_desktop/webtrek.asp*) with a standard browser (Internet Explorer, Microsoft, Inc., Redmond Wash., *www.microsoft.com*) (Davies, Stock, and Wehmeyer, 2001). Web Trek uses graphics, reduced screen clutter, audio prompts, and personalization and customization to maximize accessibility to individuals with intellectual disabilities. Twelve participants evaluated the two browsers in three tasks: searching for a Web site, saving Web sites to a favorites list, and retrieving sites from the favorites. Three measures of performance were used: independence (fewer prompts), accuracy (errors made), and task completion (completed with three or fewer prompts). All three measures showed statistically significant differences favoring the Web Trek browser, indicating that Internet access for persons with intellectual disabilities is feasible.

Concept Organization and Decision Making. Concept organization strategies and software packages facilitate the organization, storage, and retrieval of related ideas/facts. An example is *Inspiration*, a software package for organizing concepts related to a central theme. Devices in this category may be used as a memory aid or as a tool to help with writing. For example, the interconnections drawn between various items are useful for creating a logical flow of thoughts when it comes to writing, or alternatively the graphical representation may be a helpful tool for committing things to memory.

Individuals with intellectual disabilities have a very high unemployment rate. The increasing complexity of the work environment is one of the major reasons for this high rate. People with intellectual disabilities are often not able to learn complex decision-making skills that are essential for work. Davies, Stock, and Wehmeyer (2003) carried out a pilot study with a PDA-based device (Pocket Compass, AbleLink Technologies, Colorado Springs, Col., *http://www.ablelinktech.com/_handhelds/pocketcompass.asp*) specifically designed to assist in decision making. The *Pocket*

Compass uses graphic and audio prompts to guide a user through a decision-making process when participating in complex tasks. The decision-making process contains a branching sequence of cued steps with decision points based on a task analysis of the desired job activity. In the setup mode the work supervisor or care provider creates cueing sequences described by pictures and recorded audio instructions. Decision points in a decision-making process can be identified with these pictures and audio labels. Once a setup has been entered into the device, the user can move through the sequence of instructions and decision points by using the graphic and auditory prompts and making entries (beginning with START and then NEXT after each choice is presented) through a touch screen on the PDA. Up to four pictures can be presented at decision points. Forty participants who had intellectual disabilities participated in a pilot study of Pocket Compass in an activity developed from a task in which different pieces of software were packaged for shipping (Davies, Stock, and Wehmeyer, 2003). Participants using the device made fewer errors performing the task and fewer errors in decision points, and less assistance was required using the PDA than when they had only a job coach. Davies, Stock, and Wehmeyer concluded that technology can significantly assist persons with intellectual disabilities in accomplishing relatively complicated work-related tasks independently.

The Planning and Execution Assistant and Trainer (PEAT) (Attention Control Systems, Mountain View, Calif., *www.brainaid.com/*) is a PDA-based personal planning assistant designed to assist individuals with cognitive disorders resulting from brain injury, stroke, Alzheimer's disease, and similar conditions (Levinson, 1997). PEAT uses artificial intelligence to automatically generate plans and also to revise those plans when unexpected events occur. PEAT uses a combination of manually entered schedules and a library of stored scripts describing activities of daily living (e.g., morning routine or shopping). Scripts can be used for both planning and for execution. Planning involves a simulation of the activity with key decision points presented and necessary prompts (auditory and visual) supplied to aid the individual through the planning process. The plan to be executed can be either the stored script or a modified script based on the simulation. The PEAT artificial intelligence software generates the best strategy to execute the required steps in the plan (LoPresti, Mihailidis, and Kirsch, 2004). PEAT also automatically monitors performance and corrects schedule problems when necessary.

Language Tools.   Many forms of assistive technology are *language tools* that assist with reading or writing. Many devices focus on the memory requirements of language. For example, word completion programs (see Chapter 7) are useful for people who are poor at spelling. They predict whole words on the basis of the first few letters typed by the user. A list of possible word choices is presented, and the user need only recognize the intended word from that list. Dictionaries and thesauruses are low-tech alternatives to word completion programs because they also operate on the basis of using word recognition to rectify deficiencies in word retrieval. For TBI, word prediction software programs have all shown to be useful in clinical trials (Kim et al, 1999; Van Hulle and Hux, 2005).

Word prediction has been shown to be a promising strategy for improving text entry speed of students with learning disabilities as they move from hand writing to computer writing by using a word processor (Lewis, 2005). Word prediction programs written specifically for students with learning disabilities (for example, Co-Writer, Don Johnston, Inc, Volo, Ill., *www.donjohnston.com*) include features that make them more effective. In addition to simple word prediction, these programs often include dictionaries to suggest alternatives that increase the richness and interest of the writing on the basis of the topic being discussed, and they can be personalized for an individual student. Another program is WordQ (*http://www.synapseadaptive.com/quill-soft/WQ/wordq_description.htm*), which takes into account phonetic spelling mistakes.

Studies of the impact of word prediction on writing abilities of students with learning disabilities have led to mixed results (Sitko, Laine, and Sitko, 2005). In small sample studies, word prediction programs have been shown to improve writing by addressing word finding problems. When coupled with speech synthesis, the results are improved further. Results vary for word completion versus word prediction (see Chapter 7), with word prediction being more effective because it includes the context of the sentence as well as that of the word.

Spell checking programs are helpful to students with learning disabilities as editing tools, but grammar checkers are not (Lewis, 2005). Spell checking programs are designed to primarily detect typographical errors, not misspellings resulting from phonetic errors (Ashton, 2006). Thus, the target word for a student with a leaning disability, who is spelling phonetically, is often not the first word listed by the

spell checking program. Despite this limitation, students with learning disabilities were able to detect their target word 95% of the time, even if it was not the first word listed (Ashton, 2006). The reason for the lack of success with grammar checkers is that they often rely on text to have correct spelling (Lewis, 2005). When evaluated on the basis of types of spelling errors made by students with learning disabilities, spell checkers vary widely in effectiveness (Sitko, Laine, and Sitko, 2005). Spell checking programs are most effective when they are integrated into a word processing program.

Concept mapping is a process of conceptualizing information by using graphics and text. The Inspiration concept mapping software (Inspiration Software, Inc, Beaverton Ore., *http://www.inspiration.com/*) is designed to help students in grades 6 through 12 to plan, organize, and write research papers (Figure 10-11). Its alternative format for representing ideas with both text and graphics, its ability to import concepts from the Internet and other sources, and the provision of a large number of templates make Inspiration useful to students who have learning disabilities (Ashton, 2005; LoPresti, Mihailidis, and Kirsch, 2004). Inspiration also allows the student to toggle between text and concept map as they develop their reports. With use of Inspiration, eighth grade students who had LDs produced essays that were significantly above their pretest levels in number of words, concepts included, and holistic writing scores (Sturm and Rankin-Ericson, 2002).

Alternative Input.   **Alternative input** technologies offer the user different modalities for providing input commands or information to a device. One example is voice recognition software (see Chapter 7). Voice recognition can be useful for generation of text input by individuals with cognitive disabilities that limit their ability to write (LoPresti, Mihailidis, and Kirsch, 2004). Users are able to enter information or commands to a computer through voice dictation instead of mouse and keyboard. For TBI, speech recognition programs have all shown to be useful in clinical trials (Kim et al, 1999; Van Hulle and Hux, 2005). Voice recognition can be very effective in improving writing for students with LDs (Sitko, Laine, and Sitko, 2005). A person with an LD may be able to verbally articulate thoughts very well but, because of visual processing problems, may have trouble getting words down on paper: "the words jump all over the page." Automatic speech recognition provides an alternative for this type of individual.

Voice memo recorders are used in a similar manner, replacing pen-and-paper or keyboard entry as a means of storing messages for future reference. For those who are unable to make the fine motor movements required for handwriting, a portable notebook computer (e.g., Neo by AlphaSmart, *www.alphasmart.com/*) with abbreviation expansion or word completion/prediction (see Chapter 7) may be more efficient.

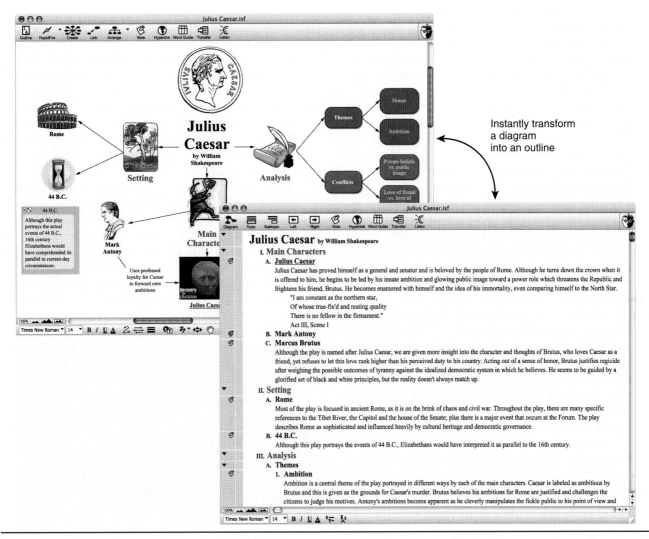

Figure 10-11 Inspiration software allows the development of ideas in a graphical format and automatic conversion to text. (Courtesy Inspiration Software, Inc, Beaverton, Ore., http://www.inspiration.com/.)

Buttons with descriptive pictures and text may make the function of input controls more obvious.

The Aurora (AUtonomous RObotic platform as a Remedial tool for children with Autism) Project investigated the feasibility of robotic toys serving therapeutic roles in improving social interaction in autistic children (Dautenhahn and Werry, 2004). Children were presented with an interactive robot toy, which was programmed to sense and imitate the children's movement. Although the long-term therapeutic effect of the toy is still unknown, preliminary findings and anecdotal reports from the project suggest that robots can potentially serve as a mediator in facilitating interaction between autistic children and their peers or other adults (Dautenhahn and Werry, 2004; Robins et al, 2004) and encouraged playing. Robins et al (2004) reported an increase in mutual gaze and gaze following among three autistic children and the experimenter during

interaction with a robotic toy, suggesting that joint attention was established. The Aurora Project is an innovative application of alternative input using robotics as an intermediary through which a person with autism can communicate with others. Because individuals with autism often demonstrate deficits in interpreting and predicting human behavior, interactions with robots can provide a relatively simplified, safe, predictable, and reliable environment.

Alternative Output. **Alternative output** technologies offer users a nontraditional means of acquiring feedback or information from a device. Some individuals are more visually oriented, and print or screen displays work well for them. For others information is easiest to access in auditory form. Synthesized or digitized speech output is often used for auditory information. The principles of electronically generated speech and its application in augmentative communication systems are discussed in Chapter 7. Many devices that were originally developed for individuals who have limited vision make use of synthesized speech to enhance or replace a typically visual output. Examples of these devices include text-to-speech screen readers for computer applications, talking calculators, a tape measure with speech output, and bar code scanners (see Chapter 8).

Synthesized speech and digitized speech (see Chapter 7) are both used to provide auditory information to children and adults with intellectual disabilities (see prompting and cueing section in this chapter). Synthesized speech associated with a word processor (for example, Write Outloud, Don Johnston, Inc, Volo, Ill., *www.donjohnston.com*) for students with LDs can provide an additional modality that is helpful in writing and editing. The greatest benefit may be in reducing the most common misspellings (i.e., those that are "non-real" words such as "thar" for "there" as opposed to word substitutions such as "to" for "two") (Lewis, 2005). Synthetic speech output also was useful when the spell checker could not suggest any words because of gross misspelling. The impact of speech output is more significant for younger learners than for secondary students. In some cases, the impact of speech synthesizers in providing writing assistance to students with LDs is less significant than the effective use of spell checkers and word prediction (Lewis, 2005). However, as illustrated by the following case study, auditory output by speech synthesis is an effective tool for students with reading or writing difficulties associated with LDs (Sitko, Laine, and Sitko, 2005). Students can often detect errors in their writing more easily if they hear the words as opposed to reading them in written form. Adding speech synthesis to the presentation of screen-based text provides a multimodal output that also assists in reading and writing.

CASE STUDY

LEARNING DISABILITY AND ALTERNATIVE INPUT FOR READING

Daniel is a student in a regular educational program. He has an LD that makes it difficult for him to read printed material. The system provided for Daniel allows him to have an alternative input modality for his reading. He completes the printed lesson that requires him to fill in blanks on a worksheet by using a scanner that digitizes his lesson and puts it into a word processor. He listens to the text using on earphones so as not to disturb the other students. With this system he is able to mark and copy the text using a reading program like those described in this section. He also makes use of word prediction, spell checking, and grammar checking in completing his assignments.

Because many individuals with LDs have greater comprehension of auditory than written information, synthesized speech output in "talking books" or "e-books" has been shown to be effective in improving reading abilities (Ashton, 2005). E-books have a number of features that are useful for students who have LDs. For example, words can be highlighted in the text as they are spoken or the document can be presented in an enlarged font. For students who need spelling practice, a spelling activity can be selected that uses the words from the story. Using software and on-line tools, teachers can create their own e-books (Ashton, 2005).

The Readingpen (WizCom Technologies, Ashton, Mass., *www.wizcomtech.com/*), an assistive reading device (Figure 10-12), is a hand-held scanner that is designed specifically for school-age reading levels. As the pen is moved across a word or full line of text, the text is spoken aloud. Using a children's dictionary and thesaurus, the device also provides information to the student about word meaning and alternative words through a three-line built-in display. The pen provides

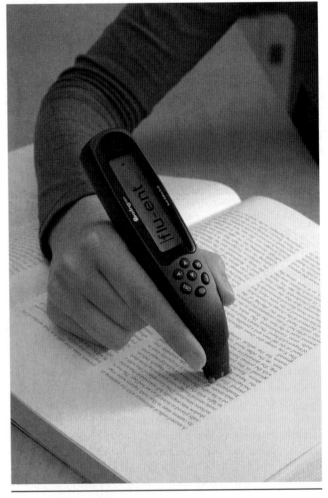

Figure 10-12   The Readingpen. Text is scanned into the pen's memory. (Courtesy WizCom technologies, Ashton, MA, www.wizcomtech.com/.)

a portable way for people with reading difficulties, LDs, or dyslexia to get immediate word support when they are reading. The scanned text may be spoken word by word or line by line. An earphone connection is available for privacy.

Altering the visual appearance of the computer screen can also aid individuals with disorders such as dyslexia (LoPresti, Mihailidis, and Kirsch, 2004). Changing features such as font size; background/foreground color combinations; contrast; spacing between words, letters, and paragraphs; and use of graphics can all improve access to screen-based information.

Tracking and Identification.   This final category consists of technologies that involve the **tracking and identification** of people or items. Such devices often provide an extra degree of safety for users who might not have the cognitive skills required to work their way out of problematic situations. For instance, the SmartChip *(www.smartchip. com/)* ID is a wearable electronic device that stores critical information about the user. If the user became lost, the stored information can be made available to someone who could make use of this information to ensure the user got home safely.

Another method of tracking is home monitoring systems that can keep track of the status of a person with cognitive disabilities. These systems include monitoring of the environment within a house (e.g., gas or smoke detectors), cardiac parameters (heart rate, arrhythmias), objects, and people (e.g., sensors that determine whether a person has left his or her bed by monitoring the weight applied to a pressure sensor place under the bed frame), and emergency call (a button that is pushed and automatically dials a central station). The suppliers (for example, in Canada, *www.lifeline.ca/*, in the United Kingdom, *http://www. tunstall.co.uk/home.asp*, and in the United States, *http:// www.lifestation.com/?ASK=Medical-Alert*) of these systems describe many case examples on their Web sites that illustrate how these systems can make it possible for persons with memory loss, wandering, and other cognitive limitations to continue to live at home (see the following case study). These systems are often incorporated into the Smart House concept discussed in this chapter.

Cognitive Assistive Technologies With Multiple Functions

The preceding sections discussed assistive technologies that are designed primarily for one function, although some may be useful for multiple needs. There are also devices designed for multiple functions. These devices are often designed to provide a more comprehensive assistance to persons with certain disorders.

A design concept and prototype for a cognitive prosthesis was developed by the Rehabilitation Engineering

---

CASE STUDY

DEMENTIA AND WANDERING

Tito is 70 years old and has recently been diagnosed with Alzheimer's dementia. He lives with his wife Betsy in the small house in which he raised his family. His son comes by and checks up on his parents three to four times a week and is readily available should necessity arise. Because of Tit(o's condition, he has acquired a forgetfulness to turn things off which require vigilance and has been found taking "walks" late at night. Unfortunately, Tito has had problems finding his way home during his outings and his son has received calls from the local police on two occasions regarding this problem. Betsy helps him remember to take his medicine and makes sure he doesn't forget the time of his weekly bingo game, and he still has no problem remembering old friends' names or solving his morning crossword puzzles. Given this profile, what types of assistive technologies that might benefit Tito?

Research Center (RERC) on Mobile Wireless Technologies for Persons with Disabilities at Georgia Tech University (Jones, 2006). The prototype was developed on a PDA platform and included three broad mobile wireless technology applications that support community re-entry for people who have cognitive impairments resulting from TBI: These are (1) time management, (2) way finding in the community with use of GPS navigational tools, and (3) prompting and cueing to initiate and sustain engagement in activity. The user interface design was critical to ensure that it was understandable and usable to people with significant cognitive impairments (Haberman, Jones, and Meuller, 2005). A drawing of the user interface is shown in Figure 10-13. The major features of the prototype were an event reminder system, a contact database, a location finder, a list tracker, image capture capability, a medical manager, a money manager, and messaging capability.

The European Union Telematics Applications Supporting Cognition (TASC) project developed a device that focused on the areas of need for persons with cognitive disability in guidance, information provision, communication, environmental control, and planning and time management (Fagerberg, 1999). TASC consists of five software modules implemented with Java components that run on standard computers. Information can be presented with text, pictures, symbols, and sound. The guidance module (TASC Prompter) guides the user through steps of daily activities such as clothes selection or meal preparations and reminds when it is time to do a specific activity like catch a bus or go to work. Information such as television or bus schedules and weather

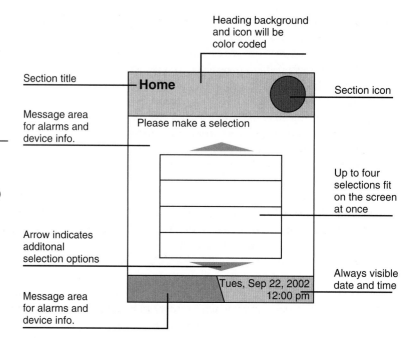

Figure 10-13   User interface for a prototype mobile cognitive prosthesis. (Courtesy Rehabilitation Engineering Research Center for Wireless Technologies, http://www. wirelessrerc.gatech.edu/projects/development/d5_index.htm.)

forecasts can be introduced directly into the system or can be downloaded from the Internet through the TASC Information Provider presented in the user's chosen format. The user can receive and make phone calls with the Communicator module, which also supports FAX transmission and allows either dialing in the standard fashion number-by-number or pressing a key labeled with a picture. For environmental control the TASC Supervisor carries out the appropriate action by using data from sensors combined with user instructions. The TASC Planner supports the independent development of plans and schedules by keeping track of details such as time and length of an activity. The user can then schedule and reschedule activities while the Planner keeps track of the details. All the modules can be programmed to fit the needs of the user. Personalized information such as photographs and voice input can easily be introduced into the system. The benefits of the TASC system are that persons with cognitive disabilities can achieve increased independence and self-assurance, improved social contacts, reduction in the need for help from others with daily activities, increased quality of life, and reduced costs for assistance and institutional care.

SUMMARY

Individuals who have cognitive disabilities of various types and severity can benefit from the use of assistive technologies. The implementation of these assistive technologies and strategies is based on the augmentation of or substitution for cognitive skills that are required for the completion of specific functional tasks. Cognitive disabilities represent a wide variety of skill levels and severity, and an equally wide range of types of assistive technologies are available to ameliorate these conditions.

Study Questions

1. Pick a specific cognitive disability, an activity, and a context and describe how the HAAT model (as described in Chapter 2) would be applied to determine the best assistive technology approach (hard and soft technologies) for that individual.

2. How do assistive technology approaches differ for congenital and acquired cognitive disabilities?

3. Pick a specific disorder and describe both the cognitive skills that are likely to be available for use of an assistive device and those that may need to be replaced or augmented by such a device.

4. List the major characteristics of mild cognitive disabilities as they relate to the use of assistive technologies.

5. List the major characteristics of intellectual disabilities as they relate to the use of assistive technologies.

6. List the major characteristics of dementia that may be aided by cognitive assistive technologies.

7. In terms of recommendation of assistive technologies, how do CVA and TBI differ from other acquired cognitive disabilities and from each other?

8. How do the considerations for mild cognitive disability, intellectual disability, and acquired disability differ?

What are the implications of these differences for the application of assistive technologies?

9. Why is ADHD not considered an LD?

10. What interventions are commonly applied to the treatment of LDs?

11. Describe the differences between remediation and compensation as they apply to cognitive disabilities.

12. How do the terms remediation and compensation differ when applied to sensory (Chapter 8 and 9) or motor (Chapter 7, 11, or 12) disabilities as opposed to cognitive disabilities?

13. What are the currently available assistive technologies that are beneficial to children with ASD? What are the efficacies and feasibilities of these technologies in replacing or augmenting skill deficits?

14. What are the characteristics of PDA-based time management systems for persons with intellectual disabilities?

15. Describe the general characteristics of memory aids.

16. Contrast the use of memory aids in intellectual disabilities, dementia, and TBI.

17. Describe how systems designed to provide prompting, cueing, or coaching are applied to assist persons with intellectual disabilities.

18. How do applications of prompting, cueing, or coaching systems differ between applications for individuals with intellectual disabilities and those with dementia.

19. What is meant by the term *stimuli control*, and how is this concept applied to Web page design?

20. What are the major challenges in using assistive technologies to address the problems faced by individuals with dementia?

21. How can word completion and word prediction benefit students who have LDs? What are the limitations in this application?

22. What are the most commonly used alternatives to printed text output?

23. What is *concept mapping* and how can it benefit students who have LDs?

24. What should be considered when recommending a time management device for a stroke patient?

25. What is a cognitive prosthesis? Describe how these devices are applied to assist individuals with TBI.

References

American Psychiatric Association: *Diagnostic and statistical manual of mental disorders, DSM-IV*, ed 4, Washington DC, 2000, American Psychiatric Association.

Anderson JR: *Cognitive psychology and its implications*, New York, 2000, Worth Publishers.

Ashcraft MH: *Fundamentals of cognition*, New York, 1998, Addison-Wesley.

Ashton TM: Students with learning disabilities using assistive technology in the inclusive classroom. In Edyburn D, Higgins K, Boone R, editors: *Handbook of special education technology research and practice*, pp 229-238, Whitefish Bay, Wis., 2005, Knowledge by Design, Inc.

Atkinson RC, Shiffrin RM: Human memory: a proposed system and its control processes. In Spence KW, Spence JT, editors: *The psychology of learning and motivation: advances in research and theory*, vol 2, pp 89-195, New York, 1968, Academic Press.

Bergman MM: The benefits of a cognitive orthotic in brain injury rehabilitation, *J Head Trauma Rehabil* 17: 431-445, 2002.

Bower B: Mind-expanding machines: artificial intelligence meets good old-fashioned human thought, *Sci News* (Aug 30, 2003): http://www.findarticles.com/p/articles/mi_m1200/is_9_164/ai_108050570. Accessed May 5, 2005

Bruno AA: Motor recovery in stroke: http://www.emedicine.com/pmr/topic234.htm. Accessed April 6, 2005.

Chakrabarti S, Fombonne E: Pervasive developmental disorders in preschool children, *JAMA* 285:3093-3099, 2001.

Chen Z, Sanchez RP, Campbell T: From beyond to within grasp: the rudiments of analogical problem solving in 10- to 13-month-olds, *Dev Psychol* 33:790-801, 1997.

Cherry EC: Some experiments on the recognition of speech, with one and with two ears, *J Acoust Soc Am* 25:975-979, 1953.

Cicerone KD et al: Evidence-based cognitive rehabilitation: updated review of the literature from 1998 through 2002, *Arch Phys Med Rehabil* 86:1681-92, 2005.

Cole E, Dehdashti P: Cognitive prosthetics and telerehabilitation: approaches for the rehabilitation of mild brain injuries, computer-based cognitive prosthetics: assistive technology for the treatment of cognitive disabilities. In: *Proceedings of the Third International ACM Conference on Assistive Technologies, ACM SIGCAPH*, Marina del Rey, CA, 1998, The Conference.

Cole E, Matthews MK: *Proceedings of Basil Therapy Congress, Basel, Switzerland*, pp 111-120 (June 1999): http://www.brain-rehab.com/pdf/cpt1999.pdf. Accessed July 27, 2006.

Coyle C, Cole P: A videotaped self-modeling and self-monitoring treatment program to decrease off-task behavior in children with autism, *J Intellect Dev Dis* 29: 3-15, 2004.

Daley D: Attention deficit hyperactivity disorder: a review of the essential facts, *Child Care Health Dev* 32:193-204, 2006.

Dautenhahn K, Werry I: Towards interactive robots in autism therapy: background, motivation and challenges, *Pragmatics Cognition* 12:1-35, 2004.

Davies DK, Stock SE, Wehmeyer ML: Enhancing internet access for individuals with mental retardation through use of a specialized web browser: a pilot study, *Educ Train Ment Retard Dev Disabil* 36:107-113, 2001.

Davies DK, Stock SE, Wehmeyer ML: Enhancing independent time-management skills of individuals with mental retardation using a palmtop personal computer, *Ment Retard* 40:358-365, 2002.

Davies DK, Stock SE, Wehmeyer ML: A Palmtop computer-based intelligent aids for individuals with intellectual disabilities to increase independent decision making, *Res Pract Persons Severe Disabil* 4:182-193, 2003.

Dawodu SY: Traumatic brain injury: Definition, epidemiology, pathophysiology, WebMD: e-medicine: http://www.emedicine.com/pmr/topic212.htm#top. Accessed August 27, 2006.

Demaerschalk B, Hachinski V: Stroke (brain attack), *Griffith's: 5-minute clinical consult: a reference for clinicians:* http://www.5mcc.com/Assets/SUMMARY/TP0175.html. Accessed August 27, 2006.

Edyburn DL: Assistive technology and students with mild disabilities: from consideration to outcome measurement. In: Edyburn D, Higgins K, Boone R, editors: *Handbook of special education technology research and practice*, pp 239-270, Whitefish Bay, WI, 2005, Knowledge by Design, Inc.

Edyburn, DL: Remediation vs. compensation: a critical decision point in assistive technology consideration (2002): http://www.connsensebulletin.com/edyburnv4n3.html. Accessed August 3, 2006.

Erlandson RF, Stant D: Polka-yoke process controller: designed for individuals with cognitive impairments, *Assist Technol* 10:102-112, 1998.

Fagerberg G: Support software for persons with cognitive disabilities, *Proceedings CSUN Technology And Persons With Disabilities Conference* (1999): http://www.csun.edu/cod/conf/1999/proceedings/session0275.htm. Accessed July 18, 2006.

Galotti KM: *Cognitive psychology: In and out of the laboratory*, Belmont, Calif., 2004, Wadsworth.

Goldsmith T, LeBlanc L: Use of technology in interventions for children with autism, *J Early Intens Behav Intervent* 1:166-178, 2004.

Golisz KM, Toglia JP: Perception and cognition. In: Blesedell Crepeau E et al, editors: *Willard and Spackman's occupational therapy*, ed 10, pp 395-416, Philadelphia, PA, 2003, Lippincott Williams & Wilkins.

Gorman P et al: Effectiveness of the ISAAC cognitive prosthetic system for improving rehabilitation outcomes with neurofunctional impairment, *Neurorehabilitation* 18:57-67, 2003.

Granlund M et al: Assistive technology for cognitive disability, *Technol Disabil* 4:205-214, 1995.

Haberman V, Jones ML, Meuller JL: Design of a mobile wireless technology for individuals with cognitive impairment, *Proceedings 2005RESNA Conference:* http://resna.org/ProfResources/Publications/Proceedings/2005/Research/Other/Hamberman.php. Accessed August 3, 2006.

Haigh KZ, Kiff LM, Ho G: The independent lifestyle assistant: lessons learned, *Assist Technol* 18:87-106, 2006.

Hunt RR, Ellis HC: *Fundamentals of cognitive psychology*, ed 6, Boston, 1999, McGraw-Hill College.

Johnson E, Mellard DF, Byrd SE: Alternative models of learning disabilities identification, *J Learn Disabil* 38: 569-572, 2005.

Jones M: Index—a design concept and prototype for a cognitive prosthesis, Wireless RERC: http://www.wirelessrerc.gatech.edu/projects/development/d5.html. Accessed August 3, 2006.

Kautz H et al: Opportunity knocks: a community navigation aid, University of Washington (2004): http://www.cs.washington.edu/homes/kautz/talks/access-symposium-2004.ppt. Accessed July 27, 2006.

Kim HJ et al: Utility of a microcomputer as an external memory aid for a memory-impaired head injury patient during in-patient rehabilitation, *Brain Injury* 13:147-150, 1999.

Levinson RL: The planning and execution assistant and trainer, *J Head Trauma Rehabil* 12:769-775, 1997.

Lewis RB: Classroom technology for students with learning disabilities. In: Edyburn D, Higgins K, Boone R, editors: *Handbook of special education technology research and practice*, pp 325-334, Whitefish Bay, WI, 2005, Knowledge by Design, Inc.

LoPresti EF, Mihailidis A, Kirsch N: Assistive technology for cognitive rehabilitation: state of the art, *Neuropsychoall Rehabil* 14:5-39, 2004.

Mann WC: *Smart technology for aging, disability and independence*, New York, 2005, John Wiley.

McKelvey M et al: Performance of a person with chronic aphasia using a visual scene display prototype, *J Med Speech Lang Pathol*. In press.

Mihailidis A: The efficiency of an intelligent cognitive orthosis to facilitate hand washing by persons with moderate to severe dementia, *Neuropsychol Rehabil* 14: 135-171, 2004.

Mihailidis A, Fernie GR, Barbenel JC: The use of artificial intelligence in the design of an intelligent cognitive orthosis for people with dementia, *Assist Technol* 13: 3-29, 2001.

Newell A, Simon H: *Human problem solving*, Englewood Cliffs, NJ, 1972, Prentice-Hall.

Novack T: What to expect After TBI, *Presented at the Recovery after TBI Conference* (September 1999): http://images.main.uab.edu/spinalcord/pdffiles/tbi3pdf.pdf. Accessed October 31, 2006.

O'Sullivan SB, Schmitz TJ: *Physical rehabilitation: assessment and treatment*, Philadelphia, 1994, FA Davis.

Piras MR et al: Longitudinal study of cognitive dysfunction in multiple sclerosis: Neuropsychological, neuroradiological, and neurophysiological findings, *J Neurol Neurosurg Psychiatry* 74:878-885, 2002.

Rabins PV, Lyketsos CG, Steele CD: *Practical dementia care*, ed 2, Oxford, 2006, Oxford Press.

Reed SK: *Cognition: theory and applications*, Belmont, CA, 2000, Wadsworth.

RESNA: Clinical application of assistive technology (1998): http://www.rehabtool.com/forum/discussions/94.html. Accessed April 6, 2005,

Robins B et al: Robot-mediated joint attention in children with autism: a case study in robot-human interaction, *Interaction Stud Social Behav Commun Biol Artificial Syst* 5:161-198, 2004.

Schuck SEB, Crinella FM: Why children with ADHD do not have low IQs, *J Learning Disabil* 38:262-280, 2005.

Shabani DB et al: Increasing social initiations in children with autism: effects of a tactile prompt, *J Applied Behavior Analysis* 35:79-83, 2002.

Shimura AP: Priming effects in amnesia: evidence for a dissociable memory function. *Q J Exp Psychol* 38A:619-644, 1986.

Sitko MC, Laine CJ, Sitko CJ: Writing tools: technology and strategies for the struggling writer. In: Edyburn D, Higgins K, Boone R, editors: *Handbook of special education technology research and practice*, pp. 571-598, Whitefish Bay, WI, 2005, Knowledge by Design, Inc.

Sternberg RJ: *Cognitive psychology*, ed 3, Belmont, CA, 2003, Wadsworth.

Sturm JM: Rankin-Erickson JL: Effects of hand-drawn and computer-generated concept mapping on the expository writing of middle school students with learning disabilities, *Learn Disabil Res Pract* 17:124-139, 2002.

Szymkowiak A et al: A memory aid with remote communication: preliminary findings, *Technol Disabil* 17:217-225, 2005.

Taber TA et al: Use of self-operated auditory prompts to decrease off-task behavior for a student with autism and moderate mental retardation, *Focus Autism Other Dev Disabil* 14:159-166, 1999.

Taylor BA, Levin L: Teaching a student with autism to make verbal initiations: effects of a tactile prompt, *J App Behav Anal* 31:651-654, 1998.

Taylor BA et al: Teaching teenagers with autism to seek assistance when lost, *J Appl Behav Anal* 37:79-82, 2004.

Tulving E: Episodic and semantic memory. In: Tulving E, Donaldson W, editors: *Organization of memory*, New York 1972, Academic Press, pp. 381-403.

Tulving E: *Elements of episodic memory*, New York, 1983, Oxford University Press.

Van Hulle A, Hux K: Improvement patterns among survivors of brain injury: three case examples documenting the effectiveness of memory compensation strategies, *Brain Inj* 20:101-109, 2005.

Wehmeyer ML, Smith SJ, Davies DK: Technology use and students with intellectual disability: universal design for all students. In: Edyburn D, Higgins K, Boone R, editors: *Handbook of special education technology research and practice*, pp. 309-323, Whitefish Bay, WI, 2005, Knowledge by Design, Inc.

Wehmeyer ML et al: Technology use and people with mental retardation, *Int Rev Res Ment Retard* 29:291-337, 2004.

Willingham DB: *Cognition: the thinking animal*, Princeton, NJ, 2001, Prentice-Hall.

World Health Organization: *International classification of functioning, disability and health (ICF)*, Geneva, Switzerland, 2001, World Health Organization.

CHAPTER 11

Augmentative and Alternative Communication Systems

Chapter Outline

Learning Objectives

On completing this chapter, you will be able to do the following:

1. Describe the different communicative needs of persons with disabilities
2. Discuss the basic approaches to meeting these differing needs

3. Recognize the needs that individuals have for conversation and for graphical output such as writing, mathematics, and drawing
4. Describe the major characteristics of alternative and augmentative communication devices
5. Describe current approaches to speech output in assistive technologies
6. List and describe the major approaches to rate enhancement and vocabulary expansion
7. Describe the major assessment questions that must be asked and answered in determining the most appropriate augmentative and alternative communication device for an individual user
8. Discuss the major goals for and the significance of training in augmentative and alternative communication device use and communicative competence
9. Delineate the steps and procedures involved in implementing an augmentative and alternative communication device for an individual consumer

Key Terms

Amyotrophic Lateral Sclerosis
Aphasia
Apraxia
Augmentative and Alternative
 Communication
Autism Spectrum Disorder
Complex Communication Needs

Context-Dependent Communicators
Dynamic Communication Displays
Dysarthria
Emergent Communicators
Icon Prediction
Independent Communicators
Language

Selection Set
Speech
Speech-Generating Devices
Traditional Orthography
Visual Scene Displays

This chapter is devoted to **augmentative and alternative communication (AAC)**, an area of clinical practice designed to ameliorate the communication problems of people who have severe speech and language impairments across the age span. Communication is a set of very complex behaviors and the very essence of being human. When someone is not developing speech and language skills or has lost the ability to speak or understand spoken or written language, then AAC intervention approaches are required to meet their **complex communication needs (CCN)**. Communication is not a solitary activity, and people communicate differently with different partners and under different conditions by using a variety of tools, techniques, and strategies. Thus, AAC interventions are dynamic and include not only the individual with a disability but also his or her primary communication partners and are focused on augmenting communication in ways the person values (Figure 11-1).

There are many tools, strategies, and techniques available to help individuals meet their daily communication needs. AAC interventions acknowledge the importance of body-based modes (e.g., gestures, eye gaze, and facial expressions), nonelectronic aids (e.g., communication boards and books, paper and pencil), and electronic communication devices (e.g., speech-generating devices, talking frame, computers, etc.). Thus, the term *AAC system* refers to all the means and modes a person uses to communicate including the use of

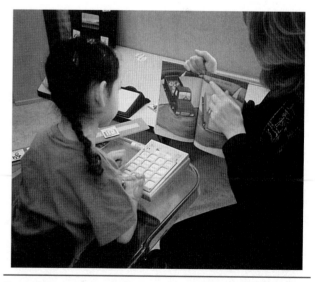

Figure 11-1 In conversations between speaking and AAC-using partners, the speaker may dominate the conversation unless careful selection, implementation, and training in use of the AAC system occurs.

both AAC and mainstream approaches to communication (e.g., phones, e-mail, computers, etc.). Table 11-1 and the case studies of Joyce and Eileen illustrate this concept.

Speech-generating devices (SGDs) produce digitally recorded or synthesized speech output. They are AAC tools

MEETING A CONGENITAL NEED FOR AUGMENTATIVE AND ALTERNATIVE COMMUNICATION

Joyce is 39 years old. She has cerebral palsy, and she currently lives with her parents. Her speech is dysarthric, and she is unable to use a pen or pencil for writing. Her communication systems are listed in Table 11-1. Unaided communication modes include head nods and eye gaze. Joyce currently uses a tread switch (see Chapter 7) mounted near her knee to control her scanning communication device, which has synthesized speech output and a small word processing program for writing. To meet Joyce's need to activate a call device for emergency help over the telephone, she uses an alarm tied into a 24-hour surveillance company and activated by a wobble switch (see Chapter 7) using her left arm. She uses her arm for the emergency call device because this movement is less limited by being supine in bed than is knee movement. Also, when she is seated in her wheelchair, arm use does not interfere with either her powered mobility or her communication because they use other control sites.

AUGMENTATIVE AND ALTERNATIVE COMMUNICATION AFTER A STROKE

Eileen is a 62-year-old woman who has sustained a brainstem stroke and now requires maximal assistance for daily living. Eileen's unaided communication modalities, shown in Table 11-1, include isolated words, facial expressions, yes/no responses, and inflectional vocalizations. She also has two AAC devices. The first of these is a letter board, accessed by her eye gaze, that she uses to indicate her needs and choices (Figure 11-2). All these systems have limitations. The unaided systems require significant amounts of interpretation by the partner, and the manual eye gaze device is slow because it relies on spelling and interpretation by her partner. These limitations are partially overcome by Eileen's electronic AAC device, which she accesses by using head movement to make selections with a light pointer mounted on a headband on the side of her head (Figure 11-3). This device includes vocabulary storage, so she can use whole words and phrases, and it provides synthesized speech output. These features allow Eileen to converse with more people, and they make it easier on the communication partner. Each of these devices contributes to the quantity and quality of her communication interactions.

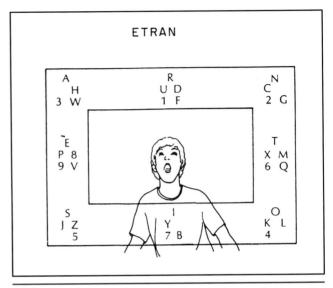

Figure 11-2 This communication system is based on the user and partner facing each other. Two eye movements are required. The first movement selects the group, and the second movement selects the letter. For example, to select the letter *A*, the user first looks to the upper left, then to the upper center. Eye gaze using pictures or other symbols is also common. (From Blackstone S: *Augmentative communication*, Rockville, MD, 1986, American Speech Language Hearing Association.)

that can significantly improve communication for individuals with CCN. SGDs and their accessories are commercially available and currently funded by governments and third-party payer programs in many countries. SGDs have a variety of features that have changed over time to meet the needs of individuals with CCN. Today, people with CCN are using SGDs to attend schools and universities,

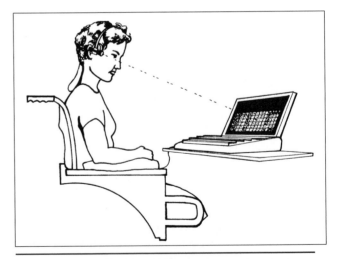

Figure 11-3 In this device a light is attached to the user's head. When the light beam is aimed at the panel of the device, it is detected and an entry is made. (From Blackstone S: *Augmentative communication*, Rockville, MD, 1986, American Speech Language Hearing Association.)

TABLE 11-1 Augmentative and Alternative Communication Case Study Examples

Subject	Communication Need	Modality	Activation/Control
Joyce	Conversation/writing	Unaided	Eye gaze or head nod
		Electronic AAC device	Knee/tread switch
	Emergency call	24-hour service	Hand/wobble switch
Eileen	Conversation	Unaided	Vocalizations, head nods, facial expression
		Letter board	Eye gaze
		Electronic AAC device	Optical pointer/head movement

work, carry on chats, participate in listservs, shop, order in restaurants, talk on the phone, and so on. People with severe disabilities and CCN who rely on AAC are living independently, getting married, and are active members of their communities. Individuals with CCN who do not gain access to AAC interventions are at high risk for abuse, crime, unemployment, and having limited social networks (Bryen, Cohen, and Carey, 2004; Collier, 2005). Infants, toddlers, and preschoolers with CCN require AAC interventions that support the development of language, communication, and emerging literacy skills. School-aged children with CCN need AAC interventions that enhance participation in their education, enable them to make friends, develop literacy and other academic skills, and engage with family members and people in their communities. Individuals who acquire disabilities later in life need AAC to help them sustain employment and maintain their relationships and social networks, independence, and dignity. As Daniel Webster said in 1822, "If all my possessions were taken from me with one exception, I would choose to keep the power of communication, for by it I would soon regain all the rest."

This chapter is devoted to a discussion of the major aspects of AAC that are important in enabling individuals with CCN to communicate across the life span, recognizing that each individual has unique needs, goals, preferences, skills, and abilities. The material presented in Chapters 3, 4, and 7 is applied to AAC here.

DISABILITIES AFFECTING SPEECH, LANGUAGE, AND COMMUNICATION

There are many disabilities that can affect an individual's communication skills and abilities. The description of cognitive function and development in Chapter 3 serves as a backdrop for discussions in this chapter. In addition, some individuals are born with or acquire conditions that interfere with their ability to make sounds or control the muscles of the chest, diaphragm, mouth, tongue, and throat and

produce intelligible speech. **Dysarthria** is a disorder of motor speech control resulting from central or peripheral nervous system damage that causes weakness, slowness, and a lack of coordination of the muscles necessary for speech production (Anderson and Shames, 2006). Verbal **apraxia** is a disorder affecting the coordination of motor movements involved in producing speech caused by a central nervous system dysfunction (Anderson and Shames, 2006). Limb apraxia may impair the ability to write. When speech or writing is severely impaired, AAC approaches are required.

There is a difference between speech disorders and language disorders. In Chapter 3 we defined **language** as any conventional system of arbitrary symbols organized according to a set of rules. **Speech** is the oral expression of language. AAC interventions for children with severe language delays or disorders are designed to support the development of receptive and expressive language and literacy skills. In adults, **aphasia** is a type of language disorder that often occurs as a result of a cerebral vascular accident or traumatic brain injury (TBI). Aphasia can affect both expression and reception of spoken and written language. For example, some people may lose the ability to recall vocabulary (e.g., names, places, events), and others may lose the ability to understand spoken language, organize language into meaningful utterances, and speak and write meaningful utterances. The degree to which various language functions are impaired is variable. AAC interventions for severe aphasia often focus on strategies that help individuals compensate for a severe loss of *language* function in ways that support functional communication.

Among the disabilities affecting communication that are ameliorated by AAC interventions are developmental conditions such as cerebral palsy (CP) and autism, acquired conditions such as TBI, stroke/cerebral vascular accident (CVA), and high-level spinal cord injury and degenerative diseases such as **amyotrophic lateral sclerosis (ALS),** progressive aphasia, and multiple sclerosis. Estimates indicate that approximately 2 million people in the United States and from 0.3% to 1.0% of the total world population of school-aged children have a need for AAC (Beukelman and Mirenda, 2005). Not all the people in this population are served equally. Blackstone (1990) conducted a survey to determine how well various populations were served and reported that in the early 1990s children with CP, individuals with good cognitive skills, and adults with some degenerative diseases (i.e., ALS) receive more attention from AAC practitioners than individuals with intellectual disabilities and children and adults with autism, dual sensory impairment, TBI, and the elderly (Blackstone, Williams, and Joyce, 2002).

Approaches to AAC interventions differ depending on the severity, type, and onset of an individual's disability. There are significant differences, for example, between meeting the needs of children who have never spoken or used written language (congenital disabilities) and adults who have developed language, speech, and writing and then lost these skills because of a disease or injury. For example, young children with severe motor impairments and CCN are learning language at the same time they are learning to "talk" and "write" by using AAC approaches. Thus, conventional means of communication (i.e., speaking and using a pencil) are unavailable to them. In addition, they have few, if any, opportunities to interact with competent AAC users who might serve as models and help them learn how to communicate using AAC. On the other hand, someone in whom ALS develops at age 46 years typically has years of experience using multiple forms of communication and intact language skills; thus, AAC interventions likely focus on providing AAC technologies and strategies so they can continue to communicate effectively with preferred partners.

What Is Augmentative and Alternative Communication?

There are many ways of looking at AAC systems. *Unaided communication or body-based modes* describe communication behaviors that require only the person's own body, such as pointing and other gestures, pantomime, facial expressions, eye-gaze and manual signing, or finger spelling. These modes are often used concurrently with each other and with speech. Even unaided modes of communication are typically culturally bound. Thus, when individuals have significant sensorimotor impairments, communication partners frequently misinterpret their nonverbal behaviors because eye gaze, facial expression, body movements, posture, traditional head nods, and pointing or reaching may be inaccurate, leading to communication misunderstandings (Kraat, 1986). Rush (1986) gives an example when he describes the difficulty his cerebral palsy causes him in delivering his line (a yell) in a play: "When a person with cerebral palsy wants to do something, he can't and when he wants not to do something, he involuntarily does it. So getting my vocal cords to cooperate with the cue was as hard as memorizing a Shakespearean play [for a nondisabled person]" (p. 21).

Aided AAC components may include a pen or pencil, a letter or picture communication board, a computer, a cell phone, and an SGD. Aided AAC may be either electronic or nonelectronic. Although a paper letter board (nonelectronic) differs from a computer-based SGD (electronic), both nonelectronic and electronic devices require that the person use a symbol system and have a way to select messages. All forms of AAC require consideration of how communication partners will participate in the communication process.

Multiple Communication Modes

Everyone uses multiple communication modalities and devices when communicating to meet a full spectrum of needs. Competent communicators use speech, a range of body-based modes, and low- and high-tech aids and devices so they can interact with multiple partners across multiple contexts. However, when someone is first taught to use AAC, decisions about what modes to teach or emphasize may require consideration of multiple factors. The two case studies of Joyce and Eileen illustrate this concept. In one published study, two young children (3 years 6 months and 4 years 6 months) with cognitive disabilities illustrate why professionals should exercise caution when introducing multiple AAC approaches at the same time (Iacono, Mirenda, and Beukelman, 1993). Each child used either (1) an electronic device coupled with manual signing (dual modes) or (2) signing alone (single mode) to produce two-word semantic combinations. Results showed that one child was more effective using both modes together and that the other preferred to use only one mode.

Augmentative and Alternative Communication Team

AAC interventions require a collaborative team approach. Each member of the AAC team has important roles and responsibilities:

- *The client and family* have the greatest knowledge of the daily communication needs of the person with CCN. Family members are often the individuals' primary communication partners and serve as advocates and facilitators.
- The *speech-language pathologist* has the greatest general understanding of communication in general and can assess language, and communication needs, abilities and skills; select AAC materials and technologies; and teach the individual, family, and staff to use AAC system components effectively.
- The *teacher* sets educational goals and oversees classroom implementation of each child's AAC system and has knowledge of literacy, social interaction, and education.

- The *physical therapist (PT) or occupational therapist (OT)* carries out the motor evaluation, addresses seating and positioning, evaluates physical access to the AAC system, and has knowledge of how to support writing, drawing, and other activities of daily living.
- The *teacher's aide/job coach* is also critical to the success of implementation. This individual supports the person in the school/work setting. Key team members are often referred to as "natural supports" because they have a continuing relationship with the individual (e.g., family, friends, coworkers, and employer). On occasion, physicians, psychologists, vision specialists, and other professionals also play an important role on AAC teams.

Role of Augmentative and Alternative Communication in the Lives of People With Complex Communication Needs

Christopher Nolan (1981), a man with cerebral palsy, wrote in the third person (as Joseph) about the importance of attentive and responsive communication partners. "Such were Joseph's teachers and such was their imagination that the mute boy became constantly amazed at the almost telepathic degree of certainty with which they read his facial expression, eye movements, and body language. Many a good laugh was had by teacher and pupil as they deciphered his code. It was moments such as these that Joseph recognized the face of God in human form. It glimmered in their kindness to him, it glowed in their keenness, it hinted in their caring, indeed it caressed in their gaze" (p. 11).

AAC systems can enhance interaction, but they can also become the center of attention, as Rush (1986) noted:

My new friend (Wendy) was good looking. She was just over five feet tall and had brown eyes that matched the color of her shoulder length hair. Her skin showed a summer tan and she had a dynamite smile. "Did he show ya all his electronic stuff?" one of my dorm mates asked her. "Go on, Bill, show her." So I demonstrated the controls for my lights and clock radio. I showed off my door opener, which I could control via a radio transmitter attached to the Plexiglas tray on my wheelchair. She was impressed with the space-age technology. "Hey, show her your wheelchair and how it works. I'll never understand how it works. It baffles me," another dorm mate said. So, wondering if I should sell tickets, I wheeled about the room. I demonstrated how I went straight, reverse, and turned left and right. I was angry at my dormmates because I was a man, not a side show freak. My wheelchair was a tool for my mobility, not a novelty. Why couldn't they see that? And why couldn't they see that I was trying to get to know Wendy. Why didn't they understand I had a right to my privacy just as they did? As I was wheeling around the room, I noticed that Wendy was typing something. I was disappointed in her.

I thought she knew that I could hear and that she didn't have to write things to me. Apparently I was wrong. When I was done showing my electric marvels to her and the guys, I rolled back to my typewriter to read, "I wish they would go, so we could talk by ourselves." They finally left and we finally got to talk. Our friendship had started. (p. 137)

The loss of speech can also occur later in life. Doreen Joseph (1986) lost her speech after an accident. Here's what she said, "I woke up one morning and I wasn't me. There was somebody else in my bed. And all I had left was my head. Speech is the most important thing we have. It makes us a person and not a thing. No one should ever have to be a 'thing'" (p. 8). Sue Simpson (1988) lost her speech after a stroke at age 36 years. She wrote: "So you can't talk, and it's boring and frustrating and nobody quite understands how bad it really is. If you sit around and think about all the things you used to be able to do, that you can't do now, you'll be a miserable wreck and no one will want to hang around you long" (Simpson, 1988, p. 11).

Dowden and Cook (2002) defined three types of AAC communicators. **Emergent communicators** have no reliable method of symbolic expression, and they are restricted to communicating about here-and-now concepts. **Context-dependent communicators** have reliable symbolic communication, but they are limited to specific contexts because they are either only intelligible to familiar partners, have insufficient vocabulary, or both. **Independent communicators** are able to communicate with unfamiliar and familiar partners on any topic. Each of these communicators has different needs and goals.

Partners of People With Complex Communication Needs Who Rely on Augmentative and Alternative Communication

Communication almost always involves a partner who may be in the room, on the phone, or a continent away on e-mail. Some "partners" may be merely imagined, as when someone writes a story. The Circle of Communication Partners (Figure 11-4) is helpful in defining the range of partners that a person with CCN who relies on AAC might encounter (Blackstone, 2003a). The first circle represents the person's life-long communication partners. This is primarily immediate family members. The second circle includes close friends (i.e., people who you tell your secrets to). These are often not family members. Acquaintances such as neighbors, schoolmates, coworkers, distant relatives (such as aunts and cousins), the bus driver, and shopkeepers are included in the third circle. The fourth circle is used to represent paid workers such as a speech-language pathologist (SLP) or a PT, OT, teacher, teacher assistant, or babysitter. Finally, the fifth circle is used to represent those unfamiliar partners

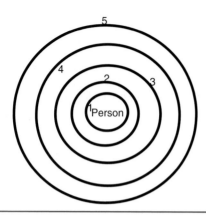

Figure 11-4   Circle of friends. *1,* Lifelong communication partners; *2,* close friends; *3,* neighbors, acquaintances; *4,* paid workers; *5,* unfamiliar partners.

with whom the person has occasional interactions. This includes everyone who does not fit in the first four circles. Thus, the familiarity with partners decreases as we move from circle 1 to 5 and the modes of communication required to communicate with people in each circle will vary. For example, Blackstone and Hunt Berg (2003) found that SGDs and low-tech displays were often used primarily with people in circle 4. They also noted that SGDs are required for successful interactions with partners in the third and

fifth circles. Gestures and impaired speech are often preferred modes in circles 1 and 2. An AAC intervention tool, *Social Networks: A Communication Inventory for Individuals with Complex Communication Needs and Their Communication Partners,* described in Box 11-1, is based on a number of theoretical frameworks including the circle of friends (Falvey et al, 1994), the field of social networks, the Participation Model (Beukelman and Mirenda, 2005), and person-centered planning.

Although the experience of the assistive technology practitioner (ATP) with individuals who have CCN may be limited to a brief encounter, the family has a long-term relationship with the individual and are key members of AAC assessment and decision-making team (Parette, Botherson, and Huer, 2000). In fact, when one family member relies on AAC, it always has an impact on the entire family (Goldbart and Marshall, 2004). Parents, spouses, and siblings need clear, jargon-free information that is presented objectively and honestly. Information about options, funding, timelines, and training in the use of the recommended AAC device or strategy is particularly important (Parette, Botherson and Huer, 2000). There is great diversity among families, of course, and this will affect the way they respond to their family member's communication needs and to AAC itself (Goldbart and Marshall, 2004). For example, parents report feeling additional pressure to use AAC in communicating

---

BOX 11-1   **Social Networks: A Communication Inventory for Individuals With Complex Communication Needs and Their Communication Partners**

Social Networks is a formalized approach to the development of communication goals, the planning of AAC interventions and measurement of progress. It is a tool that enables the perceptions of many AAC stakeholders to be considered when planning an intervention. It also provides a structure for gathering information on the basis of potential partners for communication. A pilot study of the *Social Networks Inventory* revealed some interesting features of AAC use related to the circle of partners shown in Figure 11-1 (Blackstone, 2003a). In the *First Circle,* people who use AAC tend to rely on speech, body language, and gesture. In the *Second Circle* there is a greater variety of AAC techniques that

depend on both skill and access to systems and on vocabulary and trained partners. There is more reliance on high-tech devices and less on nonsymbolic modes in the *Third Circle.* Also, emergent and context-dependent AAC communicators often need lots of support when communicating with people in this circle. Many context-dependent communicators primarily used their AAC devices with service providers in the *Fourth Circle.* When communicating with unfamiliar partners (*Fifth Circle*), a range of conventional AAC approaches is required and significant partner support is needed when the individual does not use an SGD.*

*The *Social Networks Inventory* is administered by a speech-language pathologist or someone with expertise in communication. An informant is someone in the individual with CCN's First Circle and Fourth Circle and if at all possible, the individual with CCN. It is meant to be readministered over time to track progress and includes sections on demographic and diagnostic information (see Chapter 4) and the individual's skills and abilities in motor, sensory, language, speech and cognitive areas and all current use of assistive technology. For each circle, the inventory identifies key partners (e.g., favorite partner, partner who understands the person's best, etc.) and the primary communication modes a person uses in each circle (facial expressions/body language, gestures, vocalizations, manual signs, speech writing, nonelectronic communication display, and electronic communication devices). It also collects information about the size of vocabulary the person can access and how effective, efficient, and intelligible the person's current means of communication are. Representational strategies (e.g., object, photograph, pictographic, orthographic manual signs, auditory) and selection techniques (e.g., direct selection, scanning, coding using icons, alphanumerical coding) are also identified, as are topics the individuals currently can (or would like to) talk about. The inventory also helps document which strategies communication partners rely on to support the individual's comprehension (e.g., aided language simulation, modeling AAC use, visual prompts, pictured sequences of tasks, social stories) and expression (e.g., gesture dictionaries, asking for repeat of utterance, suggesting slower speed, prompting for repair strategy use). Also included are summary sheets clinicians can use to capture this information for intervention planning.

with their child and to help others to do so (Angelo, 2000). Researchers also report that the goals of mothers and fathers may differ for their children (Angelo, Kokoska, and Jones, 1996). Mothers ranked social opportunities with both nondisabled children and other AAC users, integrating AAC into the community, and planning for future needs as their highest priorities. Fathers focused on planning for future needs, knowing how to program, repair, and maintain the SGD; integration of AAC into educational settings; and obtaining computer access with the SGD. Parents also indicated that they have to become strong advocates for their child to receive necessary services (Goldbart and Marshall, 2004).

Attitudes About and Acceptance of Augmentative and Alternative Communication

McCarthy and Light (2005) reviewed 13 research studies on the attitudes toward individuals who rely on SGDs. They identified several factors affecting attitudes: characteristics of typically developing individuals, characteristics of the person using AAC, and characteristics of the AAC system. These are elements of the social context of the human activity assistive technology (HAAT) model. Attitudes toward individuals who use AAC vary across the parameters of gender, type of disability, age, experience of the user of AAC, experience and familiarity with disability and AAC by the partner, and social context. Attitudes appear to be formed by the interaction of many of these factors.

The attitudes of children who do not have disabilities toward children who do and who use AAC is influenced by their familiarity with children who have disabilities (i.e., whether the nondisabled students had a classmate with a disability) and by age (older children are less positive than are younger children) (Beck et al, 2002). In general, girls are more positive toward disabled peers than boys are (Beck and Dennis, 1996). Although the number of conversational turns (one exchange between the speaker and partner) was almost identical in both groups, children who use AAC communicate mostly through responses and their typically developing peers initiate almost all of the requests (Clarke and Kirton, 2003). Beck et al (2002) reported that the longer the messages produced (two- vs. four-word utterances), the more positive were the peers' attitudes toward the child using AAC. Consistent with the second-circle relationship, much of the interaction among peers involves expressions of humor and intimacy (e.g., laughing, joking, teasing, tickling, etc.). In general, the attitudes of peers toward an AAC user do not appear to be affected by the type of AAC system used (Beck and Dennis, 1996). However, in one study the use of voice output led to more positive peer attitudes than when the output was only visual (letters on a display) (Lilienfeld and Alant, 2002).

Many students who use AAC are enrolled in inclusive classroom settings. Thus, the attitudes of general education teachers (circle 4) toward AAC are important to their success (Kent-Walsh and Light, 2003). Both the students who use AAC and their typically developing classmates in general education classes can develop skills and positive interactions during classroom activities. However, unequal status with classmates and dissimilar interests lead to social exclusion for students who rely on AAC. Often peers speak to the teacher or teacher's assistant rather than directly to the student. Teachers are also concerned about lack of academic gain. Some device features (e.g., speech synthesis) are perceived as disruptive to other students. School-related barriers to successful inclusion include large class sizes, the physical layout of the classroom, and the tendency of the schools to apply inclusion guidelines very liberally without a focus on educational needs. Teachers require time to adjust to the idea of having students with disabilities in class, full access to school resources for the AAC students, and availability of specialists for consultation and training.

Employers and coworkers are also influenced by workers who use AAC (McNaughton, Light, and Gulla, 2003). Benefits for the worker using AAC are social interaction, personal enjoyment, and financial gain. Benefits to the employer include positive impacts on other employees, high quality of work performance by the employee using AAC, loyalty of the employee, and the ability to fill "hard-to-fill positions." Employment challenges fall into several themes: finding a good job match to individual skills, communication challenges (e.g., noisy AAC device, speaker phone use), difficulty with typical office tasks (e.g., manipulation of paper, telephone use), education or vocational skill level too low, lack of knowledge of work culture, and physical challenges necessitating assistance from other workers and financial (e.g., insurance costs to company).

■ COMMUNICATION NEEDS THAT CAN BE SERVED BY AUGMENTATIVE AND ALTERNATIVE COMMUNICATION

When someone is unable to speak or write so that all current and potential communication partners can understand them, then an AAC system is required. As humans, we communicate in a myriad of ways depending on the circumstances. Although we rely most heavily on speaking and writing, when these modes are unavailable, then we search for (and find) other ways of communicating. People with CCN often are unable to speak and write so others can understand them. Thus, they need AAC approaches to help them communicate face to face, on the phone, and across the Internet. Use of these mainstream technologies such as the Internet and cell phones are addressed later in this chapter.

In considering writing, such activities as drawing, plotting graphs, and mathematics are included, all the things that are normally done with a pencil and paper, computer, calculator, and other similar tools. Assistive technologies for writing include not only AAC devices, discussed in this chapter, but also other approaches discussed in Chapters 15 (those primarily used for educational access) and 16 (those primarily used for vocational pursuits).

Light (1988) describes four purposes of communicative interaction: (1) expression of needs and wants, (2) information transfer, (3) social closeness, and (4) social etiquette. Expression of needs and wants allows people to make requests for objects or actions. Information transfer allows expression of ideas, discussion, and meaningful dialog. Social closeness serves to connect individuals to each other, regardless of the content of the conversation. Social etiquette is used to describe those cultural formalities that are inherent in communication. For example, students will speak differently to their peers than to their teachers.

In considering communication needs, three perspectives are addressed: (1) individuals with developmental disorders, (2) individuals with acquired conditions, and (3) individuals with degenerative conditions. Although the focus of AAC interventions may vary across these groups, there is also substantial overlap in the issues faced when communication is severely limited, no matter what the causes may be.

Augmentative and Alternative Communication for Individuals With Developmental Disabilities

Because the development of speech, language, and communication begins at birth, early intervention is important. Effective AAC intervention for children with developmental disabilities requires that AAC be integrated into the child's daily experiences and interactions and that it take into account what we know about child development (Light and Drager, 2002). For example, many young children do not have the physical or cognitive skills to learn to use current AAC selection techniques (e.g., scanning or encoding) and thus are unable to access AAC systems. Also, the design of current AAC technologies often requires a child to stop playing to use a communication device. A more desirable approach is to design AAC technologies and strategies that incorporate the use of AAC into the child's play activities so the child can talk about his or her play or interact with peers while engaged in the activity. In short, to be effective, the design, type, and layout of AAC system components should match the desires, preferences, abilities, and skills of children.

A major concern for parents is whether the use of AAC will impede their child's development of speech.

Research data put all such fears to rest (see Blackstone, 2006). The use of AAC does not interfere with speech development and may in fact enhance the development or return of speech. There are a number of possible explanations for this, including increased acoustic feedback (from voice output SGD), increased experience with conversational turns and other communicative functions, reduced pressure to speak that releases motor stress, and the development of an internal phonology as a result of AAC systems use (Blishcak, Lombardino, and Dyson, 2003).

Research shows that children with a broad range of developmental disabilities can benefit from AAC interventions. This includes children with CP, intellectual disability, Down syndrome, other genetic disorders, and **autism spectrum disorder (ASD)**. The latter is used here as an example of AAC intervention for individuals with developmental disabilities. (Intellectual disabilities and more mild disorders such as learning disabilities are discussed in Chapter 10.)

ASD is characterized by significant social communication challenges throughout life that reflect impairments in social interaction, verbal and nonverbal communication, and restricted, repetitive, stereotypical patterns of behavior, interests, and activities (Blackstone, 2003b). Early intervention (starting as young as age 2 years) improves outcomes for children with ASD. These children often have difficulty with joint attention (i.e., coordinating attention between people and objects) and understanding and using symbols. Approximately one third to one half of children with ASD do not use speech functionally (Blackstone, 2003b). The learning styles of children with ASD show a strong preference for static information and, as a result, they often benefit from the use of "visual supports." Because speech and other elements of conversations are transient, AAC devices and communication displays that use static visual symbols provide possible advantages for the child with ASD. Also, because of their dependence on rote or episodic memory, children with ASD often benefit from contextual clues and prompts, and this can lead to them becoming prompt or context dependent. Thus, AAC interventions that extend the use of language and appropriate communication behaviors across different contexts and partners are needed. Blackstone (2003b) argues that AAC can be effective for children with ASD because it addresses both their unique learning styles and their communication needs.

Children with ASD can use no-technology (e.g., manual signs) and high- and low-technology approaches to AAC (Mirenda, 2003). At this time, there is no clear evidence that one approach is superior to any other. The use of total communication (speech and manual signing) provides advantages because there is no device to worry about and because it promotes more natural forms of communication. However, not all children (or their partners) do equally well with this approach. Some children develop more functional communication using low-tech aided systems. PECS* is one widely used example. Voice output communication aids can also support interactions. For example, Schlosser and Blischak (2001) suggested that electronically generated speech might be beneficial for children with ASD who have difficulty processing natural speech. Also, computer aided instruction may help children with ASD attend to instructions and prompts when provided by electronic speech output. There are many considerations in choosing among the many available AAC approaches, including an individual's preferences, ease of learning, effect on the development of speech and language, ability to use the approach functionally across partners and contexts, and the communication tasks the person needs to accomplish. Finally, the degree of partner support and responsiveness is considered. Currently, best practice relies on clinician judgment as much as evidence because current research on the use of AAC approaches for individuals with ASD is promising but inconclusive in each of these areas.

Augmentative and Alternative Communication for Individuals With Acquired Disabilities

Adults with acquired disabilities such as TBI, aphasia, and other static conditions may require the use of AAC interventions as part of the rehabilitation process (Beukelman and Ball, 2002). Persons with recovering conditions often have changing levels of motor, sensory, or cognitive/linguistic capability that benefit from the use of human/technology interfaces, including AAC, to help them accommodate. Although many people may be unable to speak or write directly after a severe head injury or brainstem or cortical stroke, most will recover these abilities. However, over the long term, some individuals continue to benefit from the use of AAC. In this section TBI and aphasia are discussed as examples of individuals with acquired AAC needs.

Traumatic Brain Injury.   TBI can result in the loss of speech and often causes physical, cognitive, and language impairments (Beukelman and Garrett, 1988; Light, Beesley, and Collier, 1988). Although the long-term recovery of speech is variable, immediately after the injury many individuals benefit from the use of AAC interventions to support functional communication. Associated changes in motor, perceptual, cognitive, and language abilities also may have detrimental effects on communication (Carlisle Ladtkow and Culp, 1992). Thus, it is critical that the limitations associated with a severe brain injury from a car accident, gun shot wound, explosion, and so forth be identified and considered when AAC goals and interventions are determined (Beukelman and Yorkston, 1989). In a follow-up study of nonspeaking individuals with TBI 1 year after discharge, DeRuyter and Kennedy (1991) found that only 56% of those for whom an AAC device was recommended were using the device, 24% had completely discarded the device, and 20% only used it in limited environments (DeRuyter and Kennedy, 1991). In many cases, speech had returned. However, there was no indication as to why 44% of the devices were abandoned or not being used to their full potential. Beukelman and Yorkston (1989) point out that there is a need for AAC devices to be integrated and adapted into the person's living situation, outside the rehabilitation center. Frager, Hux, and Beukelman (2005) found that a group of communication partners and the continuing support of an AAC facilitator contribute to success. In a recent study, Frager, Hux, and Beukelman (2005) found that high-tech devices were favored over low-tech systems and that low-tech systems were apt to be used temporarily by people with TBI who regained speech.

Aphasia.   Persons who sustain CVAs often have language difficulties that we collectively call *aphasia*. One lasting problem these individuals have is vocabulary retrieval or word-finding difficulties. There are several AAC-related approaches with potential for aphasia rehabilitation (Jacobs et al, 2004; Kraat, 1990). For example, individuals who can recall first letters and recognize a desired word from a list may use word prediction devices/software. The individual begins typing a letter and then the device predicts several words from which to choose (see Figure 7-8). Colby et al

---

*Pyramid Educational Products, Newark, Del. The Picture Exchange Communication System (PECS) is a commercially available program developed for people with ASD that uses graphic symbols (often the Mayer-Johnson Picture Communication Symbols©) and a specific instructional method. The objective of PECS is that children or adults who are not yet initiating requests, comments, and so forth, learn to spontaneously initiate communicative exchanges. The person is initially encouraged to give something (picture/symbol) to a communication partner to complete a communication exchange. Thus, by using PECS, learners gain the attention of the communication partner to make a request. By advancing through the six phases of PECS, the student progresses from a simple exchange through increasing levels of spontaneity to sequencing words and creating sentences. No prompting is used throughout the learning process. In a study conducted by Bondy and Frost (2001) in 85 children (aged 5 years or younger), more than 95% of the children were able to exchange at least two pictures, whereas 76% began using speech with or without PECS. In other studies with smaller number of participants, positive outcomes in speech improvement, rapid mastery of the system, and decrease in destructive behavior or tantrums were reported anecdotally (Helsinger, 2001; Schwartz, 2001). Recent empirical studies on PECS have reported positive effects regarding rate of mastery of the system and improvement in general communication skills (Magiati and Howlin, 2003).

(1981) developed a microcomputer-driven device that used a specially designed database containing words, their frequency of use, and features of each word, which was specifically designed for persons with aphasia. Features included words that "go with" the desired word. This can be a sound-alike relationship; a semantic (meaning) relationship; a categorization (e.g., a piece of furniture or a fruit); and initial, middle, and ending letters. Each was shown to be effective for persons with certain types of aphasia. A similar approach was developed by Hunnicutt (1989).

Many factors must be considered when AAC is applied in aphasia rehabilitation (Kraat, 1990). Some people with severe aphasia learn to augment their speech and communication efforts by relying on gestures and an alternative symbol system (Jacobs et al, 2004). However, although persons with aphasia may be able to use graphic symbols, many find it difficult to apply them socially or to generalize their use. One commercial device designed specifically for persons with aphasia is the Lingraphica, which organizes symbols by semantic categories (e.g., places, foods, clothing) and includes synthetic speech output and animation of verbs (Steele and Weinrich, 1986). Approaches such as CHAT and TALK that model conversational flow and provide clues to word vocabulary choices based on context can also assist aphasic individuals (Kraat, 1990).

A recent development is the use of **visual scene displays** (VSDs) (McKelvey et al, 2007). VSDs use personalized photos of scenes and arrange these on a dynamic display device. The technology enables individuals with severe aphasia to use familiar photographs to engage partners in interactions about multiple topics. In addition, the design of the technology makes it relatively easy for partners to provide conversational supports. Because of the dynamic nature of the display, the user is continually prompted, reducing the individual's need to rely on recall memory. The potential for people with aphasia to benefit from the use of VSD technology is still under investigation.

The use of AAC in aphasia rehabilitation often involves the use of AAC strategies and partner training. Blackstone (1991) identified issues involved in aphasia rehabilitation that included a discussion of public policy issues (e.g., funding for assessment and therapy services) and a discussion of clinical studies involving AAC strategies and technologies. King and Hux (1995) describe the use of a talking word processor to increase writing accuracy for individuals with aphasia. The speech feedback provided additional monitoring of the written work, which helps the person to identify and correct errors. Garrett and Beukelman (1992) present a classification system for aphasic individuals that is useful in planning AAC interventions. This scheme guides intervention planning by describing five types of aphasic communicators: basic choice, controlled situation, augmented, comprehensive, and specific need. For each of these categories, the authors identify residual skills, intervention goals, and AAC skills and suggest AAC activities for both partners and the individual with aphasia. Finally, Fox and Fried-Oken (1996) propose questions related to effectiveness, efficiency, and generalization in AAC aphasiology research. One area of concern for future development in AAC is how best to represent meaning on AAC technologies for persons with aphasia (Beukelman and Ball, 2002).

Augmentative and Alternative Communication for Individuals With Degenerative Conditions

A degenerative condition in which speech or language functions are gradually lost presents a different set of challenges for the person with CCN and for AAC interventions. For many conditions, multiple AAC modes are necessary as the disease worsens. Persons with degenerative conditions often have changing levels of motor, sensory, or cognitive/linguistic capability that require the adaptation of the human/technology interfaces to accommodate their changing motor and cognitive skills. In this section ALS is discussed as an example of a degenerative condition that significantly affects communication. Dementia is discussed in general in Chapter 10.

ALS, also referred to as one of the motor neuron diseases, is a rapidly progressing neuromuscular disease that affects speech in the majority of cases (see the case study of Mr. Webster). Although persons with ALS use the same AAC systems as others, there are unique factors considered during the intervention process. For example, it is not uncommon for someone to begin using a direct-selection AAC system and later on require scanning to continue communicating. If this type of transition is not planned for initially, it can be very hard for the person to maintain effective interactions. Families differ in their desire and ability to deal with the longer term (Blackstone, 1998). Some families prefer to "plan ahead" and consider future needs, whereas others prefer to take things as they come. Some SGDs can accommodate direct selection and a variety of indirect selection modes, so these are often recommended. But they are often heavy and hard to carry and thus may be less useful at the outset when the person is still ambulatory. Patients with ALS tend to use high-tech aids with strangers and for conversation (Blackstone, 1998). No-tech approaches, including 20 questions (the person can answer yes or no by head nod, eye blink, or other means) or gestures may be most effective with family and to express basic needs. Low-tech approaches such as letter boards are more often used with strangers than with family members.

AUGMENTATIVE AND ALTERNATIVE COMMUNICATION AND AMYOTROPHIC LATERAL SCLEROSIS–CHANGING NEEDS

Mr. Webster was assessed for an AAC device shortly after he began to lose the ability to speak as a result of ALS. He received a direct-selection spelling device, which he accessed with his right index finger. This device was highly effective for him, and he was fond of making lists of tasks to be done around the house, planning menus, and creating shopping lists for his wife and son, which allowed him to maintain his role as head of the household. Unfortunately, Mr. Webster eventually lost the ability to use his finger to type and was again referred for an AAC assessment.

A new device was recommended and purchased for him. This device used single-switch scanning accessed through eyebrow movement. This system was not effective for Mr. Webster. Several factors led to the difference in results between the two systems. First, there was an 11-month period between when he was unable to use the first system and the delivery of the second system. This time without a functional communication system probably contributed to a much more dependent role in the family for Mr. Webster, and he told us that he had "nothing to say" when we asked about his nonuse of the new system. His dependent role in communication also changed his role as head of the household. The new system was also more complicated to set up and to operate. It required his wife and attendant to learn more about the system, and he had to wait for one of them to set it up for him. The effort involved on everybody's part may have been overwhelming.

Acceptance of AAC by persons who have ALS is reported by several authors. In one 4-year study, more than 96% of those given the choice of AAC accepted that choice (Ball, Beukelman, and Patee, 2004). There are several factors leading to acceptance and successful use of AAC by persons with ALS. First, it is important that clinicians provide information regarding the speech-language characteristics of ALS at the outset of intervention. There is a relationship between speaking rate and intelligibility, with 80% intelligibility occurring at about 130 words per minute (Ball, Beukelman, and Patee, 2004). Speech rate is used to determine the timing of AAC interventions. The rate continually drops as ALS progresses, and evaluation is initiated when the rate is at 90%. The second success factor is maintaining continuous contact to monitor speech rate and intelligibility along with other routinely measured motor system parameters. Finally, it is important that the family remain aware of AAC service intervention opportunities. Flexible AAC devices and strategies that will accommodate for changes over the course of the disease are important. A key reason for acceptance of AAC by persons with ALS is their desire to continue interacting with communication partners in a variety of contexts. The literature strongly supports the use of AAC as a key component of evidence-based practice in the treatment of ALS.

AUGMENTATIVE AND ALTERNATIVE COMMUNICATION EVALUATION AND ASSESSMENT

AAC assessment requires systematic consideration of many factors (Beukelman and Mirenda, 2005; Coleman, 1988; Lloyd, Fuller, and Arvidson, 1997). These factors are described by the four components of the HAAT model. The most important step is to define the goals and needs of the person with CCN and his or her current and potential communication partners through a careful analysis of the desired *activity or activities*. The Social Networks tool is useful at this stage (see Box 11-1). An evaluation of the various *contexts* in which communication will occur helps to further inform the assessment goals. The Participation Model (see below) helps to define opportunities and barriers in various contexts. Once the goals, needs (*activity* component of the HAAT model), and contexts (HAAT model) are clearly understood and agreed to by all team members (e.g., person with CCN, parent, spouse, teacher, employer, care provider, speech pathologist, OT, PT, and others), physical, sensory, cognitive, and language skills (the *human* component of the HAAT model) are assessed as they relate to augmentative communication. Finally, if a low- or high-tech AAC system component (e.g., SGD, computer) is indicated, the *assistive technology* characteristics can be matched to consumer skills and goals by systematically identifying the *human/technology interface*, the *processing* (e.g., SGD rate enhancement, vocabulary storage), and the *activity output* modes.

Assessment of Persons With Complex Communication Needs

Several types of AAC assessment may be conducted. A predictive assessment has a goal of understanding the client needs and status today, predicting future needs, and selecting a system to meet both of these. A serial assessment is a continuing evaluation to meet changing needs (e.g., as a child develops). A curriculum-based assessment is continuous in classrooms to help coordinate AAC interventions with the achievement of educational goals. In any case, the assessment process takes into consideration the individual's skills and abilities and current and future communication needs and preferences. From these, an intervention plan is developed.

The overall goals of AAC assessment are as follows: (1) to document communication needs, (2) to determine how many needs can be met through current communication methods, including speech, and (3) to reduce the number of unmet communication needs through systematic AAC intervention. Each member of the AAC team described earlier in this chapter has a specific role in the assessment process.

There are many tools available to the AAC team. However, assessment approaches designed for other populations often require adaptations of materials and procedures so that assessment results are valid and reliable, as described by Beukelman and Mirenda (2005). One tool is the *Social Networks Inventory* described earlier in this chapter. It enables the perceptions of many individuals to be considered when planning an intervention (Blackstone, 2003a) and it provides a structure for gathering of information. When used in combination, the HAAT model, Social Networks, and the Participation Model (Beukelman and Mirenda, 2005) provide a comprehensive framework for ensuring that all information needed for successful AAC implementation is obtained during the assessment process.

Assessing Barriers to Participation. In the *Participation Model, opportunity* and *access* barriers to successful AAC use are identified. Beukelman and Mirenda (2005) present detailed information regarding the implementation of the participation model, including sample assessment forms and case examples. For example, opportunity barriers are those that involve policies, practices, attitudes and knowledge, and skills of those who support the person with CCN and that interfere with successful AAC interventions. As an illustration, consider the situation where a school district purchases an SGD for a child, but the child is required to leave it at school at all times. This practice is a barrier to full societal participation and academic success. Keeping the device at school may be a policy of the district because uninformed administrators worry about the cost of the device and possible breakage or loss if it goes home. After all, schools allow students to take home band instruments, uniforms, books, and pencils. Another example of an opportunity barrier is the employer who is resistant to a worker using an AAC device. This may reflect the employer's attitudes about disability or a lack of knowledge about AAC or a lack of skill in supporting individuals with CCN.

Another key element of the Participation Model is an "activity standards inventory" in which desired communication-related activities of the person with CCN (termed "target person") are listed. The standard of desired performance is that a nondisabled peer carry out the same activity. The target person is then rated as to the level of participation (independent, independent with setup, verbal or physical assistance, or unable to participate), and the discrepancy between peer and target person (if any) are ascribed to "opportunity" or "access" barriers. These are evaluated in terms of potential needs: (1) to increase natural abilities, (2) to make environmental adaptations, and (3) to use AAC systems and/or devices. Finally, AAC potential is determined through an operational profile, a constraints profile, and a capability profile.

As described in Chapter 7, the human-technology interface evaluation is part of a capability profile. An important component of the capability assessment involves documenting the individual's speech, language, motor, sensory, cognitive, and social communication skills. Dowden (1997) describes assessment approaches for individuals with CCN who have some functional speech. There are many language tests for both children and adults. Cognitive assessments help to determine how the individual understands the world and how communication can be best facilitated within this understanding (Beukelman and Mirenda, 2005). There are no formal tests that accurately predict the ability of an individual to meet the cognitive requirements of various AAC techniques and technologies, and expressive language by use of AAC is itself required to accurately assess cognitive ability. Thus, the individual's cognitive ability is often estimated. Some cognitive skills that are important for AAC are shown in Box 11-2. Social communicative skills (e.g., degree of interaction, attention to task) are generally assessed by interviews with family, caregivers, teachers, and others and through observation during an assessment or during opportunities created specifically to encourage social interaction. One example of the information that may be required (and how it may be assessed) is delineated in the Medicare funding request for SGDs in the United States (shown in the first column of Table 11-2).

Assessing Representation. One area of assessment unique to the area of AAC is determining what types of symbols an individual can use to communicate. A variety of symbol types are shown in Figure 11-5. Clinicians may

---

BOX 11-2   **Cognitive Skills Relevant to the Use of an Augmentative and Alternative Communication System**

Alertness
Attention span
Categorization
Cause/effect
Vigilance (ability to visually and auditorily process information over time)
Express preference
Make choices
Matching
Sequencing
Sorting
Symbolic representation
Object or pictorial permanence

TABLE 11-2 Assessment of Feature Required for a Speech-Generating Device

Input Features/Selection Techniques*	Message Characteristics*	Auditory Output Features*	Additional Features	Accessory Features*
Direct selection: Keyboards/display: Dynamic/static, size and number of keys/locations Activation type: Touch or pressure sensitive, adjustable Indirect contact: Head pointing, eye gaze	Types of symbols: Words, phrase, letters, tactile, pictures (color/ black and white), pictographic Vocabulary size: number of words, phrases, etc., needed	Type: Digitized speech Synthesized speech Other sounds	Outputs: EADL (see Chapter 14) Computer access: (see Chapter 7)	Mounts Position of switches Position of device Portability Size, weight, transport/ mount, case/carrier requirements
Scanning: Display: number of elements, dynamic/static Mode: Visual/auditory Type of scan: Linear, row/column, group row/column, directed	Organization of messages: Message length, files of messages, number of different messages stored or formulated	Vocabulary expansion: Rate enhancement, prediction (word/icon), coding strategies, screens/levels	General computer-based: Laptop Tablet Palm PDA	Switch type, pressure, feedback Pointing devices Type (infrared, ultrasonic) Feedback (Visual, tactile, auditory)

*Blackstone S: Assessment protocol for SGDs, *Augment Commun News* 13:1-16, 2001.

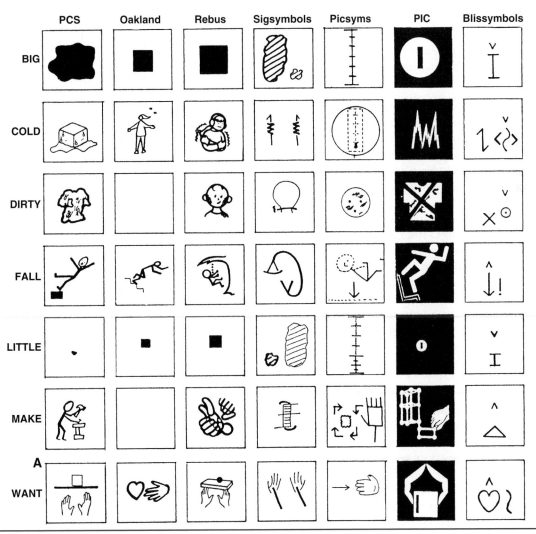

Figure 11-5 Examples of the variety of symbol systems that have been developed for AAC use. (From Blackstone S: *Augmentative communication*, Rockville, MD, 1986, American Speech Language Hearing Association.)

select from several assessment protocols (Beukelman and Mirenda, 2005). In one protocol (*functional object use)*, the evaluator shows the person a symbol and says "Show me what you do with this." The response may be a gesture (e.g., hand to mouth for "eat it") or pointing at a picture or symbol (e.g., "drink" if prompt is a soft drink can). In another approach (*visual matching)* the evaluator asks the individual to find a single stimulus item from a multiple symbol array or vice versa. The most flexible AAC systems are those that depend on spelling and require literacy skills, so word recognition and reading comprehension are often used to assess reading level, and spelling evaluations also may be conducted (Beukelman and Mirenda, 2005). There are multiple levels of spelling skills that may be useful in AAC:

1. Recognition spelling requires the client to pick the correct entry from a list of options. This can enable someone to use an SGD that presents word lists or other stored vocabulary choices and that relies on recognition memory.
2. Word completion tests evaluate the person's ability to correctly select the first letter of a word and recognize the completed word (see Chapter 7).
3. Spontaneous spelling requires the person to spell the requested word letter by letter.

Many types of symbol systems are used in augmentative communication (Lloyd, Fuller, and Arvidson, 1997; Vanderheiden and Lloyd, 1986). Several of these are illustrated in Figure 11-5. Perhaps the most concrete type of symbol is the use of real objects (full size or miniature). However, to a person with cognitive disabilities, a miniature object may not appear to represent the full-size version, and care must be taken to ensure that the association is made by the user (Vanderheiden and Lloyd, 1986). Real objects and photographs have the disadvantage that many communicative concepts (e.g., good, more, go, hurt) are difficult to portray. Pictographic symbols include provisions for more abstract communicative intents and allow much greater flexibility in developing vocabulary usage. A more flexible symbol type is the use of a symbol system possessing grammar and syntax (e.g., Blissymbols). The nature of this symbol system allows the inclusion of more linguistic functions, such as categorization by parts of language. **Traditional orthography** is the symbolic representation based on letters and words. Some individuals have reading skills that exceed their spelling skills, and they cannot rely on spelling for communication. If the person has a large word recognition vocabulary, the **selection set** should be based on words with possible "carrier phrases" that are filled in with limited spelling (e.g., "I would like a drink of ____"). Spelling is the most flexible symbol system because it can be used to create a large number of different utterances, but it can also be the slowest because of letter-by-letter entry rather than selection of whole words. Many computers,

printers, and keyboards accommodate languages other than English.

Relating Goals and Skills to Augmentative and Alternative Communication System Characteristics

Chapter 2 describes the assessment and recommendation process in assistive technology as designing a total system for a specific person. This approach is particularly true in AAC because it is necessary to define a set of system characteristics that meets the needs of the person with CCN, is consistent with his or her skills, and will support communication across multiple partners and contexts. When an SGD is a part of the recommended AAC approach for the individual with CCN, it is important to determine a match between the needs and goals of the person and the characteristics of the SGD. Table 11-2 illustrates the relationship between assessment results and device characteristics in terms of U.S. Medicare funding guidelines for SGDs. Input features, message characteristics, output features, and accessories are all specified on the basis of the assessment results. Blackstone (2001) includes several case studies that illustrate the application of this matching process for the selection of an AAC device and the preparation of a funding justification for submission to Medicare. This type of systematic approach to recommendations allows the characteristics and skills of the individual with CCN to be matched with available SGDs.

The individual or family may wish to use the SGD for a trial period, during which valuable information can be gained. For example, the person's interest in using the SGD may increase when he or she sees how effective it is in meeting needs or he or she may not like how it sounds or how friends react to it. A trial period can also help identify specific training goals for the person and his or her communication partners so that communicative competencies can be developed that enable the individual to interact effectively and efficiently. If there are special features that require learning new skills (such as storing and retrieving information), these may be assessed during the trial. For individuals who prefer a longer trial period, many companies will lease a device for a 1- to 3-month period. The outcomes of an SGD assessment should include recommendations for the SGD and any accessories or mounts and instructional strategies required to meet the person's unique needs and goals.

■ EXAMPLES OF CURRENT AUGMENTATIVE AND ALTERNATIVE COMMUNICATION APPROACHES

The HAAT model (Chapter 2) describes *activity outputs* as part of the assistive technology component. AAC is the communication activity output. As Figure 11-6 illustrates,

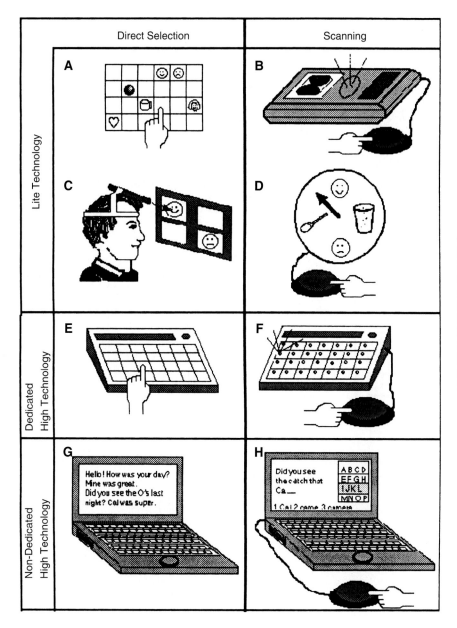

	Direct Selection	Scanning
Lite Technology	A	B
	C	D
Dedicated High Technology	E	F
Non-Dedicated High Technology	G	H

Figure 11-6 **A,** Manual communication display. **B,** Two choice voice output speech-generating device (SGD). **C,** Communication display accessed with a head-mounted light. **D,** Clock-face communication device. **E,** Direct selection SGD. **F,** Scanning SGD. **G,** Direction-selection laptop computer-based SGD. **H,** Scanning laptop computer-based SGD. (From Glennen SL, DeCoste DC: *The handbook of augmentative and alternative communication,* 1997, San Diego, Singular Publishing.)

AAC systems are composed of "no-tech" (gestures, sign language) components, nonelectronic (low-tech), and electronic (high-tech) components. Not everyone uses all these approaches, but many people do.

No-Tech Augmentative and Alternative Communication Systems

Gestures, facial expressions, and body movements help display emotional states, regulate and maintain a conversation, and support information exchange. Formal gestural codes (American Indian, Tadoma) and formal manual sign systems (e.g., ASL, SEE) are examples of more formal approaches (Beukelman and Mirenda, 2005).

Low-Tech Augmentative and Alternative Communication Systems

Chapter 1 defined low technology as inexpensive devices that are simple to make and easy to obtain. Many types of AAC approaches fit into this category. The communication vest shown in Figure 11-7, *A*, is worn by a teacher in classrooms to generate eye contact and enhance interaction with students. The activity-related symbols face the child so the teacher or child can point to them as they are discussed, which can assist in the teaching of labeling, requesting, and similar skills. The communication displays shown in Figure 11-7, *B* and *C*, are based on letters/words/phrases or graphic symbols, respectively. The communication display in Figure 11-7, *D*,

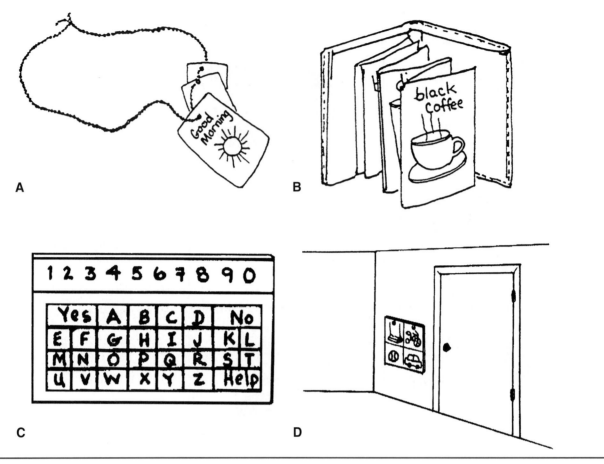

Figure 11-7   Low-tech communication aids.

is an example of an activity-specific communication display. Other low-tech approaches may include placing symbols on items around a room to develop labeling skills, using miniature objects as labels, and formal systems such as the PECS to teach requesting, as described earlier in this chapter.

High-Tech Augmentative and Alternative Communication Systems

High-tech AAC systems typically use SGDs, some of which are based on standard computers. The salient general characteristics of these devices are described in this section.

Human Technology Interface. The *human technology* or *control interface* for SGDs is the hardware by which the person with CCN accesses the low- or high-tech device (see Figure 2-6 and Chapter 7). The most commonly used control interfaces for augmentative communication devices are keyboards, single or dual switches, joysticks or multiple-switch arrays, and mouse or alternative pointing interfaces. SGDs; other AAC approaches use either direct selection or indirect selection (e.g., scanning, directed scanning, or coded access). These are discussed in Chapter 7. Most selection sets use visible symbols (e.g., letters, graphics, pictures) so individuals who have visual impairments and physical limitations requiring scanning may not be able to use visual arrays. For these individuals auditory scanning is used. Choices are presented in auditory form by a partner or an AAC and the user selects his or her choice from the auditory prompts. In some cases, both a prompting phrase and a selected auditory utterance are included and the user hears the prompting phrase through an earphone. In nonelectronic voice auditory scanning a list of vocabulary items is read aloud by the communication partner. The AAC user then chooses a vocabulary item by using a predetermined signal such as a vocalization to identify the desired vocabulary item. Kovach and Kenyon (1998) analyze a variety of approaches to auditory scanning, summarize current research in this area, and describe considerations to be included when developing an auditory scanning system for an AAC user.

Examples of Vocabulary Retrieval Techniques.   Many SGDs use the approaches to increase input rate that are discussed in Chapter 7 (abbreviation expansion, word prediction, word completion). In addition, there are several methods for storing and retrieving vocabulary that are designed specifically for SGDs.

Instant phrases are those used frequently for greetings, conversational repairs (e.g., "that's not what I meant") or similar actions; these are often included as single keystroke entries in an "activity row" or in a row of the scanning matrix, near the beginning of the scan. They can also serve as "floor holders" (e.g., "please wait while I type my question/answer.)

Coding of words, sentences, and phrases on the basis of their meanings and also known as semantic encoding or Minspeak (Baker, 1982). This approach uses pictorial representations that can have multiple meanings as codes, making recall easier. For example, when a picture of an apple is used for "food" and a sun rising for "morning." then selection of "apple" and "sunrise" could be a code for "What's for breakfast." Icons can have multiple meanings. Thus the apple symbol can take on the meaning of "eat" or "red" or "fruit" rather than food. Several examples of Minspeak sequences are shown in Figure 11-8. Baker (1986) also developed an approach based on the use of syntactical labels coupled with icons. Figure 11-9 illustrates this concept. For example, the apple icon becomes "eat" when combined with the key labeled "verb" and becomes "food" when combined with the noun key. Unity is a family of Minspeak application programs included with Prentke Romich (Wooster, Ohio, *www.prentrom.com*) AAC devices. It includes 4, 8, 15, 32, 45, 84, and 128 location overlays that differ in the pointing resolution required by the user. Sequences of icons and their locations on the keyboard are kept as consistent as possible among the overlays to account for motor skill development while allowing growth in language usage. Versions of Unity vary from a few hundred words to more than 4000 words intended to address the core vocabulary that is responsible for the majority of conversational utterances. When large numbers of sentences, words, and phrases are stored, the icon sequences can become difficult to remember. **Icon prediction** initially lights an indicator associated with each symbol that forms the beginning of an icon sequence. When one of these icons is selected, only those icons that are part

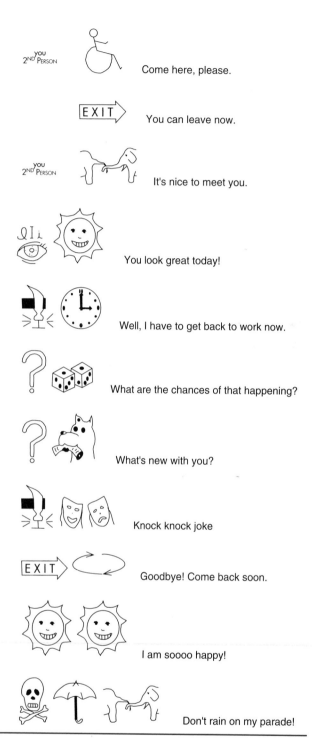

Figure 11-8   Examples of Minspeak symbol sequences. (From Romich B: *Liberator manual*, Wooster, OH, Prentke Romich.)

of a sequence light up or flash, beginning with the first selected icon. This continues until a complete icon sequence has been selected. This feature can aid recall and increase speed of selection because the device limits the number of icons that must be visually scanned for each selection.

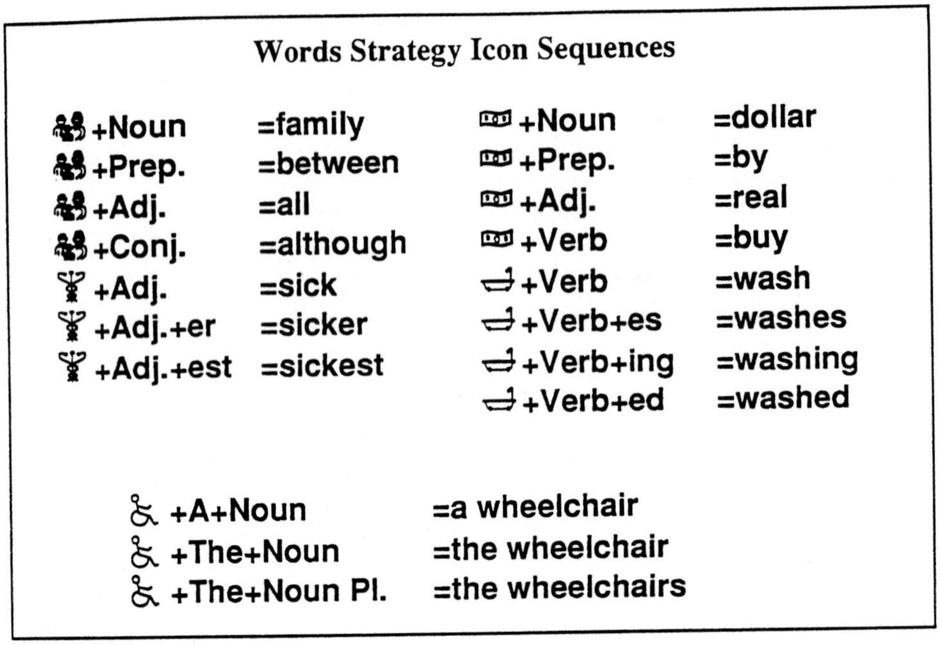

Figure 11-9 Symbols such as those used with Minspeak can be given syntactical meaning, as in this example from the Word Strategy application program. (From *Liberating the power of Minspeak*, Wooster, OH, 1991, Prentke Romich.)

Williams (1991), an accomplished user of numerical abbreviation expansion and word-based Minspeak, describes several advantages of this approach. In comparison to sentence-based Minspeak, he states that he (and most of the rest of us) does not think in sentences but in words or short phrases. This makes a word-based device easier to use. Second, he indicates that of the three encoding approaches in which he has achieved skill (each after hundreds of hours of practice), the word-based Minspeak "offers powerful advantages over the rest" (p. 133). His major reasons for this are the ease with which words are recalled during use and the large vocabularies that are possible with the use of icons rather than arbitrary codes. Williams also points out that it requires a large amount of practice and effort to become proficient with this type of device, which must be built into training programs. Williams also addresses the initial reluctance that many cognitively able but physically limited adults with CCN have to using pictorial representations as codes.

Examples of Vocabulary Programs for Language Development. The *Gateway* (Dynavox Systems, Inc, Pittsburgh, Pa., *www.dynavoxsystems.com*) series is an approach to vocabulary organizations that is based on language development in typically developing children. The levels of Gateway are designated by the number of elements in the selection set, from 12 through 75. These are intended for six distinct target user groups beginning with the 12- to 24-month language development level, progressing to two formats for mild/moderate cognitive disability for children or adults, arrays for children and adolescents/adults

with typical cognitive/language development and physical limitations, and a high-end array for augmented communicators who have well-developed syntactical skills. Pop-up menus with frequently used items (word, phrases, or sentences) are available on the larger arrays.

WordPower (Inman Innovations, available on several commercial AAC systems) combines a core vocabulary of 100 words that represent about 50% of spoken communication. It includes approximately 100 single hit words, hundreds of two and three hit words, a core dictionary for word prediction of 30,000 words, automatic grammatical endings (-ed, -ing, -s), and a QWERTY keyboard for spelling. For literate users, this approach is intuitive and leads to efficient communication. There are both direct and indirect (scanning) versions available. Picture WordPower uses labeled symbols as word cues. The same basic core vocabulary is available.

Conversationally based vocabulary storage and retrieval. Vocabulary selection can be based on conversational patterns. An early approach to this technique was CHAT (Conversation Helped by Automatic Talk) based on the premise that each keystroke should produce a complete "speech act" (an utterance with a purpose) (Alm, Newell, and Arnott, 1987). The CHAT model had five sections that could be scripted in advance: (1) greetings, (2) small talk, (3) main section, (4) wrap-up remarks, and (5) farewells. CHAT also included small talk (comments and repair). CHAT also allowed the superimposition of mood on the other features: polite, informal, humorous, or angry (Alm, Arnott, and Newell 1992).

Many conversational topics are repeated. TOPIC (Text Output In Conversation), a companion to CHAT, included a database and an intelligent user interface to hold each "conversational contribution" subject descriptors (e.g., work, family, books, science), speech act descriptors (e.g., request for information, information, disclosure), and a frequency of use counter (Alm, Arnott, and Newell, 1989). For example, a conversation about work or family or a joke is often repeated in different contexts and with different communication partners.

Dye et al (1998) combined the concepts of CHAT, TOPIC, and VSDs to develop a script-based system that used a scene-based interface. Five groups of conversational categories were included: I'm listening ("uh-huh"), openers (greetings, responses, small talk), closers (wrap-ups, farewells), feedback (comments), and control (repair of breakdowns) and were automatically presented to the user to match the flow of the conversation. Scripts can be organized in a predictive fashion as well. One example presented was a physician's office picture in which the user can click on an icon representing the receptionist to introduce himself or herself and indicate that he or she uses an SGD. The display then highlights the appointment book picture to request an appointment. The rest of the conversation is similarly scripted. These concepts have been implemented in several commercial AAC devices.

TALK (Todman, 2000) is an extension of CHAT and TOPIC based on the perspective of a typical conversation: person (me/you), queries (where, what, how, who, when, why), and tense (present, past, future). Figure 11-10 shows a typical TALK board with "where me/where/past" perspectives selected. This leads to the display of a particular set of phrases that can be chosen and spoken with one switch selection. There are also a set of comments, repair phrases along the right side, and the conversation sections similar to

CHAT along the top. These may be randomly spoken, as in CHAT, or the user may choose which phrase to use. The bottom of the screen has an area for letter-by-letter text entry. Using TALK and similar systems, the AAC user can obtain conversational rates of 30 to 60 words per minute. One version of TALK is available with Speaking Dynamically Pro (Mayer Johnson, Solana Beach, Calif., *www.mayer-johnson.com*). When individuals who have limited experience with conversations are introduced to systems such as TALK, significant training specifically oriented toward conversational flow is required (Todman, 2000).

Frame Talker (Higginbotham et al, 2005) is an AAC approach that allows the selection of natural language utterances by using a schematic format that represents the situational structure of communication events. The situational structure of communication events is represented by a communication frame. Frames can be used to semantically and functionally organize related conversational utterances. A communication frame consists of component frames, utterance constructions and lexical fields, a topic domain, and a frame hierarchy. The communication frame can be viewed as an utterance-based augmentative communication device designed to enable a person with CCN to communicate quickly and effectively. The internal structure of a communication frame consists of component frames and utterance constructions. Component frames uniquely identify typical subtopics or distinct situational portions within the larger communication frame (e.g., "severity" versus "cause" of pains) with utterance constructions located within them. A potentially large number of different utterances can be generated by each utterance construction in combination with its associated lexical field (i.e., group of semantically related terms). Topic domains are organized as clusters of individual communication frames that share similar generic topic interests.

Augmentative and Alternative Communication System Outputs. Dynamic communication displays

create greater flexibility in selection sets by changing the selection set displayed when a choice is made, as shown in Figure 11-11. For example, a general selection set may consist of categories such as work, home, food, clothing, greetings, or similar classifications. If one of these is chosen, either by touching the display surface directly or by scanning, then a new selection set is displayed. For example, a variety of food-related items and activities (eat, drink, ice cream, pasta, etc.) would follow the choice of "foods" from the general selection set. The symbols on the display can be varied, and this changes the targets for the user. Because each new selection set is displayed, the user does not have to remember what is on each level. This approach, illustrated in Figure 11-12, also avoids having to squeeze several pictures into one square on a static display. It also relies on recognition memory rather than recall for identification of

Me	Greet	Stories	Storage	Switch	Finish	Ques	F'back
You						Sympa	Hedge
	Our first house was in Carnoustie	Most of my childhood we lived in Dundee	I was away at college in Motherwell for two years			Saying	Sorry
Where						Uh huh	More
What	I don't remember it at all	We lived mainly in Charleston and Menziehill	It was really different living on the west coast			Agree	Disagree
How						Dunno	Thanks
When	Carnoustie is well known for its golf course	I really liked living there	I like the west coast of Scotland better than the east			Wait	Interrupt
Who						Good!	Bad!
Why	The first flat I had on my own was at Blackwood Court					Yes	No
						Oops!	Random
Past	It was a real adventure living on my own for the first time					Repeat	Quit
Present						Edit Last	
Future						Edit Text	Go Edit
							Speak

Figure 11-10   TALK board. (Courtesy Mayer-Johnson.)

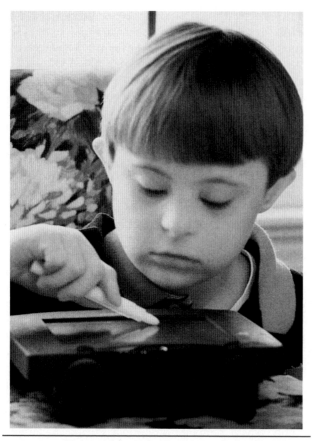

Figure 11-11 Dynamic display devices are often accessed with touch screen interfaces, making them accessible and providing a cognitively concrete user interface. (Photo courtesy Dynavox.)

the selection set elements, which can make it easier to use. A dynamic passive display requires the user to select the next page to be displayed. The dynamic active display automatically branches to the selected new page once the item is selected.

Two types of dynamic displays were used in a matching task in a case study of a 16-year-old girl with a severe cognitive disability who had several years of experience in using fixed and dynamic displays (Reichle et al, 2000). There were no differences in accuracy of the matching tasks between the three types of display for a small number (15) of symbols. However, as the number of symbols increased (to 30 in dynamic and 60 in passive) the dynamic active display was significantly better than the other two. The response time was fastest for the passive display because all possible choices were displayed at once.

Blackstone (1994) describes a number of key features of dynamic displays. The nature of these devices allows the user to quickly change the screen and to configure the size, color, and arrangement of the symbols to match the topic. Dynamic displays reduce memory requirements because the user is prompted by the display after each choice. The constant vigilance to the screen requires a high level of visual attention and constant decision making. The user must also have mastered the concept of object permanence (Chapter 3). These may be challenging for some individuals who have cognitive limitations.

Visual scene displays (VSDs) take advantage of the graphical user interface (see Chapter 7) to create displays

Figure 11-12 Dynamic display devices change the selection set presented to the user each time an entry is made.

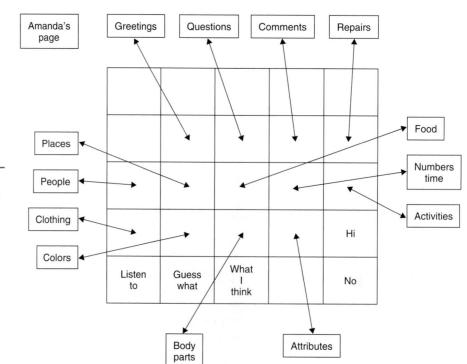

TABLE 11-3   Comparison of Visual Scene Displays and Traditional Grid Displays

Variable	Typical AAC Grid	VSD
Type of representation	Symbols, TO, line drawings	Digital photos, line drawings
Personalization	Limited	High
Amount of context	Low	High
Layout	Grid	Full or partial screen, grid
Display mgmt	Menu, pages	Menu pages, navigation bars
Concept retrieval	Select grid space, popups	Hotspots, speech key, select grid space

Based on Blackstone S: Visual scene displays, *Augment Commun News* 16:1-5, 2004.

that capture events in a person's life on the screen with "hot spots" that can be accessed to retrieve information (Blackstone, 2004). They also offer the AAC user and his or her partner a greater degree of contextual information to support interaction. The richness of the display and the information content also enables communication partners to participate more actively in a conversation. VSDs may represent either a generic or personalized context. The former includes drawings of places (e.g., house, schoolroom), whereas the latter is specific to user (e.g., a picture of his house, a family outing). Table 11-3 illustrates the difference between a traditional AAC display (referred to as a grid) and a VSD (Blackstone, 2004). The traditional grid supports communication of needs and wants and information exchange well. This type of display is usually restricted to symbols, text, or static drawings (although some animation is used with dynamic display items) and the vocabulary items are separated from any context to maximize their versatility. Figure 11-13 illustrates the differences between a typical grid display and a VSD (Blackstone, 2004). Personalization is also limited. The VSD is developed for conversational support as a shared activity. Because it uses a range of information media, including video and family pictures in addition to text, symbols and line drawings, it can be highly personalized, as shown in Figure 11-14 (Blackstone, 2004).

In addition to communication of needs, wants and information exchange, VSDs also support social closeness. Because of the dynamic nature of the VSD approach, it can also serve as a learning environment. VSDs can stimulate conversation between interactants in which they play, share experiences, and tell stories. The dynamic nature of VSDs facilitates active participation of interactants during these shared activities. VSDs can also provide instruction, specific information, or prompts to help the user interact effectively. The populations expected to be served by VSDs are those with cognitive (e.g., Down syndrome) or language (e.g., aphasia, autism) limitations.

Young (2½ years old) typically developing children did significantly better at a birthday party communication task when using a schematic VSD layout (based on activities) than when using a grid layout (schematic or taxonomic) (Drager, 2003). One explanation is that the provision of a more meaningful context in the VSD reduced the language demand on the child. The VSD was organized around scenes of rooms: living room (arrival of children for party), kitchen (eating cake), family room (opening presents), and playroom (playing games); this reduces the demands on the child's working memory because the location of the item required fewer demands on the VSD. The grid was organized around the activities, which required more language processing by the child (e.g., categorizing, remembering the symbols). For example, the topic of play could be illustrated by a digital photograph of the child's room including the toy box in the VSD and as a symbol for play on the grid. Clicking on the hot spot associated with the toy box in the VSD or on the grid element for play resulted in branching in both formats to more detailed information.

Speech Output.   The two major types of speech output use in SGDs are digitized and synthesized. These are both described in Chapter 7. Speech output allows use with partners who cannot read (e.g., small children or cognitively impaired persons). It is also the only type of output that can be used conveniently for speaking to groups (including use in classroom discussions) or speaking over the telephone (unless both the user of the device and the partner each have special TTY equipment; see Chapter 9). Typical additional

Traditional grid display   Visual scene display

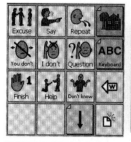
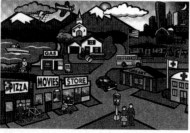

Figure 11-13   Visual scene display versus grid. (From Blackstone S: Visual scene displays, *Augment Commun News* 16:1-5, 2004.)

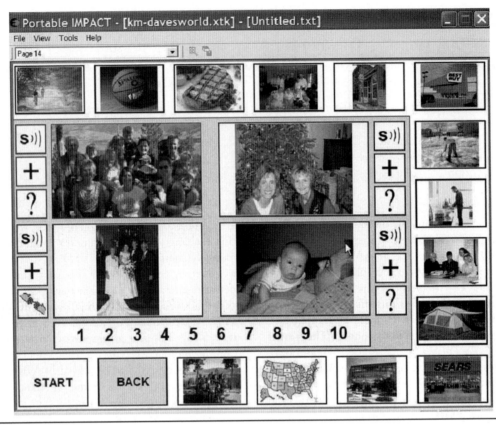

Figure 11-14   VSD layout for family outing or wedding (personalized). (From Blackstone S: Visual scene displays, *Augment Commun News,* 16:1-5, 2004.)

outputs that are available on AAC devices are printers, computer access, and electronic aids to daily living (EADL) (primarily appliance control). These are discussed in Chapters 7 and 14, respectively.

Access to Mainstream Technologies. Specialized assistive technologies such as EADL (Chapter 14) and power wheelchairs (Chapter 12) are also often of use to individuals with CCN. Many SGDs either provide the functions of EADL or interface with them through wireless connections. The use of an SGD interface to control a power wheelchair is a common application as well. The real power in connecting people with CCN to the rest of the information society lies in access to mainstream technologies. This includes entertainment (e.g., DVD, CD players) and other electronic devices such as electronic games. However, two technologies with enormous potential to create greater connectivity for people with CCN are the Internet and the cell phone.

Internet access.   The Internet provides significant resources from the computer desktop. Quick, easy, and low-cost communication with individuals around the world is routine by use of e-mail. Many people who have disabilities use e-mail to communicate with friends, business associates, and organizations (see the case study of Heidi). Many individuals with CCN access the Internet with their SGDs. Any stored

vocabulary or special access methods are available for use while on-line. Some commercial SGDs are actually portable computers with AAC software that can also function as Internet workstations. The Internet also provides access to information through company, organization, and individual Web sites (see Resources, page 556) By accessing this information, AAC users can learn about new technologies, conduct business independently, carry out research for academic pursuits, book airline reservations, and many other activities. Access to the Internet can provide many opportunities for reading and writing, and this can have a positive impact on literacy skills for AAC users (Blackstone 2003c). It is also used to train mentoring individuals who rely on AAC as demonstrated by 2 weeks of intensive training at Temple University *(http://disabilities.temple.edu/programs/assistive/ aces/index.htm)* and 1 year of follow-up through the Internet. Program graduates now mentor new students in the program. The benefits of using the Internet are not available to everyone. Those without an Internet connection or the ability to use an SGD and those who are not literate, however, can still depend on friends or family to support their participation by reading Internet content (e-mails, Web sites) and typing responses on the basis of input from the AAC user (e.g., using symbols or pictures). However, this strategy has implications for the privacy of the user.

AUGMENTATIVE AND ALTERNATIVE COMMUNICATION IN POSTSECONDARY EDUCATION

Heidi (Figure 11-15) is a doctoral student studying English at a major university. She has cerebral palsy, which limits her ability to speak and to use her hands for writing. She uses her computer to complete writing assignments and has written two plays (one for her master's degree thesis) and one book for teenagers who have cerebral palsy. She uses her notebook computer with a speech synthesizer for conversation and a word processor for writing. She also uses e-mail to communicate with her PhD thesis advisor, colleagues, students, and friends. This technology allows her to keep in touch with people without the use of the telephone, which is difficult with her AAC device. Her computer system allows her several modes of communication, as well as providing the opportunity for her to work at home much of the time and avoid the hassles of special transportation arrangements. Her e-mail contacts also prevent her from being isolated in her home environment.

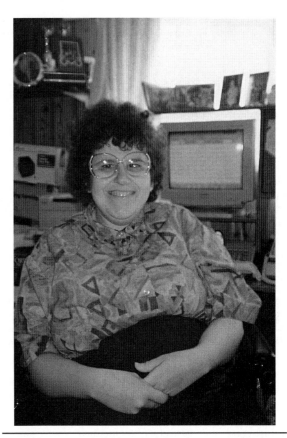

Figure 11-15   Access to the Internet provides Heidi with the tools necessary to pursue her PhD. She contacts her professors and students by e-mail, conducts literature searches over the Internet, and participates in Web-based courses and discussion groups. This access is all obtained with the same laptop computer that she uses as an AAC device in face-to-face conversations.

E-mail allows composition at a slower speed because the recipient reads it at a later time (Blackstone, 2003c). E-mail also allows an AAC user to communicate with another person without someone else being present. Because the person's disability is not immediately visible, AAC users report that they enjoy establishing relationships with people who experience them first as a person and then learn of their disabilities.

Internet chat rooms where people who have common interests can exchange information in a real-time format can help AAC users establish advocacy groups, share information, and engage in leisure pursuits. Listservs, which consist of a group of individuals with common interests but are more like bulletin boards, also provide rich sources of information and friendly interaction. A popular AAC listserv is ACOLUG hosted by Temple University.

Cell Phones.   Issues facing people with CCN in accessing cell phones are very similar to those faced by individuals who have low vision or blindness (see Chapter 8). Four changes in cell phone technology described in Chapter 8 will increase access: (1) increased processing power, (2) ease of downloading into the phone, (3) wireless connection to a worldwide network, and (4) low cost and reachable by persons with disabilities because these features will be built into standard cell phones (Fruchterman, 2003). The move away from proprietary software to an open source approach, much like personal computers of today, will lead to greater diversity of software for tasks such as text-to-speech output, voice recognition, and downloadable user profiles that allow customization for a particular activity or task. For example, a specific stored vocabulary, word prediction/completion list, and key word index for

text messaging could be resident on the Internet and downloaded as needed. Because the operating system will be open source, many applications for people with CCN can be downloaded from the Internet. An additional advantage is that features such as speech synthesis will be useful to individuals who are blind as well as to those with CCN, so the number of potential customers for software developers will rise and the cost of applications will fall. Features that were developed for people with disabilities (e.g., word completion/prediction, voice recognition, abbreviation expansion) are also being found to be useful for the general public. This will further increase their availability to individuals with CCN. Digital photography built into cell phones also increases utility for persons with CNN. In addition to the mainstream use (i.e., photography for recording family events, business, or school), the camera features can be used as an additional AAC option, reducing the descriptive information required to convey a message.

Configurations of Commercial Speech-Generating Devices.   To describe current SGDs, we have created seven categories of the major commercially available devices, shown in Table 11-4. The categories reflect different groupings

TABLE 11-4 **Feature Categories Commonly Combined in Commercial Augmentative and Alternative Communication Systems**

Category	Speech Output*	Message Type*	Message Formulation Techniques*	Access Method*	Examples (Manufacturer)
Simple scanners	None	Pre-stored	NA	1,2,4, or 5 switch scanning	All-Turn-It (A) Steeper (ZYGO) ZYGO 16 ZYGO 100
Simple speech output (8 minutes or less) SGD, K0541*	Digitized	Prestored Coverage vocabulary only	NA	Scan or direct selection, multiple methods	Advocate (ZYGO) Cardinal, (Saltillo) Mini Messagemate (Words+) Hawk series (AdamLab) Tech/Four(AMDi) TechTalk (AMDi) TechScan(AMDi) Parakeet (ZYGO) iTalk, BigMAc, Step by Step, Talk-Trac (A)
Simple speech output (greater than 8 min) SGD K0542*	Digitized	Prestored Coverage vocabulary only	Minimal rate enhancement or vocabulary expansion	Scan or direct selection, multiple methods	Bluebird, VocaFlex Chat Box series (Saltillo) Dynamo, MightyMo, MiniMo (DV) Messagemate (Words+) SuperHawk12/Plus (AdamLab) SuperTalker (A) TechSpeak (AMDi) Tech128 (AMDi) SpringBoard (PRC) Talara, Macaw (ZYGO)
Direct selection, writing only Spelling only SGD, SGD K0543*	No speech output Synthesized	Message formulation Message formulation	Spelling, rate enhancement Spelling	Direct selection Direct selection	AlphaSmart 3000, Neo, Dana (Alpha Smart) Dynawrite (AV) Polyana (ZYGO) Light Writer (ZYGO)
Multiple selection method with rate enhancement, SGD, K0544*	Synthesized	Message formulation	Spelling and rate enhancement	Variety of selection methods and control interfaces	Delta Talker (PRC) DV4, MT4 (DV) EZ Keys (Words+) Freedom 2001 (Words+) Light Writer (ZYGO) Tuff Talker (Words+) Dialect (ZYGO) Tablet XL, PalmTop (DV) Light Writer (ZYGO) Dialect, Optimist (ZYGO) Vantage, Vantage, Pathfinder (PRC) Vanguard (PRC)
Software-based Multiple selection method with rate enhancement, uses standard computer hardware as operating system, SGD, K0545*	Synthesized	Message formulation	Spelling and rate enhancement	Variety of selection methods and control interfaces	Dynavox (DV) e-Talk series (GTB) Impact (DV) Windbag, Grid (ZYGO) Pathfinder (PRC) Scan Writer (ZYGO) Vanguard (PRC) Say it Sam, EZ keys Say it Sam, EZkeys, Talking screen (Words+)

TABLE 11-4	Feature Categories Commonly Combined in Commercial Augmentative and Alternative Communication Systems—cont'd				
Category	Speech Output*	Message Type*	Message formulation Techniques*	Access Method*	Examples (Manufacturer)
Mounts SGD, K0546	NA	NA	NA	NA	Daessy List some manufacturers + many AAC manufacturers provide own
Accessories, SGD K0547*	NA	NA	NA	NA	Keyguards, head trackers, expanded keyboards, symbol system software, carrying cases, switches, joysticks†

*Categories, funding codes and features included in U.S. Medicare funding for "speech-generating devices"; elements adapted from Blackstone S: Assessment protocol for SGDs, *Augment Commun News* 13:1-16, 2001. Note: restrictions on software options required for Medicare funding.
†Vary by manufacturer; examples shown.
A, Ablenet; *ACS,* Adaptive Communication Systems; *DJ,* Don Johnston Developmental Systems; *DV,* Dynavox; *IC,* Innocomp; *PRC,* Prentke Romich Co., *D,* Daessy, *GTB,* Great Talking Box Company.

of the characteristics discussed earlier in the section on AAC characteristics as well as the funding codes and categories for Medicare reimbursement of SGDs in the United States (Blackstone, 2001). Table 11-4 also includes accessories and mounting systems for AAC devices. We have opted for a few large categories on the basis of the most essential features, resulting in variability within each category. The format in Table 11-4 appropriately groups devices serving distinct populations. Within each category there is still significant opportunity for decision making that is based on a thorough assessment of skills and needs. The commercial devices listed in each category are examples and, although a variety of manufacturers, models, products, and varying device features are included, Table 11-4 is not inclusive.

Simple scanners, the first category in Table 11-4, are generally operated by a single switch, although some can have dual-switch scanning and others allow four- or five-switch directed scanning. The devices in this category are distinguished by the use of a light to indicate the output selection, very limited vocabularies (32 items or less), no rate enhancement or vocabulary, and the general absence of voice output as a standard feature.

The devices categorized as *simple speech output* are further delineated by length of recorded digital speech. They were all developed to provide a limited-vocabulary, easy-to-use output for very young children or individuals with limited language abilities. In general, they require direct selection, but some also allow scanning. Rate enhancement in this category varies from none, to levels, to simple codes or key sequences. Vocabulary storage varies from a low of a few seconds to several minutes.

The devices in the *direct selection, writing only* category are distinguished by their small size and focus on features that support writing. Some may have a built-in printer. Several devices in this category provide direct file transfer to

a desktop computer, and several also have rate enhancement (generally abbreviation expansion, instant phrases, or word completion).

The devices in the *spelling only* SGD category are primarily distinguished by their dependence on spelling for message formulation. They also generally are a small size and use direct selection through a keyboard or touch screen.

The last two categories in Table 11-4 represent the highest level of sophistication in currently available devices. They incorporate all the rate enhancement approaches discussed in Chapter 7. Those in the multiple selection method with rate enhancement category are based on SGD hardware that is specifically designed for AAC. The devices in the last category are software applications that are designed to run on general-purpose computers such as laptops, tablets, or PDAs. Vocabulary storage capacity varies from a few hundred utterances to thousands of utterances. Interaction with other devices (e.g., computers, Chapter 8; power wheelchairs, Chapter 12; or EADLs, Chapter 14) and peripherals such as printers is possible for most of the devices in this group using either serial or parallel ports (generally USB). Within these two categories are devices that can meet the needs of a variety of consumers, from very young children who cannot spell to quantum physicists who make full use of sophisticated rate enhancement techniques. In some cases the same device can serve a wide range of needs because the software and vocabulary stored can be customized. In other cases the devices are relatively inflexible.

Devices in the last two categories provide great flexibility in control interfaces and selection methods. Several of the direct selection types allow both standard size and expanded or contracted keyboards as control interfaces. Several devices in these two categories allow scanning with single-switch or four- or five-switch directed scanning. Some also provide both one- and two-switch Morse code, and some provide direct selection by head pointing. For direct selection by head pointing, some devices use light pointers or sensors attached to the head, whereas others use reflective systems requiring the attachment of only a reflective dot. Some light pointers can also be held in the hand.

The flexibility provided by devices in these categories is particularly useful in dealing with degenerative diseases such as ALS. Initially a person may use direct selection with the hand. As this ability is lost, direct selection by head control is feasible. However, because the device has not changed, the stored vocabulary, rate enhancement strategies, and operational characteristics of the device remain the same. If direct selection by head control becomes impossible, scanning or Morse code can be used. Once again the device is not changed, and the vocabulary, rate enhancement, and operational features remain the same. This is a great advantage over having to learn a new device at each stage of the disease.

What distinguishes the last two categories is the hardware platform. The human/technology interface may use either a static or dynamic display with a variety of ways in which each of these user interfaces is implemented on the various devices listed in Table 11-4. The devices in this category allow for a variety of physical and cognitive skills on the part of users.

In summary, the categories shown in Table 11-4 are intended to provide a rough framework with which to view SGDs. It is important for the ATP to remain current regarding technologies. One of the easiest ways to do this is to attend conferences that feature assistive technologies. If the ATP will be charged with making recommendations for AAC systems and approaches, it is also important to have his or her name placed on the mailing lists for the manufacturers of these devices. Most SGD manufacturers also maintain home pages on the Internet. There are several Web sites that provide links to SGD manufacturers.

■ IMPLEMENTATION OF AUGMENTATIVE COMMUNICATION SYSTEMS

As discussed in Chapter 4, in the total process of delivering assistive technologies, the recommendation of a communication device based on a formal assessment is only the beginning of the process. Once funding is obtained and the device is procured, implementation begins. Other steps that may be required include customization to integrate components from different manufacturers (e.g., a communication device from one manufacturer and a control interface from another), programming of a device to include vocabulary specific to the individual consumer, fitting of the device to the consumer's wheelchair, and mounting a control interface in an accessible location. It is impossible in one chapter to cover all the issues related to AAC implementation.

Beukelman and Mirenda (2005); Beukelman, Yorkston, and Dowden (1984); Kraat (1985, 1986); Musselwhite and St. Louis (1982); and Riechle, York, and Sigafoos (1991) are sources rich in practical information and case studies related to AAC implementation. There are also frequent case studies presented in journals such as *Augmentative and Alternative Communication* and newsletters such as *Communication Matters* and *Augmentative Communication News*. These case studies vary from anecdotal reports written by individual who use AAC devices or those working with them. They include formal case studies and single-subject research designs. This section discusses the most basic considerations related to training and follow-up. It is important to note that things do not always progress smoothly through the implementation phase. Fields (1991) presents a case study indicating the steps that one family went through to implement an AAC system for their son. There is also a listserv for those who rely on AAC at *http://listserv.temple. edu/archives/acolug.html*.

Vocabulary Selection

AAC is unique among the needs served by speech-language pathologists in that the vocabulary must be supplied by the clinician or the individual with CCN. It is not "built-in" cognitively. Once an AAC system is selected for an individual, it is necessary to create an initial vocabulary set for programming into the device or for use on a nonelectronic system. The conversational categories shown in Table 11-5 provide a useful framework for initial vocabulary selections.

Several categories of messages are used by people who rely on AAC (Beukelman and Mirenda, 2005). Conversational messages begin with greetings and then often involve small talk as a transition between the greeting and information sharing; small talk often uses scripts for initiating and maintaining conversations. In general, SGDs do not support small talk well. Generic small talk can be used in different conversations with different people and includes topics such as "How is your family?" "What's happening?" "Isn't that beautiful?" "Good story!" and "She is great." Specific small is more focused: "How is your wife?" "What are you doing?" "That is a beautiful flower," "Good story about your vacation," and "She is a great teacher." A common form of conversational interaction for adults, particularly older adults, is story telling. Stories entertain, teach, and establish social closeness. An important role for the ATP or AAC facilitator is to assist those who rely on AAC to capture stories and assist with programming the device (e.g., to replay one sentence at a time to allow the pace of the story to be controlled by the individual).

Vocabulary needs vary by the context, communication mode, and individual characteristics. Beukelman and Mirenda (2005) compiled a composite list of 100 most frequently used words for a variety of categories including age and gender.

TABLE 11-5   Categories to Be Included in Conversational Augmentative and Alternative Communication Systems

Category	Sample Vocabulary
Initiating and interaction	Hey, I've got something to say.
	Check this out.
	Come talk to me.
	May I help you?
Greetings	Hello, I'm pleased to meet you.
	Where have you been? I've been waiting forever.
	What's happening?
Response to greetings	I'm fine.
	Great, how are you?
	Not so hot, and you?
Requests	I'd like a _____. (object, event)
	I'd like to go to _____. (place, event)
Information exchange	What time is it?
	I have a question.
	The concert begins at 8 PM.
Commenting	I agree (disagree).
	What a great idea!
	Uh-huh.
	OK.
Wrap-up/farewell	Well, gotta go. See you later
	Bye, nice talking to you.
Conversational repair	Let's start over.
	That's not what I meant.
	You misunderstood me.

Preliterate individuals require a coverage vocabulary to communicate essential messages. Because generation of novel utterances by spelling is not possible, the AAC team must ensure that as many messages as possible are stored in the device for easy retrieval. The specific vocabulary is highly dependent on the individual's needs. Most often, the coverage vocabulary is organized by context with separate displays or pages for different activities. Preliterate individuals also need a developmental vocabulary that includes words and concepts that are not yet understood. These are selected on the basis of their educational value, not for functional purposes, and they encourage language and vocabulary growth. New words can be added around special events or activities, especially when an activity is to be experienced for the first time (e.g., going to the circus). The developmental vocabulary also encourages the use of different language structures reflecting semantic categories.

Required vocabulary resources for literate individuals include a core vocabulary that is used with a variety of situations and partners and occurs frequently. There are word lists based on successful general patterns, the needs of a specific individual, and the performance of natural speakers or writers in similar contexts *(http://aac.unl.edu/)*. A list of 500 words covered 80% of total utterances for individuals who are operationally and socially competent with AAC systems (see training section of this chapter) (Beukelman and Mirenda, 2005). Words and messages that are unique to the individual are included in a fringe vocabulary that includes names of people, places, activities, and preferred expressions. This approach personalizes the AAC system by complementing the core vocabulary list. The fringe vocabulary content is often identified by family and friends as well as the individual. The initial items are those that are of high interest to the user and have potential for frequent use. It is important to include items that denote a range of semantic notions and pragmatic functions. To ease learning, the vocabulary should reflect the "here and now" and have potential for later multiword use. Ease of production by the individual and interpretation by the partner is also essential.

Environmental inventories are another form of identifying vocabulary. Some formal procedures for these are available (Beukelman and Mirenda, 2005). These inventories document the individual's experiences by noting precipitating events and subsequent consequences. The documentation includes words used by peers with and without disabilities. The identified pool of vocabulary items is reduced to a list of most critical words that the individual can manage. Communication diaries and checklists are records of words and phrases needed by an individual for AAC that are kept by informants such as family members. There are some published lists that can also act as a shortcut to vocabulary selection (Beukelman and Mirenda, 2005).

Yorkston et al. (1988) studied 11 vocabulary lists compiled from various sources. They found that most lists were unique because they contained mostly content words (those related to a specific topic) rather than function or structure words (e.g., articles, pronouns, conjunctions). The authors also compiled these 11 lists into one large list that can be used as a starting point for developing individual vocabularies for AAC devices. This list was then applied to a case study to illustrate the process of selecting vocabulary for a person who cannot read and is severely physically disabled (Yorkston et al., 1989). The list developed for this person contained words that were not on even the largest of the 11 lists of the earlier study. This finding indicates how unique the needs of each individual are. Beukelman, McGinnis, and Morrow (1991) describe the factors that need to be considered in selecting vocabulary for AAC devices. These include the need to have vocabularies for different contexts (e.g., small talk, school, and home) and considerations regarding acceleration vocabularies versus coverage vocabularies. They also analyze the factors that differ in developing AAC vocabularies for individuals who can spell (and therefore have access to a large vocabulary with only the alphabet) and those who cannot spell (and who need a large coverage vocabulary).

Participants in adult programs (day care and residential) who have learning disabilities have unique needs for vocabulary (Graves, 2000). The vocabulary needs of this population differ from those of typical adults or children (with or without disabilities). With use of diaries compiled by staff working with adults who needed AAC, more than 80% of the conversational topics were functional (e.g., physical needs and daily activities) for those with the most severe disabilities. For individuals with more moderate disabilities, the percentage of functional topics was twice that of physical needs. Emotional (feelings of anger, anxiety, fear, love) amounted to only 3.4% of all topics. Possible reasons for this low response may relate to the cognitive difficulties in expressing feelings and to cultural factors that limit the degree to which staff are able to provide emotional support to residents. These results differ from standard vocabulary lists in content and emphasis, and they reinforce the need for care in applying standardized vocabulary lists to AAC vocabulary selection.

Because most AAC devices are programmable, it is possible to continually add or amend vocabulary as needs change. The choice of additional vocabulary items is generally made on the basis of needs that occur frequently; input from family, care providers, and other communication partners and new situations that arise. In the majority of cases, vocabulary development (after the initial set is implemented) is relatively slow and occurs over a long period. Some devices (e.g., word completion or prediction systems) automatically add items to the stored vocabulary on the basis of the frequency of use.

Beukelman and his colleagues and students at the University of Nebraska at Lincoln have compiled a large number of resources relating to vocabulary selection and messaging in AAC. This information can be accessed through their Web site *(http://aac.unl.edu/vbstudy)*. Included in this resource are core vocabulary lists consisting of high-frequency words for preschool and school-age children, young adults, and older adults. They also include unabridged vocabulary lists (with use statistics) for nondisabled persons (20- to 30-year-old adults, older adults, and preschool children) and AAC users (four volumes). Vocabulary lists of small talk for children and adults, as well as context-specific messages suggested by AAC specialists, are also included. This site also provides vocabulary lists for school settings (preschool activities and classroom activities). Finally, vocabulary lists for use as initial recommendations in AAC are reported, as are references for AAC messaging and vocabulary selection. This site is a rich source of information for the ATP charged with developing vocabulary for individuals who use AAC.

Physical Skill Development

AAC devices require physical skill, whether direct selection or scanning, to operate them effectively. It takes practice to

develop this skill, and it can be useful to separate the physical skills required for the use of an augmentative communication device from the communication skills required. This aspect of training is described in Chapter 7.

If the individual has insufficient motor skill to make reliable selections but is expected to develop the necessary motor control, it is important that this *physical competence* be developed separately from the *use* of the physical skill for communication. If the ATP attempts to teach motor skills by using the communication device, it is possible that errors in selection caused by lack of motor skill will be misinterpreted as lack of communicative skill; for example, the person may have intended to select the picture of the apple (signifying "eat") but missed the mark and selected the picture of the cup ("drink"). Conversely, errors caused by communication or language inability may be interpreted as motor selection difficulties. In the previous example the person may have been capable of physically choosing apple but chose cup because he or she did not understand either the question or the communication task.

Training System Use: Developing Communicative Competence.   Figure 11-16 shows a completed installation of an SGD. When the installation is completed, the

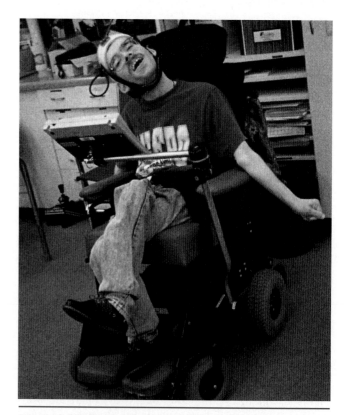

Figure 11-16   Implementation of an AAC system includes proper mounting of the AAC device and control interface to the wheelchair if necessary. Here is a completed installation ready for checkout.

individual and those working with him (e.g., care providers, family, teachers, employers, therapists, and speech-language pathologists) can begin the process of learning to use the device. Depending on the complexity of the device and the sophistication of the features included, this process can take from a few hours to several months.

The development of communicative competence is most effective when a comprehensive program is used. One such approach is the System for Augmenting Language (SAL) (Sevick, Romski, and Adamson, 2004). SAL involves a multimodal approach to training of individuals who rely on AAC, their partners, and continuing follow-up. Sevick, Romski, and Adamson (2004) illustrate the application of SAL through a case study of a preschool child who used both a VOCA and a manual display consisting of PCS symbols. For young children with cognitive and language disabilities, the development of both expressive and receptive vocabulary can be developed by using a VOCA in an exercise to teach requesting (Brady, 2000). Children were taught to request objects using PCS symbols on a VOCA. After learning these symbols, the children's comprehension was evaluated. The use of the VOCA during the labeling instruction appeared to increase later comprehension of the symbols.

Scripts that are programmed into an AAC device can be used in a training paradigm. One formal approach is called "Script Builder" (Linda J. Burkhart, Eldersberg, Md., *www.Lburkhart.com*). The scripts are a way of training individuals to achieve greater social competence and more effective interactions. The scripts are coplanned and oriented toward the development of social closeness by encouraging social purposes and a sense of belonging. Typical topics of trivia, sports, gossip, hanging out, and "who's cute" allow the individual to display aspects of his or her personality through humor, teasing, whining, and joke telling. Scripts change perceptions of individuals who use AAC because greater social competence is evident. Some scripts focus on information content, others on conversation scripts (new information plus social closeness). Example scripts are shown in Box 11-3. There are three roles in the training: the individual who is developing AAC skills, his or her partner, and a "prompter" who prompts only when necessary in an unobtrusive way. The partner's role is communicating as naturally as possible, pausing when necessary, and not prompting at all. All social scripts start with a greeting and include a range of communicative functions such as positive and negative comments, teasing, and questioning. They provide for multiple turns and use topic maintainers like "tell me more." They need to be designed to ensure that the individual doesn't get "backed into a corner." The vocabulary chosen is appropriate to the individual's age and setting and personality.

Communicative competence depends on many factors (Light, 1989). The context in the HAAT model affects

---

BOX 11-3   Scripts

THE SURPRISE
Hey come here. Want to know a secret? It's here in my bag. It's one of my favorites. I don't think you've seen this before. Take a guess. Want to see it now? Nah—take another guess. Oh you've waited long enough. Oops—can't get it out. Oh all right—here it is. Have you ever seen anything like this before? I've got a ton of things in this bag. Let's tell everyone but the teacher!

THE PROM—GETTING READY
Hey, Mom. Come here! Oh no! I've got to do my makeup for the Prom! It's getting late. Hurry, Mom! Remember, my dress is blue. Let's do lipstick first. Please...not purple! Keep my lipstick on my lips. Don't get it on my teeth. I don't want to look like Bozo. I have that red hair! I want to look like Britney Spears. She's beautiful. Could I have a little more mascara, please? Thanks! I can't wait to get to the Prom! Mom, you did a great job. I don't want to miss the dance. Let's go!

---

competence in several ways. The partner and his or her skill in listening, the environment of use, and cultural factors all contribute to or detract from communicative competence. The degree of competence is also variable, and complete mastery of an AAC device is not necessary to have functional communication interactions. Light (1989) describes four areas of competence required for successful use of AAC devices: (1) operational, (2) linguistic, (3) social, and (4) strategic.

Operational competence requires the physical skills described earlier and an understanding of the technical operation of the AAC device. Once again, the degree of operational competence can be quite variable, from very basic operation to advanced features. An AAC device is like a musical instrument that can be played by an accomplished AAC communicator. Operational competence includes the cognitive demands dictated by rate-enhancement techniques. Training operational competence requires a systematic introduction of technical features, coupled with ample opportunities for practice in their use, as shown in Figure 11-17. The individual's facilitators must also be trained in certain operational features of the device (e.g., battery charging, connecting control interfaces), even though they will not develop the same level of competence as the individual.

The second phase, basic operation, includes how to connect the device to the control interface, how to charge batteries, how to attach it to a wheelchair, how to add vocabulary using rate-enhancement techniques (e.g., codes), and an introduction to troubleshooting in case the device fails to operate properly.

The last features to be introduced are those related to storage of new vocabulary, input acceleration techniques,

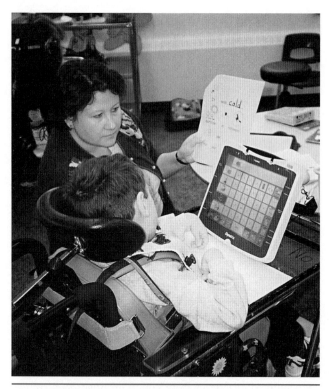

Figure 11-17   Development of operational competence with an AAC device requires a structured training program in which the device features are carefully explained and skill in their use is developed.

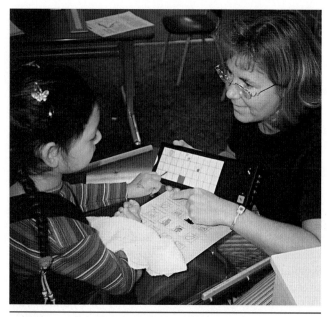

Figure 11-18   Development of linguistic competence is often taught in conjunction with other functional tasks, such as the one shown here.

and vocabulary manipulation features such as text editing and reformatting the output. Often the first two phases are accomplished in one session. However, in some cases, they may require multiple training sessions, and the process is often a lengthy one that may be integrated with the other aspects of training in communicative competence.

Linguistic competence requires that the symbol system and rules of organization be understood by the individual using the AAC system. As Light (1989) points out, the individual often must be competent in two languages: the spoken language of the community and the language of the AAC device. It is likely that the individual also lacks models of proficient use in the language of the device. Development of competence in this area may require many hours of practice. Often this practice is built around a functional reading task, such as that shown in Figure 11-18.

In contrast to the typical "drill and practice" approach to developing vocabulary and AAC use, Mirenda and Santogrossi (1985) used a prompt-free strategy to teach a young child to use a picture-based communication board. The approach involved a four-step process, which began with a picture of a soft drink being available to the child during her regular therapy session. A drink was visible to her, as was the picture of the drink. The child was not told that touching the picture would result in her getting a drink,

nor was she prompted in any way to touch the picture. If she touched the drink directly, she was told that she could have some later. If she accidentally or deliberately touched the picture, she was immediately given the drink with the explanation, "Yes, if you touch the picture, you may have the drink." Once the deliberate response had been established over several sessions, Mirenda and Santogrossi proceeded to shape the pointing behavior by progressively moving the picture farther away, until it was out of sight and the child had to actively find it. As the child became proficient in this task, the number of pictures was increased to four and the process repeated for the other choices. Eventually the child was able to generalize to a language board of 120 pictures. The advantage of this approach is that the child learns the meaning and significance of the symbolic representation by discovery rather than by drill, which leads to greater generalization and more functional use of the AAC system.

Many people who use AAC devices have little or no experience in social discourse. Even individuals who have used natural language for communication and who have sustained a disease or injury are faced with a very different mode of interaction when an AAC device is used. Rules of conversation are altered, and the perception of the individual by his or her communication partners is different. To be socially competent, the individual must have knowledge, judgment, and skills in both sociolinguistic (e.g., turn taking, initiating a conversation, conversational repair) and sociorelational areas (Light, 1989). The latter term describes the understanding of interaction between individuals. The effective communication device user is described (Light, 1988) as

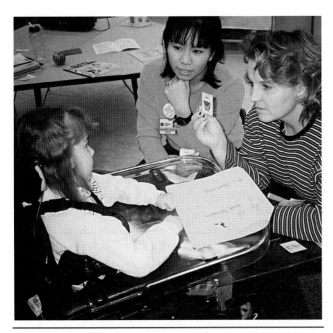

Figure 11-19 AAC users need to learn about conversational conventions and strategies. Training of these skills is often done in simulated situations. Here an aide is teaching the child how to use her AAC tools to interact with another adult partner.

having a positive self-image, interest in his or her partner, skill at drawing others into the conversation, ability to put a partner at ease, and active participation in the conversation. These are sociorelational skills, and the degree to which they are understood and used is one measure of social competence. These skills are best taught in the contexts in which they are to be used. One example of such training is shown in Figure 11-19, in which the child is being taught strategies for interacting with an adult partner. Self-determination is difficult for people who rely on AAC (Collier, 2005). They must know what they want, know how to get it, and have a sense of self-worth. To achieve these goals, they need the "language of negotiation" and negotiation skills that require transactional language to supplement requesting, information exchange and conversational control vocabulary and skill. Without these skills, individuals who rely on AAC are dependent on others for the determination of their life goals and direction. They also need these skills to avoid abuse and harassment by care givers and others or to report incidents if they do occur.

Every person who uses an AAC system develops strategies to make that use more effective. Examples include letting the partner guess the next letter on a spelling board and using gestures (e.g., waving to indicate that a misunderstanding has occurred) in conjunction with an electronic device. Strategic competence describes the degree to which the person is able to develop adaptive strategies to make the most of the system. These may differ in different contexts.

For example, a child's speech may be better understood at home than at school. He or she will rely on the electronic SGD more in school but will also develop strategies to make maximal use of both systems.

Just as the individual using the AAC system must develop several types of competencies, there are many ways of carrying out the training. One approach, shown in Figure 11-19, is to simulate a situation, model the types of interaction likely to occur, and have the user "practice" the strategies and skills necessary to make it a success. This step can be followed by an actual situation in which the ATP accompanies the user as he or she encounters the situation. The ATP can then prompt the user at appropriate times, add encouragement, and help to clarify when necessary. This combination of clinic-based practice and community-based skill development is often very effective.

For training to be effective, staff must have sufficient skill and experience to assist the AAC user, which requires training for those who are supporting AAC use. Schepis and Reid (2003) identified seven basic steps in competence- and performance-based training for staff. These include specifying desired outcomes, roles for staff to support individuals in achieving these outcomes, providing both written and oral expectations and instructions to staff, demonstration of how to perform duties, and observation of staff performing the duties with corrective feedback as necessary.

Training of the individual who relies on AAC is only effective if communication partners are also trained. For children, the training of parents to recognize communication attempts and to understand the operational, linguistic, strategic, and social competencies is also important. Bruno and Dribbon (1998) evaluated a parent training program conducted as part of an AAC summer camp experience where parents attended the camp with their children. The camp featured structured therapy sessions, activities with nondisabled campers, and activities planned for families. The parent training had both device (conducted by manufacturers' representatives) and interaction training aspects. Parents reported making positive changes in both operational and interactional skills during the camp (Bruno and Dribbon, 1998). These changes were reflected in gains made by the children in skills related to the use of pragmatic functions (e.g., giving and requesting information, requesting assistance, responding, and protesting) over the course of the camp. The camp training significantly increased the degree to which parents gave their children access to the AAC system. In some cases, skills in these areas remained constant at the 6-month follow-up, and in some there was a decrease. The areas of social exchange and giving of information continued to increase at the 6-month follow-up evaluation.

AAC training can be both complicated and lengthy (Beukelman and Mirenda, 2005). Light and Binger (1998) have developed a seven-step process for developing AAC communication competence: (1) specify the goal, do baseline observations; (2) select vocabulary; (3) teach the facilitators how to support development of the target skill; (4) teach the skill to the target individual; (5) check for generalization; (6) evaluate outcomes; and (7) complete maintenance checks. Light and Binger provide data collection and assessment forms and strategies for implementing this program. ACETS (Augmentative Communication Employment Training and Supports) (Institute on Disabilities, Temple University, Philadelphia, Pa., *http//:disabilities.temple.edu*) has been developed specifically to assist those who rely on AAC in seeking employment. A formal training manual is available for this program that is based on three principles: (1) immersion in the workplace culture, (2) acquiring a broad base of employment-related skills and experience, and (3) support of individualized goals.

Follow-up: Measuring Short- and Long-Term Outcomes.   The evaluation of communicative competence in the four domains (operational, linguistic, social, and strategic) will identify areas in which the AAC system is and is not adequately meeting the individual's needs. Periodic re-evaluation of the individual's skills and needs may also result in changes in the training or the AAC system(s). The re-evaluation may lead to new training goals in one or more of the four areas of communicative competence. In other cases the care givers, family, or other support staff may require additional training to facilitate the use of the AAC device.

The AAC device as it is configured may also be inadequate to meet the individual's needs. It may be possible to adjust some of the features (e.g., scanning rate, stored vocabulary), or it may be necessary to consider a completely new device. The magnitude of the changes in the device dictates the amount of additional operational training required. In some cases the individual's skills may decrease (e.g., degenerative disease) or increase (e.g., a young child who develops greater language skills). In either case a reevaluation and adjustments in the AAC system (device plus training and support) will be required.

Murphy et al (1996) identified obstacles to effective AAC system use in a study of 93 users of AAC systems and 186 partners (93 formal and 93 informal). The formal partners were speech-language pathologists (the majority), care providers in the day or living program, and teachers. Informal partners were family, friends, and others selected by the AAC users as those with whom they felt most comfortable using their AAC systems. In some cases one partner filled both the formal and informal roles. The majority of low- and high-tech AAC system use was in the day placement (90%), residential (70%), and leisure (60%) settings. Use was limited to organized therapy sessions in general.

AAC systems were only available to 48% of the users while shopping, 62% during outings such as day trips during their program, and 66% where they lived. SLPs were the most frequent (80%) formal partners, and residential or day care staff were the most common informal partners (62%). Friends and family were both reported as the primary informal partner in less than 10% of the cases. Only 57% of the low-tech and 59.4% of the high-tech AAC system users were able to independently access their systems (e.g., get a system out of a back pack on a wheelchair and set it up for use without a partner's help). Knowledge of the system sufficient to interact with the AAC user was reported in less than half of the formal partners and one third of the informal partners. Eighty-eight percent of the users received training from their formal partners. However, for the majority of the users, the training consisted of 60 minutes or less (or 40 hours per year on the basis of sessions conducted). This number is low compared with other types of therapy and training such as that for second language instruction (estimated by Murphy et al to be more than 200 hours per year).

Murphy et al found that basic vocabulary required for daily interactions (see Table 11-5) was not included in the AAC systems. Few users had greetings, wrap ups, or conversational flow vocabulary (e.g., comments, repair vocabulary). Thus, for these areas, the users most commonly used other modes of communication (e.g., eye gaze, gestures, facial expressions) rather than their AAC devices.

The preponderance of formal partners also reinforces the need for inclusion of both useful vocabulary and multiple modes of communication. The development of strategic competence is vital to increase the likelihood that an AAC user will be able to independently carry out conversations in a variety of settings and with a variety of partners. Availability and accessibility of AAC systems can be addressed by appropriate mounting of systems on wheelchairs and training to ensure that care providers understand the need to have the system available to the user at all times. The results reported by Murphy et al also emphasize the importance of multiple modes of communication by AAC users.

Assessment of AAC outcomes can use the general measures (MPT, PIADS, Quebec User Evaluation of Satisfaction with Assistive Technology [QUEST]) described in Chapter 4. Because of the nature of communication, there are additional considerations. Because the major goal of AAC is the provision of expressive language capability, one of the most important considerations is the determination of communicative intent by the individual evaluating outcomes (typically SLP or special education teacher). Special education teachers tend to overassess intentionality (i.e., to assign intentionality more often than experienced researchers), whereas SLPs do so less often (Carter and Iacono, 2002). Individuals with different disorders are also assessed differently relative to intentionality, and observations are inconsistent across populations, sessions, and professional groups. These results are disturbing because intentionality is a key measure of communicative competence and effectiveness.

The MPT model (Chapter 4) has been adapted to AAC use as the *AAC Acceptance Model* (Lasker and Bedrosian, 2001). This model focuses on the prediction of acceptance of AAC by adults with acquired communication impairments. Although the technology may play a small role in acceptance or nonacceptance, other factors are more important. Among these other factors are the following: (1) the communication partners' acceptance of the technology; (2) the rate (sudden or gradual) of onset of the communication impairment; (3) affective, behavioral, and cognitive components of a user's attitude toward AAC technology; (4) perception of the user and other people toward the device, and (5) how other people view the person using the device. It is not clear whether this measure can be generalized to other populations (e.g., children with developmental disabilities).

There are a number of key reasons that provision of AAC systems may not achieve the goal of a "better life" for the AAC user (Beukelman and Mirenda, 2005): (1) payer resistance to or lack of acceptance of measures that reflect quality of life rather than more concrete functional outcomes, (2) increased costs of intervention necessary to achieve broader goals, (3) time limits set by payers on length of the intervention, (4) high demands on professionals to achieve and maintain skills, (5) family and user response to increases in their responsibilities in assuming a leadership role, (6) difficulty by families in envisioning the future for the AAC user, and (7) cultural differences between the user and professionals.

We can relate meaningful AAC outcomes to the three levels of the World Health Organization ICF classification system (see Chapter 2) (Beukelman and Mirenda, 2005). At the level of body structures and functions the degree to which AAC intervention compensates for lost or absent speech or language function can be determined. Evaluations related to activity focus on the quality and quantity of communication interactions and the degree to which these meet the goals and needs of the individual. Evaluations related to participation focus on the socially defined role and tasks within a sociocultural and physical environment. Some "Big Picture" AAC outcomes are shown in Box 11-4 (Beukelman and Mirenda, 2005). There are several types of measures for AAC system outcome. Operational measures evaluate the user's ability to interact with the system itself (operational competence), whereas representational measures

---

BOX 11-4 | Big Picture Outcomes for Augmentative and Alternative Communication Intervention

Has the AAC system resulted in increased:
Self-determination for the user
Inclusion of the user in social groups
Independence, to the degree the AAC user wants it
Participation in the community
Gainful employment
Academic achievement
Social connectedness
Educational inclusion or decreased special class placement

Data from Beukelman DR, Mirenda P: *Augmentative and alternative communication: management of severe communication disorders in children and adults*, ed 3, Baltimore, 2005, Paul H Brookes.

---

evaluate symbol and grammatical capability by the AAC user (Beukelman and Mirenda, 2005).

The most important result of the follow-up phase is to evaluate the outcomes of the AAC interventions to determine their effectiveness, including both the hard and soft technologies, and the appropriateness of the match between the originally specified needs and the resulting system. The principles of outcome measurement discussed in Chapter 4 apply to AAC system evaluation as well.

■ SUMMARY

Augmentative and alternative communication systems serve needs for both writing and conversation for individuals who have difficulties in these areas. Low-technology AAC systems provide quick and easy help for meeting communication needs, whereas high-technology devices offer great sophistication in available vocabulary, speed of communication, and flexibility of access. The latter features allow persons who have very limited physical skills to use AAC systems. AAC systems also have great flexibility in required user cognitive skills, allowing for persons with a diversity of intellectual abilities to benefit from AAC. Thoughtful assessment, careful training, and thorough follow through are essential to effective AAC intervention.

Study Questions

1. What are the two major communicative needs normally addressed by augmentative communication systems?
2. Distinguish between aided and unaided communication.
3. What are the major goals for augmentative communication systems designed for conversational use?
4. What AAC needs do parents have for their non-speaking children? Do mothers and fathers have the same needs for their children?
5. Describe differences in the conversational rules that apply between two speaking persons and those between

one speaking person and one augmentative communication user.

6. Describe the relationship between the Social Networks model and the Participation Model. How do each of these relate to the HAAT model described in this text?

7. How do attitudes of the communication partners differ for the five circles of the Social Networks model?

8. What factors influence the attitudes of children toward their peers who use AAC?

9. What features distinguish competent augmentative communicators from those who are not successful?

10. Select three discourse functions from those listed in Table 11-5. Now pick an augmentative communication device (e.g., electronic, direct selection, with voice output; or a language board with letters and words) and develop a vocabulary and set of strategies for the implementation of each of the discourse functions that you choose.

11. What are the three types of graphical communication? List three ways in which they differ.

12. In what ways does the formal writing of adolescent AAC users differ from that of nondisabled adolescent writers?

13. Distinguish between formal writing and note taking in terms of the characteristics AAC devices must have to meet each need. What is the most important feature in each case?

14. What two factors must be included for a math worksheet to be effective for both arithmetic and higher math (e.g., algebra)?

15. List three features that a drawing system should have to be of use in creative expression.

16. How do drawing systems differ in structure and function from systems for scientific plotting?

17. Describe auditory scanning. Give an example of both a low-tech or no-tech approach and an electronic AAC approach. What are the essential features for the AAC auditory scanning device?

18. List three encoding methods used in AAC devices, and give one advantage and one disadvantage of each.

19. What are the major types of abbreviation approaches used in AAC devices, and what are the major advantages and disadvantages of each?

20. Pick three discourse functions and develop a logical coding scheme for each using (1) numerical codes, (2) abbreviation expansion, and (3) Minspeak codes.

21. Compare word completion and prediction with abbreviation expansion and Minspeak encoding.

22. What are the major approaches used to increase conversational rate when the individual is using scanning?

23. What are dynamic displays, and what advantages do they provide?

24. What are visual scene displays and what unique features do they have?

25. What populations might benefit most from visual scene displays? Why?

26. Describe the major challenges and approaches for AAC intervention of individuals whose primary disorder is language or cognitively based? How does this compare with individuals whose primary disorder is motor or physical?

27. List and discuss three advantages that the Internet provides for communication by AAC users.

28. What are the major advantages of conversationally based communication devices such as CHAT and TOPIC?

29. What are the four types of competencies acquired in AAC training? Pick an AAC system for an individual and design the training. You must make assumptions regarding the person's skills, her needs, and other people available to help facilitate the training.

30. For each of the categories of devices described in the section on current technologies, define a user profile (skills and needs) that would lead you to focus on that category in selecting a device for that person.

References

Alm N, Arnott JL, Newell AF: Database design for storing and accessing personal conversational material. In *Proceedings of the 12th Annual Conference on Rehabilitation Engineering,* pp 147-148, 1989, Washington, DC.

Alm N, Arnott JL, Newell AF: Prediction of conversational momentum in an augmentative communication system, *Commun ACM* 35:46-57, 1992.

Alm N, Newell AF, Arnott JL: A communication aid which models conversational patterns. In *Proceedings of the 10th Annual Conference on Rehabilitation Engineering,* pp 127-129, 1987, Washington, DC.

Anderson NB, Shames GH: *Human communication disorders: An introduction,* Boston, 2006, Allyn and Bacon.

Angelo DH: Impact of augmentative and alternative communication devices on families, *Augment Altern Commun* 16:37-47, 2000.

Angelo DH, Kokoska SM, Jones SD: Family perspective on augmentative and alternative communication: families of adolescents and young adults, *Augment Altern Commun* 12:13-20, 1996.

Baker B: Minspeak, *Byte* 7:186-202, 1982.

Baker B: Using images to generate speech, *Byte* 11:160-168, 1986.

Ball LJ, Beukelman DR, Patee GL: Acceptance of augmentative and alternative communication technology by persons with amyotrophic lateral sclerosis, *Augment Altern Commun* 20:113-122, 2004.

Beck AR, Dennis M: Attitudes of children toward a similar-aged child who uses augmentative communication, *Augment Altern Commun* 12:78-87, 1996.

Beck AR et al: Influence of communicative competence and augmentative and alternative communication technique on children's attitudes toward a peer who uses AAC, *Augment Altern Commun* 18:217-227, 2002.

Beukelman DR, Ball LJ: Improving AAC use for persons with acquired neurogenic disorders: understanding human and engineering factors, *Assist Technol* 14:33-44, 2002.

Beukelman D, Garrett K: Augmentative and alternative communication for adults with acquired severe communication disorders, *Augment Altern Commun* 4:104-121, 1988.

Beukelman DR, McGinnis J, Morrow D: Vocabulary selection in augmentative and alternative communication, *Augment Altern Commun* 7:171-185, 1991.

Beukelman DR, Mirenda P: *Augmentative and alternative communication: management of severe communication disorders in children and adults*, ed 3, Baltimore, 2005, Paul H Brookes.

Beukelman D, Yorkston K: Augmentative and alternative communication application for persons with severe acquired communication disorders: an introduction, *Augment Altern Commun* 5:42-48, 1989.

Beukelman D, Yorkston K, Dowden P: *Communication augmentation: A casebook of clinical management*, San Diego, 1984, College Hill Press.

Blackstone S: Populations and practices in AAC, *Augment Commun News* 3:1-3, 1990.

Blackstone S: Persons with aphasia: What does AAC have to offer, *Augment Commun News* 4:1-6, 1991.

Blackstone S: Dynamic displays, *Augment Commun News* 7:1-6, 1994.

Blackstone S: Amyotrophic lateral sclerosis, *Augment Commun News* 11:1-15, 1998.

Blackstone S: Assessment protocol for SGDs, *Augment Commun News* 13:1-16, 2001.

Blackstone S: Social networks, *Augment Commun News* 15:1-16, 2003a.

Blackstone S: Autism spectrum disorder, *Augment Commun News* 15:1-6, 2003b.

Blackstone S: The Internet and its offspring, *Augment Commun News* 15:1-3, 2003c.

Blackstone S: Visual scene displays, *Augment Commun News* 16:1-5, 2004.

Blackstone S: False beliefs, widely held, *Augment Commun News* 8:1-6, 2006.

Blackstone SW, Hunt Berg M: Social networks: a communication inventory for individuals with complex communication needs and their communication partners—inventory booklet, Monterey, CA, 2003, Augmentative Communication.

Blackstone SW, Williams MB, Joyce M: Future AAC technology needs: consumer perspectives, *Assist Technol* 14:3-16, 2002.

Blishcak DM, Lombardino LJ, Dyson AT: Use of speech-generating device: in support of natural speech, *Augment Altern Commun* 19:29-35, 2003.

Bondy A, Frost L: The picture exchange communication system, *Behav Modif* 25:725-744, 2001.

Brady NC: Improved comprehension of object names following voice output communication aid use: Two case studies, *Augment Altern Commun* 16:197-204, 2000.

Bruno J, Dribbon M: Outcomes in AAC: evaluating the effectiveness of a parent training program, *Augment Altern Commun* 14:59-70, 1998.

Bryen DN, Cohen K, Carey A: Augmentative communication employment training and supports: Some employment outcomes, *J Rehabil* 70:10-18, 2004.

Carlisle Ladtkow M, Culp D: Augmentative communication with traumatic brain injury. In Yorkston K, editor: *Augmentative communication in the medical setting*, pp. 139-244, Tucson, AZ, 1992, Communication Skill Builders.

Carter M, Iacono T: Professional judgments of the intentionality of communicative acts, *Augment Altern Commun* 18:177-191, 2002.

Clarke M, Kirton A: Patterns of interaction between children with physical disabilities using augmentative and alternative communication systems and their peers, *Child Lang Teach Ther* 19:135-151, 2003.

Colby KM et al: A word-finding computer program with a semantic lexical memory for patients with anomia using an intelligent speech prosthesis, *Brain Lang* 14:272-281, 1981.

Coleman CL: *Augmentative communication training modules*, Sacramento, 1988, Assistive Device Center, California State University.

Collier B: When I grow up...supporting youth who use augmentative communication for adulthood. In *Proceedings of the 2005 Alberta Rehabilitation and Assistive Technology Consortium Conference*, Edmonton, Canada (2005): www.acrat.ca. Accessed August 2007.

DeRuyter F, Kennedy M: Augmentative communication following traumatic brain injury. In Beukelman D, Yorkston K, editors: *Communication disorders following traumatic brain injury: management of cognitive, language, and motor impairments*, pp 317-365, Austin, TX, 1991, PRO-ED.

Dowden P, Cook AM: Choosing effective selection techniques for beginning communicators. In Reichle J, Beukelman DR, Light JC, editors: *Exemplary practices for beginning communicators*, pp 395-432, Baltimore, 2002, Paul H. Brookes.

Dowden PA: Augmentative and alternative communication decision making for children with severely unintelligible speech, *Augment Altern Commun* 13:48-58, 1997.

Drager KDR: Light technologies with different system layouts and language organizations, *J Speech Hear Res* 46:289-312, 2003.

Dye R et al: A script-based AAC system for transactional interaction, *Natl Lang Eng* 4:57-71, 1998.

Falvey M et al: *All my life's a circle: Using the tools of cirles, MAPS and PATHS*, Toronto, 1994, Inclusion Press.

Fields C: Finding a voice for Daniel, *Team Rehabil Rep* 2: 16-19, 1991.

Fox LE, Fried-Oken M: AAC aphasiology: partnership for future research, *Augment Altern Commun* 12:257-271, 1996.

Frager S, Hux K, Beukelman D: AAC acceptance and use by 25 adults with TBI. *CSUN Conference on Technology and People with Disabilities* (2005): http:/aac.unl.edu. Accessed August 2007.

Fruchterman JR: In the palm of your hand: a vision of the future of technology for people with visual impairments, *J Vis Impair Blindness* 97:585-591, 2003.

Garrett K, Beukelman D: Augmentative communication approaches for persons with severe aphasia. In Yorkston K, editor: *Augmentative communication in the medical setting*, Tucson, 1992, Communication Skill Builders.

Goldbart J, Marshall J: "Pushes and pulls" on the parents of children who use AAC, *Augment Altern Commun* 20:194-208, 2004.

Graves J: Vocabulary needs in augmentative and alternative communication: a sample of conversational topics between staff providing services to adults with learning difficulties and their service users, *Br J Learning Disabil* 28:113-119, 2000.

Helsinger S: Teaching the Picture Exchange Communication System to adults with pervasive developmental disorder/autism. Presented at the Picture Exchange Communication System Exposition, Philadelphia, 2001.

Higginbotham DJ et al: The Frametalker project: building an utterance-based communication device, *Proceedings of the 2005 CSUN Conference on Technology For Persons With Disabilities*, 2005, Los Angeles.

Hunnicutt S: ACCESS: A lexical access program. In *Proceedings of the RESNA 12th Annual Conference*, pp 284-285, 1989, Washington, DC.

Iacono T, Mirenda P, Beukelman D: Comparison of unimodal and multiple modal AAC techniques for children with intellectual disabilities, *Augment Altern Commun* 9:83-94, 1993.

Jacobs B et al: Augmentative and alternative communication for adults with severe aphasia: where we stand and how we can go further, *Disabil Rehabil* 26:1231-1240, 2004.

Joseph D: The morning, *Commun Outlook* 8:8, 1986.

Kent-Walsh JE, Light JC: General education teachers' experiences with inclusion of students who use augmentative and alternative communication, *Augment Altern Commun* 19:102-124, 2003.

King JM, Hux K: Intervention using talking word processor software: an aphasia case study, *Augment Altern Commun* 11:187-192, 1995.

Kovach T, Kenyon P: Auditory scanning: development and implementation of AAC systems for individuals with physical and visual impairments, *ISAAC Bull* 53:1-7, 1998.

Kraat AW: *Communication interaction between aided and natural speakers: a state of the art report*, Toronto, 1985, International Project on Communication Aids for the Severely Speech Impaired.

Kraat AW: Developing intervention goals. In Blackstone S, Bruskin D, editors: *Augmentative communication: an introduction*, Rockville, MD, 1986, American Speech-Language and Hearing Association.

Kraat AW: Augmentative and alternative communication: does it have a future in aphasia rehabilitation? *Aphasiology* 4:321-338, 1990.

Lasker J, Bedrosian J: Promoting acceptance of augmentative and alternative communication by adults with acquired communication disorders, *Augment Altern Commun* 17: 141-153, 2001.

Light J: Interaction involving individuals using augmentative and alternative communication systems: state of the art and future directions, *Augment Altern Commun* 4:66-82, 1988.

Light J: Toward a definition of communicative competence for individuals using augmentative and alternative communication systems, *Augment Altern Commun* 5:137-144, 1989.

Light J, Beesley M, Collier B: Transition through multiple augmentative and alternative communication systems: a three year case study of a head injured adolescent, *Augment Altern Commun* 4:2-14, 1988.

Light JC, Binger C: *Building communicative competence with individuals who use augmentative and alternative communication*, Baltimore, 1998, Paul H Brookes.

Light JC, Drager KDR: Improving the design of augmentative and alternative technologies for young children, *Assist Technol* 14:17-32, 2002.

Lilienfeld M, Alant E: Attitudes toward an unfamiliar peer using an AAC device with and without voice output, *Augment Altern Commun* 18:91-101, 2002.

Lloyd LL, Fuller DR, Arvidson HH: *Augmentative and alternative communications: a handbook of principles and practices*, Boston, 1997, Allyn and Bacon.

Magiati I, Howlin P: A pilot evaluation study of the Picture Exchange Communication System (PECS) for children with autistic spectrum disorders, *Autism* 7:297-320, 2003.

McCartthy J, Light J: Attitudes toward individuals who use augmentative and alternative communication: research review, *Augment Altern Commun* 21: 41-55, 2005.

McKelvey M. et al: Performance of a person with chronic aphasia using a visual scene display prototype, *J Med Speech Lang Pathol* In press.

McNaughton D, Light J, Gulla S: Opening up a "whole new world": employer and co-worker perspectives on working with individuals who use augmentative and alternative communication, *Augment Altern Commun* 19:235-253, 2003.

Mirenda P: Toward functional augmentative and alternative communication for students with autism: manual signs, graphic symbols and voice output communication aids, *Lang Speech Hearing Serv Schools* 34:203-216, 2003.

Mirenda P, Santogrossi J: A prompt-free strategy to teach pictorial communication system use, *Augment Altern Commun* 1:143-150, 1985.

Murphy J et al: AAC system use: obstacles to effective use, *Eur J Dis Commun* 31:31-44, 1996.

Musselwhite CR, St. Louis KW: *Communication programming for the severely handicapped: vocal and non-vocal strategies*, Houston, 1982, College Hill Press.

Nolan C: *Dam-burst of dreams*, New York, 1981, St. Martin's Press.

Parette HP, Botherson MJ, Huer MB: Giving families a voice in augmentative and alternative communication decision-making, *Educ Train Ment Retard Dev Disabil* 35:177-190, 2000.

Reichle J et al: Comparison of correct responses and response latency for fixed and dynamic displays: performance of a learner with severe developmental disabilities, *Augment Altern Commun* 16:154-163, 2000.

Riechle J, York J, Sigafoos J: *Implementing augmentative and alternative communication*, Baltimore, 1991, Paul H Brookes.

Rush WL: *Journey out of silence*, Lincoln, NE, 1986, Media Productions and Marketing.

Schepis M, Reid D: Issues affecting staff enhancement of speech-generating device use among people with severe cognitive disabilities, *Augment Altern Commun* 19:59-65, 2003.

Schlosser RW, Blischak DM: Is there a role for speech output in interventions for persons with autism? *Focus Autism Other Dev Disabil* 16:170178, 2001.

Schwartz IS: Beyond basic training: PECS use with peers and at home. Presented at the Picture Exchange Exposition, Philadelphia, 2001.

Sevick RA, Romski MA, Adamson LB: Research directions in augmentative and alternative communication for preschool children, *Disabil Child* 26:1323-1329, 2004.

Simpson S: If only I could tell them, *Commun Outlook* 9:9-11, 1988.

Steele RD, Weinrich M: Training of severely impaired aphasics on a computerized visual communication system. In *Proceedings of the RESNA 8th Annual Conference*, pp 320-322, 1986, Washington, DC.

Todman J: Rate and quality of conversations using a text-storage AAC system: Single-case training study, *Augment Altern Commun* 16:164-179, 2000.

Vanderheiden GC, Lloyd LL: Communication systems and their components. In Blackstone S, Bruskin D, editors: *Augmentative communication: an introduction*, Rockville, MD, 1986, American Speech-Language and Hearing Association.

Williams MB: Message encoding: a comment on Light et al, *Augment Altern Commun* 7:133-134, 1991.

Yorkston KM et al: A comparison of standard vocabulary lists, *Augment Altern Commun* 5:189-210, 1988.

Yorkston KM et al: Vocabulary selection: a case study, *Augment Altern Commun* 5:101-114, 1989.

CHAPTER 12

Technologies That Enable Mobility

Chapter Outline

Learning Objectives

On completing this chapter, you will be able to do the following:

1. Discuss needs underlying evaluation of the consumer for a mobility system
2. Describe the three categories of mobility systems on the basis of the need served by each
3. Describe the two primary structures of wheelchairs
4. Identify the major characteristics of manual wheelchairs

5. Identify the major types of power mobility systems and their characteristics
6. Understand the influence of the relationship between the center of gravity of the user and the center of mass of the wheelchair on the function of the wheelchair
7. Describe the implementation phase for personal mobility systems

Key Terms

Anti-Tip Devices	Independent Powered Mobility	Smart Wheelchair
Armrests	Lightweight Wheelchair	Standard Wheelchair
Bariatric Chairs	Low-Shear Systems	Standing Frame
Bariatrics	Manual Wheelchair	Standing Wheelchair
Camber	Nonproportional Control	Supporting Structure
Center of Gravity	Propelling Structure	Tilt
Center of Mass	Proportional Control	Transitional Mobility Device
Dependent Mobility System	Push Handles	Ultralightweight Wheelchair
Electrically Powered Wheelchair	Recline	Wheel Lock
Front Rigging	Rigid Ultralightweight Wheelchair	
Independent Manual Mobility	Scooter	
System	Shear	

Mobility is fundamental to each individual's quality of life and it is necessary for functioning in each of the performance areas: self-care, work or school, and play or leisure. As described earlier for other activity outputs, limitations to functional mobility can be either augmented or replaced with assistive technologies. The activity output of ambulation can be augmented with low-tech aids such as canes, walkers, or crutches or replaced by wheeled mobility systems of various types. In addition to the functional gain of increased independence in mobility, such other goals as positive self-image, social interaction, and health maintenance are achieved. This chapter focuses on wheeled mobility systems to enhance an individual's mobility, including manual and power wheelchairs. Our emphasis is on the total process of delivering these systems to those who need them, from initial need and goal setting, through assessment and recommendation, to implementation and training.

■ HISTORY OF THE WHEELCHAIR

The first wheeled vehicle was likely made more than 20,000 years ago by placing two logs under a sled. The first reference to a wheelchair in literature was in 1588 in mid Europe (Trujillo, circa 1960). Artists' drawings in the early 1500s show persons with disabilities still being transported in litters and carts. The first wheelchairs were wooden with solid wood wheels. They were too cumbersome to be self-propelled. King Phillip V of Spain used a wheelchair in 1700. His device had wooden wheels with wooden spokes, a reclining back, and an adjustable leg rest. This design was used for more than 200 years.

Wheelchairs were not used much in the United States until the Civil War. At that time chairs similar to King Phillip's were used. These wheelchairs had cane seats and backs and wooden wheels; however, by the end of the war they had metal rims on the wheels. In the late 1870s wire-spoked wheels came into use, probably as a technology transfer from the bicycle industry. This design dominated wheelchairs until the 1930s. In 1932 Mr. H. A. Everest, a mining engineer who had sustained a spinal cord injury in a mining accident, teamed up with Mr. H. C. Jennings, a mechanical engineer. They developed the first folding wheelchair by using an X-brace construction. This design was considered lightweight (less than 40 pounds) for the times and only measured 10 inches wide when folded, which allowed it to be placed behind a car seat. The collaboration between Everest and Jennings led to the formation of the E & J Wheelchair Company. This design, with some modifications in materials and accessories (e.g., removable armrests, reclining features) dominated the industry for quite some time.

After World War II, wheelchair sports started as a part of the rehabilitation program at Stoke Mandeville Hospital in the United Kingdom. The purpose was to provide exercise and a recreational outlet for the many individuals who had been injured during the war. The success of this program spread to other countries and eventually led to the first international wheelchair sporting competition, which was held in 1952. Athletes with disabilities competed for the first time in the same venues as Olympic athletes in 1960 (Cooper, 1998). The popularity of wheelchair sports has grown considerably since this time and has had a significant effect on wheelchair design and performance.

Advances in medicine and medical technology also followed World War II, leading to a significant increase in the numbers of individuals with paraplegia or quadriplegia surviving an accident or a disease who before that time would have died or lived a very short life. People with mobility impairments began to participate more actively in life roles and saw to it that improvements were made in mobility technology, which allowed them to maximize their participation in everyday life activities. As wheelchair users became more active and empowered, they started modifying their own chairs to suit their needs (Cooper, 1998). These needs led to the development in the late 1970s of lighter, more maneuverable wheelchairs that could be used in racing, basketball, tennis, and other sports. These needs also led to the development of the rigid or box frame style, which provided a better ride and was stronger. The advances made in sports and ultralight wheelchairs eventually became available in chairs for everyday use.

Power wheelchairs are a much more recent development. Although a patent was issued in 1940, these systems did not come into common use until 1957 (Hobson, 1990). The first models were standard folding wheelchairs with automobile motors and batteries added that functioned at a single speed. Gradually engineers began to develop new designs specifically intended for powered use. The revolution in electronics and computer technology also had an influence on power mobility systems. The use of solid state electronics for control systems increased reliability over previous electromechanical (relay) systems. Improvements in microcomputers allowed flexibility in control and provided the ability to alter the mobility system characteristics to match the users' needs more closely. These advances have made it possible for individuals who have difficulty controlling a standard joystick to operate a power wheelchair.

Changes in wheelchair technology over the last century allow individuals with limitations in mobility to become more independent and to actively participate in society. Today many of these early inventions still are evident in current designs, but dramatic advances in materials, electronic controllers, and mechanical design have led to a proliferation of types, styles, and approaches to both manual and powered mobility. Changes in wheelchair technologies are expected to continue. Thus it is imperative that the assistive technology practitioner (ATP) remains current with new technologies as they become available and know how to define the user's needs and skills so that a match can be made to the appropriate technology.

▰ MOBILITY NEEDS SERVED BY WHEELCHAIRS

There has been a significant increase in the number of individuals using mobility systems; this change is related to

three different trends. The population of most developing countries is aging with proportions of older individuals (65 years and older) expected to reach more than 20% of the population by 2030 in the United States (Bureau of the Census, 2004) and earlier in Canada (Belanger, Martel, and Caron-Malenfant, 2005). Age-related physical changes such as arthritis result in mobility impairments that require the use of mobility devices. The proportion of morbidly obese individuals is increasing in North America, which has resulted in the development of mobility devices that are specifically designed to support the increased size and weight of these individuals. **Bariatric chairs** are now available for these individuals whose mobility is impaired by obesity and related chronic diseases. Accessibility legislation in many countries has reduced physical and institutional barriers to the community participation of individuals with disabilities, with the result that more people are using mobility devices for instrumental activities of daily living (IADLs).

Data collected in the 2000 U.S. census indicate that 20.9 million U.S. families have at least one individual with a disability living in their households (Wang, 2005), and of these, 16.6% report a physical disability that results in a functional limitation. The Profile of Disability in Canada indicates that 13.7% of the Canadian population reports a mobility impairment (Cossette, 2002).

Kaye, Kang, and LePlante (2002) provide information on the number of Americans who use mobility devices. These data are derived from the 1994-1995 National Health Interview Survey on Disability. The survey indicated that 1.6 million Americans who live outside an institutional setting use a mobility device. The majority of these individuals (1.5 million) use a manual wheelchair (Kaye, Kang, and LePlante, 2002). Elderly individuals have the highest rate of mobility use, with 57.5% of manual wheelchair users and 69.7% of powered wheelchair uses reportedly 65 years of age or older (Kaye, Kang, and LePlante, 2002).

Disorders Resulting in Mobility Impairments

There are many causes of mobility impairment. Disorders that result in mobility impairment may be neurological, musculoskeletal, or cognitive. Not all individuals with a given diagnosis have a similar impairment in mobility. The onset of the disorder, whether it was acquired or congenital, also affects the individual's mobility needs.

Kaye et al (2002) present the top 10 conditions in the United States that result in use of a wheelchair or scooter. Individuals who have sustained a cerebral vascular accident are the leading group of mobility device users (11.1%) (Kaye et al, 2002). Additional neurological disorders that may result in mobility impairment include cerebral palsy, Guillain-Barré syndrome, Huntington's chorea, traumatic brain injury, muscular dystrophy, Parkinson's disease, poliomyelitis, spinal cord injury, spina bifida, and multiple sclerosis. Symptoms commonly seen in these neurological disorders are muscle weakness or paralysis, sensory deficits, and abnormal muscle tone. All these disorders can lead to limitations with joint range of motion, postural control, and mobility. The individual may also have cognitive and behavioral problems as a result of the disorder.

Orthopedic and rheumatological conditions account for another large group of mobility device users. Some of the symptoms commonly seen in individuals with arthritis include painful, swollen, and stiff joints; muscle wasting around the affected joints; and, in later stages, joint contractures resulting in range-of-motion limitations. Other disorders that affect the musculoskeletal system and may result in mobility impairments include ankylosing spondylitis, osteogenesis imperfecta, osteoporosis, Paget's disease, and scoliosis. Individuals with an amputation may also use a mobility device.

Diabetes, cardiorespiratory conditions, and obesity are final chronic conditions that may require the use of a mobility device. Frequently, fatigue or restrictions related to energy expenditure are the reasons for use of a mobility device with this population. Amputations resulting from complications from diabetes may also lead to the use of a mobility device.

Disorders that affect an individual's cognitive functioning and ability to learn, such as Alzheimer's disease and mental retardation, can also be the cause of mobility impairments. Although the onset of mental retardation is at birth, the onset of Alzheimer's disease is later in life. Consequently, there are unique aspects to each of these disorders that need to be considered by the ATP; some of these are discussed in this section.

Functional Limitations of Mobility

Limitations to mobility can also be viewed as functional limitations of an individual rather than as conditions related to specific diagnoses (Warren, 1990). The degree of limitation in mobility varies across a broad scope, as shown in Box 12-1. At one end of the range are individuals who are considered *marginal ambulators*. At the opposite end of the range are those individuals who have severe mobility limitations and are dependent in manual mobility, with powered mobility being their only option for independence.

Warren (1990) describes marginal ambulators as able to move independently in their environment but functional only at a slow rate or for short distances. Persons who have marginal ambulating skills can benefit from part-time use of a powered mobility device such as a scooter, which allows them to walk inside the home using a walker or cane and use a powered device outside the home to augment ambulation. Next are individuals who are exclusive users of manual wheelchairs. Either they are dependent in the use of a

---

BOX 12-1   **Scope of Mobility Limitations**

Full ambulator: No mobility impairment

Marginal ambulator: Can walk short distances; may need wheelchair at times, particularly outside the home

Manual wheelchair user: Has some method of propelling a manual wheelchair, whether it is with both upper extremities, both lower extremities, or one upper and one lower extremity

Marginal manual wheelchair user: May have upper extremity injury caused by overuse or manual wheelchair mobility may not be the most efficient means of mobility for the person; manual wheelchair used part of the time and power wheelchair part of the time

Totally/severely mobility-impaired user: Unable to propel self independently in a manual wheelchair; dependent mobility base or powered mobility base the only option for independent mobility

---

manual wheelchair or they propel a manual wheelchair by one of three methods: (1) using both upper extremities, (2) using both lower extremities, or (3) using an upper and lower extremity on the same side of the body (e.g., a person who has had a stroke). There are also *marginal manual wheelchair users,* who are able to propel a wheelchair manually but have upper body weakness, respiratory problems, or postural asymmetry as a result of pushing that limits their ability to propel a manual chair for a prolonged time (Warren, 1990). Marginal manual wheelchair users may also include individuals who formerly used a manual wheelchair for their mobility needs and have sustained an overuse injury from propelling the chair. Propelling a wheelchair for any length of time depletes the energy of these individuals and compromises their productivity in other areas of life. Marginal manual wheelchair users can benefit from powered mobility on a full-time or part-time basis.

At the extreme end of the range are those individuals who have a severe mobility limitation; their only means of being independent in mobility is through the full-time use of a powered mobility system. These individuals typically have a manual wheelchair, propelled by a caregiver, as a backup chair. Individuals with severely limited motor control, who are physically unable to move around in their environment without equipment, are the ones traditionally considered for powered mobility and for whom the benefits are clear. With the provision of powered mobility, these individuals can independently participate in work, school, and recreational activities. The control interfaces (see Chapter 7) that are available today make it possible for someone with only one or two movements to operate a powered wheelchair; however, perceptual, cognitive, and behavioral impairments may prevent individuals from using a power wheelchair even if they have the necessary motor skills. Frequently, these individuals also use other devices such as an augmentative communication system or an adapted van, which requires that the integration of all these devices be considered at the time of selection of the most appropriate mobility device. All mobility device users will require a system to support their seating needs (see Chapter 6).

Mobility Issues Across the Life Span

Mobility needs differ across the life span, with children having much different mobility needs than adults. Although there are many life span issues to consider, we focus on two issues that warrant special attention: (1) powered mobility for young children and (2) mobility for older adults.

The use of powered mobility by young children is an area that has received a great deal of attention in the last decade. In the past, powered mobility was deemed inappropriate for young children for a number of reasons. These concerns were related to the ability of children to operate a power wheelchair safely, the initial cost of the wheelchair and the cost of replacing it as the child grows, and possible detrimental effects on physical development if the child depends on a powered system instead of his own locomotion (Kermoian, 1998). Recent studies have demonstrated that children as young as 18 to 24 months can safely operate powered vehicles (Magnuson, 1995; Trefler and Cook, 1986). Powered vehicles allow disabled children to experience movement and control and can facilitate their social, cognitive, perceptual, and functional development (Butler, 1997; Trefler, Kozole, and Snell, 1986).

Like other areas of assistive technology use, it is suggested that a child be given access to multiple modes of locomotion and be allowed to select the one that is most convenient and most efficient for the given activity (Butler, 1997). By augmenting a child's self-locomotion with wheeled mobility devices, normal childhood development can be simulated. There are an increasing number of powered mobility devices available that can be used to augment a young child's mobility. A **transitional mobility device** can provide the young child with the means for independent locomotion without the complexity and expense of a power wheelchair. Transitional mobility devices include motorized toy cars and powered standing frames. Frequently, parents who resist standard powered mobility devices for their child are more accepting of motorized toy cars that facilitate play with their peers (Deitz, 1998). Deitz (1998) discusses the many factors that should be considered in the design and evaluation of mobility devices that facilitate self-locomotion in young children.

At the opposite end of the life span is a population that also deserves special attention when it comes to designing and recommending assistive technologies for mobility impairment: the older adult. Older adults represent a large proportion of individuals who use mobility devices. As the number of people in this group increases, so will the people with mobility impairments. Wheelchair users over the age of 60 years tend to have limited mobility associated with the aging process, osteoarthritis, and cardiorespiratory disease and typically are occasional wheelchair users (Ham, Aldersea, and Porter, 1998).

Some needs that are specific to the older adult wheelchair user have been identified in the literature. The older adult wheelchair user often depends on another person to push the wheelchair. Therefore, a mobility device that can be used easily by an attendant is important (Ham, Aldersea, and Porter, 1998; Trefler et al, 1993). Comfort, safety, and security have been identified as important needs related to seating and mobility for residents of long-term care facilities (Lacoste et al, 1998, Mortenson et al, 2005; Mortenson et al, 2006). Safety and security were deemed important for the user of the wheelchair, as well as for the care provider. For instance, it is important that the care provider be able to transfer a person in and out of the wheelchair safely. Both the user and the care provider will be more inclined to use a wheelchair that is comfortable, safe, secure, and "attendant friendly." Because the ultimate goal of wheeled mobility is to allow individuals to participate in their environment, taking these factors into consideration will ensure that the older adult with a mobility limitation is not prohibited from being a part of society.

Wheelchairs that target the bariatric client are a recent development in wheelchair design. **Bariatrics** is a term that describes the practice of medicine concerning individuals who are significantly overweight. It is derived from the Greek "baros" meaning weight and "iatrics" meaning medical treatment. In some situations, the client's obesity is the cause of the mobility impairment. Obesity has become a major health problem in North America. The Centers for Disease Control and Prevention (CDC) (2006) report a growing trend in the prevalence of obesity (generally defined as a body mass index [BMI] of 30 or more). In 1995, the prevalence of obesity was less than 20% in all states. In 2000, 28% of states reported obesity prevalence of less than 20% and by 2005 this incidence had dropped to only four states. The 2005 figures further indicate that 17 states report a prevalence of obesity of equal to or greater than 25% and three a prevalence rate of equal to or greater than 30% (CDC, 2006). Diabetes is a serious chronic health condition that is associated with obesity. All these factors limit the individual's ability to move independently in the environment. Typical wheelchairs have standard weight limits up to 300 pounds. Chairs for bariatric clients are capable of supporting weights up to 600 pounds and in some cases up to 1000 pounds. Examples of these chairs will be described later in this chapter. Clients who are morbidly obese present specific challenges when measuring for a wheelchair, as will be discussed later.

■ EVALUATION FOR WHEELED MOBILITY

Needs Assessment

The goal of wheeled mobility intervention is to support the user's ability to move in the environment (i.e., the mobility output of the activity component of the human activity assistive technology [HAAT] model). Consistent with the HAAT model described in Chapter 2, the evaluation to determine the most appropriate wheeled mobility base starts with an assessment of the activities in which the individual wishes to engage while using mobility technology. Will the mobility device be used primarily to move from one place to another in the community or will the individual use it as the primary means of mobility and consequently perform most activities (e.g., ADLs, work and leisure occupations) while seated in the device? The ATP should determine which activities are important and necessary for the device user to complete as well as those in which he or she wishes to engage. Further, the level of assistance individuals require to complete these activities is also an important consideration. Will they complete these activities on their own, with the assistance of another person, or using other technology such as an augmentative communication system?

Evaluation of the Human Factors

Box 12-2 identifies the factors that should be considered when selecting a mobility base for a consumer. It is important to know what the person's disability is so that its influence on the person's level of functioning can be ascertained. It is important to know whether the disability is temporary or permanent and whether the person's condition is expected to improve, progressively deteriorate, or remain stable. For example, an individual who has recently had a stroke may be expected to regain functional ambulation, but for the short term requires a system for mobility. In this situation the rental of a wheelchair would be warranted. On the other hand, an individual with amyotrophic lateral sclerosis is expected to lose functional abilities and requires a mobility system that will accommodate this deterioration in functional status. An individual with a complete spinal cord injury at the C6 level will not typically demonstrate significant changes in mobility after injury and requires a mobility system on a long-term basis.

The individual's physical and sensory skills are evaluated for range of motion, strength, motor control, skin integrity, vision, and perception. This assessment also includes determining the user's optimal control site and interface for propelling the wheelchair. All these factors are discussed in Chapters 4, 6, and 7. Information on the person's weight and size is gathered to determine the size and capacity of the wheelchair. Measurements of the person's leg length, thigh length, back height to base of scapula, back height to top of shoulder, and hip breadth are taken while the person is sitting. A very large person will need a bariatric wheelchair. Clients who are obese should be measured in sitting because adipose tissue spreads when they lie down, resulting in an inaccurate measurement (Daus, 2003). If the consumer is a child and is expected to grow, that expected change needs to be reflected in the decision making as well.

The person's functional abilities are also evaluated. Two elements are important. The first is evaluation of different ADLs and instrumental ADLs. In addition to identifying in which occupations the individual wishes to engage, this evaluation will determine how he or she completes those activities. The second element involves evaluation of wheelchair skills. The Wheelchair Skills Test (Kirby et al, 2002, 2004) is a well-developed, standardized measure of various wheelchair skills. This test assesses the individual's ability to perform basic wheelchair skills such as removal of an armrest and application of the brakes to more complex, advanced skills such as performing a wheelie to negotiate a curb. This test is one of the few that has had extensive research in all phases of its development. In addition to the evaluation, a training program has also been developed and evaluated. Information about this test and the training program are available at *www.wheelchairskillsprogram.ca*.

Environmental Factors

Physical Context. The ATP needs to explore the physical contexts in which the mobility device will be used. Will the device be used both indoors and outdoors? How accessible are these environments? Width of doorways, floor surfaces, bathroom layout, and access to the structure (e.g., ramp, stairs) all need to be considered. On what type of surfaces will the consumer travel when using the device outdoors? Does the user expect or need to transport the device between different locations such as home, school, or work? How will the user and the mobility device travel (e.g., will he or she use a private vehicle or

---

BOX 12-2	Factors to Consider When Selecting a Wheelchair

Consumer profile: Disability, date of onset, prognosis, size, and weight
Consumer needs: Activities, contexts of use (e.g., accessibility, indoor/outdoor), preferences, transportation, reliability, durability, cost
Physical and sensory skills: Range of motion, motor control, strength, vision, perception
Functional skills: Transfers and ability to propel (manual or powered)

public transportation)? Does the user access other modes of transportation such as trains or airplanes?

Just as the climate was a factor in the recommendation concerning a seating system, it also influences the recommendation of a mobility device. A different recommendation for a device may be made if the consumer lives in a climate where snow is a typical part of winter and he or she expects to use the device outdoors versus a consumer who lives in a climate where snow and cold temperatures are not a routine expectation.

Social Context. Family members, peers, and others in the social environment can influence the choice of a mobility device. Peers with experience with various mobility devices can be a great source of information and can share their knowledge of what works and what does not. Conversely, peers and families may exert pressure in the choice of a manual versus a power wheelchair. The individual may prefer to use a powered chair because it allows him or her to conserve energy for other occupations but may be viewed as lazy by others if this technology is chosen. The willingness or ability of decision makers in the school, workplace, and other community environments to accommodate various types of mobility devices also needs to be considered.

Institutional Context. Institutional regulations and policies influence the recommendation of a mobility device. The ATP needs to be aware of the criteria for funding these devices in his or her jurisdiction. The ATP needs to consider the client's future needs and the implications that a current recommendation will have on the ability to access an appropriate mobility device in the future. For example, some funding programs have a specified time during which a new system will not be funded. Further, some stipulate that if a person receives one type of mobility device, a second one will not be funded or not funded for a period of years (e.g., 5-year life of the system). Funding agencies, in particular those funded with public money, produce criteria that identify functional abilities of the individual and stability of the medical condition that determine whether funding will be available to assist with the purchase of a device. Each ATP is responsible for knowing the regulations and policies regarding access to mobility devices in his or her jurisdiction.

■ CHARACTERISTICS AND CURRENT TECHNOLOGIES OF WHEELED MOBILITY SYSTEMS

This section discusses the major characteristics of manual and powered mobility systems. Table 12-1 lists the major manufacturers of personal mobility systems. Modern mobility

CASE STUDY

WHEELCHAIR ASSESSMENT

Matthew is a 5-year-old boy who just started kindergarten. He has severe cerebral palsy. His teacher referred him to you for a wheelchair and seating evaluation. He currently does not have a wheelchair. At home Matthew is either carried from place to place, placed in a high-density foam positioning seat, or stands in his vertical stander. Outside the home he is pushed in an umbrella baby stroller. The parents have agreed to go along with the evaluation, although they are hesitant about getting a wheelchair for Matthew at this time. They are still hoping he will walk and feel that putting him in a wheelchair will hinder his progress in ambulating. They are also afraid that he will be kept in the wheelchair for long periods without a change in his position.

Your evaluation findings indicate that Matthew has mixed tone. At rest his tone is low. When excited or when completing an activity, his tone increases. His head control is fair. He is unable to sit independently. He has a slight startle reflex to loud noises. Matthew has some right hand function, as evidenced by his ability to play computer games by using a four-position switch array. Matthew is nonverbal and communicates with facial expressions, gestures, sounds, yes/no signals, and a picture board. His functional vision appears to be intact.

Matthew lives with his parents and a younger sister in a single-story house. The flooring in the main living area of the home is linoleum with area rugs. The bedrooms are carpeted with a low shag carpet. Doorways inside the home are all wheelchair accessible. The front doorway to the home is wide enough for a wheelchair but has two steps leading up to it. The family has two mid-size sedans and cannot afford to purchase a wheelchair van at this time.

QUESTIONS

1. Is there other information that you need about Matthew before making a recommendation for a mobility system? If so, what is that?
2. Given the information that you know about Matthew at this time, what types of mobility systems would you potentially consider for Matthew? What might be some features needed in a mobility system for Matthew?

systems are more flexible and more capable of being adapted to a variety of functional tasks. These adaptations may include height adjustment, recline, axle position adjustment, and combinations of all these. The selection of a wheelchair is based on the evaluation discussed in the

TABLE 12-1 **Major Wheelchair Manufacturers**

Manufacturer	Type of Wheelchairs	Web Address
Alber (in the United States) Frank Mobility Systems, Inc. 888-426-8581	Stair-climbing wheelchair; add-on power unit	www.ulrich-alber.de/en/index.php
Altimate Medical, Inc. 800-342-8968	Standing systems	www.easystand.com
Amigo Mobility International, Inc. 800-692-6446	Scooters	www.myamigo.com
Bruno Independent Living Aids 800-882-8183	Adult and pediatric scooters, sedan and van wheelchair lifts	www.bruno.com
Columbia Medical 800-454-6612	Dependent mobility bases	www.columbiamedical.com
Convaid, Inc	Dependent mobility bases, transport chairs	www.convaid.com
ConvaQuip	Bariatric wheelchairs	www.convaquip.com
Etac (in the United States) Balder USA, Inc. 888-422-5337	Independent manual wheelchairs for children and adults	www.etac.com
Frank Mobility Systems, Inc. 888-426-8581	Stair-climbing wheelchair, add-on power unit	http://www.frankmobility.com
Freedom Designs 800-554-8044	Pediatric wheelchairs, tilt-in space wheelchairs	www.freedomdesigns.com
Gendron, Inc 800-537-2521	Bariatric manual and power wheelchairs	www.gendroninc.com
Graham-Field Health products 888-426-5881	Dependent and independent manual, sports wheelchairs, adult and pediatric chairs, tilt chairs	http://www.grahamfield.com/ Channels/Home.aspx?MenuID=1
Innovative Products, Inc. 800-950-5185	Pediatric powered mobility	www.mobility4kids.com
Invacare 800-333-6900	Manual, power, and sports wheelchairs	www.invacare.com
Levo USA, Inc. 888-538-6872	Manual and powered stand-up wheelchairs for adults and children	www.levo.ch
Life Stand (Vivre-Debout) (in the United States) Frank Mobility Systems, Inc. 888-426-8581	Manual and powered stand-up wheelchairs for adults and children	www.lifestand-usa.com
Motion Concepts 888-433-6818	Specialty powered wheelchairs	www.motionconcepts.com
Mulholland Positioning Systems, Inc. 800-543-4769	A variety of standing systems, pediatric wheeled bases, and tilt bases	www.mulhollandinc.com
Otto Bock 800-328-4058	Pediatric seating and positioning, adult positioning, manual and power wheelchairs	www.ottobockus.com
PDG 888-858-4422	Wheelchairs for individuals with special needs, such as bariatric chairs; high agitation and manual tilt wheelchairs	www.pdgmobility.com
Permobil, Inc. 800-736-0925	Stand-up power wheelchairs; power wheelchair with elevating seat; sports wheelchairs; lightweight manual wheelchairs	www.permobil.com
Pride Mobility Products Corp. United States 800-800-8586 Canada 888-570-1113	Manual and electrically powered wheelchairs, scooters	www.pridemobility.com
Snug Seat 800-336-7684	Specialty bases for children and adults, car seats, dependent and independent mobility bases, pediatric wheelchairs	www.snugseat.com
Sunrise Medical 800-333-4000	Dependent and independent manual bases, sports wheelchairs, lightweight manual wheelchairs, power wheelchairs, add-on power unit; adult and pediatric wheelchairs, tilt wheelchairs and scooters	www.sunrisemedical.com
TiLite 800-545-2266	Adult and pediatric titanium wheelchairs; manual wheelchair; sports wheelchair	www.tilite.com www.titaniumsports.com

previous section and is a process of matching characteristics to the consumer's needs and skills. This section discusses the characteristics of mobility systems, starting with the wheelchair's two basic structures: a supporting structure and a propelling structure. To meet the varied needs of individuals with mobility impairments, there are three broad categories of wheeled mobility systems: dependent mobility, independent manual mobility, and independent powered mobility.

Dependent mobility systems, which are propelled by an attendant, include strollers and transport chairs. A dependent mobility system is chosen when (1) the individual is not at all capable of independently propelling a wheelchair (likely because of cognitive, perceptual, or behavioral deficits) or (2) a secondary system is needed that is lightweight and easily transported.

An **independent manual mobility system** is for those individuals who have the ability to propel a wheelchair manually. These bases have two large wheels in the back and two smaller front wheels that allow the user to propel independently.

Independent powered mobility systems are required when the user has difficulty propelling a **manual wheelchair.** These are **electrically powered wheelchairs** that are driven by the user. Within each of these categories there are many commercial options available to meet the needs of the individual user. This section discusses the characteristics of mobility systems, starting with the wheelchair's two basic structures: a supporting structure and a propelling structure. Figure 12-1 shows the anatomy of a manual wheelchair.

Supporting Structure

The **supporting structure** of the wheelchair consists of the frame and attachments to it. Specialized seating and positioning (see Chapter 6) are often considered part of the supporting structure. Accessories to the frame (e.g., armrests, footrests) are also a part of the supporting structure. In some wheelchairs these accessories are manufactured as part of the frame. Some supporting structures are unique in that they are adjustable to allow for changes in the orientation of the user in space, which includes systems that tilt, those that change the seat-to-back angle, and those that provide support in a standing position.

Frame Types.   Three underlying factors will be discussed before different classifications of manual wheelchairs are described: type of frame (rigid or folding), adjustability of the position of the axle of the rear wheel, and material used to construct the wheelchair frame.

Frames may be either folding or rigid (Figure 12-2), and there are three common frame styles (Cooper, 1998). Rigid frames are available in a box, cantilever, and T or I frame style (Figure 12-3). Typically the box frame construction has a rectangular shape that provides a strong and durable base to which the seat and wheels are attached. Lighter weight designs are accomplished by replacing the box with a single bar extending between the wheels, forming a cantilever structure. Upright tubes from this main support are used to attach the seat and back. The footrests are extensions of the seat rails. As shown in Figure 12-3, the T construction uses a bar similar to the cantilever design but has a single bar attached to the center of the cantilever that

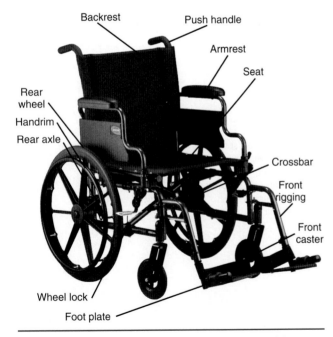

Figure 12-1   Manual wheelchair showing the major parts of the supporting and propelling structures. (Courtesy Invacare Canada.)

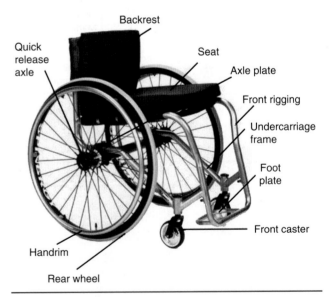

Figure 12-2   Rigid frame wheelchair showing the major parts of the supporting and propelling structures. (Courtesy Invacare Canada.)

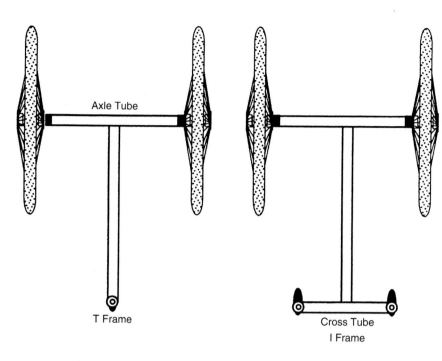

Axle Tube

T Frame

Cross Tube
I Frame

Figure 12-3   T and I frame styles. (From Cooper RA: *Wheelchair selection and configuration*, New York, 1998, Demos Medical Publishing.)

connects to a single front caster. This configuration forms a T shape under the seat. If two front casters are used, then the T becomes an I shape. For transportation, the wheels on all these chairs are removed, and in some cases the back folds down. The choice between rigid or box frame and folding frame styles involves a number of elements

including the consumer's needs, functional ability, method of transfer, and level of activity (Cooper, 1998).

The position of the axle of the drive wheel relative to the user's **center of gravity** affects the stability and maneuverability of the wheelchair. Figure 12-4 displays this relationship. The center of mass of an empty wheelchair is located

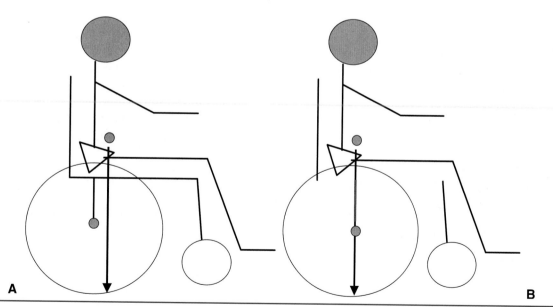

A

B

Figure 12-4   Relationship of the center of mass of the user to the axle of the wheel affects the mobility and stability of the chair. **A,** When the user is seated with his center of mass ahead of the axle of the wheelchair, the chair is more stable. **B,** When the user is seated with his center of mass directly above the axle of the wheelchair, the chair is more mobile

under the seat, in front of the drive wheels (Engstrom, 2002). When the user is seated in the wheelchair, the center of mass moves above the seat and forward and backward, depending on the seated position of the individual and the drive wheels. When the center of mass is forward of the axis of the drive wheels, more weight is placed on the castors, making it more difficult to lift them (Engstrom, 2002). The chair is more stable but less maneuverable in this configuration. As the center of mass moves backward, closer to the axis of the drive wheel or even slightly behind it, stability decreases and maneuverability increases. Understanding this relationship is important when setting up the chair. An active user will want a configuration that is easily maneuverable and allows him or her to perform a wheelie (i.e., lift the castors up, to clear curbs and other barriers). A less confident wheelchair user will be most comfortable with a chair that does not tip backward easily, allowing him or her to feel secure in the chair.

Another fairly recent advancement in the wheelchair industry is the material used to form the chair frame. Much of the advancement in materials comes from the cycling industry. Wheelchair frames are made from many different materials, including steel, aluminum, steel/aluminum alloy, titanium, and carbon fiber composites. These materials vary in their weight, strength, cost, how they conduct vibration, method of attaching components together, and how they are formed. Understanding the benefits of each material in combination with the user's needs will help determine whether the functional benefit is worth the cost of the higher end materials.

Wheelchairs are classified according to a number of parameters, including weight, adjustability, and available options. **Standard wheelchairs** are generally useful for very short-term use such as rentals at an airport or shopping mall (Schmeler and Bunning, 1999). They are folding chairs, with very limited adjustment; in particular the axle of the rear wheel is fixed. Features such as footrests and armrests may be fixed or detachable. There is limited choice of seat width and depth. They are the heaviest of the manual wheelchairs and therefore are not useful for long-term use because they require a great deal of energy to propel on a regular basis.

Lightweight chairs (Schmeler and Bunning, 1999) weigh less than the standard chair, as their name would suggest. Otherwise, they tend to have similar features. These chairs offer more flexibility in choice of seat width and adjustment of back height. Both the standard and lightweight chairs are available with a lower seat-to-floor height that allows the user to propel the chair with the feet.

An **ultralightweight wheelchair** is substantially lighter than the standard chair. Schmeler and Bunning (1999) suggest that the chairs in the standard and lightweight categories are not suitable for use over the long term. The ultralightweight chair is one they consider useful for an individual who uses a manual wheelchair as the primary means of mobility. It retains the folding frame and is available with a lower seat-to-floor height for individuals who propel with their feet. The axle of the rear wheel is adjustable relative to the center of gravity of the user.

Rigid ultralight wheelchairs (Schmeler and Bunning, 1999) are a huge growth area for the wheelchair industry. The primary difference between these and the previous categories is the rigid frame. These chairs have quick release rear wheels and the back of most folds down to facilitate transfer and storage of the chair in a vehicle. The axle of the rear wheel of these chairs can be adjusted relative to the center of gravity of the user.

Accessories. **Armrests** on conventional wheelchairs may be manufactured as a fixed part of the frame, flip back out of the way, or be completely removable. Nonremovable armrests decrease the width of the wheelchair slightly and do not get lost because they cannot be removed. In general it is advantageous to have armrests that flip back or are removable to facilitate transfers and other activities. Two lengths of armrests are available. Desk-length armrests are shorter in the front to allow the consumer to move close to a desk or table. Full-length armrests, which provide more support, extend to the front of the seat rails. Armrests may be fixed or adjustable in height. Armrests that are height adjustable can be moved up or down to accommodate the length of the user's trunk and provide the proper amount of support for the arms. A clothing guard on the armrests prevents clothing and body parts from rubbing against the wheels. Leg rests and footplates support the legs and feet. Taken together, these two components are often called the **front rigging** of the wheelchair. Angle options are often available for the leg rests with either 90- or 70-degree hangers. These options increase the comfort of the user by accommodating the preferred knee flexion angle, but they can also add to the turning radius, which may be a factor for mobility in some environments. Leg rests may be fixed (built into the frame) or removable (swing away). Styles that swing away make it easier to transfer in and out of the wheelchair. Footplates are attached to the leg rests and are available as a single plate to support both feet or as two separate units, with individual height adjustment. The height of the footplate should support the desired position of the lower extremities. The angle of the footplate can also be adjusted to accommodate ankle flexion or extension. Heel loops can be attached to the back of the footplate to prevent the foot from sliding backward (see Figure 12-1). **Wheel locks** are the devices that prevent the wheels from moving, during transfers and other stationary activities. They are available in a number of configurations such as push or pull to lock, with lever extensions for individuals with limited reach, under the seat mounts, hill holders, and

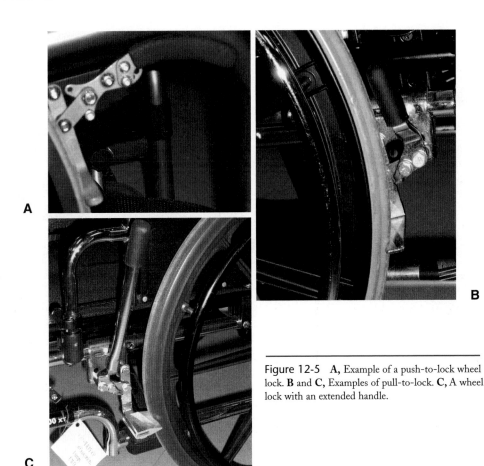

Figure 12-5 **A,** Example of a push-to-lock wheel lock. **B** and **C,** Examples of pull-to-lock. **C,** A wheel lock with an extended handle.

attendant controlled. Figure 12-5 shows some of the various wheel lock styles. When determining the type of wheel lock for the chair, consider how the user transfers in and out of the chair, his or her ability to access the wheel lock, the most reliable method available to manipulate the wheel lock, and the ability of the user or caregiver to maintain this component. As with the brakes of a motor vehicle, proper maintenance of the wheel locks is an important safety consideration.

Antitip devices are small wheels attached to a rod and mounted at the back of the chair. These devices prevent the chair from tipping backward. When the drive wheels are located forward on the chair, antitip devices are recommended, particularly when the individual cannot safely perform a wheelie. Because these devices limit backward tipping of the chair, they can interfere with travel over some obstacles such as curbs. Antitip devices can be removed or rotated so they do not interfere with such travel when an attendant is pushing the chair. However, they must be returned to their original position when the user resumes propelling the chair (Engstrom, 2002).

Push handles are another option on a manual chair. These are the handles used by an attendant or caregiver to

maneuver the chair. Some of these are height adjustable to accommodate the different heights of individuals who push the chair. Extended handles are available for pediatric chairs to avoid low back strain for the individual pushing the chair. Push handles have different shapes and are of different materials to assist with grip and handling in difficult situations such as inclement weather or traveling up or down a hill.

The upholstery of most wheelchairs that are intended for regular long-term use is designed to be used with a seating system. The option exists for most chairs to remove the upholstery completely and replace with a back or seat that is attached directly to the frame of the chair. Generally, only those chairs that are for occasional use come with a hammock style upholstery attached to the frame.

Frames for Recline and Tilt.   **Tilt** and **recline** features are available on both manual frames and power bases. Figure 12-6, *A* and *B,* shows examples of these systems. These features recognize that sitting is not a static activity and that we need to provide the opportunity to change position for individuals who cannot do so independently. Tilt refers to the ability to rotating a specific seating position

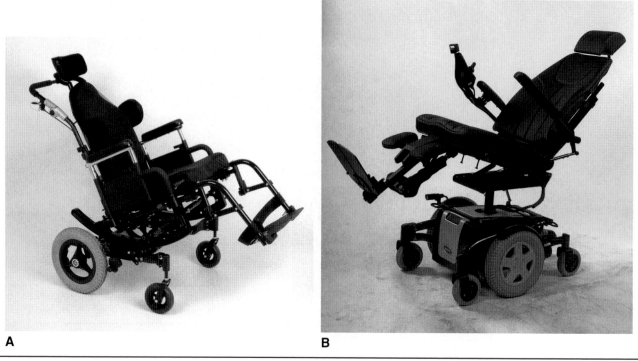

A **B**

Figure 12-6 Tilt-and-recline wheelchair supporting structures. **A,** Supporting structure with tilt feature (Courtesy Sunrise Medical.) **B,** Supporting structure with recline feature (Courtesy Motion Concepts.)

around a fixed axis, changing the orientation in space. Recline refers changing the seat to back angle, resulting in a seat to back angle greater than 90 degrees (Lange, 2000). The seat-to-back angle typically ranges from upright to nearly horizontal. Tilt and recline have some common benefits to the user. Both provide a change of position and improved circulation, thus bringing pressure relief and greater comfort (Lange, 2000; Smith, 2004; Wilson and Miller Polgar, 2005). They have the potential to improve head and postural control, providing an improved functional position and influence muscle tone (Engstrom, 2002, Kreutz, 1997; Lange, 2000, Smith, 2004). They have the potential to improve respiratory function, provide a better visual field, regulate blood pressure, ease transfers and allow rest during the day (Kreutz, 1997; Lange, 2000). Recline or tilt can be used to achieve a more typical spinal alignment, for example, to reduce a thoracic kyphosis (Engstrom, 2002).

Recline is also useful for individuals who become fatigued when sitting upright for a length of time. A chair with a recline feature allows rest without the need to transfer to bed. Recline also can accommodate cases in which more than 90 degrees of hip flexion is required, either because of structural limitations or when a hip flexion angle

of greater than 90 degrees helps the user maintain spinal extension. Recline provides passive range of motion of the hips and knees (when elevating legrests are also provided). It can alleviate orthostatic hypotension (Kreutz, 1997; Lange, 2000) and improve bowel and bladder function. Recline may be preferred to tilt in a work or social environment because it is considered to be less obtrusive by the user (Lange, 2000). Recline does not raise the knees during the position change, which allows the user to work at a desk or table. When elevating legrests are included, there is a potential to reduce edema in and improve circulation to the lower extremities (Lange, 2000).

Recline is not a good option for some consumers. Opening the hip angle will cause excessive extensor tone in some individuals, particularly children with cerebral palsy or individuals who have sustained a head injury. Obviously, it is not useful when the user has limited hip extension range of motion. Individuals who use a custom contoured seating system should not use a recline system because of the shear forces that are inevitably present when changing the seat to back angle.

Shear is of concern when changing the seat-to-back angle. In Chapter 6 shear is defined as the friction that occurs when two surfaces slide across each other. Shear has the potential to tear skin, which can lead to a pressure ulcer. Most recline systems are designed to minimize shear, referred to as **low-shear systems.** These systems follow the user as the system reclines, resulting in a reduction of shear but not its elimination (Smith, 2004). Low-shear systems are available in both manual and power options.

Tilt systems are recommended when it is desirable to maintain the seating position for function or for control of other devices mounted to the wheelchair, such as augmentative and alternative communication devices (Lange, 2000). Because the whole seat pivots around an axis, shear is not of concern as it is with a recline system. In addition to rearward tilt, some systems also provide lateral tilt, which again maintains the seating position but tilts the user in the sagittal plane. The combination of anteroposterior and lateral tilt gives the user control to change position as he or she wishes.

Tilt systems do pose disadvantages that recline systems do not. Most systems increase the seat-to-floor height. Further, when the user is in the tilt position, the knees are raised, sometimes higher than the level of the head. The seat-to-floor height and position may interfere with the ability to work at a table or desk and poses a risk for injury if the user attempts to move into a tilt position while seated at a desk or table. As the seat tilts and the knees are raised, the lower extremity may be impinged between a desk and the system (Lange, 2000). Because tilt maintains the hip angle (typically 90 degrees), bladder constriction may occur, causing problems with fully emptying the bladder (Kreutz, 1997). Extreme degrees of tilt may cause the user to feel posturally insecure, which has the potential to increase muscle contraction, thus defeating the purpose of alleviating fatigue. Finally, tilt may interfere with the use of a tray: objects will slide off a tray when in tilt.

Center of mass shifts are a consideration when evaluating a wheelchair that incorporates a tilt-in-space option. The relationship of the center of mass of the seat to the center of mass of the base must be considered. The center of mass moves posteriorly as the seat tilts on some systems. This movement can cause rearward instability if the center of mass of the seat is shifted too far back with respect to the center of mass of the base. Most wheelchair designs compensate for this concern with mechanisms that maintain the center of mass of the seat over the center of mass of the base.

Consumers who use either a tilt-in-space or a recline system frequently also have other assistive technology whose use must be integrated with these positioning options, specifically, control of a power wheelchair with a head array, use of a ventilator, and use of an adapted van. Head array controls should be turned off when the user is in the tilt or recline position so that he or she can fully rest the head. When a ventilator is mounted on the wheelchair, care must be taken to ensure that the tilt or recline mechanism

does not impinge on the unit and that the ventilator retains its proper position (Lange, 2004). Finally, evaluation of the user's method of transportation must be considered when tilt and recline options are used. Tilt increases the seat to floor height, which may prevent the user from transferring into an adapted van. Both have the potential to increase the overall length of the system, which may limit the maneuverability of the user and the chair once in a van (Lange, 2000; Phillips, Fisher, and Miller Polgar, 2005). Integration of wheelchairs with adapted vans will be considered in Chapter 13 when transportation is discussed.

Frames for Standing.   We normally think of mobility in terms of wheelchairs; that is, the user is seated. There are, however, many advantages to placing an individual in a standing position (Eng, 2004; Mogul-Rotman and Fisher, 2002; Walter and Dunn, 1998). Among the positive effects of standing are physiological improvement in bladder and bowel function, alleviation of orthostatic hypotension, prevention of decubitus ulcers (see Chapter 6), reduction in muscle contractures and osteoporosis, and improved circulation. In addition, there are psychological benefits from being able to interact face to face with other people. Standing frames and standing wheelchairs are two different types of supporting structures that allow the individual to stand.

Standing frames are categorized as prone standers, supine standers, upright standers, and mobile standers (Mogul-Rotman and Fisher, 2002). Prone standers, such as the one shown in Figure 12-7, are the most common type.

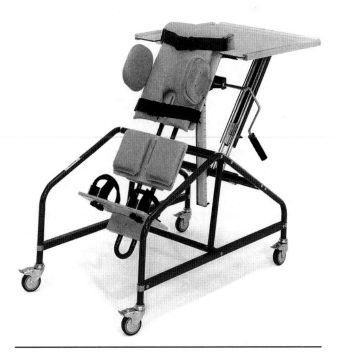

Figure 12-7   Large prone stander. (Courtesy Rifton.)

They provide support on the anterior side of the body. Weight bearing on the long bones and lower extremity joints is a major benefit. Often a lap tray is added to the stander, which serves two purposes. First, it provides a supporting surface for the upper extremities as the user leans on it. Second, it provides a work surface for activities such as writing, playing with toys, or using a communication device. Prone standers are generally tilted forward to use gravity for keeping the body upright in the stander. Some types have fixed angles and others are adjustable. Adjustment for growth is incorporated into some designs. This type of standing frame does not give the individual the option of moving into a seated position, as does the stand-up wheelchair, which is discussed below.

Supine standers are less common, and there are fewer options. This type of stander provides support for the posterior surfaces of the body. Because the user is leaned back, hand use is less functional. This type of stander is useful for persons who do not have good head control because the stander supports the head and neck. *Upright standers* provide for complete weight bearing on the lower extremities. People who have good upper body strength can use stationary models. Mobile versions are often sit-to-stand wheelchairs that allow changes in position from sitting to standing throughout the day. The change from sitting to standing and vice versa can be either powered or manual. When the user is in a vertical position, these units generally function like a prone stander.

Standing wheelchairs have both functional and social benefits. Many tasks of daily living, such as cooking, are simplified with the use of a standing wheelchair. Additionally, the use of a standing wheelchair may make it possible to avoid having to make modifications to a home or work setting. For example, a person cooking dinner while using a standing wheelchair is able to reach items in upper cabinets and reach the surface of cabinets and stoves without requiring modifications. Individuals who use a standing wheelchair report positive psychological benefits when they are at the same level as others (Eng, 2004).

Standing wheelchairs (Figure 12-8) are available in three basic configurations: manual driven with a manual lifting mechanism, manual driven with a power lifting mechanism, and power driven with a power lifting mechanism. Standing wheelchairs with manual lifting mechanisms consist of a hydraulic system that uses either a pump or a lever to raise the person to the standing position. With a powered system, the person activates a button to move into the upright position. When standing, the person is supported with padded bars at the knees and torso. Stability in the upright position is a concern with standing wheelchairs because movement into the standing position moves the client's center of gravity forward in the chair, ahead of the center of mass of the base. For this reason not all standing wheelchairs are mobile while in the upright position.

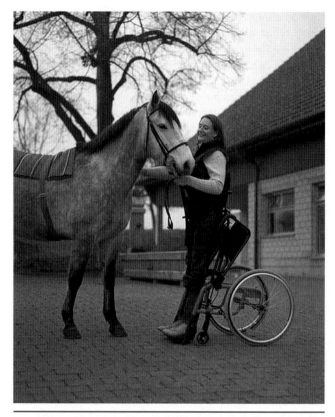

Figure 12-8   Stand-up wheelchair. (Courtesy Levo AG.)

Those that are designed to be mobile in the standing positioning have a wider-than-normal base of support.

Although there are significant benefits to be gained from the use of standing frames and standing wheelchairs, their cost and size often limit usefulness, especially in a home environment. Selection must be based on a systematic evaluation, and the requirements of the individual consumer for a standing system are determined during the needs assessment. Fitting a consumer to a standing wheelchair poses some unique challenges in that the individual will be changing positions from sitting to standing; these dynamic positioning needs should be taken into consideration. Cooper (1998) offers some suggestions for fitting an individual for a standing wheelchair.

Frames That Provide Variable Seat Height.   Another available option on power wheelchair frames is a seat that can be lowered or raised. The person remains in a seated position, and when the mechanism is activated, the wheelchair seat raises and lowers within a given range. The mechanism to change the height of the wheelchair seat may be operated manually or with power. A seat that lowers near the floor is particularly useful for small children. Being at floor level allows the child to play on the floor and interact at a level with children his or her age. There are also benefits to raising the height of a seat. As with a standing wheelchair, a seat elevator is useful because it raises the person up and can make it easier for the individual to participate in certain self-care, work, and educational activities. As with standing wheelchairs and tilt in space and recline systems, the location of the center of mass has implications to safety. Some systems have a power lockout that prevents the chair from moving when the seat is raised to a certain height. Stability when traveling around corners may be compromised if the center of mass is too high relative to the footprint of the chair.

Frames That Accommodate Growth.   A major requirement of the supporting structure of the wheelchairs for children is that they accommodate growth. Two approaches are commonly used. The first of these is to design the supporting structure so that it can be adjusted directly. Kits are provided in the second option that allows replacement of various tubes on the frame increasing seat width and length, seat-to-floor height, and other important components.

Access to the drive wheels is another consideration when pediatric chairs are recommended. One strategy to improve this access is to set the drive wheels in slight camber. A second approach, for very young children, is to reverse the configuration of the drive wheels, placing them at the front of the chair with the casters at the back. Stability of the chair, rearward, must be carefully assessed with this configuration.

Push handles are a final consideration for a pediatric frame. Extended handles are available so that the caregiver does not need to lean or bend forward to grasp the push handles. This configuration greatly reduces the load placed on the caregiver's lower back by allowing an upright position during this activity.

Propelling Structure: Manual

For manual or *body-powered* wheelchairs, the **propelling structure** consists of two main parts: (1) wheels (including tires and casters) and (2) an interface that the consumer uses to move the wheelchair (Ragnarsson, 1990). Each of these components is discussed in this section.

Tires.   There are three main types of wheelchair tires: solid, semipneumatic, and pneumatic (Robson, 2005). Solid tires require less maintenance of all types but are the least versatile. They generally perform well on smooth indoor surfaces but are less efficient when used on carpeted surfaces or other rough, uneven terrain. Solid tires typically have a smooth surface.

Pneumatic tires may have an inner tube or a flat free insert. Although they are useful over more varied terrain than solid tires, they require maintenance to maintain proper tire pressure and can be punctured, resulting in a flat. Sawatsky,

Denison, and Kim (2005) found that rolling resistance and energy expenditure were significantly decreased when tires were inflated to 50% of their recommended pressure. They report clinical evidence that wheelchair tires are commonly found to be inflated to only 25% of their recommended pressure. In addition to maintaining tire pressure, the user should inspect the tires regularly for any cracks or imperfections that may lead to a flat. These tires are available with different tread depths; deeper treads are useful on rough terrain but create more rolling resistance when used on smoother surfaces.

Wheels.   Rear wheels are of two basic types: composite or spoke, shown in Figure 12-9 (Robson, 2005). Composite wheels tend to be more economical than spoke wheels and require less maintenance. There is less risk of the user getting a hand caught in the wheel. These wheels tend to be more rigid than spoke wheels and thus may give a more uncomfortable ride (Robson, 2005). Spoke wheels do have more maintenance because it is more difficult to clean them and the spokes should be readjusted. These wheels tend to transmit less vibration from the surface to the user than do more rigid composite wheels (Robson, 2005). They are lighter in weight than composite wheels. High-performance wheels, such as the Spinergy wheel, are available for active users. These wheels use lightweight materials that provide better strength and greater shock absorption. Wheels range in size from 18 to 26 inches in diameter. Power wheelchairs typically have 18-inch wheels, and conventional manual types have 24-inch wheels.

Many wheelchairs allow adjustment of the location of the drive wheels forward or rearward on the chair. Figure 12-10 shows a mounting plate that allows adjustments of the position of the drive wheels. The location of the wheels relative to the center of gravity of the user affects the mobility and stability of the chair. When the axle of the wheel is located either directly under the user's center of gravity or anterior to it, the result is a more maneuverable, responsive chair, one that is desired by the active user. More novice wheelchair users or those with less control will feel most comfortable with the axis of the wheel located behind the center of gravity, resulting in a more stable chair (Engstrom, 2002). A quick-release feature (see Figure 12-9) makes it possible to remove the wheel easily for transportation.

Wheel camber affects the responsiveness of the chair. **Camber** refers to the degree to which the wheel is mounted off vertical, usually 1 to 4 degrees. Camber tips the wheel so the top is closer to the user's body. When the wheels are set this way, the wheelchair becomes more stable and propulsion is more efficient. There is greater access to the wheels. Camber increases the overall width of the chair and lowers the rear seat to floor height (Robson, 2005). Wheel alignment also affects the ease with which the chair can be propelled. *Alignment* refers to the degree to which the

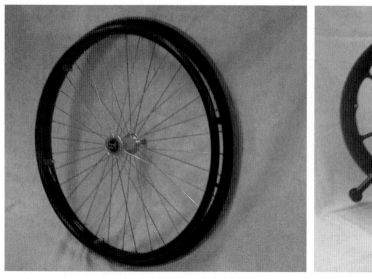
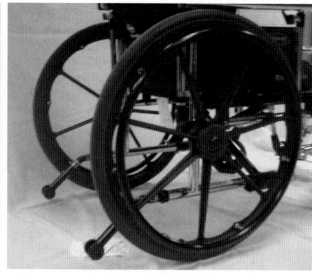

Figure 12-9   Types of rear wheels for a manual wheelchair. **A,** Spoked wheel, **B,** Composite mag wheel.

two wheels are parallel to each other. If they are not parallel and at equal distance from each other, there is greater rolling resistance for the wheelchair.

Casters. The front wheels on wheelchairs are referred to as *casters.* They range in diameter from 2¾ to 8¼ inches (Fields, 1992). Larger casters give a smoother ride but are less responsive and can interfere with foot placement (Robson, 2005). Smaller casters are more responsive,

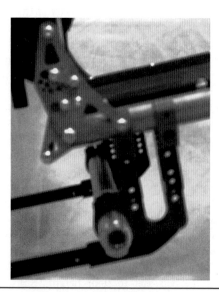

Figure 12-10   Axle plate of manual wheelchair that allows adjustability of the position of the rear wheels.

contribute to more efficient propulsion, and allow more flexibility in position of the feet, but these benefits are compromised by a rougher ride (Engstrom, 2002; Robson, 2005). Solid semipneumatic casters are available. The relationship of the user's center of gravity to the chair's center of mass is important here. If the user is seated too far forward in the chair, excess weight is placed on the casters (i.e., front loading the casters), making it more difficult to propel because the force required to overcome inertia is greater (Engstrom, 2002). This situation may also result in loss of forward stability.

Shimmy is one of the major problems with casters (Fields, 1992). This term refers to the rapid vibration that is often felt when pushing a shopping cart. Smaller casters tend to have less shimmy than larger ones, but larger casters offer a smoother ride and are less likely to be caught on uneven surfaces. The major factors resulting in shimmy are the position of the caster fork and stem, the shape of the wheel, and the tension in the caster axle and swivel mechanism where they attach to the frame. Caster float occurs when one of the casters does not touch the floor when the wheelchair is on level ground (Cooper, 1998), which can result in reduced stability and performance. Excessive wear on one caster or unequal camber in the rear wheels will bring about caster float. Replacing the caster, adjusting the rear wheel camber, or lowering the caster that floats with a spacer can eliminate the problem (Cooper, 1998).

Caster placement affects the performance of the chair. Trailing casters are located with the caster behind the front vertical tube of the chair. Casters in this position reduce the overall length of the chair and improve the chair's responsiveness but result in less forward stability of the chair. Leading casters are located ahead of the front vertical tube.

Casters in this position increase forward stability and are less sensitive to front loading (as described previously). They do contribute to a longer wheelbase and are less responsive (Robson, 2005). Like other features on a chair, it is clear that the needs of the consumer in the various activities, for which he or she will use a wheelchair, need to be matched with the performance features of the casters. Similarly, maintenance is required to ensure that the casters are properly aligned and loaded.

Hand Rims.   The human/technology interface for a manual wheelchair is most commonly a ring attached to the wheel, called a *hand rim*. Hand rims are made from a variety of materials, including titanium, aluminum, and stainless steel. They may have a vinyl coating. Knobs or extensions can be added for individuals who have difficulty gripping hand rims (Figure 12-11). Ergonomically designed hand rims use a material that spans the space between the wheel rim and the hand rim, thus allowing a natural fit with the user's palm. If an individual has the use of only one arm and hand, two hand rims are put on the intact side and a linkage is attached between the inner hand rim and the opposite wheel, as shown in Figure 12-12 (Wilson and McFarland, 1990). By grasping both hand rims, the user can move forward. Turning is possible using one hand rim at a time.

Propelling Structure: Powered

The **propelling structure** of power wheelchairs has more variability than do manual systems. The major components are a wheeled mobility base with a power drive to the wheels, a control interface that the consumer uses to direct the movement of the wheelchair, an electronic controller, and powered accessories (e.g., recline, tilt). This section discusses current approaches.

Drive Wheels.   Electrically powered wheelchairs have undergone a tremendous change in the last decade. The development of microprocessing capabilities enables developers of powered mobility technology to include a wide range of functions in these devices. One of the most significant developments is the change in the location of the drive wheels. Power is delivered to one pair of wheels in mobility technology with the additional sets of wheels providing stability. Direct drive systems also often provide dynamic or active braking of the wheelchair by providing a voltage that stops the motor. This action offers more

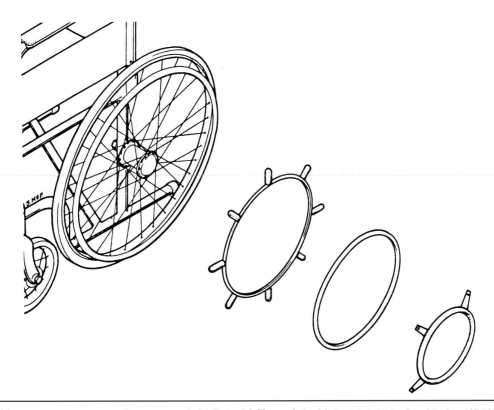

Figure 12-11   Examples of hand rims. (From Wilson B, McFarland S: Types of wheelchairs, *J Rehabil Res Dev Clin Suppl* 27:104-116, 1990.)

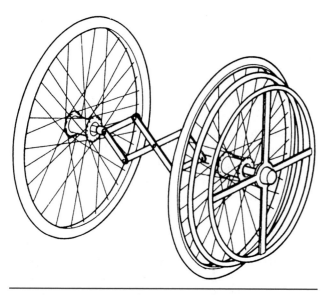

Figure 12-12   One-hand drive mechanism. (From Wilson B, McFarland S: Types of wheelchairs, *J Rehabil Res Dev Clin Suppl* 27: 104-116, 1990.)

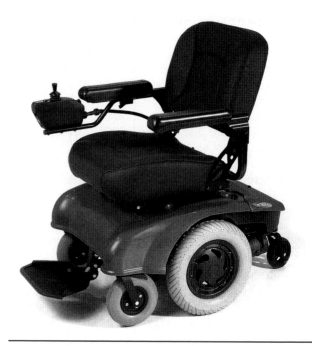

Figure 12-13   Electrically powered wheelchair with mid-wheel drive system. (Courtesy Sunrise Medical.)

control than the common situation of letting the chair coast to a stop after the voltage is turned off to the motor. Most motors used are direct current types in which the speed is proportional to the voltage applied and the torque is proportional to the applied current. Cooper (1998) describes in detail the engineering considerations in wheelchair drive systems.

Electrically powered wheelchairs are generally classified as rear-, mid-, or front-wheel drive, depending on the location of the wheels that propel the chair. Rear- and mid-wheel drive chairs are the most common. In addition to castors, antitipping devices may also be present on a power chair. Figure 12-13 shows a typical mid-wheel drive electrically powered wheelchair, with the housing for the motor and batteries located underneath the seat.

Recently, Denison and Gayton (2002) proposed a different classification on the basis of the relationship of the drive wheel to the center of gravity of the user and the ratio of weight on the drive wheels to that on the castors. The drive wheels of a rear-wheel drive chair are located behind the center of gravity of the user. These are well behind the center of gravity in a low-ratio rear-wheel drive. The front wheels are castors and antitipping wheels may or may not be present. The drive wheels of a high-ratio rear-wheel drive are closer to the user's center of gravity. In addition to front castors, antitipping wheels are located behind the drive wheels. The drive wheels of a mid-wheel drive chair are located directly under the user's center of gravity. Castors are located both in front of and behind the drive wheels. These castors are intended to be in contact with the surface when the chair is in motion. The drive

wheels of a front-wheel drive chair are located ahead of the user's center of gravity, with the high-ratio front-wheel drive wheels being closer to the center of gravity than with the low ratio. The location of the drive wheels affects the performance of the chair, making it an important consideration when recommending a chair to a client.

Evaluation of the client's physical and cognitive abilities and examination of his or her mobility needs are important steps in determining which type of powered wheelchair is most suited to the client's needs and lifestyle. There is limited literature that evaluates the function of powered wheelchairs to assist the client and clinician in making a power mobility decision. Because the purchase of a powered wheelchair is a significant financial investment, a trial period of use of a potential chair is necessary. Rentschler et al from the Rehabilitation Engineering Research Center on Wheeled Mobility at the University of Pittsburgh used the American National Standards Institute (ANSI)/ Rehabilitation Engineering Society of North America (RESNA) standards to evaluate five power chairs that were commonly recommended for clients in the Veterans Affairs health care system (Rentschler et al, 2004). They examined two rear-wheel drive chairs, two mid-wheel drive chairs, and one front-wheel drive chair. Outcome measures included static and dynamic stability, braking distance, energy consumption (i.e., range of a single battery charge under standard conditions), static, impact and fatigue strength, and performance under different climatic conditions.

Stability tests were conducted under two conditions: chair configured in most stable manner and chair configured in least stable manner. Their results did not point conclusively to the benefits of one chair over another but did give a good initial foundation with which to compare a chair's performance with the consumer's needs.

Control Interfaces for Powered Mobility Systems.

There are a number of ways in which a power wheelchair can be controlled. Two control distinctions need to be made first before the various technologies are discussed: proportional versus nonproportional control. **Proportional control** with 360-degree directionality means that the chair moves in whichever direction the joystick is displaced, and the greater the displacement, the faster the chair moves (Lange, 2005). The joystick controls fewer degrees of movement with **nonproportional control** and, regardless of the displacement, the chair travels at a preselected speed. If the user wishes to change direction, he or she must release the joystick in one direction and activate it in the direction of the change (Lange, 2005).

Many options exist that provide access to power wheelchair controls. The ATP's assessment includes the determination of movements that the client is able to make reliably. A similar process can be used to determine the most appropriate method of access, as was described in Chapter 7 regarding computer and augmentative and alternative communication access. An important difference between assessment for computer access and powered wheelchair control is that the ATP needs to determine that the movement used to control the power wheelchair is safe and reliable (i.e., the user must be able to initiate or cease a movement as required because he or she is controlling a moving vehicle).

Many of the types of switches that are described in Chapter 7 are also useful for powered mobility control. These switches can be mechanical or electronic (Lange, 2005). Mechanical switches must be physically activated to initiate a control command. For example, they must be moved, depressed, touched, or released. Electronic switches do not require physical contact from the user. Proximity switches activate when the user is close to the switch, but not necessarily touching it. Fiberoptic switches emit an invisible beam that initiates an action when interrupted (Lange, 2005).

The most common method of control of a power wheelchair is direct selection through the use of a four-direction joystick. Typically, a joystick can be positioned on either side of the chair or in midline to be controlled with the hand or forearm. It can also be fixed or mounted on a swing-away plate that facilitates transfers. It can be positioned to be used with the, chin, foot, leg, or head. When a chin joystick is used, an additional switch (often activated by a shoulder shrug) can be used to control a powered arm

that moves the joystick into position for use and swings it out of the way for eating, talking, or mouthstick use.

Most joysticks have a ball on top. However, many different types of tops are available for users with different grasping abilities (Lange, 2005). For example, a U-shaped cuff that supports the person's hand on the sides may enhance control of the joystick. Other variations include smaller or larger balls, a T-bar, and an extended joystick.

Sip-and-puff switches are a common control interface for individuals with a high spinal cord lesion. A small tube is placed in close proximity to the person's mouth. The user controls the switch with either a puff (blowing air out of the mouth) or a sip (sucking air into the mouth). A hard puff causes the chair to move forward while a hard sip causes it to move in reverse. A soft puff turns the chair right; a soft sip turns it left. The forward direction is latched (i.e., once the user activates forward movement, the chair will continue to travel in that direction until reverse is activated). Good oral motor control is required to use a sip-and-puff system. Figure 12-14 shows a sip and puff system for controlling a wheelchair.

Various head control systems are available, arranged in a head array in a headrest. Figure 12-15 shows an example of this type of control interface. These are electronic, not mechanical, switches. Typically the user has access to three switches: moving the head backward causes the chair to move forward, tilting it to the right moves the chair right, and the opposite initiates travel to the left. Tilting the head forward stops the chair (Lange, 2005). Control can be either proportional or nonproportional depending on the head control of the user. Individuals who tend to move into extension when their neck is extended may not be good

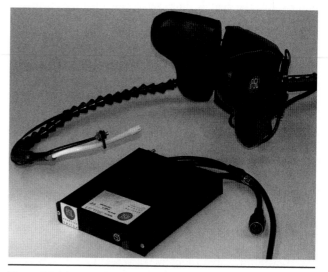

Figure 12-14   Sip-and-puff controller. (Courtesy Adaptive Switch Laboratories.)

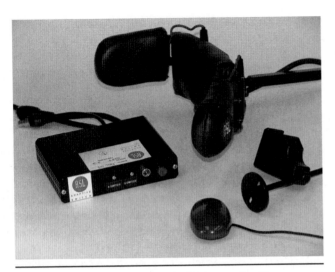

Figure 12-15 Head array, power wheelchair controller. (Courtesy Adaptive Switch Laboratories.)

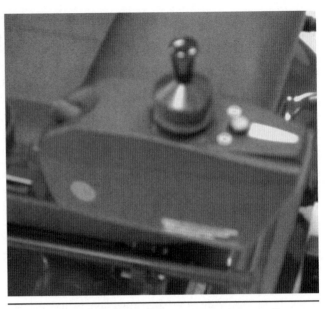

Figure 12-16 Electrically powered wheelchair controller.

candidates for this type of system because they may not be able to reliably stop or reverse the chair if extensor tone inhibits forward flexion of the neck.

Magitek (*www.magitek.com*) produces a head control system that uses a 360-degree tilt sensor mechanism (Cole, 2004). These sensors detect tilt in the lateral and anterior/posterior planes. It is usually attached to a headband, but it can be attached to other body parts. This system is a useful alternative for an individual with adequate head control who tends to go into extension with neck extension.

Indirect selection using scanning is also available for consumers who can only use a single switch. In this case there are four lights, one for each direction, arranged in a cross pattern. The lights scan around the pattern until the user presses the switch. The wheelchair then moves in the direction selected. Other functions (e.g., high-low range) are also scanned. Single-switch scanning is time consuming and cognitively demanding and should be considered for power wheelchair control only after other options have been excluded.

Controllers. A *power wheelchair controller* connects the control interface to the drive system. This component is the processor in the assistive technology component of our HAAT model. Figure 12-16 shows a typical wheelchair controller. In a proportional drive system the controller determines the amount of voltage to supply to the motor by the amount of deflection in the joystick, and this voltage is directly related to motor speed. In a switched control system this type of proportionality is not obtained from the control interface. To allow the wheelchair to accelerate gradually (as the user with a proportional control would do),

the controller provides a gradual acceleration when any direction is selected. In most controllers the rate of acceleration can be adjusted to meet the consumer's needs. For example, an expert power wheelchair user could have the acceleration set on the high end so that the chair is highly responsive, whereas a novice user could set the rate of acceleration slower to allow for a slower start. The rate of deceleration (braking) can also be adjusted. Deceleration is the swiftness with which the wheelchair comes to a stop once the control interface is deactivated. With these two features on a controller, it is possible to set one rate for acceleration and a different rate for braking.

Controllers also provide either momentary or latched switch control. In *momentary control* the motors are activated only while the switch is pressed, which provides the greatest control for the user. Some consumers are unable to maintain switch activation, but they can press and release quickly. In this case *latched control* is used. In this mode, when the switch is pressed once, the motors turn on and remain on. When the switch is pressed again, the motors turn off. It is important that the consumer be able to activate the switch reliably and rapidly when it is in the latched mode, so as to stop quickly when necessary. This feature is often used with sip-and-puff switches. It allows the user to give a hard puff once to latch the control for the wheelchair to move either forward or backward and then use soft sips and puffs to turn left or right (Taylor and Kreutz, 1997).

Most powered wheelchair controllers are programmable by the user to some extent, which gives them much more flexibility and adjustability. Forward and reverse maximal speeds can be independently adjusted. On some devices the ratio of forward to reverse speed is selected. It is more difficult to control the wheelchair when turning than when going straight, and the controller feature that allows turning speed to be set independently of (or as a function of) forward speed is useful.

Some consumers have difficulty controlling their movements because of tremor, which can make the use of a joystick or other wheelchair control interface difficult. To accommodate for tremor, an averaging feature is incorporated into some controllers. The averaging system effectively damps out the tremor by ignoring small rapid movements and responding to larger, slower ones (Aylor et al, 1979). The disadvantage of this approach is that the system can become sluggish, resulting in reduced capability to respond to obstacles quickly. This feature is sometimes referred to as the *sensitivity* or *tremor dampening* of the controller.

Another adjustment allowed by the controller is the ability to alter the degree of range of motion required for an individual to operate a control interface. This is called the *short throw adjustment* and is most commonly used with joysticks. This feature is useful for consumers who have limited range of motion at the control site that is being used. Some current controller models have an LED display that visually represents the different functions and the results of adjustments as they are made.

Computer-based controllers allow the storage of a set of values for parameters such as those described earlier. These parameters can then be recalled for use in a particular situation (e.g., outdoors on a hill or indoors on a smooth floor). A therapist working with a consumer to gradually develop driving skills can also store the setups and recall them when needed. In training or assessment settings where several consumers may use one powered wheelchair, there can be different configurations stored for each consumer. Most power wheelchair controllers also have provision for the attachment of an "attendant control," which is very useful for training. This control can override the user's control interface in an emergency situation.

Another feature of many controllers is the ability to operate different functions of the wheelchair or other devices with the same control interface. Generally, an output from the controller is connected to the external device (e.g., an augmentative communication system or electronic aid to daily living). These outputs may be called *auxiliary* or *ECU* on different commercial wheelchair controllers. By using a switch, the user is able to transfer the output of the controller from the motors to the external device. The control interface is then able to control the external device directly. A visual display identifies which function is being used. For example, if a joystick were being used for mobility, then switching to communication would allow directed scanning (see Chapter 7) to be used for selections on an augmentative communication device.

A switch would allow the user to change between these two operations.

Batteries.   The power for a power wheelchair is supplied by a pair of batteries that are mounted under the seat of the chair. The batteries used are rechargeable lead-acid types. The name comes from the suspension of lead plates in a solution of sulfuric acid. There are two plates. The positive terminal is called the cathode and the negative plate is the anode; the size of the plates determines how much current can be drawn from the plate. When the wheelchair controller and motors are attached to the battery and turned on, current is drawn out of the battery, which causes current to flow from the negative terminal to the positive terminal. Inside the battery, chemicals from the acid solution are deposited on the plates. When a majority of the chemicals have moved out of the solution, the battery is discharged. Applying an external current to the battery terminals with a battery charger reverses the process and causes the deposited materials to move back into solution, which recharges the battery.

Batteries differ in several ways. Automobile batteries require a high current for a short period to start the car. Wheelchair batteries, on the other hand, require smaller amounts of current for a longer time. This difference is reflected in the use of *deep-cycle* lead-acid batteries for power wheelchairs. These have thicker plates, which allow them to provide current for longer periods. The chemicals inside the battery may be in a liquid form, called a *wet cell*, or in a semisolid form, called a *gel*. Wet-cell batteries are less expensive and last longer; however, they are more hazardous and require more maintenance than gel batteries so are less commonly used for powered wheelchairs. The fluid in wet-cell batteries is subject to spilling and evaporation. Replacement of the fluid with distilled water is required at regular intervals. Gel (often called *sealed*) batteries will not spill, which makes them more desirable for transportation. They do not require any maintenance other than keeping them charged. These batteries are typically allowed on public transportation systems, whereas the wet cell batteries often are not. They do not need to be fully discharged before they require recharging. They do not have a "memory," which means that the battery capacity is not limited by previous recharges. Battery power between charges is determined by the capacity measured in ampere-hours. At room temperature, wheelchair batteries commonly have 30 to 90 ampere-hours capacity at 12 volts (Cooper, 1998). The type of motors, environmental conditions (e.g., extremes of temperature), and amount of regular maintenance can all affect battery life and performance. Different batteries require different types of chargers, and it is imperative that the correct battery charger be used. The technology for wheelchair batteries has changed very little over the years.

Smaller, lighter-weight batteries with an increase in capacity would help to decrease the weight of power wheelchairs and increase the distance that the user can travel on one charge.

ANSI/RESNA standards identify a test method for determining the capacity of wheelchair batteries on a single charge. This test requires the chair to be driven at maximum speed around a 54.5 m track 10 times in each direction. Amperes per hour are measured and the theoretical maximum distance is calculated from this measurement (ANSI/RESNA, 1998). Rentschler et al (2004) indicate that this test does not take into account the varying draw on battery power when the user travels up hill, in different weather conditions or across different terrains, for example. Information on the theoretical distance of a battery is vital information because serious injury or death could result from a power wheelchair user who is stranded by a dead battery.

Ventilators.   Consideration must be given to the placement and movement of a ventilator when the power wheelchair user is dependent for respiratory support. Like many other products, ventilators have become much more compact and streamlined in recent years, yet they still affect the overall length, weight, and center of mass of the chair. Ventilators can be mounted low on the base of the chair or on a frame that is attached to the vertical uprights of the back. Mounts for ventilators can be fixed or articulating. The orientation of the ventilator is congruent with that of the wheelchair seat in a fixed mount. An articulating mount is required with tilt or recline features of the seating system. This option maintains the vertical orientation of the ventilator as the seat moves in tilt or recline modes. Further, it keeps the ventilator out of the way of the chair batteries.

Specialized Bases for Manual Wheelchairs

The major wheelchair characteristics have been described; now dependent mobility bases that have unique structural and propelling characteristics will be discussed. Because an attendant or care provider is responsible for pushing the consumer in a dependent-mobility wheelchair, special attention is given to making this action as easy as possible. Items normally required for independent manual mobility (e.g., large rear wheels with hand rims) are often omitted in these systems. Bases for dependent mobility are commonly lighter in weight and lower priced than wheelchairs for independent manual mobility (Trefler et al, 1993).

Stroller Bases.   *Strollers,* similar to those used for transporting very young children, are typically of two types: (1) umbrella folding with a sling seat and (2) full-sized units with solid seats (Trefler et al, 1993). Although originally designed for children, there are now strollers that accommodate consumers who weigh up to 200 pounds. The umbrella type generally does not provide good sitting support, but it folds easily for storage in a vehicle. Consumers who use strollers should not be transported in the stroller unless it has been crash tested (Kemper, 1993). The lightweight construction of some units makes the attachment of solid seating systems difficult; however, on other units it is possible to attach seating components. Some of these seating components can be removed from the stroller base and used as car seats.

More solidly built stroller bases that can accommodate specialized seating systems (see Chapter 6) are available from several manufacturers. In some cases these systems have provision for growth. The most common approach is to use a frame large enough to accommodate a few years' growth and then add components that keep the child in a stable and functional position.

Another attraction of stroller bases is that they resemble standard strollers in appearance, which can be appealing to parents. One feature that appeals to parents is the ease with which they can be transported. The small wheels and short wheelbase of most strollers makes them easily maneuverable by an attendant. One disadvantage of the stroller is that the child is often in a reclined position, which may limit his ability to carry out functional tasks. Strollers are sometimes purchased as a second wheelchair to facilitate transportation, with a standard wheelchair used for functional tasks.

Transport Wheelchairs.   Transport wheelchairs are designed for occasional use, often available for transporting patients in hospitals or in short-term situations such as traversing an airport or shopping mall. They typically have upholstery seating and four small wheels. They do not have any adjustability nor is it anticipated that seating systems will be used. They are lightweight, durable, and relatively maintenance free. These chairs provide a dependent mobility option and are not intended to provide seating and positioning in the long term.

Wheelchairs for Use by Older Clients. The setup of a manual wheelchair for regular use by an older client is different from that of a younger, more active user. Age-related disabilities such as arthritis, osteoporosis, and osteopenia contribute to reduced muscle strength and range of motion. Further, older clients may feel less secure in their movements. Age-related visual changes, including disorders such as age-related macular degeneration and glaucoma, are further considerations for setup of a chair for use by an older client. Care should be taken to ensure that the center of gravity ratio of the client to the axis of the drive wheel provides an optimal stability and mobility balance. Access to the drive wheels and hand rims relative to range of motion and strength in the upper extremities needs to be considered along with rolling resistance. Effects of visual-perceptual changes resulting from a cerebral vascular accident will affect the user's ability to navigate in the environment and will need to be considered when providing training in wheelchair skills.

Some manufacturers are producing chairs that have a rocking feature. Often these chairs have a tilt feature as well. A mechanism on the chair allows the user to rock the seat of the chair. This mechanism can be disengaged in some situations, such as transportation, when it is not desired. This feature is recommended for clients who become agitated with the view that the rocking motion is calming for the client.

Wheelchairs for Bariatric Clients.

Bariatric clients, those individuals with a BMI of 30 or greater, were identified as a population with an increasing prevalence in North America. These individuals require frames that are designed to accommodate their weights and their larger sizes. Most typical wheelchairs have a maximum weight capacity of 300 pounds. Chairs for bariatric clients accommodate a maximum weight of 600 pounds, with some manufacturers offering chairs that will accommodate up to 1000 pounds (Daus, 2003). The location of the mechanics of electrically powered wheelchairs beneath the seat allows the use of a larger seat while still maintaining as narrow a width as possible. Some chairs provide user adjustable seat depth and width. Tilt is also an option that can be provided for the bariatric client. The Eclipse (Figure 12-17) is an example of a chair designed for bariatric clients.

Fitting a wheelchair for a bariatric client has special considerations because soft tissue distribution and accumulation are varied, resulting in different body sizes and shapes

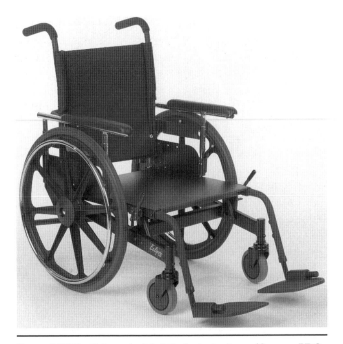

Figure 12-17 Eclipse wheelchair for bariatric clients. (Courtesy PDG Mobility.)

(Daus, 2003). Measurement should be done with the client in the seated position, on a firm surface. If there is significant soft tissue accumulation around the buttocks, the configuration of the seat back must be considered because the buttocks may protrude further than the shoulders, requiring the individual to lean back if the upper back is to be in contact with the seat back. Some manufacturers produce a back that provides support along the entire back surface. A change in the width of the back from hip to shoulder to accommodate a different shape is another accommodation made by some manufacturers.

Specialized Bases for Electrically Powered Wheelchairs

iBOT Mobility System.

A significantly different approach to powered mobility is incorporated in the INDEPENDENCE 4000 iBOT mobility system, shown in Figure 12-18. In this approach an electronic balance system is used, which allows the mobility system to be customized for a user's size, weight, and center of gravity. By use of a complex set of gyroscopes and computer-controlled electronics, the INDEPENDENCE 4000 constantly adjusts its position to ensure that the user remains balanced and stable regardless of the terrain, movements of the user, or functions of the device. There are five functions for the device: standard, four-wheel, stair, balance, and remote. In its standard function the INDEPENDENCE 4000 drive wheels are in the rear position. In its four-wheel function (Figure 12-18, *A* and *B*), the INDEPENDENCE 4000 can navigate uneven surfaces, travel through sand and gravel, and climb over street curbs. In each of these activities the user is kept in a horizontal position and is balanced and stable. This function significantly expands the recreational options for users because they can visit the beach, go over hiking trails, and cross grass fields. Uneven pavement, cobblestone sidewalks, and other similar obstacles can also be navigated with the INDEPENDENCE 4000 in four-wheel function. In the stair function (Figure 12-18, *C)* the INDEPENDENCE 4000 is able to go up or down flights of stairs, although users must have sufficient upper extremity strength to stabilize themselves with handrails. If the user lacks this capability, a trained assistant can provide the necessary help for stair climbing.

The most unique feature of the INDEPENDENCE 4000 is its balance function (Figure 12-18, *D*). In this function the INDEPENDENCE 4000 uses its control system to balance the system on two wheels, which has several advantages. First, the user is raised to eye level, a significant factor for many individuals with mobility needs. Second, the balance function allows the user to reach objects on shelves, to reach the back of counters, and to generally function in a manner closer to that of standing. While in balance function, the INDEPENDENCE 4000 can be controlled by the joystick interface, just like a power wheelchair.

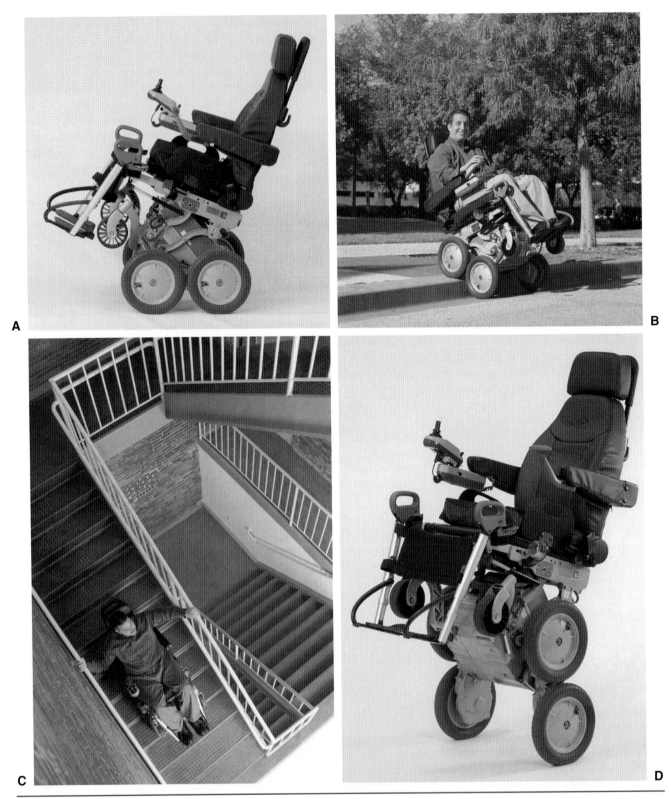

Figure 12-18   INDEPENDENCE® iBOT® Mobility System. **A,** Standard function. **B,** Four-wheel function. **C,** Stair function. **D,** Balance function. (Courtesy Independence Technology, a Johnson & Johnson Company.)

Finally, remote function allows the user to transfer out of the INDEPENDENCE 4000, fold down the seat, and unlatch the control interface (joystick, keypad, and display). The INDEPENDENCE 4000 is tethered to the control with a cable and can be "driven" slowly, which allows the user to drive the INDEPENDENCE 4000 into the rear of a van (up a ramp with up to a 25-degree slope) for transportation.

Eligibility criteria have been established for purchase of the INDEPENDENCE 4000 on the basis of physical needs either required to operate the device or that exclude the safe use of the device (i.e., physical needs of the consumer that cannot be accommodated by the device). Requirements for safe operation of the device include a weight range of 75 to 250 pounds and ability to operate a push button telephone and control a joystick. Needs or functions of the user that exclude their use of the iBOT mobility system include need for tilt and recline, use of a ventilator, inability to sit upright and reach the foot plates, and bone conditions that place the individual at high risk for fracture (Independence Technology, 2005).

A small study has been completed that evaluated the ability of individuals with disabilities to safely and effectively use the device and to determine whether it improved

function (Uustal and Minkel, 2004). Twenty subjects with a variety of disabling conditions who regularly used a mobility device participated in the study. The INDEPENDENCE 3000 was used for a period of 2 weeks after successful completion of a training program for the device. Outcome measures included the number of reported adverse events and the Community Driving Test, which was designed for this study. Comparison was made between performance with the iBOT mobility system and their typical devices. No difference was found for reported adverse events. The four-wheel drive and stair-climbing options provided significantly better function than the users' typical devices (Uustal and Minkel, 2004). This study provides preliminary support for the benefits of this device. A large multicenter evaluation is currently in progress.

Customizable Electrically Powered Wheelchairs. The range and combinations of features available on electrically powered wheelchairs is rapidly increasing. Some of these features, such as tilt, recline, elevating seats, and footrests have been mentioned already. The Attitude and the Latitude systems (Figure 12-19, *A* and *B*) both provide power

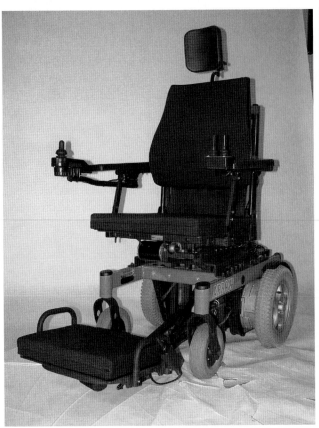
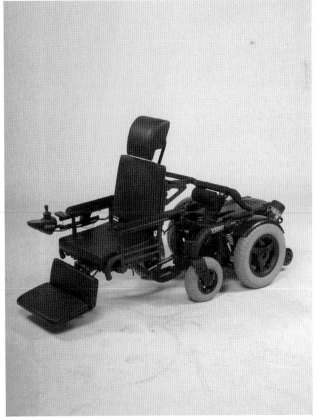

A   **B**

Figure 12-19   Attitude and Latitude electrically powered wheelchair systems that allow the user to transfer independently from the floor to the chair. **A,** Attitude. **B,** Latitude. (Courtesy Motion Concepts.)

options to enable independent transfers. The Attitude has a foot platform that lowers to the ground and then raises up to seat height, allowing an individual to transfer independently. To transfer into the chair, the foot platform is lowered to the floor; the user transfers onto the foot platform, raises it to seat height, and then transfers on to the seat. The Latitude system is similar, but the entire seat moves forward and down to the floor.

Smart Wheelchairs.   Smart technology is being incorporated into wheelchairs to provide additional options for individuals who are unable to control a wheelchair in other ways. **Smart wheelchairs** are defined as "either a standard power wheelchair to which a computer and a collection of sensors have been added or a mobile robot base to which a seat has been attached" (Simpson, 2005, p. 424). These technologies are useful for wheelchair users who have low vision or a severely restricted visual field, motor impairments such as excessive tone or tremor, or cognitive impairments that limit their ability to navigate a wheelchair safely. Smart technologies can be integrated into the available power system or built as an add-on feature (Simpson, 2005).

Smart wheelchairs typically provide three functions: collision avoidance, navigation along walls or through doorways, and navigation from one place to another. In the latter situation, the wheelchair has an internal map of the individual's environment, allowing the user to move from one programmed start place to an end point. The user must have some control of the chair because collision avoidance is not a feature with this navigation function. Input to the system is through a joystick or other control interfaces as described earlier, voice input, or more sophisticated means such as perception of head position or eye gaze. The NavChair (Levine et al, 1999) is one example of a wheelchair that uses smart technology. It has three functions: collision avoidance, navigation through a doorway, and travel along a wall.

Four main types of sensors are used to guide the chair: infrared (see Chapter 14 for a further explanation of this type of sensor), sonar (sound wave technology), laser range finders, and computer vision (Simpson, 2005). As might be anticipated, the cost of these systems is extremely high and consequently they are very limited in their commercial availability. Most of their use is in a research setting at this time. Like the sophisticated sensor and navigation technology for the automobile, however, this technology is becoming increasingly more accessible, so we can anticipate that these functions will be available in the future.

Scooters.   **Scooter** wheelchairs (Figure 12-20) comprise a large proportion of the electrically powered systems on the market. Individuals who are marginal ambulators and need mobility to conserve energy most often use the scooter. For this reason, it is most commonly used by the consumer outside the home. Grocery stores and shopping malls often provide scooters for customers who may need them. The propelling structure of the scooter includes the drive train, the tires, the tiller, and the battery. There are a number of models available, in either three- or four-wheel versions, with front-wheel drive or rear-wheel drive. Scooters with front-wheel drive do better on level terrain and are more maneuverable. For this reason, they perform better in small spaces. In rear-wheel drive scooters, the rider's weight is positioned over the motor, so there is better traction and more power. The bases of rear-wheel drive scooters are wider and longer than the other powered chairs. These scooters are better able to handle inclines and uneven or rough terrain and therefore are preferable for outdoor use.

A tiller-type control is used to steer the wheelchair, and acceleration is accomplished by either grasping a lever on the tiller with the fingers or pressing with the thumb. When the accelerator is released, the scooter eases to a stop. On some scooters the height and angle of the tiller is adjustable. Depending on the model, scooters can have either proportional (variable speed) control or switched (constant speed) control. There is a separate control setting for adjusting the speed of the scooter. Some scooters have a dial that provides a range of settings, whereas others have a toggle switch for high and low.

The seat of the scooter is mounted to a single post coming up from the base. Typically the seat is a bucket type that has few options for seat width, depth, or back height (Toonstra and Barnicle, 1993). The seats come in padded or unpadded versions, and several types of armrest styles (fixed, flip-up, or none) are available. In the past, if a person needed a specialized seating or positioning system, it was not possible to interface it to a scooter. There are now some scooters that can accommodate specialized seating equipment. On most scooters there is a mechanism that releases the seat so it can swivel to the side and then locks it in place again. This feature is helpful for transfers in and out of the seat and for accessing a table surface.

Some of the advantages of scooters are that they are lighter in weight, can be disassembled for transportation in a car, are easy to maneuver, are less costly than other power wheelchairs, and are more acceptable than other types of power wheelchairs. The primary disadvantage of scooters is that they do not provide flexibility in control interfaces. The consumer needs to have a fair amount of trunk and upper extremity control to operate the tiller of the scooter. Scooters also have very little flexibility in terms of speed, braking, or turning control. Finally, the seat of a scooter typically does not provide adequate postural support, and many types of seating systems needed by individuals with postural control problems cannot be interfaced to a scooter.

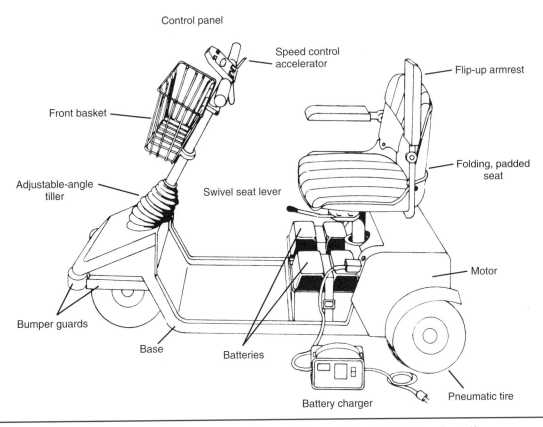

Control panel

Speed control
accelerator

Flip-up armrest

Front basket

Folding, padded
seat

Adjustable-angle
tiller

Swivel seat lever

Motor

Bumper guards

Base

Batteries

Battery charger

Pneumatic tire

Figure 12-20   An electrically powered scooter. (Courtesy National Rehabilitation Hospital.)

Power-assist Mechanisms. Considerable attention has been given to the shoulder injuries that result from prolonged propulsion of a manual wheelchair (for example see Boninger et al, 2002, 2005; Cooper et al, 1997b; Sawatsky et al, 2005; Veeger et al, 2002). One option for individuals with shoulder pain that limits the ability to propel a manual wheelchair but for whom an electrically powered wheelchair is not desirable is push rim–activated power-assist wheels. These wheels are interchanged with those of a manual wheelchair. A motor is located in the hub of the rear wheels that is linked to the hand rims (Algood et al, 2005). These units supply power to the manual wheelchair as needed by the user. When the user applies force above a preset level to the hand rims, such as when going up an incline, the motors engage and help to propel the wheelchair. Propulsion and braking assistance are provided for both forward and rearward motion. The unit can also be turned off, which allows the manual wheelchair to function in the usual manner. These units add considerable weight to a manual chair, which is a consideration in their selection.

A new product on the market with a similar purpose is Magic Wheels, which provides geared technology for manual wheelchairs (Figure 12-21). Magic Wheels gives the user a

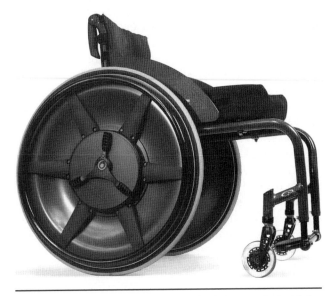

Figure 12-21   Magic Wheels multigear wheels for manual wheelchair. (Courtesy Magic Wheels, Inc.)

selection of two gears, similar to the concept of bicycle gears, with the second gear providing a 2:1 mechanical advantage. The user selects the second gear by moving the housing of the gear, located on the hub of the wheel. Changing gears does not require grip or substantial strength. Magic Wheels are most useful on inclines, where they provide assistance propelling upward and braking when traveling downward. Finley et al (2006) completed a pilot study of the effect of Magic Wheels use on shoulder pain, length of time the user was able to sustain uphill travel, and perceived exertion during this task. An A-B-A design was used, with baseline being use of consumer's typical wheels. After 4 months of use, shoulder pain was stable or reduced, and users were able to travel uphill for a longer time with no change in perceived exertion.

Wheelchair Standards

As discussed in Chapter 1, *standards* can be used to provide manufacturing guidance to ensure product quality. One area of assistive technologies in which standards have been developed is for wheelchairs. Both the International Standards Organization (ISO) and ANSI and RESNA have published standards for manual and power wheelchairs, seating systems, and wheelchair use during transportation. There is considerable overlap in these standards. A comparison of the ISO and ANSI/RESNA standards is shown in Box 12-3. Although these standards are voluntary, there are strong motivations for manufacturers to adhere to them. For example, the Department of Veterans Affairs (VA) has purchasing requirements for wheelchairs. As the largest purchaser of wheelchairs in the United States, the VA could significantly affect compliance with the standards shown in Box 12-3 by adopting them by reference, rather than developing their own standards. Some published studies exist that have applied these standards to manual and electrically powered wheelchairs and seating cushions (for example, see Cooper et al 1997a, 1999; Fass et al, 2004; Pearlman et al, 2005; Rentschler et al, 2004; Sprigle and Press, 2003).

■ IMPLEMENTATION AND TRAINING FOR MANUAL AND POWERED MOBILITY

As we have emphasized throughout this text, the assistive technology system includes much more than a piece of equipment. For the consumer to be satisfied and successful with an assistive device, proper implementation and training need to be part of the system. The same holds true to maximize the performance of consumers who use mobility systems.

BOX 12-3 — Comparison of ISO and ANSI/RESNA Wheelchair Standards

Standard	ISO	ANSI/RESNA
Nomenclature, terms, and definitions	✓	✓
Determination of static stability	✓	✓
Determination of overall dimensions, mass, and turning space	✓	✓
Determination of seating and wheel dimensions		✓
Static, impact, and fatigue strengths	✓	✓
Test dummies		✓
Determination of coefficient of friction of test surfaces	✓	✓
Requirements for information disclosures, documentation, and labeling	✓	✓
Determination of flammability	✓	✓
Wheelchairs used as seats in motor vehicles		✓
Wheeled mobility devices for use in motor vehicles	✓	
Determination of performance of stand-up wheelchairs		✓
Setup procedures	✓	✓
Maximum overall dimensions	✓	✓
Determination of dynamic stability of electric wheelchairs	✓	✓
Determination of efficiency of brakes	✓	✓
Energy consumption of electric wheelchairs and scooters for determination of theoretical distance range (ISO)	✓	✓
Determination of maximum speed, acceleration and retardation of electric wheelchair	✓	✓
Climatic tests for electric wheelchairs	✓	✓
Determination of obstacle climbing ability for electric wheelchairs	✓	✓
Testing of power and control systems for electric wheelchairs	✓	✓
Requirements and test methods for electromagnetic components of power wheelchairs and motorized scooters	✓	✓
Requirements and test methods for attendant-operated stair-climbing devices	✓	
Requirements and test methods for user-operated stair-climbing devices	✓	

Fitting of Mobility Systems

It is advisable that a fitting appointment be held with the consumer and caregiver. The purpose of this appointment is to make any adjustments needed to the wheelchair and to try the chair and determine whether it meets the original objectives outlined during the assessment. During the initial fitting, time should also be spent demonstrating to the user and the care giver important features of the chair and going through instructions for maintenance. Box 12-4 shows a checklist of items to be covered during the fitting process for either a manual or power wheelchair. Depending on the complexity of the wheelchair and whether seating components are involved, more than one fitting appointment may be necessary.

Because today's wheelchairs are often multifunctional, a number of components on the wheelchair are adjustable. Some adjustments and settings are made in the factory before shipping, but typically the provider of the wheelchair will need to make modifications to fit the chair to the user once it arrives from the factory. Adjustments to the wheelchair that can make a difference in user comfort, safety, and performance include axle position, wheel camber, and wheel alignment. Appropriate adjustment of the seat angle, back height and angle, and height and angle of leg rests and footrests are also critical to user performance. Cooper (1998) and Ham, Aldersea, and Porter (1998) describe in detail how to make each of these adjustments. Any adjustments to the chair should be made carefully and with the user's safety in mind. After adjustments are made, the user should be cautious in trying out the wheelchair until he or she becomes acclimated to the changes.

BOX 12-4   Checklist for Wheelchair Fitting Process

Seating position
Position of control interface
Transfer method
Indoors: size, obstacles, doorways, turning circle
Outdoors: curbs, soft grass, rough ground, inclines
Distance required to travel
Maneuverability in community
Lights, horn
Care provider's training
Assembly and disassembly
Charging method
Battery life and maintenance
Transport in personal and public vehicles
Storage
Maintenance and repair

Modified from Ham R, Aldersea P, Porter D: *Wheelchair users and postural seating: a clinical approach*, p. 238, New York, 1998, Churchill Livingstone.

Maintenance and Repair of Personal Mobility Systems

Wheelchairs are designed to be low maintenance, and there are few items on a wheelchair, particularly a manual wheelchair, that require maintenance by the user (Cooper, 1998). The user is responsible for keeping the chair clean, the tires properly inflated, and the brakes properly adjusted and for seeing that the wheelchair is inspected on a regular basis. The user of an electrically powered wheelchair needs to ensure that the correct battery for the wheelchair is used and that it is properly charged. A checklist of items that wheelchair users should monitor or have monitored regularly is shown in Box 12-5. The user manual for the wheelchair will also specify a schedule for periodic inspection and maintenance. A reputable assistive technology supplier should complete any maintenance that needs to be done on the wheelchair.

Developing Mobility Skills for Manual and Powered Systems

Training in mobility skills can occur before and after the delivery of the final chair to the consumer. In situations where it is undetermined which chair is most suitable for the consumer or whether the consumer will be able to operate the wheelchair, a trial period takes place. During the trial period the person is loaned or leased a wheelchair, either manual or power, which allows the consumer to test the chair and determine whether it is appropriate to meet his or her needs. Often, particularly with powered mobility, this trial involves a period of training to determine whether the person can develop the skills to use the wheelchair. For example, powered mobility may be identified as a goal, but the individual may not yet have the skills required to control a power wheelchair safely. If there is any question, it is best to delay making an expensive equipment purchase and risking the safety of the user and others. It is important that the potential user develop these skills through a training program before permanently acquiring the device. Implementation does not always end with the consumer's acquisition of the device. In many cases, further training sessions are necessary. In development of either manual or powered mobility skills, it is important to set specific, measurable objectives for training.

For manual mobility, basic skills include maneuvering the wheelchair indoors on a level surface, in and around tight spaces, and over surfaces such as carpet, tile, or linoleum. For the active user of a manual wheelchair, preparation in advanced wheelchair mobility skills is suggested. These include the ability to negotiate rough, uneven terrain; propel up and down ramps and curbs

BOX 12-5   Checklist for Basic Wheelchair Maintenance

On Receipt	Weekly	Monthly	Periodically	
				GENERAL
•			•	Wheelchair opens and folds easily
•	•			Wheelchair rolls straight with no excess drag or pull
•			•	Footrests flip up/down easily
•			•	Legrests swing away and latch easily
•			•	Backrest folds and latches easily
•			•	Armrests easy to move and latch
•			•	All nuts and bolts are snug
				WHEELS
•			•	Axle threads in easily or slides in and latches properly
•	•			No squeaking, binding, or excessive side Motion while turning
•			•	All spokes and nipples are tight and not bent or nicked
•	•			Tire pressure is correct and equal on both sides
•		•		No cracks, looseness, bulges in tires
				CASTERS
•		•		No cracks, looseness, or bulges in caster tires
•	•			No wobbling of caster wheel
•	•			No excessive play in the caster spindle
•	•			Caster housing is aligned vertically
				WHEEL LOCKS
•		•		Do not interfere with tire when rolling
•	•			Easily activated and released by operator
•	•			Hold tires firmly in place while activated
				ELECTRICAL SYSTEM
•			•	Wires show no cracks, splits, or breaks
•	•			Indicators and horn work properly
•	•			Controls work smoothly and repeatedly
•		•		Battery cases are clean and free from fluids
•			•	Motor runs smoothly and quietly
				UPHOLSTERY
•			•	No tears, rips, burn marks, or excessive fraying
•		•		No excessive stretching (e.g., hammocking)
•	•			Upholstery is clean

From Cooper RA: *Wheelchair selection and configuration*, New York, 1998, Demos Medical Publishing.

independently; and execute "wheelies." The Manual Wheelchair Training Guide (Axelson et al, 1998) provides information on basic wheelchair setup and maneuvering the wheelchair in indoor and outdoor environments.

One well-researched training program, the Wheelchair Skills Program (Kirby, 2005), is available from *www.wheelchairskillsprogram.ca*. This program was developed in conjunction with the Wheelchair Skills Test (Kirby et al, 2002, 2004). The program teaches wheelchair users basic use of the wheelchair, such as applying and releasing the brakes, removing footrests, and folding the chair.

It teaches basic propulsion such as rolling forward and backward, turning, and maneuvering through doorways. More advanced skills include propulsion on an incline, level changes, performance of a wheelie, and various wheelie skills. Skills are classified as indoor, community, or advanced (Kirby, 2005).

As with the skills required for driving an automobile, successful powered mobility use requires training and practice, which applies to everyone who uses a power wheelchair. A systematic approach that develops these skills and progresses in small increments is most likely to be successful.

As with manual mobility, the training in powered mobility skills should progress from basic skills to more complex skills and situations. Some schools purchase a power wheelchair that can be used with various control interfaces and seating systems. It is then possible to use the wheelchair with different children for training as needed. For young children, it is recommended that training be fun, starting with a toy cart and moving to a wheelchair base as appropriate (Barnes, 1991). Many children's games can be adapted to develop skills needed in powered mobility training, such as "red light, green light" for learning how to stop on command. Computer activities can also apply to the development of powered mobility skills; these are discussed in Chapter 7.

The development of powered mobility skills in young children can be described as progressing in three stages: stage I, exploratory; stage II, directive; and stage III, purposeful (Janeschild, 1997). In stage I, the exploratory stage, the child is encouraged to explore mobility in an environment that is safe and motivating. The goal is for the child to explore and learn how to control the mobility device. The trainer gives verbal feedback as it relates to what the child is doing at the moment and only to reinforce simple mobility concepts; for example, "You are moving *closer* to your mommy." The purpose of this stage is to minimize the amount of verbal direction given to the child and to maximize the child's interest in interacting with the environment. During stage II, the directive

stage, the goal is for the child to use the mobility device to move in the general area of a target. In the purposeful stage (stage III), the skills learned by the child are applied to home and school contexts in which more constraints are placed on the situation. Janeschild (1997) presents a tool for documenting the child's progress through the three stages.

■ SUMMARY

Mobility is very important for participation in self-care, home, work, school, and leisure activities. Mobility needs for individuals with disabilities vary depending on the age and the disability status of the user. In this chapter we describe the general characteristics of personal mobility systems and the various types of mobility devices available to meet individual needs of the user. Personal mobility devices fall under the categories of independent manual, dependent manual, and powered mobility. Both manual and electrically powered wheelchair options were described. With the plethora of personal mobility options that are available, the ATP requires thorough assessment and evaluation processes, considering all the elements of the HAAT model, to ensure the most appropriate initial recommendation for and the continuing utility of the mobility device.

Study Questions

1. On the basis of consumer needs, what are the three categories of mobility bases?
2. What factors are considered as part of a wheelchair evaluation?
3. In what situations may powered mobility be considered?
4. What are the two major structures of a wheelchair?
5. Describe and contrast the advantages and disadvantages of tilt versus recline systems. What are the indications for the recommendation of each?
6. Discuss the relationship of the center of mass of the user to the center of mass of the wheelchair as it was described in the various sections of this chapter. What are the implications of this relationship to function?
7. What are the ways in which pediatric wheelchairs can accommodate growth?
8. List the four types of standing systems and give an advantage and disadvantage of each. What are the major benefits of these systems?

9. Describe the major considerations in choosing manual wheelchair tires, wheels, and casters. List the major options available for each.
10. Define camber and describe indications for its use and how it affects the function of a manual wheelchair.
11. Define bariatrics and discuss the implications of wheelchair prescription and configuration for this population.
12. Discuss the considerations of wheelchair prescription and configuration for elderly clients.
13. Identify the different locations of the drive wheels of an electrically powered wheelchair and describe how each affects the function of the chair.
14. What types of control interfaces are typically used for powered wheelchairs?
15. Delineate the major functions of a wheelchair controller. What additional features do computer-controlled units provide?
16. What special considerations are important in considering the inclusion of ventilators on a wheelchair?

17. What types of batteries are used in power wheelchairs? How do they differ from automobile batteries? What is the difference between wet cell and gel batteries?

18. Why are wheelchair standards important? Name three major elements covered in the wheelchair standards.

19. Describe what should happen during the implementation phase for a powered mobility device.

References

Algood SD et al: Effect of a pushrim-activated power-assist wheelchair on the functional capabilities of persons with tetraplegia, *Arch Phys Med Rehabil* 86: 380-386, 2005.

American National Standards Institute/Rehabilitation Engineering and Assistive Society of America: *Wheelchair standards: additional requirements for wheelchairs (including scooters) with electrical systems*, vol 2, New York, 1998, ANSI/RESNA.

Axelson P et al: *The manual wheelchair training guide*, Santa Cruz, CA, 1998, Pax Press.

Aylor J et al: Versatile wheelchair control system, *Med Biol Eng Comput* 17:110-114, 1979.

Barnes KH: Training young children for powered mobility, *Dev Disabil Spec Interest Sect Newsl* 14:, 1991.

Belanger A, Martel L, Caron-Malenfant E: *Population projections for Canada, provinces and territories, 2005-2031*, Ottawa, ON: 2005, Ministry of Industry.

Boninger M et al: Propulsion patterns and pushrim biomechanics in manual wheelchair propulsion, *Arch Phys Med Rehabil* 83:718-23, 2002.

Boninger M et al: Pushrim biomechanics and injury prevention in spinal cord injury: recommendations based on CULP-SCI investigations, *J Rehabil Res Dev* 42:9-20, 2005.

Bureau of the Census: U.S. interim projections by age, sex, race, and Hispanic origin, Table 2a, Projected population of the United States, by age and sex: 2000 to 2050 (March 2004): www.census.gov/ipc/www/usinterimproj/natprojtab02a.pdf. Accessed October 29, 2006.

Butler C: Wheelchair toddlers. In Furumasu J, editor: *Pediatric powered mobility: developmental perspectives, technical issues, clinical approaches*, Arlington, VA, 1997, RESNA Press.

Centers for Disease Control and Prevention: State-specific prevalence of obesity among adults—United States, 2005, *Morb Mortal Wkly Rep* 55(36):985-8, 2006.

Cole E: Selecting controls for power wheelchairs. In *Proceedings of the 20th International Seating Symposium*, pp. 179-187, 2004, Vancouver, British Columbia.

Cooper RA: *Wheelchair selection and configuration*, New York, 1998, Demos Medical Publishing.

Cooper RA et al: Performance of selected lightweight wheelchairs on ANSI/RESNA tests, *Arch Phys Med Rehabil* 78:1138-44, 1997a.

Cooper RA et al: Methods for determining three-dimensional wheelchair pushrim forces and moment—a technical note, *J Rehabil Res Dev* 38(1): 41-55, 1997b.

Cossette L: *A profile of disability in Canada, 2001*, Ottawa, ON, 2002, Ministry of Industry.

Daus C: The right fit, *Rehabilitation Management* (2003): http://www.rehabpub.com/features/892003/4.asp. Accessed October 31, 2006.

Denison I, Gayton D: Power wheelchairs selection (2002): http://www.assistive-technology.ca/newdef2.htm. Accessed October 28, 2006.

Deitz JC: Pediatric augmented mobility. In Gray DB, Quatrano LA, Lieberman ML, editors: *Designing and using assistive technology: the human perspective*, Baltimore, 1998, Paul H Brookes.

Eng JJ: Getting up goals, *Rehabilitation Management* (2004): http://rehabpub.com/features/1022004/5.asp. Accessed October 28, 2006.

Engstrom B: *Ergonomic seating: a true challenge*, Sweden, 2002, Posturalis Books.

Fass MV et al: Durability, value and reliability of selected electric powered wheelchairs, *Arch Phys Med Rehabil* 85:805-14, 2004.

Fields CD: Groundwork: Casters, *Team Rehabil Rep* 3:22-23, 33, 1992.

Finley MA et al: Effect of 2-speed manual wheelchair wheel on shoulder pain in wheelchair users: Preliminary findings. In *Proceedings of the 22nd International Seating Symposium*, 2006, Vancouver, British Columbia.

Ham R, Aldersea P, Porter D: *Wheelchair users and postural seating: a clinical approach*, New York, 1998, Churchill Livingstone.

Hobson DA: Seating and mobility for the severely disabled. In Smith RV, Leslie JH, editors: *Rehabilitation engineering*, Boca Raton, FL, 1990, CRC Press.

Independence Technology: iBOT Mobility System: FAQ: http://www.ibotnow.com/ibot/faq.html. Accessed November 4, 2006.

Janeschild M: Early power mobility: evaluation and training guidelines. In Furumasu J, editor: *Pediatric powered mobility:*

developmental perspectives, technical issues, clinical approaches, Arlington, VA, 1997, RESNA Press.

Kaye S, Kang T, LaPlante MP: Wheelchair use in the United States, *Disab Stat Abst* 23:1-4, 2002.

Kemper K: Strollers: a growing alternative, *Team Rehabil Rep* 4:15-19, 1993.

Kermoian R: Locomotor experience facilitates psychological functioning: implications for assistive mobility for young children. In Gray DB, Quatrano LA, Lieberman ML, editors: *Designing and using assistive technology*, Baltimore, 1998, Paul H Brookes.

Kirby RL: Wheelchair skills program v. 3.2 (2005): www.wheelchairskillsprogram.ca. Accessed October 30, 2006.

Kirby RL et al: The wheelchair skills test: a pilot study of a new outcome measure, *Arch Phys Med Rehabil* 83: 1298-1305, 2002.

Kirby RL et al: The Wheelchair Skills Test (version 2.4): measurement properties, *Arch Phys Med Rehabil* 85: 41-50, 2004.

Kreutz D: Power tilt, recline or both, *Team Rehabil Rep* 8:29-32, 1997.

Lacoste M et al: Identifying elderly wheelchair users' needs: results of a focus group. In *Proceedings of the RESNA '98 Annual Conference*, pp 158-160, 1998, Washington, DC, RESNA.

Lange M: Tilt in space versus recline: new trends in an old debate, *Tech Spec Int Sec Quart* 10:1-3, 2000.

Lange M: Power wheelchair access: assessment and alternative access methods. In *Proceedings of the 21st International Seating Symposium*, pp. 87-88, 2005, Orlando, FL.

Levine S et al: The NavChair assistive wheelchair navigation system, *ISEE Trans Rehabil Eng* 7:443-451, 1999.

Magnuson S: Annotated bibliography: powered mobility for young children with physical disabilities, *Phys Occup Ther Pediatr* 15:71-79, 1995.

Mogul-Rotman B, Fisher K: Stand up and function, *Rehabilitation Management* (2002): http://www.rehabpub. com/features/892002/3.asp. Accessed October 28, 2006.

Mortenson B et al: Perceptions of power mobility use and safety within residential facilities, *Can J Occup Ther* 72: 142-52, 2005.

Mortenson B et al: Overarching principles and salient findings for inclusion in guidelines for power mobility use within residential care facilities, *J Rehab Res Dev* 43: 199-208, 2006.

Pearlman JL et al: Evaluation of the safety and durability of low-cost non-programmable electric powered wheelchairs, *Arch Phys Med Rehabil* 86:2361-70, 2005.

Phillips K, Fisher K, Miller Polgar J: Thinking beyond the wheelchair. In *Proceedings of the 21st International Seating Symposium*, pp. 97-98, 2005, Orlando, FL.

Ragnarsson KT: Prescription considerations and a comparison of conventional and lightweight wheelchairs, *J Rehabil Res Dev Clin* (Suppl):8-16, 1990.

Rentschler et al: Evaluation of select electric-powered wheelchairs using the ANSI/RESNA standards, *Arch Phys Med Rehabil* 85:611-19, 2004.

Robson M: 25 Choices: Manual wheelchair configuration and new technology. In *Proceedings of the 20th Canadian Seating and Mobility Conference*, pp. 113, 2005, Toronto, Ontario.

Sawatsky BJ, Denison I, Kim WO: Rolling, rolling, rolling: *Rehabilitation Management*, (2005): http://www.rehabpub. com/features/892002/7.asp. Accessed October 29, 2006.

Sawatsky BJ et al: Prevalence of shoulder pain in adult- versus childhood-onset wheelchair users: a pilot study, *J Rehabil Res Dev* 42, 1-8, 2005.

Schmeler M, Bunning MJ: Manual wheelchairs: Set-up and propulsion biomechanics (1999): http://www.wheelchairnet. org/wcn_wcu/SlideLectures/MS/5WCBiomech.pdf. Accessed September 8, 2006.

Simpson R: Smart wheelchairs: A literature review, *J Rehab Res Dev* 42: 423-435, 2005.

Smith ME: The applications of tilt and recline (2004): http://www.wheelchairjunkie.com/tiltandrecline.html. Accessed October 28, 2006.

Sprigle S, Press L: Reliability of the ISO wheelchair cushion test for loaded contour depth, *Assist Tecnol* 15:145-150, 2003.

Taylor SJ, Kreutz D: Powered and manual wheelchair mobility. In Angelo J: *Assistive technology for rehabilitation therapists*, Philadelphia, 1997, FA Davis.

Toonstra M, Barnicle K: Focus on scooters, *Team Rehabil Rep* 4:24-26, 1993.

Trefler E, Cook H: Powered mobility for children. In Trefler E, Kozole K, Snell E, editors: *Selected readings on powered mobility for children and adults with severe physical disabilities*, Washington, DC, 1986, RESNA Press.

Trefler E, Kozole K, Snell E, editors: *Selected readings on powered mobility for children and adults with severe physical disabilities*, Washington, DC, 1986, RESNA Press.

Trefler E et al: *Seating and mobility for persons with physical disabilities*, Tucson, AZ, 1993, Therapy Skill Builders.

Trujillo EF: *History of the wheelchair*, ca. 1960, California Wheelchair Athletic Club.

Uusatal H, Minkel JL: Study of the Independence IBOT 3000 Mobility System: an innovative power mobility device, during use in community environments, *Arch Phys Med Rehabil* 85:2002-2010, 2004.

Veeger HEJ, Roxendaal LA, van der Helm FCT: Load on the shoulder in low intensity wheelchair propulsion, *Clin Biomech* 17:211-218, 2002.

Walter J, Dunn R: Taking a stand, *Team Rehabil Rep* 9:31-34, 1998.

Wang Q: *Disability and American families: 2000*, Washington, 2005, US Census Bureau.

Warren CG: Powered mobility and its implications, *J Rehabil Res Dev Clin Suppl* 27: 74-85, 1990.

Wilson B, McFarland SR: Types of wheelchairs, *J Rehabil Res Dev Clin Suppl* 27:104-116, 1990.

Wilson K, Miller Polgar J: The effects of wheelchair seat tilt on seated pressure distribution in adults without physical disabilities. In *Proceedings of the 21st International Seating Symposium*, pp. 115-116, 2005, Orlando, FL.

CHAPTER 13

Technologies That Aid Transportation

Chapter Outline

Learning Objectives

On completing this chapter you will be able to do the following:

1. Describe the correct use of child restraint systems for passenger safety
2. Describe the correct use of child restraint systems designed for children with special needs
3. Understand the basic features of standards for crashworthiness of wheelchairs and seating systems
4. Understand the use and basic features of standards for wheelchair tie-downs and occupant restraint systems
5. Identify the major components of driver evaluation
6. Identify the major components of driver retraining programs
7. Discuss major design features to consider when making a vehicle purchase
8. Discuss vehicle access issues for individuals with disabilities
9. Describe vehicle modifications to promote access for individuals with disabilities
10. Describe primary and secondary driving controls

Key Terms

Booster Seat
Child Vehicle Restraint System
Crashworthiness
Driving Evaluation
Forward-Facing Child Seat
Large Accessible Transit Vehicles

Original Equipment Manufacturer
Primary Driving Controls
Rear-Facing Infant Seat
Secondary Driving Controls
Universal Docking Interface
 Geometry

Vehicle Seat Belt Assembly
Wheelchair Tie-Down and Occupant
 Restraint System
Wheelchair Tie-Down System

Robert Murphy, a social anthropologist who described his experience with a spinal tumor in the book *The Body Silent*, eloquently describes how the loss of the ability to drive deprived him of the spontaneity to go places when he wanted. This chapter explores issues and technologies related to transportation.

> The inability to drive was more than a retreat from mobility, for it was one step away from spontaneity and the free exercise of will. Where as I could once act on whim and fancy, I now had to exercise planning and foresight. This was true of even the simplest of actions. (Murphy, 1990)

Chapter 12 focused on personal mobility systems, specifically manual and electrically powered wheelchairs, that afford individuals the ability to move within their immediate environments and for short distances between local environments. This chapter considers mobility systems that afford movement over longer distances, such as movement between home, school, work, and community sites such as shopping and leisure venues, as well as travel between communities. Our focus is on safe personal (car, van, etc.) and public transportation across the life span, including travel as a passenger or a driver. The technology aspects of driving will be considered here, but this chapter is not intended to provide a comprehensive discussion of driving assessment and rehabilitation.

■ SAFE TRANSPORTATION FOR CHILDREN

Legislation exists in most jurisdictions that requires children of certain weights and heights to travel in a **child vehicle restraint system.** The majority of jurisdictions require children weighing less than or equal to 40 pounds to be properly secured in a vehicle restraint system. An increasing number are also requiring the use of booster seats for children who weigh more than 40 pounds (e.g., the majority of the United States, three provinces in Canada, and the United Kingdom; legislation is pending in Australia). Many children with mild to moderate seating needs can safely sit in vehicle restraint systems that are produced for typical children who have no special seating needs, so these products will be discussed first, including their proper use and installation. The array of products is vast and constantly changing. The following discussion is general and readers should review specific requirements in their own jurisdictions, particularly those related to booster seats.

Vehicle Restraint Systems for Children

There are three main types of vehicle restraint systems for children: **rear-facing infant seats, forward-facing**

child seats, and **booster seats.** A number of Web sites provide access to up-to-date information on the proper use and installation of these devices for their specific jurisdictions (Box 13-1). The Canada Safety Council has the *Buckle Up Bears* education program. Daimler-Chrysler offers the Fit for a Kid program that provides free car seat inspections and determination of whether the vehicle restraint system is properly installed. In the United States, the National Highway Traffic Safety Association maintains current information on vehicle restraint systems. The American Academy of Pediatrics also provides current information on vehicle restraint systems, including those specifically for children with disabilities. Federal regulations exist that govern the structure and testing of vehicle restraint systems, including those for children with disabilities. In the United States, the Federal Motor Vehicle Safety Standards (FMVSS) group produces these regulations and in Canada they are produced by the Canadian Motor Vehicle Safety Standards (CMVSS) organization. Restraint systems that meet these regulations are labeled with a sticker identifying either FMVSS or CMVSS and the specific standard that the system has met. These regulations can be found at *http://www.nhtsa.dot.gov/cars/rules/rulings/ChildRestrSyst/Index.html* and *http://www.tc.gc.ca/acts-regulations/GENERAL/M/mvsa/regulations/rssr/rssr.htm* for U.S. or Canadian standards, respectively.

Rear-facing infant seats (Figure 13-1, *A*) are intended for use from the time the infant leaves the hospital after birth to the time he or she reaches 12 months and 22 pounds (10 kg). Although most vehicle restraint systems indicate a height and weight limit for the child, rear-facing infant vehicle restraint systems have an age and weight limit, which means that the child must be 12 months of age before he or she is turned to the forward-facing position. Infants younger than this age do not have sufficient head control and their bones are not sufficiently developed to withstand even a minor crash (American Academy of Pediatrics, 1996). A common error on the part of parents is to move a child to the next type of child vehicle restraint system too early (Ebell et al, 2003; Winston et al, 2000; Winston et al, 2004; Yakupcin, 2005). Many children reach the

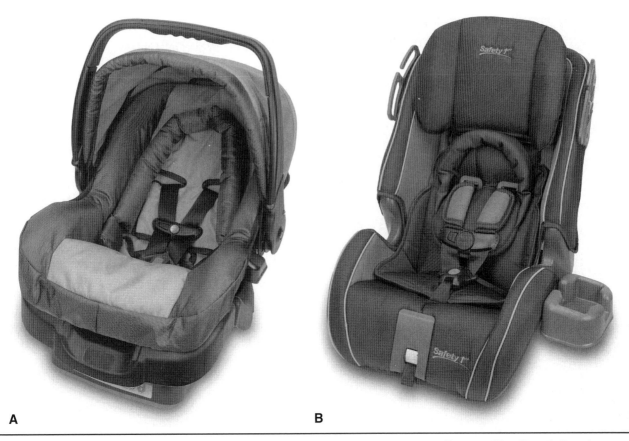

Figure 13-1   **A,** Rear-facing infant restraint system. **B,** Forward-facing child restraint system. (Courtesy of Dorel Juvenile Group.)

22 pound/10 kg weight limit well before their first birthdays. In this instance, they should be moved to a vehicle restraint system that will accommodate their heavier weight but will allow them to remain in the rear-facing position. Rear-facing infant seats are typically not left in the vehicle. Rather, the child is transported in the infant seat between the vehicle and destination. The car seat belt system provides restraint for the child and the seat inside the vehicle. Some seats secure into a base that remains installed in the vehicle over the long term.

Forward-facing vehicle restraint systems (Figure 13-1, *B*) are intended to be installed in a vehicle and remain for the long term. These systems accommodate children up to and including 40 pounds and 40 inches. Proper installation of these systems is critical. A biomechanical study of the demands of installation of a forward-facing vehicle restraint system found that proper installation required efforts that exceeded maximal force output for many participants and postures that limited the force that could be produced, particularly in the shoulder. Further, the configuration of the vehicle interior resulted in postures that put parents at risk for low back injury (Fox, Sarno, and Potvin, 2004; Sarno, Fox, and Potvin, 2004).

Two errors are common when installing the forward-facing car seat: (1) nonuse or misuse of the tether strap and

(2) improper use of the strapping system of the restraint system (Kohn, Chausme, and Flood, 2000; Lang, Lui, and Newlin, 2000). These seats all fasten to the vehicle frame with a tether strap. All new vehicles are equipped with tether anchors. The tether strap must be fastened and tightened so that an excursion of the restraint system of no more than ½ inch is allowed. The strapping component of the restraint system should be snug to the seat with the chest buckle about two fingerwidths below the child's neck. Often these straps are loose, allowing the child to wiggle free of them. Since 2002 vehicles have been equipped with Lower Anchor Tethers of Children (U.S. name) and lower universal anchorage systems (Canadian name) that make installation of forward-facing car seats simpler. Clasps attached to the restraint system are attached to anchors that are fixed at the level of the seat. These systems are tested to a weight of 48 pounds (21 kg).

Once a child reaches 40 pounds and 40 inches, he or she can be moved to a booster seat. These seats position the child so that the vehicle seat belts fit properly. The vehicle seat belt provides restraint when a booster seat is used. Figure 13-2 shows the proper positioning of the seat belt, coming over the shoulder, not across the neck, and across the lap, not the abdomen. Booster seat laws are relatively recent and do not necessarily have the same provisions for when

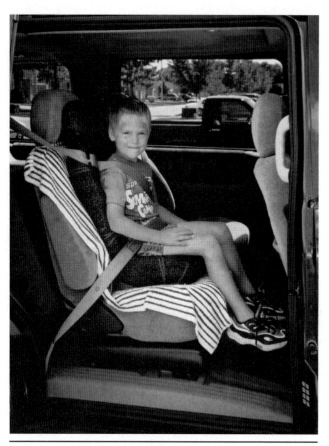

Figure 13-2   Proper positioning in a booster seat.

the child is ready to move to use the vehicle seatbelt assembly alone. Usually, a child is ready to move to use of the vehicle seat belt only when he or she reaches 80 pounds and is at least 4 feet 9 inches in height.

Location in the Motor Vehicle

The safest location for the child in a motor vehicle is the center rear seat (American Academy of Pediatrics, 1996, 1999a). When this seat is not available, the right outboard seat is preferred because this seat is usually on the side of the lane that borders the road shoulder rather than the side that faces oncoming traffic. Booster seats require the use of a three-point seat belt assembly (i.e., one that has both a shoulder and a lap portion), which sometimes precludes locating the child who uses a booster seat in the rear center seat because the restraint system in this location does not always include the shoulder portion. Children under the age of 12 years should not travel in the front passenger seat of a vehicle that has passenger side airbags. The airbags can seriously injure or kill a young child when they deploy. Some auto manufacturers have "smart" airbags that sense the weight of the occupant of the front passenger seat and either adjust the force of the airbag deployment or turn it off.

Vehicle Restraint Systems for Children With Disabilities

As previously mentioned, some children with mild to moderate seating needs are able to use a car seat that is designed for children without disabilities. This option is preferred when possible because of the costs of vehicle restraint systems that are designed specifically for children with disabilities. In some cases, the child may be able to use the child restraint system without any modification. When modifications are required, elements of the system that are provided by the **original equipment manufacturer** (OEM) cannot be altered or removed because the system was crash tested with those elements present. Alteration or removal may limit the ability of the seat to protect the child in a crash. Similarly, nothing can be placed underneath the padding or the straps. In the case of the strapping system, placing something underneath alters the direction of the pull on the child's body and may cause him or her to be ejected from the seat in a crash. However, rolls can be placed alongside the child's legs, trunk, or head to help maintain an upright position. A roll can also be placed under the child's knees to reduce extensor tone (American Academy of Pediatrics, 1999b).

Some children with disabilities cannot be safely transported in a child vehicle restraint system that is designed for children without disabilities or they do not have sufficient postural control to be safely secured by the **vehicle seat belt assembly** once they become too heavy to safely use other restraint systems. Some indicators of the need for a vehicle restraint system that is specifically designed for children with disabilities are children with tracheostomies, children with either excessive high or low tone for whom the typical restraint system does not provide sufficient support, and children who have a spica cast after hip surgery.

Commercial child restraint systems for children with special needs accommodate children up to 130 pounds and 56 inches (142 cm). The weight limit varies on these products so the assistive technology practitioner (ATP) needs to check to determine that the child can be accommodated safely. In addition to accommodating children who are heavier than 100 pounds, these systems provide more postural support and have the option for greater tilt of the system. Postural control may be achieved by the form of the seat shell, providing contouring of the seat and more integral fit with the child's body, or by padding that is supplied by the manufacturer. Some of these products have the option for the addition of a pommel to maintain leg abduction. Tilt in the system helps maintain postural control in a manner similar to that provided in mobility systems described in Chapter 12. These systems must meet federal safety standards and be crash tested for use as a vehicle restraint system.

Transportation for children who are unable to maintain a sitting position is difficult. Federal regulations exist for car beds but the companies that manufactured or distributed these devices no longer produce them. The E-Z ON Vest remains on the market as a product that will help restrain the child in the supine position. Box 13-2 lists Web sites of companies that manufacture child safety systems for children with disabilities.

SAFE TRANSPORTATION OF INDIVIDUALS IN WHEELCHAIRS

A person who routinely uses a wheelchair for mobility is safest in a motor vehicle when he or she is able to transfer into the vehicle seat and use the belt restraint systems that are supplied by the OEM. When transfers are not possible, the individual may travel in a motor vehicle while remaining seated in the wheelchair. Three factors collectively influence the increasing number of individuals who remain seated in their wheelchairs while riding in a motor vehicle: (1) legislation that promotes the rights of individuals with disabilities, (2) standards that are applied to wheelchairs and tie-down systems that relate to the design and testing of these devices for use in a motor vehicle, and (3) the increased availability of vehicle modifications that allow the wheelchair to be secured safely.

Crashworthiness of Wheelchairs and Seating Systems

Voluntary standards have been developed by the American National Standards Institute (ANSI)/Rehabilitation Engineering Society of North America (RESNA) and the International Standards Organization (ISO) that make provisions for the testing of wheelchairs and seating systems to determine their performance in a 21 g/48k m frontal impact crash simulation. These standards are *ISO 7176-19 Wheeled Mobility Device for Use in Motor Vehicles* (2001a) and *ANSI/RESNA Wheelchairs/Volume 1: Requirements and Test Methods for Wheelchairs (including Scooters)* (2000) and *ISO 16840: Seating Devices for use in Motor Vehicles* (2004). See Box 13-3 for a summary of the ANSI/RESNA

BOX 13-2 Web Sites of Manufacturers of Safety Systems for Children With Disabilities

Britax	www.childseat.com
Besi	www.BESI-INC.com
Columbia Medical	www.columbiamedical.com
E-Z-On Products	www.ezonpro.com
Q'Straint	www.qstraint.com
Sammons Preston	www.tumbleforms.com
Snug Seat	www.snugseat.com

BOX 13-3 Summary of ANSI/RESNA WC-19 Standard

The ANSI/RESNA WC-19 standard:
- Specifies general design requirements, test procedures, and performance requirements related to frontal impact performance for manual and power wheelchairs
- Applies to passengers in paratransit, transit, school bus, over-the-road coaches, and personally licensed vehicles
- Applies to securement of wheelchairs by four-point strap-type tie-down systems that are occupied by children and adults
- Applies to a wide rage of wheelchairs, including manual, powerbase, three-wheeled scooters, tilt-in-space wheelchairs, and specialized mobile seating bases with removable seating inserts
- Specifies strength and geometric requirements for wheelchair securement points and occupant restraint anchorage points on the wheelchair
- Provides requirements and information for wheelchair accessory components, seat inserts, and postural support devices with their regard to design and use in motor vehicles
- Applies primarily to wheelchairs that are retrofitted for use as a motor vehicle seat by the addition of after-market add-on components

---

WC-19 standard. The first two standards identify crash test procedures and manufacturer requirements for labeling and provision of information for a wheelchair and its dedicated seating. The use of an after-market seating system invalidates the wheelchair crash testing. Because many consumers purchase a wheelchair from one manufacturer and a seating system from another, ISO 16840 makes provisions for testing of a seating system independent of a specific wheeled mobility base. These standards are specific to a frontal impact; further development is required to test **crashworthiness** in side and rear impact crashes. Similar standards for wheelchair transportation exist or are being developed for Canada (Z605), Australia (AS-2942), and other parts of the world (ISO 10542, Parts 1 to 5). More information can be found on standards for wheelchair transportation at the Web site for the University of Pittsburgh's RERC (*www.rerc.pitt.edu*).

In addition to describing the crash test procedure, the standards set peak excursion limits for the head, the pelvis, and the hip in the anteroposterior plane. They place restrictions on the condition of the wheelchair and seating system after the crash test and provide a rating system for the ease of use and the fit of the vehicle restraint system on the consumer's body. It is important to remember that the vehicle restraint system (i.e., the vehicle seat belt) provides restraint for the wheelchair occupant, not the straps that are fixed to the wheelchair (Bertocci, Karg, and Fuhrman, 2005; Schneider and Manary, 2006). The rating system that evaluates use of the vehicle restraint system considers the following factors: the size of the opening through which the vehicle restraint system is threaded, the contact of the system with the consumer's body and where that contact is made, the angle of the pelvic portion of the restraint system, and whether the vehicle restraint system comes into contact with any sharp surfaces (ISO 2001, 2004). As was described earlier for positioning of the vehicle restraint system for a child in a booster seat, the vehicle restraint system must sit across the pelvis, not the abdomen, and rest on the shoulder, not on the neck. Further, the vehicle restraint system must not be held away from the user's body by any part of the wheelchair or seating system.

ISO 7176-19 and the corresponding ANSI/RESNA standard require manufacture of a frame that has four securement points for a **wheelchair tie-down system**. These standards apply to manual and electrically powered wheelchairs and scooters. Wheelchairs that have been successfully crash tested are commonly referred to as WC-19 chairs. As noted initially, these standards are voluntary, with the result that only a small percentage of wheelchairs have been crash tested. A number of reasons for this small proportion were identified at a recent State of the Science Workshop on Wheelchair Transportation Safety (Karg, Schneider, and Hobson, 2005). These reasons included the concern of manufacturers to assume legal liability of marketing a wheelchair as conforming to WC-19 standards, the lack of knowledge of safe transportation requirements and issues on the part of many ATPs and consumers, the added expense of purchasing a WC-19 chair, the voluntary nature of the standards, and the fact that the standards are more rigorous and conflict with federal regulations for safe transportation in a public vehicle (Schneider, Manary, and Bunning, 2005).

The requirements for manufacturers to warn users of potential hazards provide useful information regarding safe transportation for persons who travel seated in their wheelchairs. The most protected position is for individuals to be seated forward facing, yet on many public transit vehicles, the configuration for securement of a wheelchair seats the individual sideways. In addition to being unsafe in a crash, the individual feels less secure because he or she is required to adjust to the acceleration and deceleration of the vehicle. Any peripheral devices such as a communication system or a lap tray need to be removed from the chair and stored securely. Chest harnesses are recommended only when they have a quick release mechanism. Although they may be useful in aiding proper positioning of the shoulder component of the vehicle restraint system, they do have the potential to restrict the user's airway if they become loose (Bertocci, Karg, and Fuhrman, 2005). A head restraint is also recommended (Bertocci, Karg, and Fuhrman, 2005).

Wheelchair Tie-Down and Occupant Restraint Systems

The person with a disability is best protected from injury if he or she transfers to the vehicle seat and uses the standard OEM's restraint system (see Box 13-4 for summary; J2249 Guideline, version June 9, 1999, *http://www. wheelchairstandards.pitt.edu/WCS_T/WCS_T_SAE/WCS_T_ SAE_Restraints/WCS_T_SAE_Restraints.html*). However, for many individuals with disabilities, transferring to the seat of a vehicle is not possible or practical. For these individuals, the wheelchair functions as the vehicle seat. Once the person is inside a personal or public vehicle as either a passenger or a driver, both the person and the wheelchair need to be properly restrained for safety. The four-point strap tie-down system with the three-point occupant restraint system is considered to be the standard means of securing a passenger who is seated in a wheelchair in a vehicle (van Roosmalen and Hobson, 2005). It is important to view **wheelchair tie-down and occupant restraint systems** (WTORS) as separate parts of a total system designed to protect the passenger or driver who uses a wheelchair (Thacker and Shaw, 1994). The system that secures the wheelchair to the vehicle should be separate from the restraint that protects the occupant (which is the vehicle seat belt assembly as described above). The standards that specify the design, testing, and manufacturer labeling and information are: ISO 10542, Parts 1-5 *Wheelchair tiedowns and occupant restraint systems. Tie-down systems* secure the wheelchair to the vehicle floor (Figure 13-3). There are two types of tie-downs that have been crash tested: four-point strap and docking types (ISO 2001b, 2001c; Hobson, 2005). The four-belt type of tie-down, the most commonly used system in public transit vehicles, secures the wheelchair at each corner of the frame. In front the belts are attached to the frame (not the leg rests) just above the front caster pivot. WC-19 chairs have very obvious locations for the attachment of these straps. The strapping system and buckles are similar to those used in the aircraft industry for securing cargo. The major advantage of belt systems is low cost and their ability to secure most types of wheelchair frames. Their disadvantage is that use is time consuming and cumbersome and cannot be done independently by the wheelchair rider.

Docking systems have two components: a bracket that is secured to the vehicle floor and a component that is fixed

---

BOX 13-4   Principal Elements of SAE Recommend Practice J2249

1. Upper and lower torso restraint be provided
2. Restraint forces be applied to the bony regions of the body and not the soft tissues
3. Postural supports not be relied on as occupant restraints
4. The occupant faces forward in the vehicle.
5. Adequate clear space be provided around the occupants seated in wheelchairs

From: J2249 Guideline, version June 9, 1999, http://www. wheelchairstandards.pitt.edu/WCS_T/WCS_T_SAE/WCS_T_SAE_ Restraints/WCS_T_SAE_Restraints.html.

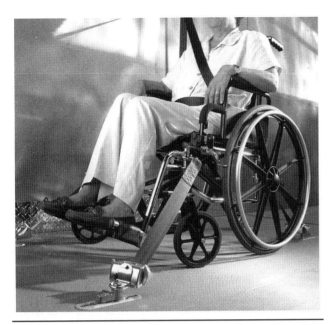

Figure 13-3 Wheelchair tie-down securement system for use of wheel-chair in a vehicle. Q-Straint wheelchair tie-down system.

to the lower portion of the wheelchair that couples with the bracket. These systems are specific to each model of wheelchair, thus limiting their use in public transit vehicles. Figure 13-4 shows the E-Z Lock system. Some of these devices have an auto engage feature; all have some feedback mechanism that tells the user that the wheelchair is properly secured (Schneider and Manary, 2006). A switch control

that is either activated by the wheelchair rider or by another vehicle occupant disengages the wheelchair from the docking component. The major advantages are quick and easy connection and independent use by the wheelchair rider. The disadvantage is that they require adding hardware to the wheelchair (which adds weight), and they are two to five times as expensive as belt systems.

For occupant restraint, variations of seat and shoulder belts used in passenger cars can be coupled with the four-belt and docking tie-downs to form a complete WTORS. The occupant restraint can be attached either directly to the van floor or to a point that is common to the tie-down attachment point. It is less likely that the wheelchair and occupant will move different distances during a collision if the occupant restraint is attached to the latter point. If they are not attached at the same point, it is likely that the wheelchair will move farther, forcing the occupant into the restraint and causing injury (Thacker and Shaw, 1994). Both the four-point strap tie-down and the docking systems described above have disadvantages. Strap systems cannot be used independently by the wheelchair rider. Current docking systems are wheelchair specific, limiting their use to private vehicles. The ISO 10542-3 describes specifications for a **universal docking interface geometry** (ISO, 2005). This standard specifies the dimensions and shape of the adaptor, location on the rear of the wheelchair and dimensions of space required around the adaptor (ISO, 2005). Researchers at the Rehabilitation Engineering Research Center on Wheelchair Transportation Safety *(www.rercwts.pitt.edu/)* are in the process of developing and testing a universal adapter that meets these criteria.

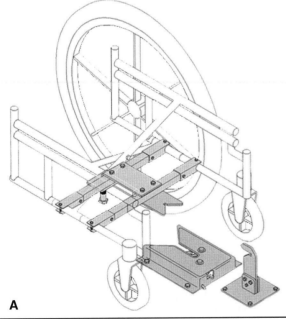

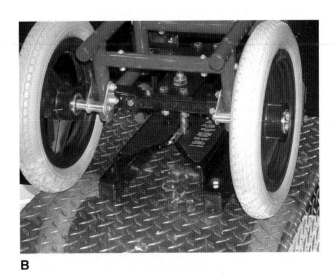

A

B

Figure 13-4 **A,** Schematic depicting the components of the E-Z lock system. **B,** Wheelchair connected to E-Z lock system in vehicle. (From Pellerito J: *Driver rehabilitation and community mobility: principles and practice,* St. Louis, 2005, Mosby.)

Another advancement in the technology for securing wheelchairs in a vehicle is a passive, rear-facing system that is being introduced in Canada, Australia, and Europe for **large accessible transit vehicles**. This technology uses a securement station based on external structures, rather than straps, to protect the passenger in the event of a crash. A padded structure that fits closely to the person's back and head protects in forward motion, the wall of the vehicle and a bar on the opposite side limit lateral movement, and the brakes of the wheelchair and the user's ability to grasp a bar limit rearward movement (van Roosmalen and Hobson, 2005). Wheelchair riders prefer this system because they can use it independently. However, problems remain, most notably the unreliability of many manual wheelchair brakes and the great variance in the ability of individuals to grasp and hold the barrier to stabilize themselves (Hobson, 2005). No industry standards exist for these stations.

■ EVALUATION AND TECHNOLOGIES FOR TRANSPORTATION AND DRIVING

Driving is a valued activity, particularly in North America where people depend more on private vehicles than on public transportation. Driving affords independence and spontaneity. People are often very reluctant to give up their driver's license even when they realize that they can no longer drive safely (Vrkljan and Miller Polgar, 2006). It is estimated that in 1997 70% of women and 92% of men over the age of 65 years held valid driver's licenses. By 2012, these numbers will change to 100% of men and 90% of women (Rosenbloom, 2004).

Evaluation for Driving

An individual may require a driving evaluation for a variety of reasons, including physical disability such as spinal cord injury, impairments resulting from a cerebral vascular accident or traumatic head injury, or age-related changes such as vision loss. A driving evaluation may be used to determine whether an individual whose license has been removed because of an illness, such as a stroke, is safe to return to driving or whether an individual who is currently driving remains safe to do so. The decision to recommend to a regulatory body that an individual is no longer safe to drive is a difficult one for two reasons: the knowledge that removing a person's driver's license frequently results in withdrawal from social activities and depression (Marottoli et al, 2000) and the concern that this conclusion is based on sound assessment procedures. Two consensus conferences on driving evaluation recently published their findings (Korner-Bitensky et al, 2005; Stephens et al, 2005). These conferences were prompted by concern that a common driving evaluation was not used.

A **driving evaluation** usually has two components: an off-road assessment that is paper or computer based and an on-road component with a trained evaluator. In some situations, performance on the off-road assessment may indicate that the client is not safe to proceed with an on-road evaluation or that the on-road evaluation should be conducted in a safer environment such as a closed-circuit course.

Both consensus groups recommended that the off-road assessment should include cognitive, physical, visual, and perceptual elements, although these were not necessarily defined in the same way. The international group (Stephens et al, 2005) also included cutaneous sensation as an element and the Canadian group (Korner-Bitensky et al, 2005) included behavior as a component. Cognitive components include attention (e.g., sustained and divided attention), memory, executive functions such as organization and planning, and higher level functions such as impulse control and judgment. Visual components include useful field of view, visual acuity, contrast sensitivity, visual fields, and visual acuity. In many cases a formal visual evaluation by an optometrist or an ophthalmologist was recommended. Motor abilities include range of motion, lower extremity strength, gross motor function, reaction time, and balance. Perceptual functions include visual scanning, proprioception, and spatial relations. The international group made suggestions for specific, standardized assessments for many of these components, with the recognition that there is limited evidence to date that these assessments are predictive of driving ability (Stephens et al, 2005).

The Canadian group went on to make recommendations for an on-road evaluation. They recommended that the individual drive a course that includes many common driving maneuvers such as stopping at a light or stop sign, making right and left hand turns, merging and accelerating into traffic, driving in reverse and driving on roads with a variety of speed limits. Behaviors scored during an evaluation include but are not limited to the ability to drive at a consistent, appropriate speed, stopping when appropriate and continuing when appropriate (i.e., not stopping at a green light), maintaining a safe distance from a lead car and from cars and other objects that are parked on the side of the roadway, proper lane position, and the ability to drive safely when additional cognitive tasks are present, such as when a passenger talks to the driver.

In addition, both groups recommended that a medical history and a driving history be taken. Further, the client's knowledge of the rules of driving should be tested. The results of these consensus groups provide an excellent start to the recognition of a consistent driving evaluation test battery. Their continued efforts to examine the relationship between driving performance and performance on the standardized tests included in the battery will provide evidence for the validity of this type of evaluation. Administration of this evaluation is very long so there remains a need for a valid screening assessment that would help clinicians determine who should proceed to a more intensive assessment when such a decision is not clear.

On the basis of the results of the evaluation, a recommendation for driving is made. The outcome of the evaluation can be one of the following: (1) the individual has the skills to continue to drive safely, (2) the individual does not have the skills required for safe driving, (3) the individual has the basic skills and continues with a driver training program, or (4) the individual has a specific impairment that limits the ability to drive with typical equipment so the individual must be assessed and trained to use adapted driving controls.

CASE STUDY

DRIVING EVALUATION

Sandra was 35 years old when she sustained an incomplete C5-6 spinal cord lesion. She has good control of her shoulder movement, the ability to flex and extend her elbows with gravity removed, and weak hand movements. Her muscles are stronger on her right side compared with her left. She has poor trunk control and flaccid lower extremities. Sensation is absent below the level of the lesion. She uses a mid-wheel drive power wheelchair that she controls with a joystick located on her right-hand side. She is now ready to return to driving and has been referred to you for driver evaluation and retraining and vehicle modifications. She still has the four-door sedan that she drove before her injury.

QUESTIONS

1. Describe the evaluation you would conduct for both driving and vehicle access.
   Would you recommend that she drive while seated in the OEM vehicle seat or in her power wheelchair? Justify your recommendation.
2. Describe your evaluation of her vehicle. What vehicle modifications would you recommend?
   Given the information you have about Sandra, what assistive technology would you recommend to enable her to drive?

Driver Training or Retraining

Driver education and training give the opportunity for the consumer to relearn driving skills or to learn driving skills in the case of an individual who is learning to drive with hand controls. This training can include classroom activities, use of a driving simulator, and on-road instruction. Many driving schools will provide driving instruction for individuals whose basic skills are no longer safe but who have the

potential to regain safe driving skills as determined by an evaluation. Classroom training is competency based and focuses on topics such as emergency driving procedures, defensive driving techniques, purchase of a vehicle, vehicle maintenance, accident responsibilities, and traffic laws. This classroom training is followed by on-road practice of basic driving maneuvers.

One well-developed driver training or refresher program is 55-Alive, which was developed by the American Association of Retired Persons in the United States and adapted for Canada by the Canada Safety Council. This program is specifically targeted to the older driver and provides off-road classes. In addition to discussing rules of the road, the program teaches safe driving strategies such as route planning, not driving at night or in bad weather, and avoiding heavily traveled freeways. Other modules talk about cognitive and visual changes that have the potential to affect safe driving, the effect of medications on driving performance, vehicle safety features, and how to judge personal fitness to drive. Although this program provides excellent information, the lack of an on-road component limits its ability to ensure that participants will be safe drivers in the actual driving situation (Bédard et al, 2004).

Driving simulators allow training of specific driving skills in a safe environment (Stephens et al, 2005). There are many different types of driving simulators. The simplest form consists of one or more computers that display a preprogrammed route. A steering wheel and brake and accelerator pedals are connected to the computer. The client may sit in a regular chair, wheelchair, or a vehicle seat. More sophisticated models project a driving route onto a screen that surrounds a vehicle on three sides. A client sits in the vehicle and uses the vehicle's controls. The vehicle is usually fixed with this type of simulator. The most complex simulators use a pod that contains a vehicle with route projected onto a screen that surrounds the vehicle. This pod is mounted on a system that provides six degrees of freedom of movement in an attempt to simulate the motion of a vehicle. Although the technology is continually refined, there is concern that the simulated motion is not sufficiently coupled with the projected image, which can produce nausea in the client.

Driving simulators are useful tools for the driver education process (McCarthy, 2005). They allow the instructor to program specific driving elements into a system and vary the demands placed on the client. Routes can be simple, straightforward driving for use when an individual is learning to use hand controls, for example. The complexity increases with the addition of driving elements, interaction with other vehicles and pedestrians, and unexpected hazards. However, there are drawbacks to these systems. One drawback is the validity of these simulations with respect to actual on-road performance. The ability to predict on-road performance from performance on a simulator is not well established (McCarthy, 2005). A major drawback is simulator sickness. Many clients, particularly seniors, cannot tolerate the simulation and develop nausea and dizziness, which obviously limits the device's usefulness.

Driver assessment and rehabilitation have the primary goals of keeping safe drivers on the road and helping those who have the potential to remain safe to regain necessary skills. Evaluation and retraining are linked components of this process. Because of the increasing prevalence of senior drivers in many developed countries, many resources are available that provide information about remaining safe behind the wheel and identifying signs for when driving is no longer a safe occupation (Box 13-5).

Vehicle Selection

A number of factors are important when selecting a vehicle for a person with a physical disability. Some of these include: whether the person will use the vehicle seat or a wheelchair, vehicle access, visual aspects, location and size of primary and secondary driving controls, and seatbelt and airbag design. Resources are available to assist with the process of selecting a vehicle. Most of these are geared to the elderly population (Box 13-6).

Ingress and egress refer to getting into and out of the vehicle. Miller Polgar and Shaw (2003) conducted semistructured interviews with seniors about their use of vehicle features.

Seniors reported a number of factors that made ingress and egress easier, including whether the height of the seat roughly matched the hip, a wide door opening, and some form of handle to help them steady themselves. Seats that have less bucketing also make transfers easy. Figure 13-5 shows an after-market modification of a passenger seat that pivots 90 degrees and then moves forward and down to come out of the vehicle to facilitate transfers. Seniors also reported that the weight of the door affected ingress and egress; a door that was too heavy was a concern because seniors felt less stable when they reached out to close it. Once in the vehicle, the driver should determine access to the steering wheel, pedals, and controls for secondary functions such as windshield wipers.

Visual aspects are another consideration when selecting a vehicle. The driver needs to determine the sightlines in the vehicle and whether there is clear visual access to the front, the side, and the mirrors. Further, the driver needs to determine whether he or she can read the information on the dashboard, both during the day and at night. A final aspect of vision relates to the location of various controls. Are controls for important features such as the temperature and wipers located in such a way that a quick glance away from the road is sufficient to guide a reach to use them?

The location and size of the controls have physical as well as visual implications. Consideration should be made of the range of motion required to reach vehicle controls for features such as wipers, turn indicators, temperature, and window defrost. Are they of sufficient size that the driver or passenger can target them accurately when reaching? What force is required to activate them? What action is required to activate them? Modifications to these controls are discussed in a later section.

Seniors who participated in the study by Miller Polgar and Shaw (2003) overwhelmingly indicated that seatbelts were problematic. They were difficult to reach, fasten, and unfasten. Participants had difficulty seeing the coupling mechanism. In some vehicles the location of the receiving part of the seatbelt is very difficult to see. Seatbelts did not fit properly (as described above), often sitting uncomfortably on the neck. Some after-market products are available which attempt to make the seatbelt more comfortable. These devices are not regulated, so there is the potential that they may invalidate any crash testing completed with the seatbelt and limit the potential of the seatbelt to protect the occupant in a crash. After-market devices should not alter the proper fit of the seatbelt.

Consideration should be made of the safe use of airbags. The driver should sit about 10 inches away from the steering wheel to avoid injury from an airbag that is activated at less than that distance. The height and weight of passengers is a further issue. Car manufacturers recommend that children under the age of 12 years should not occupy the front seat in a car equipped with passenger airbags because of

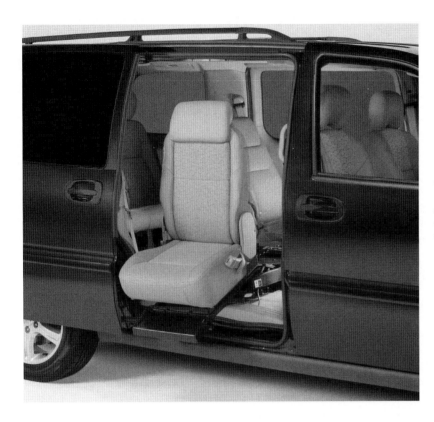

Figure 13-5 After-market seat modification that rotates seat 90 degrees and moves it toward outside of vehicle to facilitate transfer. (Courtesy Braun Corporation.)

the risk of serious injury or death. Adults who are the height or weight as a typical 12-year-old are at similar risk. Many new vehicles have sensors in the seat that vary the force with which the airbag activates or whether the airbag activates in a crash on the basis of the weight of the seat occupant.

Access to storage of a mobility device and any regularly transported equipment should be checked. If a vehicle occupant uses a wheelchair that is transported with the individual, it is important to determine whether the wheelchair will fit in the vehicle and how difficult it is to lift and position in the vehicle. This suggestion seems like a very obvious one, but it is one that can be neglected with a very frustrating outcome.

A final consideration is whether an individual who uses a wheelchair will transfer into the vehicle seat or whether he or she will be transported in the wheelchair. This discussion will focus on the driver because of access issues to driving controls, but many of the comments will be applicable to a passenger who regularly uses a wheelchair. Transfer to the vehicle seat provides the most protection for the occupant because the OEM's seat belt provides the most effective protection in a crash (Schneider and Manary, 2006). The vehicle seat back and headrest also provide better protection than that of a wheelchair seating system. The vehicle seat should put a driver in a better position to reach necessary controls. However, use of the vehicle seat does require the ability to complete a transfer relatively easily. A seating system

will provide the user with a better functional position generally than a vehicle seat will do (Phillips, Fisher, and Miller Polgar, 2005). The most important limitation of using the vehicle seat concerns individuals at risk for pressure ulcers. Vehicle seats are not designed with tissue integrity in mind and over a long trip a pressure ulcer could easily develop.

The benefits and limitations of remaining in a wheelchair during transportation are the reverse of the above with some additional factors. The wheelchair seating system is designed to give better postural control and trunk stability than a vehicle seat, which are important safety considerations for either a driver or a passenger (Phillips, Fisher, and Miller Polgar, 2005; Schneider and Manary, 2006). Any vehicle tie-down system will not be as safe a restraint as the OEM's system. A less apparent consideration is the suspension system of the wheelchair. Vehicle seats do not have suspension systems, so the seat does not move independently of the vehicle. Such is not the case with a wheelchair with a suspension system. Travel in these chairs may have the uncomfortable side effect of motion sickness (Phillips, Fisher, and Miller Polgar, 2005).

Vehicle Access

Ingress and egress issues for an individual who transfers into a vehicle seat were considered above. This section will discuss access issues for individuals who remain in their wheelchairs for transportation. In these instances, the vehicle will be a modified van. Also considered will be aftermarket devices that load and store the wheelchair once the user has transferred to a vehicle seat.

Van modifications typically involve provision of a ramp or lowered floor for access and a tie-down system to secure a wheelchair. The latter were discussed in an earlier section of this chapter. These are either side or rear loading, manual or power operated. They provide access through the sliding passenger door or the rear. Figure 13-6 shows a lowered floor that accesses the side sliding passenger door. Newer designs store the lowered floor in a recessed area on the van floor so they do not interfere with access inside the vehicle. Many car manufacturers provide reimbursement for after-market modifications required to make a van accessible. The Web addresses for the main van conversion companies are listed in Box 13-7.

Integration of the wheelchair with the van modifications is critical. A mismatch between these mobility devices is a very expensive mistake. The consumer needs to know the dimensions and configuration of his wheelchair before proceeding with van modifications. The following should be considered: (1) the width of the wheelchair for movement through the opening into the vehicle and maneuvering once inside the vehicle, (2) the height of the wheelchair for head clearance (remember that a tilt chair may increase the overall height, and (3) the length of the wheelchair and consequent turning radius; front rigging and the need for a reclined position will increase the length of the wheelchair. If a person remains in the wheelchair to drive, further considerations are made. He or she must be able to fit into the space

allocated for the driver. The seat height must not interfere with the travel of the steering wheel. He or she must be able to reach the necessary controls and finally be able to see out of the front and side windows and access the mirrors. In some situations, if the seat height is too high, the driver will not be able to see out of the front window (Phillips, Fisher, and Miller Polgar, 2005). These are important considerations; a modified van that does not accommodate the user's wheelchair is of no benefit.

If it is not possible for the individual to load the wheelchair manually into the vehicle, there are powered wheelchair-loading devices that can assist with this function. These devices pick up and store a manual wheelchair in the back seat, in the trunk, or in a carrier attached to the roof or back of the car. Figure 13-7 shows an example of a loading device that folds and stores a conventional wheelchair inside a cover that is mounted on top of the car. The other advantage of this type of loading device is that the wheelchair does not take up room in the trunk or back seat. These devices can be operated either from outside or inside the vehicle.

◼ MODIFICATIONS FOR DRIVING

The driver with a disability needs to be carefully evaluated for any modifications that are being considered. The assessment of an individual for driving modifications progresses in a logical manner, starting with an assessment of ability to operate the primary controls, followed by an assessment of the use of the secondary controls. Once modifications are recommended, only a reputable dealer should install them.

Primary Driving Controls

The **primary driving controls** are those that are used to stop (brakes), go (accelerator), and steer. Modifications are available to assist the driver to maintain a grip on the steering wheel, to access the pedals, or to control the vehicle with the hands and arms only when the driver does not have use of the legs to control the vehicle. Each of these vehicle modifications will be considered in turn.

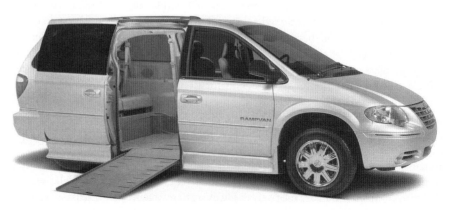

Figure 13-6 Side access lowered floor accessible minivan for transfer with wheelchair into and out of vehicle. (Courtesy Braun Corporation.)

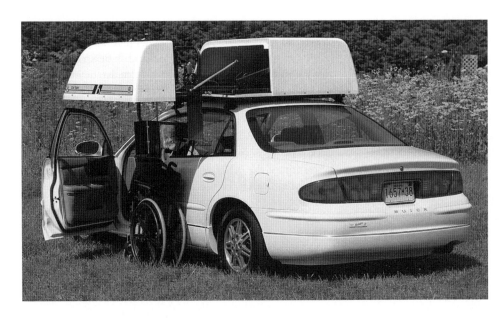

Figure 13-7   Wheelchair loading device for a sedan. (Courtesy Braun Corp.)

There are a number of options to consider for steering for drivers who use one arm or use a prosthetic arm or who have impaired arm and hand function. For a driver who uses one hand to steer, a steering device allows the driver to maintain control of the wheel at all times (Lillie, 1996). Evaluation of the client's hand function determines both the type and location of the device (Bouman and Pellerito, 2006). Steering devices attach directly to the steering wheel or to a bar that stretches across the inner diameter of the wheel and attach to each side of the steering wheel. These devices are frequently removable so that another person can drive the vehicle (Bouman and Pellerito, 2006). Steering devices (shown clockwise in Figure 13-8) include palm grip, tri-pin, fork-grip or V-grip, spinner knob, and amputee ring (for use with prosthetic hooks). Additional modifications for steering may include a reduced-effort or zero-effort steering mechanism, a steering wheel of reduced diameter, height and angle adjustments to the steering column, and reduced

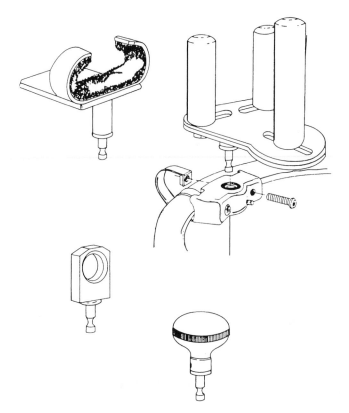

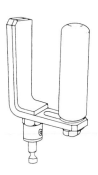

Figure 13-8   Different steering aids that accommodate a variety of consumer needs. (Courtesy Mobility Products and Design.)

gain (the number of turns of the steering wheel required to pivot the wheels from fully left to fully right). Reduced- or low-effort steering systems reduce the effort required for steering a vehicle by 40%, whereas zero-effort systems are able to reduce the effort required by 70% (Peterson, 1996).

Two primary types of pedal adaptations are available: a left foot accelerator and pedal extensions (Bouman and Pellerito, 2006). The latter are available from many OEMs and are used by individuals who are not able to reach the pedals. As the name would indicate, the left foot accelerator allows the driver to control both braking and acceleration with the left foot. This device is also removable for other drivers. It requires an automatic transmission vehicle.

Hand controls for accelerator and brake consist of a mechanical linkage connected to each pedal, a control handle, and associated connecting hardware. There are four common design approaches: push-pull, push-twist, push-right-angle-pull (Bouman and Pellerito, 2006; Lillie, 1996; Peterson, 1996), and push-tilt (Bouman and Pellerito, 2006). In each case the first designation (e.g., push) refers to activation of the brake and the second (e.g., pull or twist) is used for activation of the accelerator. By using a push control (Figure 13-9, *A*), the consumer activates the brakes by

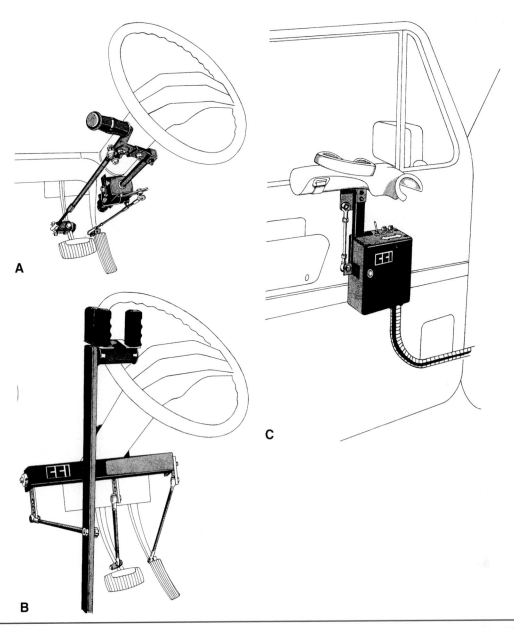

Figure 13-9   Hand control for braking and acceleration. **A,** A push-twist hand control. Pushing down applies the brakes, and twisting the lever to the left accelerates the vehicle. **B,** A mechanically assisted manual system. **C,** An electrically assisted controller and interface. (Courtesy Creative Controls, Inc.)

pushing on a lever in a direction directly away from him or her, parallel to the steering column. Acceleration is accomplished either by pulling back on the control, rotating it, or pulling downward at a right angle to the steering column. The weight of the user's hand is sufficient to maintain a constant velocity. When the accelerator control is released, it returns to the off position. These controls are easily attached to almost any vehicle by the connecting hardware, which clamps a rod to each pedal and stabilizes them by attachment of a mounting bracket to the steering column. The connecting rods are adjustable in length to accommodate different vehicles. They are normally operated with the left hand, and the right hand is used for steering; however, right-hand mounting systems are also available from a variety of manufacturers (Bouman and Pellerito, 2006).

Additional assistance is required for persons with weak upper extremities (e.g., high-level spinal cord injury). There are two basic approaches: (1) mechanical assist and (2) power assist. Mechanical assist systems use one of the approaches described above, but they provide a lever arm that affords a mechanical advantage (Figure 13-9, *B)*. Instead of connecting the hand control directly to the accelerator and brake pedals, there is a mechanical linkage that magnifies the force applied by the user. Typically this is a long arm, attached to the floor, that is pulled back for acceleration and pushed forward for braking. The arm is also linked to the pedals through connecting hardware. Power-assisted devices use either hydraulic or pneumatic assist (similar to power brakes or steering) or electronic powered systems. Electronically powered systems add servomotors that apply force to the brake and accelerator system. An electronically assisted brake and accelerator control is shown in Figure 13-9, *C*. One of the most recent developments is the use of a joystick that the driver pushes back for acceleration and pushes forward for braking.

Secondary Driving Controls

In addition to the controls necessary to maneuver the vehicle, **secondary driving controls** are needed for safe operation of a vehicle. These include turn signals, parking brakes, lights, horn, ignition, temperature control (heat and air conditioning), and windshield wipers. The knobs for operating secondary controls may not be within reach of the driver or may be of such a shape that the driver cannot operate them (Bouman and Pellerito, 2006). These knobs can be adapted by adding extensions or a differently shaped control or by relocating them so the driver can use them. A control panel that contains all these functions can also replace the standard controls. This panel is a special-purpose membrane keyboard that interfaces through a microcomputer to activate the secondary functions. It is mounted to either side of the steering wheel in a location that is within reach of the driver (Figure 13-10). Drivers who only have the use of one hand have an option of a voice-activated control panel that activates the functions above through spoken commands (Bouman and Pellerito, 2006).

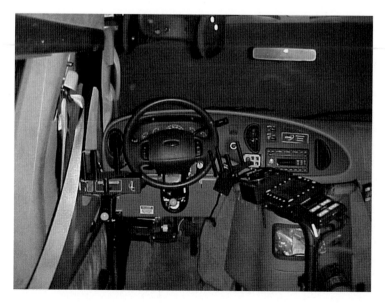

Figure 13-10   Control panel for primary and secondary driving control. (From Pellerito J: *Driver rehabilitation and community mobility: principles and practice,* St. Louis, 2005, Mosby.)

■ SUMMARY

Access to a vehicle affords independence and the ability to participate in community activities. Technology relating to occupant protection and vehicle access, either as a driver or a passenger, needs to be considered in light of its ability to provide safety when traveling in the vehicle. This chapter considered assistive technology that aids safe transportation for individuals with disabilities. A primary concern is occupant protection, which included selection and use of proper vehicle restraint systems for children who are not able to use the vehicle seatbelt assembly and for individuals with mobility impairments who remain seated in a wheelchair while riding in an adapted vehicle. The factors that need to be considered when determining whether an individual can transfer to a vehicle seat or needs to remain in a wheelchair were discussed. Further, the voluntary standards that guide the testing and labeling of wheelchairs for use during transportation and for vehicle tie-down and occupant restraint systems were also discussed. Two further main topics were covered in this chapter: vehicle access and selection and driver evaluation and retraining, including vehicle modifications for driving.

Study Questions

1. What are the three main categories of child restraint systems for vehicles? What are the indications for the use of each category?
2. What modifications can be made to a child restraint system, designed for a typically developing child, that accommodate the positioning needs of a child with a disability? What types of modifications cannot be made to these systems? Why?
3. Describe the advantages and disadvantages of transferring to the OEM vehicle seat for travel in a vehicle, rather than remaining in a wheelchair. Describe the advantages and disadvantages of remaining in a wheelchair when traveling in a vehicle.
4. Name the standards that set the criteria for crash testing and labeling of wheelchairs and seating systems. What are the requirements of these standards?
5. Define a wheelchair tie-down and occupant restraint system.
6. Describe the advantages and disadvantages of each of the two types of wheelchair securement systems for vehicles.
7. What off-road components are recommended for inclusion in a driver evaluation?
8. What on-road components are recommended for inclusion in a driver evaluation?
9. What are the advantages and disadvantages of the use of driving simulators for driving evaluation and retraining?
10. Describe the major considerations for selection of a vehicle for use by an individual with a disability, as either a driver or a passenger.
11. Discuss the elements that need to be considered to ensure that an individual's wheelchair is compatible with the modified vehicle.
12. What are primary and secondary vehicle controls?
13. How are primary mechanical hand controls designed and operated? What are the major types?
14. How are secondary driving controls used?

References

American Academy of Pediatrics, Committee on Injury and Poison Prevention: Selecting and using the most appropriate car safety seats for growing children: guidelines for counseling parents, *Pediatrics* 97:761-763, 1996.

American Academy of Pediatrics, Committee on Injury and Poison Prevention: Safe transportation of newborns at hospital discharge, *Pediatrics* 104:986-987, 1999a.

American Academy of Pediatrics, Committee on Injury and Poison Prevention: Transporting children with special needs, *Pediatrics* 104:988-992, 1999b.

ANSI/RESNA: Wheelchairs: *Requirements and test methods for wheelchairs (including scooters), Section 19: wheelchairs used as seats in motor vehicles*, vol 1, 2000, Pittsburgh, ANSI/RESNA.

Bédard M et al: Evaluation of a re-training program for older drivers, *Can J Public Health* 95:295-298, 2004.

Bertocci G, Karg P, Furhman S: Wheelchair seating systems for use in transportation. In: Karg P, Schneider L, Hobson D, editors: *State of the science workshop on wheelchair transportation safety: final report 2005*, pp. 35-56, Pittsburgh, PA, 2005, RERC on Wheelchair Transportation Safety.

Bouman J, Pellerito JM: Preparing for the on-road evaluation. In JM Pellerito, editor: *Driver rehabilitation and community mobility*, pp. 239-253, St. Louis, MO, 2006, Elsevier Mosby.

Ebell BE et al: Use of child booster seats in motor vehicles following a community campaign, *JAMA* 289:879-884, 2003.

Fox M, Sarno S, Potvin J: A biomechanical evaluation of child safety seat installation: forward facing. In *Proceedings of the inaugural Ontario Biomechanics Conference*, p 53, Barrie ON, 2004, The Conference.

Hobson D: Problem-solving the next generation of wheelchair securement for use in public transport vehicles. In: Karg P, Schneider L, Hobson D, editors: *State of the science workshop on wheelchair transportation safety: final report 2005*, pp. 57-78, Pittsburgh, PA, 2005, RERC on Wheelchair Transportation Safety.

ISO: *ISO 7176-19: Wheelchairs: wheeled mobility devices for use in motor vehicles*, Geneva, Switzerland, October, 2001a, ISO.

ISO: *ISO 10542-1: Technical systems and aids for disabled or handicapped persons—wheelchair tiedown and occupant-restraint systems—Part 1: requirements and test methods for all systems*, Geneva, Switzerland, July 2001b, ISO.

ISO: *ISO 10542-2: Technical systems and aids for disabled or handicapped persons—wheelchair tiedown and occupant-restraint systems—Part 2: four-point strap-type tiedown systems*, Geneva Switzerland, July 2001c, ISO.

ISO: ISO 16840-4: *Wheelchair seating—Part 4—seating systems for use in motor vehicles*, Geneva Switzerland, February 2004, ISO.

ISO: ISO 10542-3: *Technical systems and aids for disabled or handicapped persons—wheelchair tiedown and occupant restraint systems—Part 3: docking type tiedown systems*, Geneva, Switzerland, 2005, ISO.

Karg P, Schneider L, Hobson D: *State of the science workshop on wheelchair transportation safety: Final report 2005*, Pittsburgh, PA, 2005, RERC on Wheelchair Transportation Safety: www.rercwts.pitt.edu. Accessed December 3, 2006.

Kohn, M, Chausme K, Flood, MH: Anticipatory guidance about child safety misuse: Lessons from safety seat "check-ups," *Arch Pediatr Adolesc Med* 154:606-609, 2000.

Korner-Bitensky N et al: Recommendations of the Canadian Consensus Conference on driving evaluation in older drivers, *Phys Occup Ther Geriatr* 23:123-144, 2005.

Lang WG, Lui GC, Newlin E: The association between hands-on instruction and proper child safety seat installation, *Pediatrics* 106:924-929, 2000.

Lillie SM: Driving with a physical dysfunction. In Pedretti LW, editor: *Occupational therapy: practice skills for physical dysfunction*, St. Louis, 1996, Mosby.

Marottoli RA et al: Consequences of driving cessation: decreased out-of-home activity levels, *J Gerontol* 55: S334-S340, 2000.

McCarthy D: Approaches to improving elders' safe driving abilities, *Phys Occup Ther Geriatr* 23:25-42, 2005.

Miller Polgar JM, Shaw L: Seniors' perceptions of their safety while using a private vehicle. In *Proceedings of the 18th International Seating Symposium*, pp. 227-228, Orlando, FL, 2003, The Symposium.

Murphy RF: *The body silent*, New York, 1990, W.W. Norton.

Peterson WA: Transportation. In Galvin JC, Scherer JM, editors: *Evaluating, selecting and using appropriate assistive technology*, Gaithersburg, MD, 1996, Aspen Publishers.

Phillips K, Fisher K, Miller Polgar, J: Transportation integration: Thinking beyond the wheelchair. In *Proceedings of the 21st International Seating Symposium*, pp. 97-98, Orlando, FL, 2005, The Symposium.

Rosenbloom S: Mobility of the elderly: good news and bad news. In *Transportation in an aging society: a decade of experience. Technical papers and reports from a conference*, pp. 3-21, Washington, 2004, Transportation Research Board.

SAE Recommended Practice J2249: *Wheelchair tiedown and occupant restraint systems for uses in motor vehicles*, October, 1996, revised, January 1999.

Sarno S, Fox M, Potvin J: A biomechanical evaluation of child safety seat installation: rear facing. *Proceedings of the inaugural Ontario Biomechanics Conference*, p 54, Barrie ON, 2004, The Conference.

Schneider LW, Manary MA: Wheeled mobility tiedown systems and occupant restraints for safety and crash protection. In Pellerito JM, editor: *Driver rehabilitation and community mobility*, pp. 357-372, St. Louis, MO, 2006, Elsevier Mosby.

Schneider LW, Manary MA, Bunning ME: Barriers to the development, marketing, purchase and proper use of transit-safety technologies. In Karg P, Schneider L, Hobson D, editors: *State of the Science Workshop on Wheelchair Transportation Safety, final report 2005*, pp. 4-34, Pittsburgh, PA (2005): www.rercwts.pitt.edu. Accessed December 3, 2006.

Stephens BW et al: International older driver consensus conference on assessment, remediation, counseling for transportation alternatives: summary and recommendation, *Phys Occup Ther Geriatr* 23:103-12, 2005.

Thacker J, Shaw G: Safe and secure, *Team Rehabil Rep* 5: 26-30, 1994.

van Roosmalen L, Hobson D: Looking toward future wheelchair transportation—what should be our vision and how do we realize it? In Karg P, Schneider L, Hobson D, editors: *State of the Science Workshop on Wheelchair Transportation Safety, final report 2005*, pp. 79-94, Pittsburgh, PA (2005): www.rercwts.pitt.edu. Accessed December 3, 2006.

Vrkljan B, Polgar JM: Linking occupational performance and occupational identity: an exploratory study of the transition from driving cessation in older adulthood, *J Occup Sci* 14:42-52, 2007.

Winston FK et al: The danger of premature graduate to seat belts for young children, *Pediatrics* 105:1179-1183, 2000.

Winston FK et al: Recent trends in child restrain practices in the US, *Pediatrics* 113:e458-e464, 2004.

Yakupcin JP: Child passenger safety in the school age population, *Pediatr Emerg Care* 21:286-290, 2005.

CHAPTER 14

Technologies That Aid Manipulation and Control of the Environment

Learning Objectives

On completing this chapter, you will be able to do the following:

1. List functional manipulative tasks that can be aided by assistive technologies
2. Describe the operation of electrically powered feeding aids
3. List the features and design properties of electronic page turners
4. List the functions carried out by environmental control systems
5. Describe the basic components of environmental control systems and how they are implemented
6. Discuss the uses of robotic devices in aiding manipulation by persons with disabilities

Key Terms

Alternative
Augmentative
Desktop Robots
Electrically Powered Feeders
Electrically Powered Page Turners
Electronic Aid to Daily Living
Environmental Control Units
General-Purpose Manipulation
  Devices

Head Pointers
Infrared Transmission
Mobile Assistive Robots
Mouthsticks
Programmable Controllers
Radio Frequency Transmission
Reachers
Remote Control
Robotic Systems

Special-Purpose Manipulation
  Devices
Telephone Controllers
Trainable Controllers
Ultrasonic Transmission
Universal Remote

One of the activity outputs described in Chapter 2 (see Figure 2-5, *B*) is manipulation. At the most basic level, *manipulation* refers to those activities that are normally accomplished with the upper extremities, particularly the fingers and hand. In using assistive devices, especially those that are electronically controlled, there are many types of "manipulation" required. For example, keys must be pressed for computer entry, joysticks controlled for powered mobility, and switches activated for communication devices. This type of manipulation has been discussed in previous chapters, and it is excluded from the general discussion of manipulation in this chapter. In this chapter, manipulation is taken to be the end goal of the person's actions. For example, activities such as hand writing, food preparation, eating, and appliance control depend on manipulation of physical objects, and these types of activities are the focus.

Figure 14-1 is a characterization of assistive technology devices used for manipulation. As in many other areas of assistive technology application, we can provide manipulative aids that are either **alternative** (a different method of doing the same task) or **augmentative** (assistance in doing the task in the same manner as it is normally done). For manipulation, we can also distinguish devices as being either *specific purpose* or *general purpose*. **Special-purpose manipulation devices**

are designed for only one task, whereas **general-purpose manipulation devices** serve two or more manipulative activities. For example, an augmentative, specific-purpose approach to eating may include a modified fork with an enlarged handle. An alternative, special-purpose apparatus for eating is an electromechanical device that lifts food off the plate and up to mouth level when a switch is pressed. A robotic arm is a general-purpose alternative manipulative aid. It can be used for eating, but it also has application in work site manipulation and many other areas. A hand splint that allows gripping of any utensil serves as a general-purpose augmentative aid because it can be used to hold a fork for eating or a pen for writing. This chapter discusses all four categories of manipulation assistive technologies shown in Figure 14-1.

■ LOW-TECHNOLOGY AIDS FOR MANIPULATION

Chapter 1 defines low-technology aids as inexpensive, simple to make, and easy to obtain. Many manipulative aids fall into the low-technology category. We group these aids into general- and special-purpose devices. Within special-purpose devices, we categorize devices according to the major performance areas of the human activity–assistive technology (HAAT) model: self-care, work or school, and play or leisure. All the examples used in this section are available from mail-order catalogs.* Many of these devices are also available at drugstores and other local sources.

General-Purpose Aids

To be classified as general purpose, a manipulation aid must serve more than one need. Three general-purpose aids are

Alternative Specific Purpose	Augmentative Specific Purpose
Alternative General Purpose	Augmentative General Purpose

Figure 14-1 Assistive technologies for manipulation can be categorized in two dimensions: general purpose versus specific and alternative versus augmentative.

*Suppliers of the aids described in this section include Cleo, Inc., Cleveland, Ohio; Independent Living Aids, Plainview, N.Y.; Maddak, Inc, Pequannock, N.J.; Maxiaids, Farmingdale, N.Y.; Sammons Preston, Bolingbrook, Ill.; and Smith and Nephew Rehabilitation Products, Milwaukee, Wisc.

discussed: mouthsticks, head pointers, and reachers. The first two of these are often used as control enhancers in conjunction with control interfaces. In Chapter 7, head pointers and mouthsticks are discussed in detail, including their use as control enhancers for activating control interfaces. Both **mouthsticks** and **head pointers** are also used for direct manipulation. Turning pages is often accomplished with a mouthstick or head pointer used in conjunction with a book or magazine mounted on a simple stand. A ballpoint pen tip or a pencil can also be attached to a mouthstick for writing. Additional attachments include a pincher that is opened or closed by tongue action and a suction cup end that can be used to grip objects (e.g., a page) by sucking on the end of the mouthstick. Many tasks require sliding objects (e.g., paper, pens) around on a desk or table. Both mouthsticks and head pointers can be used for this task. Mouthsticks or head pointers can also be used for such functions as dialing a telephone, typing, and turning lights on and off.

Many individuals need to extend their physical range. Often the need for extended range is a result of being seated in a wheelchair and wanting to reach an object on a counter or in a cabinet. In other cases it is a need to reach an object on the floor when bending is difficult or stability is poor. In all these cases, **reachers** can be useful. As shown in Figure 14-2, a reacher consists of a handle grip that is used to control the jaws of the reacher to grasp an object. The grasp required to activate the grip may be of several types: squeeze with the whole hand, pistol grip with all the fingers, or trigger with the index finger. Overall length varies from 24 to 36 inches, and some models fold for ease of carrying. The gripper portion of the reacher may be circular for ease of gripping cans or pincherlike for picking up smaller objects. Rubber or other nonslip materials are often used for reacher grippers. Reachers can be used to manipulate many objects, including food (e.g., cans, packages), cooking utensils (e.g., pans, pots, plates, dishes), office objects (e.g., paper, books, magazines), and recreational or leisure objects (e.g., books, tapes, CDs).

Chen et al (1998) conducted a study of the effectiveness of reachers in meeting the needs of a population of older (over 60 years) subjects. The characteristics found to be most important were adjustable length, one-handed use, a locking system for the grip to hold objects, support for the forearm, light weight, and a lever trigger action in the grip. Chen et al (1998) also list 38 tasks for which their population uses reachers. These include food preparation, self-care, appliance control, and gardening. Chen et al (1998) also discuss the relative ease of use of reachers for a variety of tasks.

Special-Purpose Aids

Because special-purpose, low-tech aids are designed for one or two tasks only, they serve those tasks very well. However, because they are so specialized, it may be necessary to have

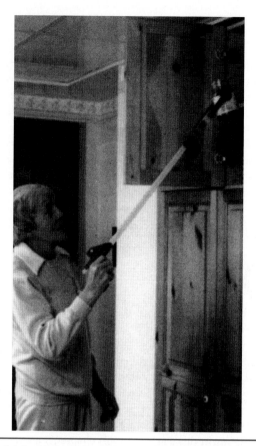

Figure 14-2   Mechanical reachers are general purpose devices. (Courtesy TASH, Ajax, Ontario, Canada.)

several of these available to meet the demands of self-care, work, and leisure.

Most special-purpose adaptations of products involve one of four things: (1) lengthening a handle or reducing the reach required, (2) modifying the handle of a utensil for easier grasping or manipulation, (3) converting two-handed tasks to one-handed ones, and (4) amplifying the force that a consumer can generate with her hands. A variety of modified handles are shown in Figure 14-3. These include enlarged grips for easier grasping, cuffs that hold a utensil and circle the fingers, angled handles for ease of scooping (for people with limited wrist movement), swivel handles that allow the end to be oriented differently for different positions in space (e.g., on a table or near the mouth), and handles requiring limited grasp (often called "quad handles").

Self-Care.   Self-care includes aids for assistance in several areas: food consumption, food preparation, dressing, and hygiene. Examples of food preparation adaptations include one-handed holders for can and jar opening, brushes with suction cups for one-handed scrubbing of vegetables, bowls with suction cup bottoms for stability while stirring with

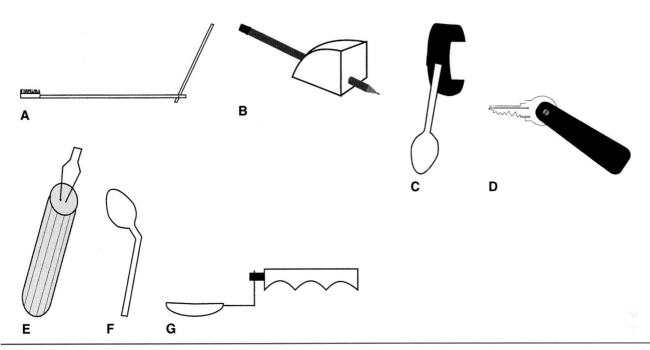

Figure 14-3 Types of handles used on low-tech manipulative aids. **A,** Brush with extended handle. **B,** Enlarged grip for pencil or pen. **C,** Spoon with cuff. **D,** Key holder with quad grip. **E,** Buttoner with enlarged handle. **F,** Spoon with bent handle for scooping. **G,** Spoon with swivel handle.

one hand, bowl and pan holders (some of which tilt for pouring), and cutting boards that stabilize food during cutting. Modified handles are available for knives and serving spoons, as well as for other utensils.

Food consumption aids include a variety of utensils with modified handles (knives, forks, spoons, and combinations called "sporks"). Modifications to plates include suction cups for stability, enlarged rims that make it easier to scoop food onto a utensil, and removable rims that attach to any plate. Drinking aids include cups with caps and "sipper" lids through which fluid can be sucked; nose cutouts that allow drinking to occur without tipping the head back; double-handled cups for two-handed use; and cups modified at the bottom with a quad grasp to allow lifting and tipping with limited hand function.

Dressing aids designed to compensate for poor fine motor control include adapted button hooks for single-handed buttoning and zipper pulls. These are available with enlarged, suction, and quad grip handles. For limited reach, there are aids for pulling on socks and pantyhose, long-handled shoe horn, and trouser pulls. A variety of dressing aids are shown in Figure 14-4.

Areas of hygiene that can be aided by special-purpose devices include hair combing and brushing, tooth brushing, shaving, bathing, and toileting. Hairbrushes and combs may have any or all of the following adaptations: modified handles of all types, extended handle lengths, and angled ends (where the comb or brush attaches). Modified toothbrushes have enlarged, quad, and offset handles. Toothpaste and shaving cream containers can be adapted with a simple device that allows one-handed dispensing of the product. For shaving, there are holders with adapted handles for both electric and manual razors. For bathing, there are long-handled sponges, curved handle brushes for washing the back, and holders for sponges or washcloths that accommodate limited grasping ability.

Other self-care items are intended for use in the home. For example, there are gripping cuffs that are used with brooms and mops, extended handles on household items such as dustpans and dusters, and key holders.

Work and School. Throughout this book we have described assistive technologies that aid consumers in accomplishing work- and school-related tasks (e.g., computers, augmentative communication devices). This section discusses low-tech aids that specifically help work and school in the areas of writing and reading.

Handwriting is a major need in work and school environments. Special-purpose manipulative aids that assist handwriting focus on one of two problems: holding the pen or pencil and holding the paper. Some consumers lack the ability to grip a standard pen or pencil. Low-tech approaches to this problem include modified grippers that attach to the hand and clamp to the pen or pencil; wire, wooden, or plastic holders that support the pen or pencil off the paper and allow it to slide across the paper; weighted pens (with variable amounts of weight) that help reduce problems associated with tremor; and pens with enlarged bodies to make

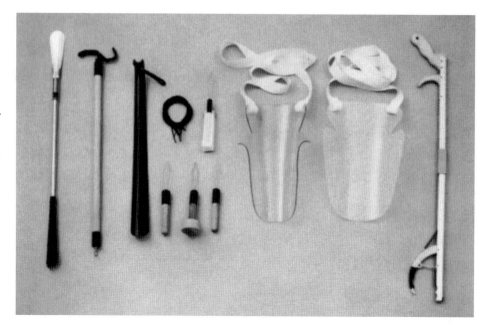

Figure 14-4 A variety of dressing aids. *Left to right:* Long-handled shoehorn, dressing stick, plastic shoehorn, elastic shoe laces, button hooks (4), stocking aids (2), and reacher. (Courtesy TASH, Ajax, Ontario, Canada.)

them easier to grasp. There are several different designs for holding paper in place for one-handed writing. Generally the paper is held to a plate using either clips or a magnet (in this case the plate is steel). Desks can also be modified using a rotating "lazy Susan" device that rotates to bring items within reach. File folders are often modified for easier grasping by putting hooks or loops on them. The loop or hook protrudes above the folder so that it can be grasped more easily. High-tech aids for writing are discussed in Chapter 11, and additional work-related assistive technology applications are described in Chapter 16.

There are also low-tech reading aids. Book holders provide support for the reading material so that the consumer does not have to hold it. Page turning is done either by hand or with a head pointer or a mouthstick. The next section discusses electrically powered page turners that aid reading.

Play and Leisure. As with other types of manipulative aids, lack of grasping ability in recreational or leisure aids is generally accommodated for by altering the type of handle. Recreation and leisure examples include cameras with modified shutter release, modified grip scissors, modified handles on garden tools, and modified grasping cuffs for pool cues, racquets, or paddles. A person with limited manipulation strength can fly a kite by adding special wrist or hand cuffs for holding the string. Pinball machines can be adapted with larger buttons to allow control by children and adults with disabilities (for example, *http://www.rehabilitystores.com/*). The paddles can be controlled by puff-and-sip or any other switches. This makes it possible for a consumer to compete in a fast-paced, interesting game. Computer access methods that were described in Chapter 7 enable an individual to play

computer games in the same way they provide access to educational materials.

One example of a holder is a gooseneck arm attached at one end to a table clamp. At the other end is a bracket that holds an embroidery frame. Using this device, an individual can embroider, crochet, or mend with only one hand. Other examples of devices designed for one-handed assistance are playing card holders, knitting needle holders, and card shufflers. For individuals with limited two-hand function, there are handheld playing card holders.

Devices that aid lack of reaching ability include a mobile bridge for holding the end of a pool cue off the table (a small bracket with wheels to allow positioning of the pool cue) and ramps for use while bowling (the ball is placed at the top of the ramp and the user releases it after aiming the ramp toward the pins). Lange (1998) describes a variety of options for reading when manipulation of the material is difficult.

■ SPECIAL-PURPOSE ELECTROMECHANICAL AIDS FOR MANIPULATION

There are two primary manipulative tasks for which electromechanical devices have been specifically designed and for which there are commercially available products: (1) feeding and (2) page turning. These special-purpose alternative manipulation devices are discussed in this section.

Electrically Powered Feeders

One area of human activity in which independence is highly desirable is eating. Anyone who has been unable to feed himself or herself (even for a brief period) knows the frustration of looking at one type of food on the plate and being fed another (e.g., expecting peas and getting potatoes). Being fed by another person can also create a feeling of dependency, and lack of independence in eating is often equated with childlike behavior. None of these stereotypes is accurate, and most persons who are fed by an attendant maintain control over the situation through direction of the attendant's actions. Nevertheless, many people would prefer to feed themselves if it were possible. Electromechanical feeders make this an option even for individuals who have very little motor control.

Use of an automatic feeder requires that the individual be able to control two separate functions. The first of these is location of the particular type of food that is to be eaten, and the second is picking up the food and moving it to mouth level. Currently available feeders require that the human operator be able to take food off a spoon, chew it, and swallow it safely. These requirements eliminate a large number of persons, but there are many who only lack the ability to pick up the food and get it to their mouths. It is this group for whom feeders are most beneficial.

Generic electromechanical feeders are shown in Figure 14-5. The first task of feeders, that of locating the desired type of food, is typically accomplished by placing the plate on a turntable whose rotation is under the control of the user. The user is able to stop the rotation when the desired food is properly positioned. The second action, moving the food to mouth level, is typically accomplished by a spoon attached to an arm whose height above the plate is variable. Two types of arms are used: (1) two-piece articulating and (2) telescoping. The articulating arm is capable of carrying greater weights and can position the spoon in more locations. The telescoping arm collapses into a smaller stored length and can be easier for transportation. Picking up the food is a process of scooping the food onto the spoon. One of two approaches can be used: moving the spoon against a fixed stop or moving a pusher against a fixed spoon (see Figure 14-5). For either of these approaches, both the spoon and the plate can be removed and washed with other dishes.

To control the feeder, the user must activate either one or two switches. The two-switch approach typically has one switch for plate rotation and one to scrape the food onto the spoon and raise and lower the spoon. In the one-switch version, activating the switch one time causes the plate to rotate; a second activation causes a complete cycle of pushing food onto the spoon and raising it to mouth level. Any single or dual switch described in Chapter 7 can be used.

The most commonly available feeder is the Winsford Feeder (Winsford Products, Pennington, NJ, available from Sammons Preston Rolyan, a Patterson Medical Company, *www.sammonspreston.com*), which is also marketed by several mail order equipment companies. This feeder has rechargeable batteries that are used to power it at many different settings. It has an adjustable height base that can accommodate varying spoon height requirements. A two-switch mode of operation is used, with one switch rotating the plate and the other scooping the food onto the spoon and elevating it to mouth level. A chin-activated dual switch is mounted on a long, solid wire. When it is pushed in one direction, plate rotation occurs, and when it is pushed in the opposite direction, food is pushed onto the spoon and elevated to mouth level. A two-position rocking switch is also commonly used with the Winsford Feeder. Other dual switches or two single switches may be adapted to work with this feeder. There is also a carrying case available for transportation of the feeder.

Another commercially available feeder is the Beeson Automaddak Feeder (Maddak, Inc., Pequannock, N.J., *http://service.maddak.com*). This feeder is powered by a 110-volt line. It is operated by two switches, one for plate rotation and the other for spoon control. In contrast to the Winsford Feeder, each switch must be held down to continue action; that is, the spoon elevation stops if the spoon switch is released. The Electric Self-Feeder (Sammons Preston Rolyan, a Patterson Medical Company, *www.sammonspreston.com*) is another powered feeder. This feeder uses a chin switch to activate the motorized pusher that fills the spoon. After the spoon is full, it automatically moves to the mouth. The plate is rotated to bring the desired food into range of the spoon.

A robotic system specially designed for feeding is the Handy 1 (Topping, 1996). The Handy 1 uses a series of seven columns or compartments on a tray. When it is activated, the Handy 1 scans through the tray, illuminating a light behind each column in succession. The user activates a single switch to choose the column, and the food in that column is bought to the mouth. An eighth light allows the user to access a cup for drinking at any time during the meal. More than 100 individuals have benefited from the use of the Handy 1 on a regular basis (Topping, 1996).

Harwin, Rahman, and Foulds (1995) compared the Handy 1 and the Winsford Feeder. They point out that the Winsford Feeder has only two degrees of freedom, whereas the Handy 1 has five. This increases the flexibility of the Handy 1 in dealing with the task of feeding, and it also allows it to perform some other tasks of daily living (e.g., self-care). The interface requirements of the Handy 1 are also more flexible than those for the Winsford Feeder. For example, the location where the food is to be transferred into the person's mouth can be changed. However, the Winsford Feeder is considerably less expensive than the Handy 1. This illustrates the tradeoff between flexibility and complexity (and hence cost) discussed earlier.

All these feeders require that the food be prepared in bite-sized portions for the user. It is also sometimes difficult to eat certain foods such as soups and those composed of

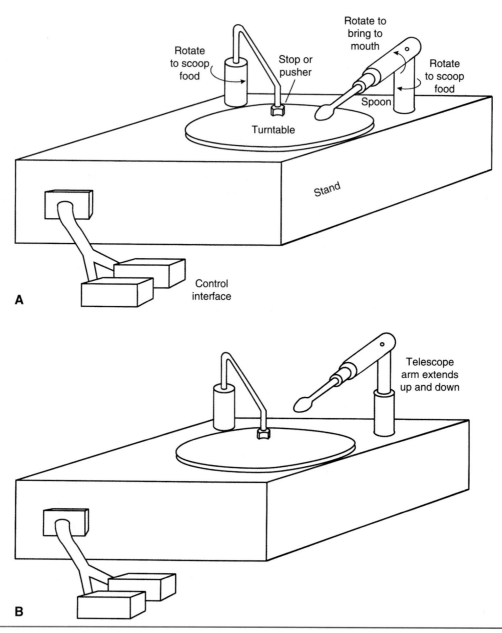

Figure 14-5 Two types of electromechanical feeders. **A,** The spoon is attached to a lever arm that is moved to mouth level. **B,** The spoon is attached to a telescoping arm that moves it to mouth level.

small pieces (e.g., rice, peas). Because of the necessity for assistance from a human aide or attendant, independence is reduced. However, the user is able to complete the eating activity independently, and this can save attendant time (and cost) and improve the user's sense of independence and control. Recall that the HAAT model discussed in Chapter 2 includes both an activity (in this case eating) and a context (defining the environment where the activity takes place). One of the most important considerations of the context is whether the environment will support the use of a feeding device. An individual may choose to use the device in one setting but not in another. For example, in the home situation where the physical and social context supports this type of technology, feeding devices might be acceptable. However, in a restaurant situation, they may draw unwanted attention to the user.

The primary safety considerations with feeders are mechanical injury from the spoon hitting the face and embarrassment caused by food falling off the spoon or plate. These devices can be messy to use and difficult to transport, and this may cause some people to restrict their use to home and to rely on a human attendant in the community.

Although they serve a restricted need and can be used by only a specific segment of persons with disabilities, **electrically powered feeders** can play an important role in increasing independence for persons whose motor limitations prevent them from using standard eating utensils.

Electrically Powered Page Turners

Access to books, magazines, and other reading material is important for the acquisition of information for school, work, or leisure. There are many individuals with disabilities who are able to read but who cannot physically manipulate the pages of the reading material. There are several approaches that can be used to assist these individuals. A book holder and mouthstick (see the section on low-tech aids in this chapter) allow independence in page turning for some persons. The major limitation of this approach is the requirement that the book be set up by an aide and properly positioned for both visual and physical access. This method also requires a high degree of head control and the ability to hold a mouthstick. A mechanical head pointer eliminates the last requirement, but there are still limitations of access.

Talking books, such as those made available for the blind, can also provide an alternative to physically manipulating pages. These are discussed in Chapter 8. By using a simple **environmental control unit**, a person with physical limitations can control the tape recorder and obtain access to the talking book at his or her own speed. Another approach is the use of books on computer disks. These can be loaded into a word processor, and the person needing access can use standard computer adaptations to turn the pages, scan through the material, find key words, and so on. This approach is also used by persons who have low vision or are blind, and it is discussed in Chapter 8. Both talking books and computer-based reading have the limitation that not all reading material is available in these formats.

An alternative to all these methods is the use of a human attendant to turn the pages. Because the turning of a page occurs every few minutes, this is not practical for any large amount of reading. The limitations in all these approaches have led to the development of **electrically powered page turners**.

From a manipulative point of view, page turning requires two primary actions: (1) separating the page to be turned from the other pages and (2) physically moving the page from one side to the other (forward or backward). Additional useful but not essential features include scanning a number of pages, turning to a specific page, and locating a bookmark and turning to that page. Currently available page turners use one of two methods to accomplish the first task of separating pages. Some devices use a vacuum pump that sucks the first page up and holds it away from the remaining pages. Other devices use a sticky roller that is placed on top of the page. When it rotates, the roller causes one page

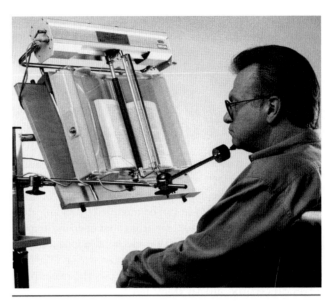

Figure 14-6   The Gewa page turner. (Courtesy ZYGO Industries.)

to be separated from the others. The roller may use putty, rubber gum (like a pencil eraser), or double-sided tape. This function is the most difficult for page turners, and its success for any page turner is a major indicator of the quality of the unit. Because reading materials differ widely in size, binding (e.g., uniform, spiral, loose leaf), and paper types (e.g., rough, slick, newsprint), it is important to evaluate any individual page turner with reading materials that vary in size, paper type, and binding style.

Once the page to be turned is successfully isolated, the page turner must move it to the opposite side of the book or magazine. The Gewa page turner (in North America, distributed by ZYGO Industries, Portland, Ore., *http://www.zygo-usa.com/*) (Figure 14-6) uses a rotating roller to separate pages from each other and then moves the entire roller from one side of the book or magazine to the other after the page has been separated. The standard control for the Gewa is a four-direction joystick. Two joystick directions cause roller rotation either clockwise or counterclockwise, and the other two cause the roller to move forward or backward. Any other four-switch control interface can also be used. An additional accessory for the Gewa page turner is a scanning selection method in which a single switch is used to select one of the four control functions as they are presented in sequence. The display of functions consists of small LED indicators, each labeled function corresponding to one joystick direction.

Other page turners have different mechanisms. The Touch Turner (Touch Turner Company, Everett, Wash., *www.touchturner.com/*) uses a rubber-coated wheel to separate the pages, and then a rotating semicircular disk pushes the separated page from one side to the other. As the disk rotates, the page is moved forward or backward, depending on the direction of rotation of the disk. The Touch Turner has both one-direction and two-direction models for standard books and a special model for paperback books and magazines. Vacuum-based systems often move the vacuum unit from side to side.

◼ ELECTRONIC AIDS TO DAILY LIVING

Many objects that need to be manipulated are electrically powered devices such as appliances (e.g., television, room lights, fans, kitchen appliances such as blenders or food processors) and others that can be modified by adding electrically powered control to them (e.g., door openers, drapery controls). The majority of these electrical appliances and controls are powered from standard house wiring (110-volt AC in North America). Figure 14-7 shows the major parts of an **electronic aid to daily living** (EADL). The user interacts with the EADL through a control interface (see Chapter 7). Feedback to the user is provided through a display that reflects the action being controlled (e.g., which appliance is to be activated, status of the system). The control interface and user display constitute the *human/ technology interface*. They are connected to the rest of the system and to each other by a block labeled *selection method*. Likewise, the appliances to be controlled are connected to the selection method through an *output distribution block*. The selection method and output distribution functions

together make up the *processor*. In some cases the human/ technology interface and the selection method are provided through an augmentative and alternative communication (AAC) device (see Chapter 11) or a computer (see Chapter 7) by a serial input, which can reduce the number of devices and also provides an identical user interface for both AAC and EADL functions. Some AAC devices also include the output distribution component. This component is connected to either a remote (wireless) linkage or a hard-wired connection or both; it produces an *activity output* by turning on and controlling the appliances.

Some devices or appliances require on-off control. Normally this is achieved by a switch that is pressed to activate the device. An example of this type of control is that used in many remote garage door openers, which require a single press and release to start the door opener. The process then proceeds automatically until the door is open. This type of appliance control device is often used by persons with disabilities to open other doors (e.g., house or apartment). This may require either that the switch on the garage door opener be adapted or that the entire function be incorporated into the EADL.

There are two switch outputs available on most EADLs: (1) momentary and (2) latched. A momentary switch closure is active only as long as the switch is pressed. In the case of the EADL, this output remains active only as long as the control interface is activated (e.g., a switch is pressed). The momentary output mode is useful for continuous functions such as closing draperies. The output can be sustained as long

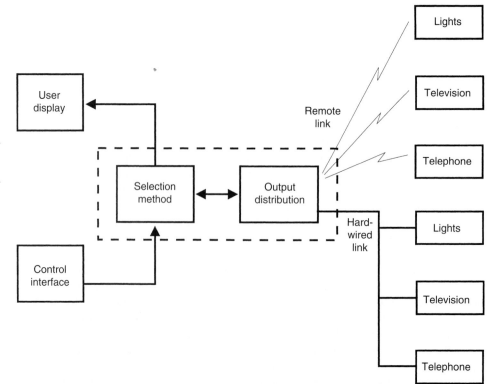

Figure 14-7 The major parts of an EADL. The *control interface* and *user display* constitute the human/technology interface. The components within the dotted box are the processor. The appliances listed on the right side of the figure are the activity output.

as the person desires it to be (e.g., to open drapes half way). In the latched mode a switch closure is turned on by the first activation and off by the next activation, and it toggles between these two states with each activation. This can be useful when turning on an appliance such as a light or radio.

Selection Methods

Chapter 7 defines several selection methods used for control of assistive technology devices. These include direct selection, scanning, directed scanning, and coded access. Each of these can be used with EADLs. Direct selection occurs when the user of the system can choose any output directly. For example, an EADL for controlling a room light, a fan, and a radio on-off control may have one control interface (possibly a key on a small keyboard or speech recognition) for each of the three functions (Figure 14-8). If the same three-unit system is to be operated by scanning access, then the keyboard can be replaced by a scanning panel and each of the three items to be controlled has a corresponding light. When the light

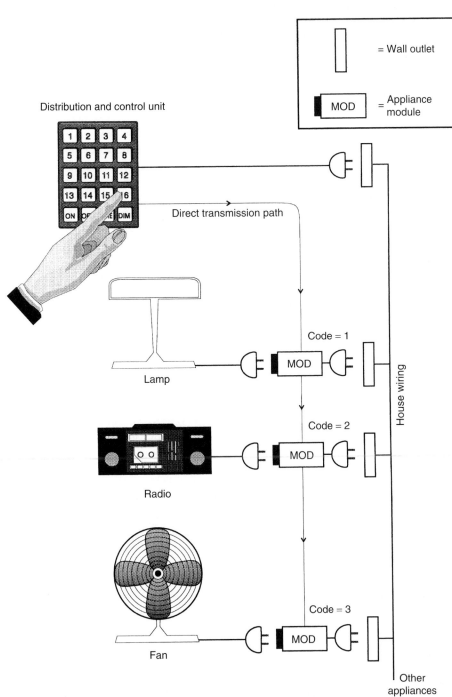

Figure 14-8   A direct-selection EADL. Each appliance has a numerical code, and the keypad is used to select the appropriate module. Control functions such as ON, OFF, and DIM are also activated by pressing the proper key on the keypad. This figure also illustrates the use of house wiring for distribution of the control signals to the appliance modules.

of the device to be activated comes on, the user activates a control interface to select that item. Finally, a code such as Morse code (see Chapter 7) can be used for one of the four output devices. The user enters a series of dots and dashes corresponding to the numerical code required to activate the desired appliance. Each of these selection systems is used in current EADLs, and some EADLs have multiple options available. Specific selection methods are discussed in the remainder of this section. Choice of a control interface for use with an EADL is based on the considerations presented in Chapter 7. Some control interfaces (e.g., speech recognition,* single switch) are commonly used with EADLs.

Control Functions Implemented by Electronic Aids to Daily Living

Chapter 7 defines the input domain for the control interface as either discrete or continuous. The most common type used in EADLs is *discrete control*, in which a device is either turned on or off or set to a specific value by activation of the EADL. Examples of on/off control include lights, television, or radio controls and starting or stopping a blender. Other EADL applications require setting a value. For example, a telephone dialer may have several stored numbers that may be selected. Each number is a discrete entry, and its selection produces a different result. Television channel selection is another example of discrete control. The other type of control function used in EADLs is *continuous control*, which results in successively greater or smaller degrees of output. Examples of EADL continuous control are opening and closing draperies, controlling volume on a television or radio, and dimming or brightening lights.

Transmission Methods

All EADL systems must transmit a signal to the appliance to be controlled. There are several methods used for this transmission. Although it is theoretically possible to connect all the appliances to be controlled directly to the rest of the EADL by wires, this method is not practical. Direct wiring requires that the controlled devices be physically close together or necessitates the installation of special wiring just for the EADL. More cost-effective and practical methods use some form of remote control. We use the term **remote control** to mean the absence of a physical attachment among the various components shown in Figure 14-7. In general, the link between the output distribution and the devices to be controlled is remote. However, it is also possible to

have remote links between the control interface and the processor.

House Wiring-X10.   One way to interconnect appliances and the output distribution function is to use the house AC wiring as a communication channel. Digital control signals are transmitted over the house wiring from the distribution control device to individual appliance modules, which are plugged into the standard electrical outlet (see Ciarcia, 1980, for a description of the operational details of these units). Figure 14-8 shows how this approach works. The distribution and control unit is also plugged into a wall outlet. This unit has a transmitter that sends out two codes over the house wiring. The first code identifies the device to be controlled, and the second selects the function to be performed (e.g., turn on or off, dim or brighten a light). Each appliance to be controlled is plugged into a module, which is then plugged into the wall. Each module contains a receiver that can interpret the codes sent out by the distribution and control unit. Most commercial systems have selector switches on the appliance modules to allow them to be set for a code from 0 to 15. In addition, both the distribution and control unit and the appliance modules can have one of 16 different "house" codes that allow two or more such systems to operate on the same wiring system. The combination of house codes and device numbers yields 256 possible controlled devices (16 × 16). Although this may seem like a large number, it can be useful to have more than a few choices, especially when the control is by computer-based software rather than manual selection of keys on the distribution and control unit. This type of appliance control was designed for use by the general population, and consequently, it is common and inexpensive. Devices are available at many consumer electronic stores (for example, the X-10 Powerhouse System, Northvale, N.J., *www.x10.com*). This type of device can become a relatively complete EADL for individuals who are able to press the buttons on the control unit. However, only binary control functions are available, (i.e., on/off) and such functions as channel selection (quantitative) or volume control (discrete) require more specialized systems.

The major advantage of house wiring transmission is the lack of installation costs because existing wiring is used (Mills, 1987). Disadvantages include (1) the lack of privacy, (2) possible interference between systems on the same electrical power system (e.g., in an apartment building), (3) the inability to transmit when multiple circuits are used for the wiring system, and (4) the lack of portability. Multiple circuits are often used in house and commercial wiring. Each circuit has a separate circuit breaker, and they are physically separate from each other, which means that a module connected to one circuit does not receive the control signals from a transmitter connected to a different circuit.

---

*For example, Simplicity Voice/Plus and All in one Plus, Quartet Technology, Inc., Tyngsboro, Mass., *www.qtiusa.com*; Butler in a Box, AVSI, Los Yorba Linda, Calif., *www.mastervoice.com*; Sicare Pilot, TASH, Ajax, Ontario, Canada, *www.tashinc.com/catalog/env_index.html*.

Ultrasound Transmission.   A second type of transmission used between the control and distribution unit and the appliances to be controlled is ultrasonic transmission. This type of transmission uses sound waves that are too high in frequency to be heard by the human ear. In general, that is any signal more than 20,000 Hz, but in practice signals of approximately 40,000 Hz are used. These signals are transmitted through the air to a receiver located up to several hundred feet from the transmitter. Because ultrasound waves are mechanical energy, they can be blocked by solid objects (including human tissue), and it is important to have a clear path between the transmitter and the receiver.

Ultrasonic transmission devices (for example, ElectraLink, TASH, Ajax, Ontario, Canada, *www.tashinc.com*) often consist of a transmitter unit, which is either handheld or mounted on a wheelchair, and a set of receivers, one for each appliance to be controlled (Figure 14-9). A latched mode is typically used. Various selection methods, including scanning and coded access, are available for these devices. The principle of operation is slightly different from that of house wiring–based systems. Each receiver has a code, and the transmitter sends a signal that corresponds to this code. When the transmitted code is received, the receiver is latched, which turns the appliance either on or off, depending on its

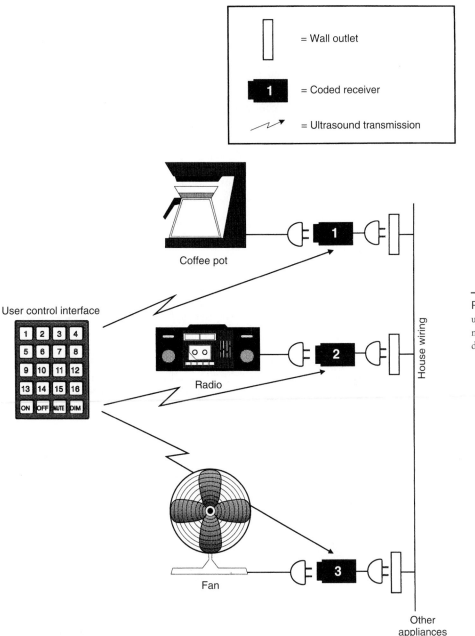

Figure 14-9   An EADL system using ultrasound transmission to discrete modules. Each module receives its signal directly from the transmitter.

state when the signal is received. Each appliance must have its own code, and most ultrasonic devices have a limited number of channels (generally four or eight).

Ultrasonic transmission is also used for some remote television controls. In this application, transmission of various codes is used for all basic television functions, such as on/off, channel change, volume control, and picture adjustments. Another use of ultrasound transmission is illustrated in

Figure 14-10. In this case the coupling between the control interface and the distribution and control unit is by ultrasonic transmission. This remote coupling enables the user to be more mobile than when the control interface is hard wired to the distribution and control unit.

The major advantage of ultrasonic transmission is that it is highly portable because it is easy to unplug the receiver modules and move them to a new location. The major

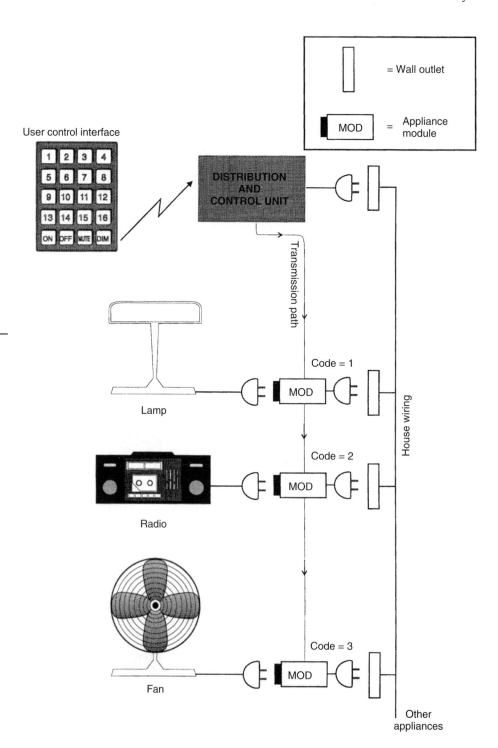

Figure 14-10 An EADL that uses ultrasound or IR transmission from the control interface to the distribution and control unit. As in Figure 14-8, house wiring is used for transmission from the distribution and control unit to the appliance modules.

disadvantages are the necessity to have the transmitter and receiver in the same room and to avoid obstacles between the transmitter and receiver that might block the signal.

Infrared Transmission.   Another mode is based on the use of invisible **infrared (IR) transmission** as the medium. This method is the most common in the control of home electronics (e.g., television set, cable television, DVD/CD player). IR remote controls are used for binary (latched and momentary), discrete, continuous, and quantitative types of control. The DVD functions of FAST FORWARD, SEARCH, and so on can also be controlled with an IR remote controller. Generally each remote device has a set of unique codes, and a remote unit manufactured by one company cannot be used with a system manufactured by someone else, which means that several remote controllers may be necessary to manage TV, cable, and other devices, unless a "universal remote" is programmed to control all these appliances.

IR remote control is also used in EADLs. The remote link between the control interface and the distribution and control unit in Figure 14-10 is often implemented by using IR instead of ultrasound. In this case the control scheme is the same as that described above for other IR remote controls. Sometimes the link between the control and distribution unit and the remote appliances is also implemented with IR transmission. The engineering, design, and construction of IR controllers are described by Ciarcia (1987b).

The major advantages of the IR devices are no installation costs (compared with hard wiring) and ease of portability. A major disadvantage is that the signal can be blocked by many materials, so a direct line of sight between the transmitter and receiver is required (Mills, 1987), which means that the transmitter and receiver must be in the same room. Because the receiver must be connected to the controlled appliances (possibly through the house wiring), the line-of-sight requirement limits the range of application (e.g., outside, inside, different rooms). Because the IR devices are light sensitive, they often do not work well in bright sunlight. Recall that the HAAT model includes a consideration of the physical context (see Chapter 2, Figure 2-4) in which a given activity is taking place. In this case the EADL is typically used in an interior location where light, heat, and sound can be controlled. However, interference from other appliances or interference caused by transmission from the EADL can affect the performance of these systems.

Radio Frequency Transmission.   A final transmission approach is the use of radio frequency (RF) waves as the link between the distribution and control unit and the control interface, the controlled appliances, or both. The most common examples of this type of remote control are garage door openers and portable telephones. The term *RF transmission* is used because the signals are in the same range as broadcast FM radio. **Radio frequency transmission** is used as the link between the control interface and the processor.

The major advantage of RF transmission is that it is not blocked by common household materials (it can be blocked by metal that is connected to the ground), and transmission can be over a relatively long distance throughout a house and yard. Because it is less restricted, it has the major disadvantages of interference and lack of privacy (Mills, 1987). The interference problem is generally approached by reducing the distance between the transmitter and the receiver and by having several transmission channels available. The user can switch between channels (or the device will automatically scan) to find the strongest signal. Privacy is generally addressed by allowing the user to select a transmission code (often with a bank of small switches) and then matching the transmitter and receiver codes.

One form of wireless technology is known as ZigBee. In addition to providing control that has all the advantages of RF transmission, ZigBee has low power consumption (meaning longer battery life) and long range of operation (range enough to control the whole home from anywhere inside it, not just the immediate room). ZigBee is ideally suited for low data rate applications (i.e., applications where the amount of information to be transmitted is small as in simple on-off controls) such as EADLs (Bessell et al, 2006). There are specifications for ZigBee applications that are made available through the ZigBee Alliance *(http://www. zigbee.org/en/about/)*. The goal of the alliance is to build wireless intelligence and capabilities into everyday devices. This will lead to companies having a standards-based wireless platform optimized for the unique needs of remote monitoring and control applications that includes simplicity, reliability, low cost, and low power (Kinney, 2006).

Trainable or Programmable Devices

Remote devices that use ultrasound, IR, or RF typically are designed for operation with only one appliance (e.g., TV, VCR). If an individual owns several remotely controlled devices, this can lead to "controller clutter," with a separate control required for each device. To reduce this problem, several manufacturers produce remote control units that can be adapted to work with any appliance. Some of these are called **trainable controllers**. These devices operate by storing the control code for any specific appliance function (e.g., on/off). As shown in Figure 14-11, *A*, the storage is often accomplished by pointing the trainable controller at the controller for the specific appliance and sending the specific function code (TV ON in Figure 14-11). The trainable device then stores this code for future use. When the stored code is sent to the appliance, it is received and used as if it had been sent by the appliance's own controller. This process is illustrated in Figure 14-11, *B*. In this manner, all the functions of the individual appliance controllers can be stored in

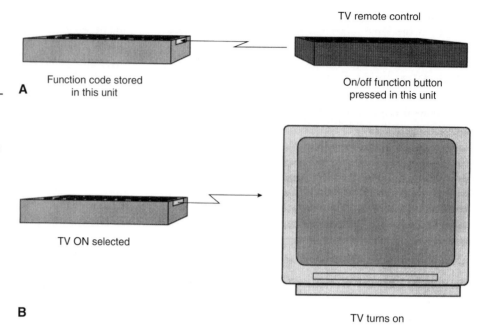

TV remote control

A   Function code stored
in this unit

On/off function button
pressed in this unit

Figure 14-11   A trainable IR controller. The trainable or programmable controller is shown on the left. **A,** Training is accomplished by aiming the device-specific control at the trainable controller and pressing the desired button (in this case, TV ON). **B,** The trained unit can then be used with the appliance to accomplish the desired function.

TV ON selected

B

TV turns on

one master controller and the user need only activate this one device. Most of these controllers have two modes: train and operate. Figure 14-12 shows a programmable EADL unit mounted to a wheelchair and used for controlling appliances such as the television.

Some controllers have codes for many appliances permanently stored in them. The user selects a code corresponding to his appliance (e.g., a television set made by a specific manufacturer). Ciarcia (1987a) describes the technical operation of trainable devices for IR controllers. These devices, like the individual appliance units, are designed using special-purpose microcomputers. In the training mode the EADL device is aimed at the individual appliance, the function

to be stored is pressed on the individual control, and the code is stored. This process is repeated for all functions and for all individual controllers. These devices are relatively small, lightweight, and battery powered, and they can be hand carried or mounted to a wheelchair.

An alternative approach is based on the storage, in the controller, of codes that are appropriate to a range of appliances. The user selects her appliance and looks up the controller code in a table. Once this code is entered into the controller, it is able to control the appliance. We refer to these as **programmable controllers.**

Trainable or programmable controllers designed for the general home electronics market can be of benefit to persons with disabilities who are able to press the small keys associated with these devices. For those persons who cannot use standard controllers, there are specially adapted trainable or programmable units that provide both direct selection and scanning selection.* Control interfaces include expanded keyboards or a built-in keyboard or single switches for scanning access. In the latter case, one of two methods is typically used: (1) small lights that are located next to each button are sequentially illuminated or (2) alphanumerical labels or numerical codes for each function are sequentially displayed. For each of these approaches, the user presses the switch when the desired choice is presented.

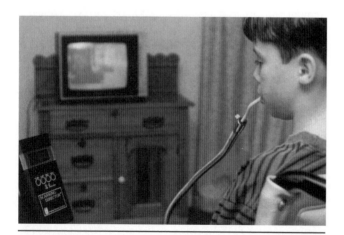

Figure 14-12   A trainable infrared EADL with scanning access. The EADL is shown mounted to a wheelchair. It is positioned so there is a line-of-sight link to the television for use of IR control. (Courtesy APT Technology, Inc., DU-IT CSG, Inc., Shreve, Ohio.)

*For example, Gewa Link, ZYGO Industries, Portland, Ore, *www.zygo-usa.com*; Imperium, Mini Relax and Relax #3, TASH, Inc., Ajax, Ontario, Canada, *www.tashinc.com*; Simplicity Switch & All-in-One, Quartet Technology, Inc., Tyngsboro, Mass., *www.qtiusa.com*; U-Control, Words Plus, Palmdale, Calif., *www.words-plus.com*.

As shown in Figure 14-11, most of the trainable or programmable EADL devices can be interfaced to other electronic devices (e.g., AAC devices, computers, power wheelchair controllers) through a serial port. To control the EADL, a code must be sent from the communication device or computer to the controller, and all specific functions and separate appliance codes must be stored in the communication device or computer. Several manufacturers include control software for EADL in their communication software programs (see Chapter 11). When the EADL is controlled by a computer or communication device, the software program generates the control signals and sends them through the serial port to the EADL.

To facilitate the control of appliances, cell phones, and other electronic devices the concept of a **universal remote** has been developed (Zimmerman et al, 2004). The universal remote standard is intended to allow users (including EADL users) to interact with networked devices and services in their environments. The universal nature of the controller specification means that all devices meeting the standard will be able to interact because they will follow predefined protocols rather than being unique to each manufacturer. The universal remote standard provides a versatile user interface description for devices and services, called a "user interface socket" to which any universal remote console (URC) can connect. Each URC can electronically "discover" remote devices or services in its range and then access and control them. Examples of services include cell phones and wireless computer networks. Devices could be any of these described for EADL control (e.g., television, CD/DVD players, standard telephones). A major advantage is that, with only one user interface description, diverse URC technologies can be supported, including connection through desktop and laptop computers and personal digital assistants.

Telephone Control

Persons with physical disabilities of the upper extremities often have difficulty in carrying out the tasks associated with telephone use. These include lifting the handset, dialing, holding the handset while talking, and replacing the handset to its cradle. Telephones differ greatly in design (e.g., portable, speaker, rotary or touch-tone dial), but all require that the listed tasks be performed. As in many other areas of assistive technology, there are a variety of ways to accomplish the same tasks. Mouthsticks or head pointers (see the section on low-tech aids earlier in this chapter) can be used to press a button to open a line on a speaker phone (equivalent to lifting the hand set), dial by pressing buttons, and hang up at the end of a conversation. There are also simple holders that position a handset for hands-free operation and mechanical switches with long handles that control the switch hook for answering a call or hanging up after a call. Finally, telephone

companies provide operator-assisted calling for persons with disabilities, so it is only necessary to press 0 for an operator, who then dials the call for the consumer. Our emphasis in this section, however, is on electronic telephone access systems, which are often integrated into EADLs.

Because modern telephones are actually sophisticated electronic devices, automation by use of electronic **telephone controllers** is relatively easy, and there are a variety of commercial products available to accomplish telephone access for persons with disabilities (for example, Relax 3 and Imperium, TASH, Ajax, Ontario, Canada, *www.tashinc.com*; Gewa IR Controlled Telephone, ZYGO Industries, Portland, Ore., *www.zygo-usa.com*). Many of the general-purpose EADLs have telephone functions built in (for example, Ezra, KY Enterprises, Belgrade, Montana, *www.quadcontrol.com*; EZ Control, Regenesis, North Vancouver, B.C., Canada; Simplicity Switch, Quartet Technology, Inc., Tyngsboro, Mass., *www.qtiusa.com*; Imperium, Sicare Pilot, Relax 3 TASH, TASH, Ajax, Ontario, Canada, *www.tashinc.com*). The functional components of a telephone controller are shown in Figure 14-13. Individual devices may group these components differently. Telephone controllers for a person with disabilities are built around standard telephone electronics. In some cases the controller is connected into the standard telephone, whereas in others the telephone is bypassed and the controller plugs directly into the telephone line. In any case, several of the important functions are common to consumer telephones. For example, the use of stored numbers (automatic dialing) and redial can save a great deal of time when the user must use scanning to select numbers. Another useful feature of currently available adapted telephones is that the user can answer electronically rather than by physically picking up the handset. This is done as an additional choice on a scanning menu or a direct selection on an EADL telephone control panel.

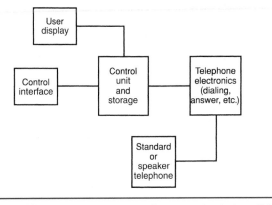

Figure 14-13 Functional components of an automatic telephone dialer. The *control interface* and *user display* constitute the human/technology interface, the *control unit and storage* and *telephone electronics* are the processor, and the *telephone* constitutes the activity output.

Other parts of the telephone controller shown in Figure 14-13 are necessary only for persons who require single-switch access to the system (e.g., the user display). The control interface is connected to a control unit that also interfaces with a display and with the telephone electronics. Although systems vary in their design, a typical approach is for the device to present digits sequentially on the display. When the digit to be dialed is presented, the user presses the switch to select the number and the scan begins again at zero. In this way, any phone number can be entered. Once the number is entered, it is sent to the telephone electronics for automatic dialing.

Many persons with disabilities respond slowly, and each switch press may take several seconds. If we assume that it takes 2 seconds to respond, then we must display each number for at least 3 seconds, which may require scanning through 10 numbers (30 seconds) just to get to the desired number. If all the desired numbers were large (e.g., 7, 8, 9), it could take almost 5 minutes (300 seconds) to dial one long-distance (11-digit) number. For this reason, all practical systems use stored numbers and automatic dialing. They also allow numbers to be entered and either stored or dialed by scanning. Redial also can speed things up, and this feature is normally included as well. Another unique feature in most telephone dialers designed for persons with disabilities is the inclusion of a HELP (e.g., a neighbor) or EMERGENCY (911) phone number that can be dialed quickly.

There are several modes of operation in automatic telephone dialers. First, the user must choose among dial, answer, or hang up. If dial is chosen, then the user must decide whether to access a stored number, redial, call for help, or dial an unstored number. For single-switch devices, this decision is generally made in one of two ways: (1) the system sequentially presents the choices to the user and the user waits until the desired choice is presented before pressing the switch or (2) a second switch is available that accesses the operational modes only (e.g., dial, answer, store) and the other switch is used for selecting numbers. In either method, if HELP is selected, it is automatically dialed with no further entry. Some units merely reserve the first place in the stored number directory for HELP, whereas others use a special selection scheme for it (e.g., a long switch press). The next place in the phone list choice is generally redial.

If redial is not chosen, then stored numbers are presented, usually by a code. Most systems have a capacity of 50 to 100 stored numbers. The user merely waits until the code for the number of the person he wants to call is presented and then presses the switch. At this point everything else is automatic. If the user wishes to dial or store a new number, he or she waits until that choice is presented and then activates the switch. Once in this mode, the method discussed above is used to enter the number, and the user then tells the controller whether to enter it into memory or to dial it.

Because the telephone controller obtains access to the telephone lines in the course of its normal operation, it is relatively easy to include other telephone-based functions in the adapted controller's operation. For example, apartment buildings often use the telephone system for the intercom and front door latch, and the adapted telephone dialer can access these by including additional codes selected by the user.

When a computer is used as part of an EADL, the telephone dialing functions can be implemented by using software programs coupled with an electronic telephone interface that connects to the telephone line. These software and electronics are common for use in modems for communication between computers (e.g., for Internet access), and they have been adapted for some EADL systems.

Configuring Electronic Aids to Daily Living

Having looked at the components that normally make up EADLs, next is a discussion of how EADLs are selected and configured to meet the specific needs of a person with a disability. The first step in this process is to carry out an assessment of the person's needs and skills.

Assessment for Electronic Aids for Daily Living Use. As discussed in Chapter 4, the initial assessment step is to determine the consumer's needs carefully, especially in the context of daily living demands (e.g., home, employment). Retrospective studies of EADL use show that such factors as employment status, lifestyle (passive versus active), and gender all play a role in the effectiveness of EADL systems (Efthimiou et al, 1981; Sell et al, 1979). Bentham, Bereton, and Sapacz (1992) discuss major considerations to be included in a careful needs assessment for EADL selection. These studies emphasize the need for a careful analysis of factors in addition to physical and cognitive ability, such as ease of use, displays, home modifications required, and equipment standardization. Several of these are discussed later in this chapter.

Holme et al (1997) conducted a survey of occupational therapists (OTs) working in spinal cord injury and disease centers. The purpose of the survey was to determine the use of EADLs by persons who have had spinal cord injuries, reasons for recommendations of EADLs (or not) by OTs, and the skills required to assess consumers for use of EADLs and recommend appropriate devices. They found that 84% of the OTs working in these centers used EADLs with their clients as part of the in-patient rehabilitation process. Consumers who had injuries at the C4 or higher level were generally viewed as able to benefit from EADLs. The top four reasons for recommending an EADL were (1) empowerment of the client, (2) improvement in the client's quality of life, (3) increased access to call systems, and (4) decreased need for attendant care. Holme et al (1997) also found that more than 50% of the EADLs recommended and purchased for clients were still in use. They identified the major reasons for *not* recommending an EADL as: (1) lack of funding (64% of respondents), (2) high cost of EADLs (47%), (3) unavailability of EADLs for trial, and (4) lack of EADL knowledge by the OT responsible for the client's rehabilitation. The major reason that clients did not use EADLs recommended for them was a preference for having another person provide the necessary assistance. Holme et al (1997) concluded that more frequent recommendation of EADLs by OTs is dependent on two factors: (1) outcome studies that identify the effectiveness of EADLs and their cost-effectiveness and (2) inclusion of knowledge and skills related to EADLs in OT training.

An Australian survey of 20 users of EADLs identified key issues for successful application (Ability Research Center, 1999). Training of the person who will use the EADL and those who support the person, reliability of the EADL, and support for such things as customization and trouble shooting in the early days of use were the top three areas of concern raised. Only about 30% of the users in this study had received training, and this influenced their use of the EADL. Nearly 50% described their EADL system as "very unreliable" or "hardly satisfactory." This is a major issue because EADLS are often recommended to allow less personal assistant time and create greater independence for the user. An unreliable system cannot be depended on for independence and may influence the safety of the user. In the Australian study only 45% of the users felt that they had received adequate support to use the EADL effectively. These findings reinforce the need for soft technologies of training and user support to make the hard technology EADL devices useful and effective.

Dickey and Shealey (1987) describe an evaluation process that follows the needs assessment and leads to the selection of EADLs. The first step in this evaluation is to determine the person's physical abilities (see Chapter 4) and the ability to use a control interface (see Chapter 7). If the person is also using an augmentative communication device (see Chapter 11) or a power wheelchair (see Chapter 12), then EADL functions may be included in one of these other devices and a separate control interface may not be necessary.

The next step in Dickey and Shealey's (1987) evaluation process is to determine the consumer's cognitive status, which includes such things as short- and long-term memory, attention, and problem-solving skills. Motor planning skills also require evaluation. These abilities are all important in understanding and effectively using an EADL. In determining the feasibility of using an EADL, Dickey and Shealey (1987) suggest that the consumer's ability to learn new tasks and the most reliable method of integrating new skills with old activities should be determined. These two areas can have a significant impact on the effectiveness of an EADL. Motivation and functional capabilities must also be assessed. In the retrospective studies, motivation was

found to be a major factor, closely coupled to lifestyle and employment status.

Dickey and Shealey (1987) also suggest that the specific tasks to be accomplished be identified both in an interview and by a home visit. Some tasks can be easily accomplished with an EADL, whereas others require different manipulation aids; a careful environmental survey can determine which tasks fall into each category. It is also important at this stage to understand the consumer's expectations of an EADL and determine whether it is possible to meet these expectations. The consumer's daily routine, the accessibility of her residence, the attendant care available, and the existence of other assistive technologies also affect the recommendation of an EADL. Finally, available funding to acquire the EADL plays a role in the selection of a system, and it may be necessary to set priorities among needs and tasks to allow for unknown funding amounts. Figure 14-14 illustrates an assessment form used in EADL evaluations (Barker, Gross, and Henderson, 1991). This form or an equivalent can be used to summarize the evaluation results, including the needs and EADL configuration, for an individual consumer.

The outcomes of an EADL assessment include (1) identification of control sites and control interfaces, (2) determination of cognitive abilities related to understanding EADL operation, (3) listing of EADL functions desired (in priority order), (4) evaluation of the consumer's motivation to use electronic environmental control, (5) a listing of other electronic devices that the consumer uses, and (6) identification of the environments in which the EADLs will be used. The listing of functions may include such things as lighting, TV, and drapery control. The listing of other electronic devices should include both consumer electronic devices, such as TV, CD/DVD player, computer, and speaker telephone (all with brand names and model numbers), and assistive technologies, such as communication devices and power wheelchairs. Armed with this information, it is then possible to work with the consumer to select an EADL that meets his or her needs.

Single-Device Binary Control Electronic Aids to Daily Living. Electonic aids to daily living that control only one appliance can be useful in developing motor control and cognitive concepts such as cause and effect (for example, the Power Link, Ablenet, Minneapolis, Minn, *www.ablenetinc.com*). Chapter 7 describes a motor training program that uses these types of EADLs. Most of these have both momentary and latched modes, and they include a timer to activate the appliance for a preset number of seconds. These devices are useful when only a single device control can be understood by the user (e.g., in the case of developmental disability) or when only one device is required (e.g., a radio or light). The cost is low (less than $200), and there can be a significant increase in independence.

DEVICES TO BE CONTROLLED / ENVIRONMENT(S)

Home, Worksite, or School Environmental Assessment

Living, Work, or School Situation
Living: alone, with family/roommate/attendant, group living
Work/School: type of facility, # people sharing room(s)

Daily Routine Within Environment(s) - How is time spent

Devices to be Controlled (type, number, how devices operated)

___ Telephone	___ * TV	___ ~ Electric Bed
___ Lights	___ * VCR	___ ~ Window Opener
___ Call Bell	___ * Stereo	___ ~ Drapes/Curtains
___ Alarm System	___ *^ Compact Disk	___ ~ Door Opener
___ Air Conditioner	Player	___ DoorLock/Unlock
___ Fan	___ ^ Tape Recorder	___ Page Turner
___ Intercom	___ ^ Tape Player	
___ Radio	Other _____
___ Computer	_____

~ Items often require momentary mode
* Items often require infrared
^ Insertion?

Where Devices Are
rooms, centers of activity within rooms, devices in room,
number & type of outlets (2 or 3 prong receptacles)

Room	Devices	#Outlets
_____	_____	____
_____	_____	____
_____	_____	____

Layout of Building & Rooms
building / room considerations _____
doors opened or closed _____

Access to EADL Needed from Different Places or Positions
power wheelchair _____
manual wheelchair _____
other chair/ position_____
bed _____

Other Equipment EADL to be Compatible With
wheelchair_____
computer _____
communication device _____
other _____

Access to Devices for Other People _____

Figure 14-14   An evaluation form used for assessing environmental needs and goals. (From Barker P, Gross K, Henderson K: Control of the environment. *In Proceedings of the '91 RESNA Pacific Reg Conference*, 1991, The Conference.)

The use of single-function EADLs often leads to the use of multiple-function EADLs or electronic communication devices (see Chapter 11). This progression is described in Chapter 7.

Matching the Characteristics of Multiple-Function Electronic Aids to Daily Living to the Needs of the User.
When an EADL is planned to meet specific needs, it is useful to group the tasks (determined during the assessment described earlier) into the five categories shown in Table 14-1. This grouping, based on the common ways of implementing specific functions, is the first step in specifying an EADL. After completing the assessment form, shown in Figure 14-14, the assistive technology practitioner (ATP) will know the type of appliances that need to be controlled. The EADL functions required can be identified in the left-hand column of Table 14-1. The corresponding information in the right-hand column identifies the methods available for EADL implementation. This allows options to be considered.

The first group in Table 14-1 is binary (on/off) latched (stays on or off until the next activation) control of appliances that operate from standard household wall current. As described previously, there are two basic ways that current EADLs control such appliances: (1) by plugging them into receivers that plug into the house wiring and transmitting

TABLE 14-1	Functions Performed by Electronic Aids to Daily Living

Functions	Methods of Implementation
Binary latched control of AC appliances (e.g., lights, radio, on-off only)	House wiring transmission Direct ultrasound control
Discrete or continuous appliance (e.g., TV, VCR, CD, cassette tape control)	IR remote transmission Ultrasound remote transmission
Momentary control of appliances (e.g., door opener, drapery control)	RF remote transmission
Telephone control	Hard-wired switch control
Switch control (any device requiring one or two switches)	Hard wiring IR link to switch box Ultrasound link to switch box

control signals over the house wiring and (2) by direct ultrasonic transmission to a receiver into which the appliance is plugged. The most common commercially available components for use with house wiring transmission are the X-10 modules and controllers (X-10 Powerhouse, Inc., Northvale, N.J., *www.X-10.com*). These modules are incorporated into many EADLs. The major direct ultrasound receiver-based control device is the ElectraLink (TASH, Inc., Ajax, Ontario, Canada. *www.tashinc.com*). The second category in Table 14-1 is appliances that require discrete or continuous control, such as television channel selection or volume control. The most common EADL control method for discrete or continuous appliances is IR remote transmission, and several EADLs use integrated trainable or programmable IR controllers. This technology allows several devices (e.g., TV, CD/DVD) to be incorporated into one package controlled by the EADL. Each of these devices must have its own IR control to be incorporated into the trainable or programmable controller. The options available to the ATP depend on what appliances the consumer has and whether he or she has IR remote control. If IR remote devices are available, then the choice is to use an EADL with a trainable or programmable IR device. If the consumer needs continuous or discrete control but does not have IR-controlled appliances, then the ATP should consider EADLs with built-in discrete or continuous control, which may require modification of the appliance or purchase of a stand-alone IR controller.

If the consumer wants to control items such as draperies, then momentary control (i.e., the appliance is turned on for a variable period of time and then turned off) is required. For example, a drapery motor or bed elevation control may be turned on long enough to move the curtain or the bed to the proper position, and then the motor must be turned off. A latched control generally presents problems in

this scenario. Very short activation times are not possible with latched control, especially if the user has delays in muscle motor response. In some cases the range of movement for the task is always the same (e.g., when opening a door), and a device that is started by the user and automatically stopped at the end of the task by the device (e.g., when the door is fully open or fully closed) can be used. This type of control is often implemented by using RF transmission. Hard-wired switch control can also be used for these functions. Common examples are the enlarged switches often placed near doors for persons with disabilities or the active floor mats or light sensors used to trigger the opening of these doors.

Telephone control is listed separately in Table 14-1 because the functions performed are different from other EADL tasks. Generally telephone controllers use switches connected directly to them (hard wired). Integrating all EADL functions is often desirable. If the consumer is also going to use IR continuous or discrete control, the ATP should consider the use of an IR-controlled telephone. This allows the consumer to control the telephone in the same way as the TV, CD/DVD, and so on.

The final category in Table 14-1 is for devices that require one- or two-switch control. Other examples of appliances requiring switch control are call signals and drapery and door controls. The simplest method to implement this type of control is hard wiring of the switch to the EADL component. However, this approach has two major disadvantages: (1) the user is forced to go to the device to be controlled and use the switch at that location, so flexibility in movement is limited and (2) it is difficult to integrate the switch control with other EADL functions into a total package controlled by only one control interface. If a consumer must use different switches for different devices, then independence can be reduced. If the individual does not have good motor control and requires careful positioning of the control interface for successful use, the problem is even more difficult.

One way to integrate switch control with other EADL functions is to use a component that can detect IR or ultrasound signals and generate a switch-type output. This type of output is sometimes referred to as *relay output*. For example, if the consumer is using a trainable or programmable IR EADL controller for TV, CD/DVD, and telephone use and needs to control a drapery motor as well, a two-output IR trainable switch box (as shown in Figure 14-15) can be used. The IR EADL can provide the equivalent of a switch output directly, and the consumer does not need to have two additional switches to control the drapes (e.g., one switch to open them and one switch to close them). Some EADLs have built-in switched or relay outputs.

Not all remote control uses IR transmission. Binary latched control of electrical appliances is often implemented by either ultrasound or RF transmission, and trainable or

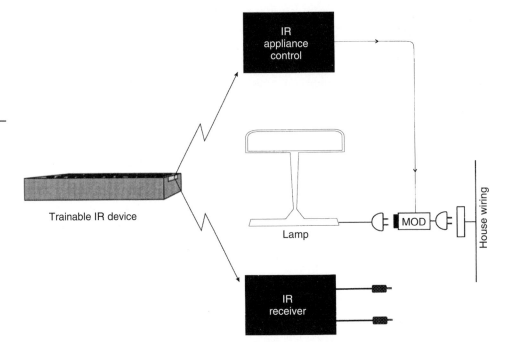

Figure 14-15 One approach to the integration of appliance control and single-switch or dual-switch control is to use an IR receiver that provides one- or two-switch closure outputs when activated. The two jacks shown in the lower right of the figure can be connected just as any switch would be.

programmable IR controllers are not usable for these functions. Two basic approaches are used to integrate binary appliance control and remote IR controllers. The first of these, shown in Figure 14-15, has a control and distribution unit that uses IR transmission. The transmitted codes are used to select an appliance (the number of appliances can vary from 4 to 256) and the function to be accomplished (on/off or dim/brighten for lights only). The trainable or programmable IR device is programmed to recognize these

codes, and the remote unit treats the appliance control and dual-switch receiver as IR-controlled devices.

The second approach to integration of discrete or continuous IR control with binary latched appliance control, shown in Figure 14-16, is to incorporate ultrasound and RF control into the trainable or programmable device together with IR transmission. In this case there is no need for a separate IR transmission distribution and control unit because the ultrasound and RF transmission is built into the trainable

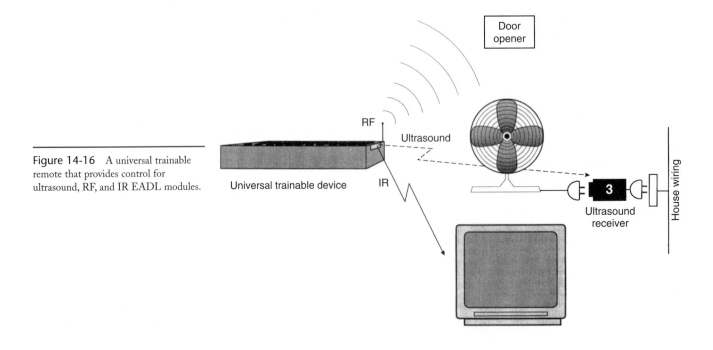

Figure 14-16 A universal trainable remote that provides control for ultrasound, RF, and IR EADL modules.

or programmable remote controller. This technology combines the trainability of the IR unit for TV, CD/DVD, and so on with the simplicity of direct ultrasound or RF transmission for binary control of appliances. This configuration allows more flexibility in the choice of individual environmental control components and allows us to focus on the needs of the EADL user rather than on the devices that may be available.

Hospital-Based Electronic Aids to Daily Living. Individuals with a high-level spinal cord injury are hospitalized immediately after the injury and remain hospitalized for many months. During this time, they have needs for environmental control that are similar to those for home use, but their needs also differ in important ways. Jones et al (1980) list four advantages of using hospital-based EADLs: (1) increased independence, (2) increase in motivation for self-rehabilitation, (3) reduction in anxiety from helplessness, and (4) increased nursing time available for more essential services. As Efthimiou et al (1981) have found, an important factor in increased postdischarge use of EADLs is experience during the acute and subacute hospital-based rehabilitation phase. This is an additional advantage of hospital-based EADLs.

There is some controversy, however, as to when an EADL should actually be recommended and obtained (Ability Research Centre, 1999). Arguments for introduction of the EADL during the acute hospital phase of rehabilitation include developing a sense of control and possible independence in the patient and providing the system while there is significant support available for set-up and training. The arguments in favor of waiting until the patient returns home are that the person needs to learn to do as many things independently as possible with minimal assistance and the simplest level of technology possible should be used to accomplish this independence. A second reason for waiting is that the exact specifications and configuration of an EADL requires an assessment of the home environment and the recommendation should wait until the person has returned home.

To achieve these advantages, it is necessary to include features not commonly found in home-based EADLs. The first of these is inclusion of access to the nurse call system of the hospital. This requires that the EADL have an interface to standard hospital nurse call systems. A variety of control interfaces must be available for the patient to use in accessing this function. As Jones et al (1980) point out, it is often necessary to have one control interface usable during the initial, acute phase of injury (approximately 6 weeks after initial admission). Because of spinal shock, the patient often has greater paralysis during this phase than in later stages, and efforts to use residual limb movement will be compromised. They recommend using above-the-neck movements to activate the control interface during this phase. Respiration may also be more significantly compromised

during the acute phase, which limits the use of puff-and-sip control interfaces. Finally, cervical traction may limit head movements during the acute phase. (Removal of the head traction apparatus often signals the transition from acute to subacute rehabilitation.) On the basis of these considerations, Jones et al (1980) have found that chin-controlled switches are the most generally useful during the acute phase of rehabilitation.

During the acute phase of rehabilitation, the patient is normally restricted to bed. EADL functions that are useful include television control (on/off, volume, and channel change), electric bed control, and appliance control (radio, lamp, fan). Although available on most hospital-based EADLs, telephone control is not frequently used during the acute phase of rehabilitation.

During the subacute phase of hospital-based rehabilitation, the patient generally has greater control because of the removal of the head traction apparatus, reduction of spinal cord swelling, and an increase in respiratory capability. These changes allow for more options in control interface selection. The patient also has greater interest in his surroundings, and telephone, television, and appliance control become more important to him. EADLs designed for hospital use generally do not have a wide range of options. For example, they may allow only one or two appliances to be controlled or they may have a small number of stored phone numbers (e.g., five). These design considerations reflect the unique requirements of the hospital situation. Other special features include very simple operation; large displays that are lighted for use in dim intensive care units; special electric bed and nurse control interfacing; and flexibility in the number of options and capabilities, depending on the needs of the user. Jones et al (1980) present design details for one computer-controlled hospital-based EADL.

Studies of Users of Electronic Aids to Daily Living

Several studies have been conducted to determine the preferred features and factors influencing successful application of EADLs. Most of the studies were conducted before some of the current features (e.g., trainable or programmable IR controllers) became available, but they still reflect basic preferences of users.

Symington et al (1986) studied the effect of EADL availability on attendant care in an institutional setting. Using a paired questionnaire for EADL users and nursing attendants in an institutional setting, they evaluated attitudes and perceptions of both users and staff regarding self-worth, independence, and usage of EADLs. The survey was administered before EADL system delivery and after EADL system use. For the users of devices, only one area (irritability) showed a statistically significant decline after EADL delivery. Perceptions of self-worth and independence increased, and users generally felt that they were less frustrated, had greater privacy, and needed to "bother" staff less frequently. The staff felt that the users had greater independence and that the staff was relieved of "extra duties" and saved time. An electromechanical counter recorded EADL usage, but no data were reported on frequency of use or usage patterns.

Woods and Jones (1990) reported on 10 years of experience with EADLs in institutional settings. They reported that EADL use can increase the independence of patients in such a setting. However, they also stressed the importance of training in proper use. Mann (1992) studied the use of EADLs by elderly nursing home residents. In this study, residents were divided into control and experimental groups. The experimental group received EADLs for use in their rooms to control lights and radios. They also received training in the use of these devices. Those in the control group did not have EADLs. Mann found that independent use of radios by the experimental group occurred at three times the rate of the control group at the end of the study. These results indicated that elderly nursing home residents will increase their environmental interaction if they have access to EADLs.

Studies have also been conducted on EADL use in community settings. Sell et al (1979) studied eight different EADLs over a 44-month period. Their subjects were persons with high-level (C4 or higher) spinal cord injuries who used the EADLs in their homes. Both groups were physically able to access the EADL functions. Features of EADLs that were judged valuable included visual and auditory selection displays, overall size and appearance (fitting into a home), ability to make confidential telephone calls with an automatic telephone dialer, direct access to telephone dialing (rather than using the operator), and reliability. Reliability was judged by the absence of failures of the device or of operational errors by the user.

Efthimiou et al (1981) studied the impact of EADLs on the postdischarge lives of persons with spinal cord injuries. Identified factors related to EADL use included gender (74% of men chose to use EADLs, whereas only 14% of the women did), exposure to an EADL during the in-hospital rehabilitation process, and availability of EADL systems (including funding) after discharge. They also looked at scales of activity and correlated these with EADL use. One substudy included 13 EADL users and 7 nonusers, all men. All the users were employed compared with only 54% of the nonusers. Another difference between the user and nonuser groups was that users more frequently participated in educational activities, phone calls, and travel, whereas nonusers spent more time in passive recreational activities. Users more frequently used assistive devices in general, and they performed more tasks independently than did the nonusers. In this study, use or nonuse was unrelated to adjustment to the disability and personality type. The major reasons given for not using an EADL were lack of space and an inaccessible home.

McDonald, Boyle, and Schumann (1989) studied EADL use by persons who had incurred high-level spinal cord injuries. In contrast to earlier studies that had used very small samples, these authors had 29 subjects accessed through the manufacturers who had provided their EADLs. More than 90% of their sample of EADL users found them to be helpful and more than 70% felt that EADLs increased their independence. The group of users also indicated that the EADL positively affected their disposition (67%) or was neutral in this regard (33%). The needs for EADL use were ranked in order of importance: communication, security/health, recreation, household tasks, employment, and education. EADL functions judged important (in rank order) were telephone, television, room lights, emergency signal, door, and computer. The 29 respondents also indicated that they were comfortable and felt secure for longer periods alone when an EADL was available.

Rigby et al (2005) investigated the psychosocial impact and functional performance of EADL use in the home by comparing a group of users (n = 16) and a group of nonusers (n = 16), all of whom had sustained cervical spinal cord injuries. They found that functional abilities were greater (as measured by standardized functional task instruments) and the psychosocial impact was positive for competence, adaptability, and self-esteem (as measured by the Psychosocial Impact of Assistive Devices Scale [PIADS]). In contrast to these studies of EADLs that reported only general opinion and did not objectively measure actual usage, Von Maltzahn, Daphtary, and Roa (1995) monitored usage of EADLs in home settings. They used a data logger that kept track of time and type of activation over a 16-week period and found that the greatest usage was in the evening and the largest activity was in television control. The small sample of subjects (five) showed great variability as well, with a factor of almost 30 times between the greatest and least number of uses of the EADL per week. Von Maltzahn, Daphtary, and Roa (1995) also used an end-of-study questionnaire to determine perceptions and attitudes of the users and their care providers. Once again the importance of training was cited, and both users and caregivers indicated that there was greater user independence and fewer demands made on the caregivers.

Jutai et al (2000) used the PIADS (see Chapter 4) to evaluate the psychosocial impact of EADLs. The goal of this study was to determine the perceived benefit of EADLs to the consumer's quality of life. Two groups were included: users of EADLs and those for whom EADLs were appropriate but who had not yet received them. Users' perceptions were measured at two points 6 to 9 months apart to determine the stability of the perception of psychosocial impact. Jutai et al found that EADLs produced similar degrees of positive impact on users and positive perceptions of anticipated impact on those without EADLs. The two measures of those using EADLs indicated that the psychosocial impact was stable over the time frame used. This study demonstrated the utility of the PIADS as an instrument for quantifying the psychosocial impact of assistive technologies.

In a similar study, user's perceptions of the benefits of EADLs were evaluated throughout the assessment and acquisition process using the PIADS (Ripat and Strock, 2004). In the preacquisition phase, potential EADL users predicted that there would be positive impact on feelings of competence and confidence and that an EADL would enable them in a positive way. One month after obtaining an EADL, the perceptions were still positive but less so than in the preacquisition phase. After 3 to 6 months the level of positive perception had returned to the preacquisition level, indicating that the original predictions were actually met. The most likely reason for the reduced positive impact perception in the middle phase is that the users were learning the new device and were adjusting to carrying out activities of daily living in a new way with the EADL.

Ripat (2006) reported results of a follow-up study. This study found that the positive benefits were sustained over time, as measured by the Canadian Occupational Performance Measure (COPM) and PIADS. (See Chapter 4 for a description of both measures.) Both new and more experienced users perceived an overall positive impact of EADLs (Ripat, 2006). Both the COPM, which measures an individual's perception of performance and satisfaction with performance in activities of daily living, and the PIADS, which measures the impact of assistive technology on an individual, yielded positive results that were highly correlated with each other. The use of EADLs for a short trial period of 2 weeks also decreased frustration, increased independence, and decreased the time to complete tasks (Croser et al, 2001).

Examples of Electronic Aid to Daily Living Application

To illustrate the process of configuring EADLs for specific needs, several case examples are described. Each of these cases is based on an actual situation faced by a person with a disability (Cook and Hussey, 1992). Gross (1992) presents a detailed case study of EADL use by a person with a high-level spinal cord injury. She also describes a process for analyzing needs and converting them into EADL specifications.

◼ ROBOTIC AIDS TO MANIPULATION

Because *robots* or **robotic systems** are intended to assist with manipulation, they are a natural alternative manipulation device for persons who have disabilities. There are, however, some significant differences between the use of

CASE STUDY

EADLs FOR INCREASED INDEPENDENCE

Joyce is 39 years old. She has cerebral palsy, and she has just moved into an apartment with an attendant. She is unable to speak, and she uses a communication device based on a laptop computer. Joyce controls her scanning communication device with a tread switch mounted near her knee. The communication device consists of a software program* running on a laptop computer. The communication and environmental control aspects of Joyce's system were integrated by using an IR trainable or programmable remote device interfaced to the serial port of the laptop computer.† The remote device is activated by the scanning communication software computer program, and it controls a TV and VCR directly. A two-channel IR receiver with switch output is used to control an automatic telephone dialer.‡ The telephone controller also allows control of four ultrasound receivers (Ultra Four), which Joyce has connected to two lamps and to a drapery control to open her curtains automatically. All the EADL functions are controlled by selecting the device from a menu and then sending a command through the IR remote unit to activate it (turn on the switch to the telephone dialer, change TV channels, and so on).

---

*Scanning WSKE, Words Plus, Lancaster, Calif., *www.words-plus.com*.
†Relax II, TASH, Inc., Ajax, Ontario, Canada, *www.tashinc.com*.
‡E.A.S.I. Dialer, TASH, Inc., Ajax, Ontario, Canada, *www.tashinc.com*.

robots by persons with disabilities and their use industrially. Industrial robots often have the role of *replacing* the human operator for reasons of strength, safety, or precision. In production line environments (e.g., automobile manufacturing), it is often necessary to lift large or heavy objects and position them for attachment to other parts. Robots are stronger than humans and are not subject to fatigue after hours of service. Many work environments are hazardous (e.g., those involving radiation or very high or low temperatures). To ensure safety of the operator, handling of objects in these environments is done by a robotic manipulator controlled by the human operator. At the opposite extreme from heavy object positioning is the repeated assembly of small parts (e.g., electronics assembly). Robots can be programmed to carry out the exact same task over and over without fatigue or loss of accuracy. In each of these cases the human is an ancillary part of the total system.

In contrast, in assistive robotics the human operator is at the center of the process. Instead of replacing the human operator, the goal is to enhance his or her ability to manipulate

Eileen, who is 62 years old, had a brainstem stroke and requires maximal assistance for daily living. She sits in a reclining chair at home for the majority of the day. Eileen is able to use head movement to make communication selections with a built-in Madentec Tracker* light pointer mounted on a headband to control a communication device.[†]

Eileen also needs a simple EADL that can control the TV (turn it on, select channels, and control volume), a lamp, and a call signal to use when her husband is out of the room. She controls a scanning trainable IR remote[‡] with a single switch mounted next to her head. This directly accesses the required TV functions. For the call system, an IR-sensitive switch is used to control an X-10 module. The module can be plugged in anywhere in the house, and her husband carries it with him when he goes outside or into a remote part of the house. In this way Eileen can summon him at any time if necessary. She can activate the switch by using head movement without having to have the light pointer taken off. This makes her communication function independent of her EADL function, and it offers a contrast to Joyce's preference of having them integrated.

*Edmonton, Alberta, Canada, www.madentec.com.
[†]Vantage, Prentke Romich, Wooster, Ohio, www.prentrom.com/.
[‡]Relax II, TASH, Inc., Ajax, Ontario, Canada, www.tashinc.com.

Dorothy, a 45-year-old woman who has amyotrophic lateral sclerosis, lives with her son, daughter, and husband and receives attendant care daily. Dorothy uses a computer for written communication and an EADL for telephone, door, and electrical bed and appliance control. For writing, she uses a trackball with a virtual keyboard software program for text entry (see Chapter 7).

Appliance and telephone control were implemented with a stand-alone EADL* accessed with a single-touch switch. This approach was taken, instead of combining the communication and environmental control functions, because Dorothy generally does not need access to the EADL functions while she is writing. Automatic telephone dialing is accomplished by the scanning approach described above. Dorothy's needs for controlling augmentative communication appliances are met by using X-10 modules plugged in to the house wiring. The EADL also plugs in to the house wiring to communicate with the modules. These can control lights, appliances, or a call signal. The electric door opener is controlled by a switch output on the EADL.

*Control 1, formerly available from Prentke Romich, Wooster, Ohio.

injury, head injury, and locked-in syndrome. On the basis of the incidence of these conditions, the authors estimated that approximately 150,000 persons in the United States have limitations of upper extremity function and could benefit from a robotic aid.

History of Powered Manipulators

Early rehabilitative manipulators were powered orthoses. An orthosis is an external brace that supports a body part. By adding motors to the joints (i.e., wrist, elbow, and shoulder) of an upper extremity orthosis, Correl and Wijnschenk (1964) developed one of the first rehabilitative manipulators. This system had four degrees of freedom (independent movements) and was controlled by a minicomputer. Another orthotic approach was the Rancho Arm (Corker, Lyman, and Sheredos, 1979). This system also used an external upper extremity splint, but it had seven degrees of freedom. This allowed control of the shoulder (abduction-adduction and flexion-extension), elbow (flexion-extension), wrist (pronation-supination, radial and ulnar deviation, flexion-extension), and fingers (grasp-release). Each degree of freedom was controlled by a bidirectional tongue-activated

objects and to function independently. This makes issues of safety more important for assistive robots. To ensure safety, forces are kept within 1 or 2 pounds (2 to 5 kg) and velocities are less than 10 cm/sec (Seamone and Schmeisser, 1985). Assistive robots perform many functions, in contrast to the relatively limited repertoire of an industrial robot. Although some tasks (e.g., feeding) are repeated, the assistive robot must be able to carry out totally unplanned movements spontaneously. This section discusses the development and application of assistive robots. In contrast to technologies discussed in other sections of this chapter, assistive robots are still largely in the research and development stage, and application of these systems is not yet widespread.

Stanger and Cawley (1996) evaluated the incidence of 12 disabling conditions associated with reduction of upper limb function. These were cerebral palsy, arthrogryposis, spinal muscular atrophy, muscular dystrophies, rheumatoid arthritis, juvenile rheumatoid arthritis, multiple sclerosis, amyotrophic lateral sclerosis, poliomyelitis, spinal cord

switch. This single-joint control made it difficult to carry out complex movements. To understand this, place a pencil or pen on the table. Now reach for it and pick it up, but only move in one of the degrees of freedom (i.e., one joint) listed above at a time. This type of movement takes great concentration. Now, reach for the pen or pencil as you normally would. This is called *end-point positioning,* and it is much easier to accomplish, but it makes the control system and robot much more complicated. The difficulties associated with controlling individual joints were a major downfall of early rehabilitation manipulators, and most current assistive robots use end-point positioning.

In the late 1970s and early 1980s, stand-alone assistive robots began to be developed. These devices were generally table mounted, but some were mounted to wheelchair frames or lap trays. These robots were more versatile because they did not have to support and move the user's limb, but they created new challenges because they were not attached to the body. The user had to develop a new coordinate system for controlling the robot, one related to the workspace of the robot rather than to his own body. The rapid development of microcomputers allowed miniaturization of the controllers while adding more sophistication. These systems also were capable of being "trained" to carry out repeated tasks. These advances made everyday use of assistive robots more feasible.

The remainder of this section discusses currently available assistive robots and their application. Three types of applications are discussed: (1) fixed workstations, which are built around assistive robots; (2) mobile robots for use in work, home, and school settings; and (3) robots developed and used to meet the educational goals of children. Each of these systems is a general-purpose manipulation device, as opposed to special-purpose manipulation devices such as the feeders and page turners described earlier. In some cases there is a blurring between these two categories. For example, we describe the Handy 1 (Topping, 1996) under electrically powered feeders, but it is actually a special-purpose robotic arm.

Robotic Workstations

A *workstation* can be defined as an area dedicated to the performance of a specific job or activity. Examples of activities are design (e.g., a computer workstation for engineering students), reading (e.g., a library-based workstation), and clerical tasks (e.g., a workstation for word processing, telephone answering, and manipulation of files). These workstations involve manipulation of papers, books, and other devices. When the user of the workstation has difficulty with upper extremity function and manipulation, **desktop robots** can play a major role in creating full access to the workstation. Because the workstation is fixed in one location, the design of the robotic system can focus on manipulation of objects only, rather than movement to the object and then manipulation

of it. Two robotic workstations that have been evaluated in the workplace are described. Both these systems were developed by the Veterans Administration.

Applied Physics Laboratory Robot Arm Worktable System.   The Applied Physics Laboratory Robot Arm Worktable (APL RAWT) system is built around a powered upper extremity prosthesis that has four degrees of freedom: (1) shoulder flexion-extension, (2) elbow flexion-extension, (3) wrist pronation-supination, and (4) hand grasping (Seamone and Schmeisser, 1985). In the workstation the prosthetic arm is mounted on a turntable, which allows a fifth degree of freedom comparable to internal-external shoulder rotation. Finally, the entire arm and turntable assembly is mounted in a track that allows it to be moved from front to back of the work surface. This results in a total of six degrees of freedom for the arm. The movements of this arm are shown in Figure 14-17, together with the total size of the reachable workspace. There are three motors for the six degrees of freedom. One DC motor controls elbow flexion-extension, wrist pronation-supination, or shoulder flexion-extension, depending on the commands sent. The second motor controls turntable rotation or hand grasping. Any joint not being activated is kept in place with a solenoid lock. This allows one motor to serve several functions at different times, but it prevents multiple joint movements simultaneously. The third motor is a geared servomotor used for positioning the arm in the front-to-back track.

The APL RAWT was designed for use by persons with high-level spinal cord injuries (SCI). This limited the choice of control sites to the head, neck, and voice. Chin control was chosen over other control modes (e.g., speech recognition or sip-and-puff) because of its compatibility with power wheelchair control. Because many persons with SCI

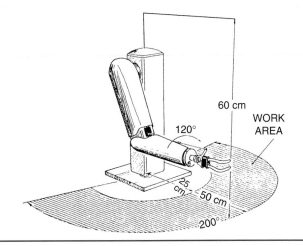

Figure 14-17   The coordinate system and working envelope of the APL RAWT system. (From Seamone W, Schmeisser G: Early clinical evaluation of a robot arm/worktable system for spinal-cord-injured persons, *J Rehabil Res Dev* 22:38-57, 1985.)

have experience using chin control for wheelchairs, training in the use of the RAWT would be decreased. Lateral movement of the modified chin control allows wheelchair steering. Reverse is activated by a microswitch located on the chin control lever. When the user approaches the RAWT in the wheelchair, contact is made between the RAWT and the wheelchair by an optical (IR) link. The user lifts the chin control briefly and control is transferred from the wheelchair to the RAWT. The user controls the RAWT with the chin joystick (left/right, in/out) and two additional switches (up/down).

Two basic modes of control are provided. First, the user may activate any one degree of freedom and control the arm in that axis. As discussed, this can be tedious and difficult, but it is sometimes necessary for precise movements. The second and most common method of control is to select one of the prestored specific tasks. Examples of some of these tasks are given in Box 14-1. As is shown in the box, the APL RAWT combines the high technology of the robot with the low technology of a mouthstick for some tasks. For example, the robot can bring the mouthstick holder into position for the user and then bring the telephone into position. The user can dial the telephone using the mouthstick. Likewise, a book or magazine can be positioned in a reading stand by the robotic arm, and the mouthstick can be used to turn pages. To select a prestored task, the user activates a menu of choices using the chin joystick and then searches through a list of tasks on the display screen to select the one wanted. Once the task is chosen, the arm automatically executes it. For some tasks such as feeding, there are intermediate points at which the user must reactivate the control. For example, a spoon of food is brought to mouth level and the arm is stopped. The user takes the food off of the spoon and then initiates a new cycle. Tasks such as self-feeding require the use of additional components, such as adapted bowls and utensils.

A block diagram of the total APL RAWT system is shown in Figure 14-18. The entire system is controlled by a special-purpose computer microprocessor. A keyboard is provided for programming new movements and general interaction with the system. It can be used by either the consumer or an attendant or therapist. Function keys on the keyboard specify robot motions. Prestored movements can be edited by use of the keyboard. This increases the flexibility because a new movement task can be created by editing an existing task that is similar.

The APL RAWT was clinically evaluated at three Veterans Administration centers. A total of 20 evaluators with high-level SCIs participated in clinical trials. The RAWT was typically set up in the evaluator's residence. Often this was the evaluator's home, but for some evaluators

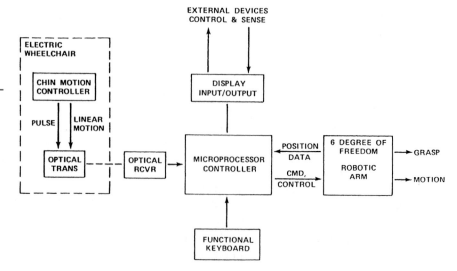

Figure 14-18   Block diagram showing the component parts of the APL RAWT system. (From Seamone W, Schmeisser G: Early clinical evaluation of a robot arm/worktable system for spinal-cord-injured persons, *J Rehabil Res Dev* 22:38-57, 1985.)

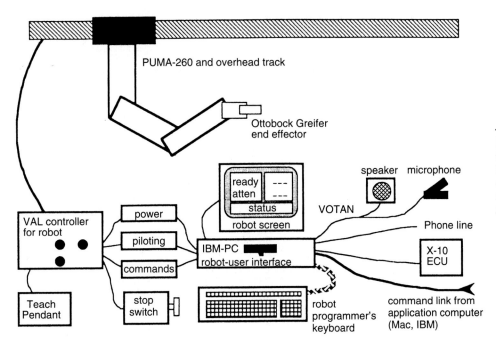

Figure 14-19 Basic components of the Desktop Vocational Assistant Robot (DeVAR). (From Hammel JM et al: Clinical evaluation of a desktop robotic assistant, *J Rehabil Res Dev* 26:1-16, 1989.)

the residence was a Veterans Administration medical center, nursing home, or state institution. The most popular features were self-feeding and computer and telephone use. Inadequacies of the chin controller were the most frequently cited negative feature. Seamone and Schmeisser (1985) discuss the evaluation of the APL RWAT in detail. The overall impression of the system was that it had the potential to be very effective for individuals with SCIs, but it needed further development and refinement.

Desktop Vocational Assistant Robot. The Desktop Vocational Assistant Robot (DeVAR-IV) system is built around an industrial-grade, low-payload robotic arm (PUMA-260) mounted on an overhead track (Figure 14-19) (Hammel, Van der Loos, and Perkash, 1992). This system has a primary goal of vocational assistance. DeVAR-III used a table-mounted PUMA arm, and the emphasis was on completion of tasks of daily living (Hammel et al, 1989). The DeVAR *human/technology interface* includes speech recognition (Votan VPC-2100) and multiaxis joystick control, coupled with a color monitor and voice synthesis. The voice synthesis is for user feedback (e.g., to confirm a task selection) and for warning messages. The monitor displays command prompts and robot status during task completion. The *processor* is a dedicated computer with appropriate software. A task-oriented programming language (VAL-II) is used. Using this language, routines can be developed for specific tasks. Example tasks for self-feeding are listed in Table 14-2 (Hammel et al, 1989). Once a task is initiated, commands are issued by the user for specific functions within the task. Examples of these are shown in Table 14-3 for the task of eating soup listed in Table 14-2. Note that

some commands (e.g., SOUP) have different meanings at different times during the task. Other commands (e.g., USE) are repeated many times to recycle through a subtask under the user's control. The user can also pilot the arm by using basic commands such as RIGHT, LEFT, BACKWARD, FORWARD, UP, DOWN, STOP, GO, OPEN, and CLOSE (gripper). As shown in Table 14-3, these direction commands can also be used within a prestored task. All the commands are spoken by the user and entered by the voice recognition system. The user must train the speech recognizer (see Chapter 7) to recognize her speech. For a typical vocabulary of about 60 commands, this takes approximately 10 minutes (Hammel et al, 1989). Similar tasks and command sequences can be developed for other applications (e.g., vocational work site tasks).

Outputs include environmental control (by an X-10 system) and the robotic arm. Examples of tasks that various versions of DeVAR have performed are listed in Box 14-2

TABLE 14-2	Desktop Vocational Assistant Robot Tasks and Their Commands
Task	Command
Prepare a bowl of soup	SOUP
Eat the soup with standard spoon	SPOON
Brush teeth with electric toothbrush	TOOTHBRUSH
Wash and dry face with adapted washcloth	WASH
Shave face with electric shaver	SHAVE

Modified from Hammel J et al: Clinical evaluation of a desktop robotic assistant, *J Rehabil Res Dev* 26:1-16, 1989.

TABLE 14-3 Desktop Vocational Assistant Robot Commands Used to Prepare and Eat Soup

Command	Action
SOUP	Robot takes soup out of refrigerator, puts in microwave, closes door, sets time, heats soup.
SOUP	Robot brings soup from microwave to table.
SPOON	Robot gets spoon from tool holder and brings to neutral point in front of user. User says direction commands to bring spoon near mouth (UP, DOWN, LEFT, RIGHT, BACKWARD, FORWARD). Robot remembers this point and returns to it each time.
USE	Robot scoops a spoonful of soup and brings to user's mouth. User says USE for each mouthful until finished eating.
BACK	Robot returns soup to refrigerator to finish later
CLEAN	Robot puts bowl in dirty dish container to be cleaned

Modified from Hammel J et al: Clinical evaluation of a desktop robotic assistant, *J Rehabil Res Dev* 26:1-16, 1989.

BOX 14-2 Tasks Performed by the Desktop Vocational Assistant Robot

MEAL PREPARATION AND FEEDING
Prepare meal
Open or close microwave
Manipulate bowls
Set timer
Pour liquids
Set timer
Beat eggs
Toss salad
Cook and serve soup
Heat and serve dinner
Serve pudding, fruit
Bake cake
Use standard utensils
Get drinks
Mix drinks

VOCATIONAL
Write with pen
Retrieve books
Set up books
Retrieve mouthstick
Type on keyboard
Adjust keyboard
Operate telephone
Turn pages
Insert floppy disk
Insert audio tapes
Open or close drawers
Operate printer
Manipulate printouts

HYGIENE
Wash or dry face
Brush teeth
Shave face
Comb or brush hair

RECREATIONAL
Arrange flowers
Paint
Play video game
Play board game
Light candle

Modified from Hammel J et al: Clinical evaluation of a desktop robotic assistant, *J Rehabil Res Dev* 26:1-16, 1989.

(Hammel et al, 1989). The use of an industrial-grade robotic arm has the benefit of providing more precise control, proven safety features and reliability, and greater payloads, but the cost is significantly higher than robotic manipulators designed for educational or assistive uses. The gripper is a modified Otto Bock prosthetic hand (Otto Bock, Minneapolis, Minn., *www.ottobock.com*).

Two versions of the DeVAR have been field tested. DeVAR-III was evaluated by Hammel et al (1989). Twenty-four male evaluators were either inpatients or outpatients of the Palo Alto Veterans Administration SCI Center. Twenty-one of the evaluators had SCIs at the C4 or higher level, and all had little or no functional upper extremity movement. Each subject was given training by both an OT and an engineer. The speech recognition system was trained to recognize 60 command words. Both preprogrammed movements (e.g., those in Table 14-3) and directional movements were used by the participants. Pretests and posttests were administered using voice commands on the computer to evaluate the user's perception of the usefulness of the robotic system. Participants indicated a high degree of satisfaction with the performance of the robot in the tasks shown in Table 14-3. They also expressed a preference for the robot over attendant care for these tasks. The major concerns expressed were about reliability, the amount of space the robot occupied, and safety with children. Overall pretest ratings were lower than posttest ratings, reflecting a lack of knowledge of how well the robot would perform and a degree of skepticism in the pretest. Hammel et al (1989) discuss the evaluation results in more detail.

DeVAR-IV, the version developed for a work environment, has also been evaluated (Hammel, Van der Loos, and Perkash, 1992). A single-subject research design was used with two components (R = robot assistance; A = attendant assistance). The workstation used by the evaluator also included a speech recognition keyboard and mouse-emulating device for access to his computer workstation (see Chapter 7). The evaluator was a 50-year-old man with a C4-C5 SCI. He was employed full time as a database programmer for a utility company. He used the DeVAR-IV system for his normal office activities and for some daily living tasks (e.g., serving lunch, emptying his leg bag, dispensing medications). The DeVAR-IV system was installed in his office for 6 months before data collection. This ensured that the evaluator was fully trained in and comfortable with the use of DeVAR-IV. During the first phase of data collection, the robot was used for six 10-hour days (corresponding to his normal workday of 10 hours). During the second phase (A) the robot was turned off and the attendant performed its tasks. All sessions were videotaped and observed by two project staff members. The evaluator expressed a preference for the robot over attendant assistance for all activities except feeding. When the robot was used, attendant assistance could be replaced for two 5-hour periods during the workday. Complete replacement was not possible because of required setup tasks (e.g., meal preparation for feeding by the robot). The replacement of personal assistant care is a major factor in determining the economic feasibility of the robot system. Hammel, Van der Loos, and Perkash (1992) show a projection (based on $7 per hour attendant care and a $50,000 robot) that makes the robot less expensive after a period of 5.5 years. Installation, training, and continuing maintenance costs for the robot are included in their analysis.

Birch et al (1996) carried out a study to determine actual costs of using a robotic assistant compared with using a personal assistant for office-related tasks. They used a simulated office environment and standardized tasks. They found that, although the robotic assistant did reduce assistant time and therefore cost, it also resulted in decreased productivity by the user. They attributed this reduction in productivity to waiting times necessitated by robotic movements, which were slower than the corresponding human attendant actions.

Mobile Assistive Robots

Because we rarely do all our manipulation from a fixed location, **mobile assistive robots** have been developed. These fall into one of two general classes: (1) wheelchair mounted and (2) mounted on a mobile base that is controllable by the user. The major limitation of the first approach is that the most functional robot arms are relatively large. This large size, coupled with the other apparatus that must be attached to the wheelchair, makes attachment of the arm to the wheelchair impractical in many cases. Recent miniaturization of these arms has solved this problem. The separate mobile base approach solves these problems, and it is practical in the home or at the work site. However, this approach also has disadvantages. The mobile robot requires that the user add "steering" to the required control commands. Because the user of a robot most likely has a restricted set of control signals available, the addition of these steering commands may be impossible. It is also difficult to transport the mobile base from one location to another. It is like having

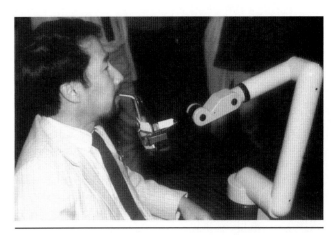

Figure 14-20 The Manus wheelchair-mounted robotic arm. (Courtesy C.W. Heckathorne, Northwestern University Rehabilitation Engineering Research Center, Chicago, Ill.)

two powered wheelchairs to transport. Thus the most practical application of mobile robots is within one location. This location can, of course, include all rooms in a house or any location within a school, factory, or office.

Wheelchair-Mounted Robotic Arms. The Manus manipulator, pictured in Figure 14-20, is a robotic arm mounted to a wheelchair (Verburg et al, 1996). It was designed to serve as a general-purpose manipulative aid for people who have severe upper extremity limitations. The robotic arm has eight degrees of freedom, can lift a 1.5-kg (3.3-pound) weight when the arm is fully extended, and can exert a gripping force of 20 N. The arm weighs 20 kg (9.09 pounds). Verburg et al (1996) describe the development of the Manus system, including several clinical and community-based trials that were used to gain user feedback. Clinical trials of early versions of the Manus arm identified two major problems: (1) the limited interface options and (2) the fact that when the Manus arm was mounted to the wheelchair, the weight and width of it were increased too much.

Since these trials, several generations of this arm have been developed and multiple user interfaces have been tried. These include a multidimensional joystick, head control using either a joystick or the frontalis muscle electromyograph, enlarged keyboard, and foot control. There has also been work to integrate the Manus control into the wheelchair control system. The latter was strongly recommended by user trials and provides a major improvement in integration of functions for the user. These changes have addressed the first of the early clinical trial concerns. A new mounting system, which includes moving the Manus out of the way when other activities are to be carried out, has addressed the second concern.

A technology assessment to determine the requirements for prescription and funding of the Manus system was carried out in the Netherlands from 1992 to 1993. This review included criteria for both the user skills required and the development of a set of prescription indicators. The report recommended that potential users should have minimal or no hand function or limited coordination of the upper extremities, inability to lift their arms against gravity, limited reach, use of an electric wheelchair, inability to feed or drink independently, and inability to manipulate objects. Indicator diagnoses included spinal cord injury, multiple sclerosis, rheumatoid arthritis, progressive dystrophies, and severe spasticity (e.g., cerebral palsy). User activities that were determined to be important for use of a Manus system included the need to engage in activities at different locations, an inability to function without assistance for large parts of the day, a living setting in which absence of a system like Manus would constitute an unacceptable load for family, and the ability to begin or resume work or school if a Manus were available. Motivational and cognitive criteria included general motivation to use Manus, ability to understand and remember the technical commands, and general familiarity with computers. The technology assessment also recommended that a 3-month trial period in the community occur before final prescription approval. Criteria for evaluating the outcomes of the trial to determine whether final funding would be approved included whether the Manus was being used in the locations and for the purposes specified in the evaluation, whether the Manus had increased the user's independence, and how the Manus had affected the roles of aides and family members (e.g., increased or decreased time required for assistance and by how much). On the basis of this technological assessment, the Manus was approved for funding in several European countries.

Use of the Manus system was also evaluated by 14 individuals in six European countries (the Netherlands, Germany, Norway, France, Italy, and Switzerland) (Oderud, 1997). These community-based evaluations demonstrated that the Manus manipulator was frequently used at home for activities of daily living (e.g., fetching objects, eating and drinking, preparing food in a microwave oven). Limitations in this home environment included the added size and weight of the wheelchair when the Manus was mounted to it (despite its redesign) and the need for training of the user and significant others. In these studies the Manus was not frequently used for vocational tasks. The major limitation in this context was that the Manus could not be preprogrammed for repetitive tasks, which added to the cognitive load of the user in the work environment, where speed of task performance was more critical.

There are still relatively few (less than 100) Manus systems in daily use by persons with disabilities. Cost, lack of understanding of the potential value of robotics, minimal infrastructure for marketing and support, and the need for training of users and professionals are the most often cited reasons for this slow growth in consumer base for this technology (Oderud, 1997; Verburg et al, 1996).

Ivlev et al (2005) added sensors to the Manus arm to attempt to overcome its relative inaccuracy and to make it more autonomous. The basic approach was to detect the location of objects to be manipulated and to automate the manipulation process, relieving the person from complex instructions. They called their robots FRIEND I and FRIEND II. Cameras were mounted to the back of the wheelchair above the person's head to visualize the work envelope and in the gripper to detect that the object to be manipulated was in range. A scale and touch pad were mounted in a lap tray to give additional information about object location and weight. The FRIEND robot is shown in Figure 14-21. By providing information about location and

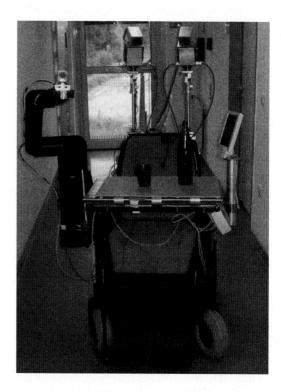

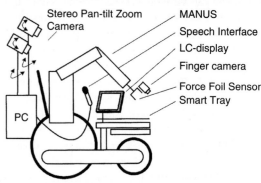

Figure 14-21 The FRIEND robotic arm system. (From Ivlev O, Marterns C, Graeser A: Rehabilitation robots FRIEND I and FRIEND II with the dexterous and lightweight manipulator, *Technol Disabil* 17:111-123, 2005.)

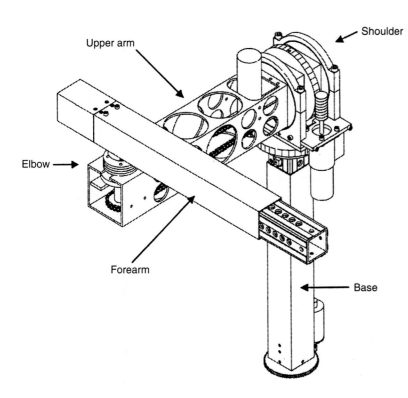

Figure 14-22   Engineering drawing of the Middlesex rehabilitation robot. (From Parsons B et al: The Middlesex University rehabilitation robot, *J Med Eng Technol* 29:151-162, 2005.)

weight of objects, it was possible to program the system to identify specific objects (e.g. a bottle and glass) and to execute a task with those objects (e.g., pour from the bottle into the glass). This allowed the user to issue commands like "find glass" rather that having to manipulate the arm through more primitive commands of moving up/down/left/right to reach the glass. Thus, with the automated system a task that required 20 instructions without automation was reduced to 5 instructions with the FRIEND robot. FRIEND II differed form FRIEND I in hardware (a pneumatically control gripper with individual fingers was added) and more sophisticated positioning software.

The Raptor robotic arm is the first such assistive technology device to be approved by the U.S. Food and Drug Administration (Mahoney, 2001). The Raptor is similar to the Manus in function with four degrees of freedom and attachment to the wheelchair frame (giving two additional degrees of freedom). A joystick, keypad, or sip-and-puff switch can control it. The Raptor emphasizes mobility, payload, and reduced precision with a 48-inch extension and it can lift up to 4 pounds. The Raptor requires cognitive skill to position the gripper because some positions and orientations can only be achieved by moving the wheelchair (and the user). The intended user population is the same as for the Manus.

Another wheelchair mounted arm that is under development is the Middlesex University rehabilitation robot (Parsons et al, 2005). The design goals for this prototype focused on low cost, general-purpose applicability, function driven by user prioritization of tasks to be completed, wide range of input options, and a variety of control modes and safety. The resulting prototype used a design that reduced the number of joints that oppose gravity, reduced the weight of the arm (by holes drilled in the material that were not weight bearing), and used telescoping components to reduce overall size while increasing rang of operation. The engineering drawing for the Middlesex arm is shown in Figure 14-22. The control software provides for cartesian coordinate positioning in space (as opposed to requiring that each joint be controlled separately) and a "teaching" function that records a trajectory or routine for later replay.

The FRIEND and Middlesex robots offer improvements on earlier robots, but they have yet to be thoroughly evaluated in a daily living setting. Their development does help identify the major limitations that users and engineers have addressed on the basis of evaluation of earlier commercial robots such as the Manus and the Raptor.

Mobile Vocational Assistant Robot.   The Mobile Vocational Assistant Robot (MoVAR) represents a specially configured robotic system developed for assistive applications. Many of the components of DeVAR are included in MoVAR (Van der Loos, Michalowski, and Leifer, 1988). These include the PUMA-260 robotic arm, a speech recognition control interface (Votan), a multiaxis joystick control, a task-oriented programming language (VAL-II), and a host-computer menu command interface. To meet the goals of mobility, two major additional components are added to the system. The first of these is a mobile base that is specially designed to allow easy movement in any direction in a small space. Specially designed and built wheels allow this flexibility in movement. Second, an expanded sensing system is added. A small camera is mounted on the robotic arm. This camera image is displayed directly to the user, and its image is used in modeling the environment for task-level programming. Touch-sensitive bumpers that can determine whether to stop (e.g., at a wall) or to push harder (e.g., to open a door) are also included in the MoVAR. The MoVAR is about the same size as a powered wheelchair. The systems described in this section are examples chosen because of their design goals and their clinical evaluations. Several other robot systems are under development.

Use of Robotics in Education

Most rehabilitative robotic systems have been designed for adults (e.g., those with high-level spinal cord injuries), and their control requires relatively high-level cognitive skills that exceed the developmental level of younger children (Van Vliet and Wing, 1991). Severe physical disabilities may also limit the access to standard rehabilitation robots (Eberhardt, Osborne, and Rahman, 2000). The educational setting places additional constraints on the robot system. First, the user may be very young, which necessitates simplified, age-appropriate control schemes and user interfaces. Second, a robot that is intended for use by young children has added safety demands because school children cannot be expected to exercise the same caution as adults.

For young children, manipulative tasks contribute to the development of cognitive and language skills (see Chapter 3). Robotic devices that aid manipulation can help young children with limited physical capabilities to develop these cognitive and language skills as well as directly aid manipulation. Cook, Liu, and Hoseit (1990) carried out a study to determine whether very young children would interact with a small computer-controlled robotic arm. Six disabled and three healthy children, all less than 38 months old, were used in the study.

The system consisted of a microcomputer for control and data collection, a small robotic arm (about half the adult human scale), and a guidance unit used to train the arm to make specific movements (Cook et al, 1988). The arm can rotate around its base; flex and extend at the elbow and shoulder; extend, flex, supinate, and pronate the wrist; and open and close the gripper. The guidance unit used a joystick to train the arm by moving the joystick in the desired direction of arm movement. This made it intuitively simple for a teacher, therapist, or parent to train a specific movement that was of interest to the child. Three phases were used: (1) training the arm for a specific movement, (2) playback of the movement by the child using a single switch, and (3) monitoring the child's behavior during arm movement. Training of the arm was done by either using the guidance unit or by entering a series of text commands to train the arm.

Using the guidance unit, the teacher, therapist, or parent moves the arm through the desired movement with the joystick, and the movement is stored for later playback. In the text training mode, commands such as 100 FORWARD (move the arm forward 1 inch) were typed and combined to form a complete task (e.g., bringing a cracker within reach of the child or dumping the contents of a cup).

In a typical task a child used the robot arm as a tool by pressing the switch only when it was necessary to bring an object closer to him or to uncover a hidden object (e.g., by tipping a cup containing an unknown object), and the child did not press the switch when he or she could reach the object. This tool use is unique to a robotic arm compared with toys or computer graphics used as contingent results, and it provides additional information over these simpler modes of interaction regarding the child's skills. Fifty percent of the disabled children and 100% of the healthy children interacted with the arm and used it as a tool to obtain objects out of reach. All the disabled children with a cognitive developmental age of 7 to 9 months and older did interact with the arm, whereas those below this developmental level did not. Gross and fine motor skill levels were less related to success in using the robotic arm than were the levels in cognitive and language areas. This study showed that very young children will use a robotic arm to accomplish tasks that are of interest to them.

Open-ended tasks such as drawing have also been carried out using single-switch scanning with the Handy 1 Robot (Smith and Topping, 1996). In this case, selection of the color of a pen, the position of the pen, up (move) or down (draw), and the pen's movement are accomplished with single-switch scanning. Tasks such as these are cognitively demanding, and widely varying levels of success were reported for the three subjects included in the study.

To facilitate the development of more complex tasks, it is necessary to move beyond single-switch playback for a movement. Cook et al (1988) developed a hierarchy of robotic movements that sequentially increased the complexity of the tasks the child needs to accomplish. These are related to the cognitive developmental levels described in Chapter 3. The child progresses from understanding simple playback of complete movements, to segments of movements, to complete control of the end point. Nof, Karlan, and Widmer (1988) used a two-level system for developing a child's interaction with a robotic arm. At the first level, the arm functions to carry out complete tasks. Sublevels included by Nof, Karlan, and Widmer were one- and two-step sequences, each used to carry out the same task. At the second level, the robotic arm allows the child to control component actions and incorporate these into more complex sequences.

Cook et al (2000) used a robotic arm to determine whether children (aged 4 to 7 years) who have severe physical disabilities would be able to understand a sequence of motor actions and to use them to find buried objects of interest. The robot was adapted to allow control by children with severe disabilities (Cook et al, 2000). The system was programmed to (1) carry out preprogrammed movements when the child hit a switch, (2) execute three-dimensional cartesian coordinate movements when activated by one of six switches or keyboard keys, and (3) move any of the six degrees of freedom and open or close the gripper when one of 14 switches or keyboard keys was pressed. Enlarged keyboards that reduced the physical demands for high-resolution movements by the child could be used instead of single switches. Three specific robotic arm movements, each executed by a single switch press, were programmed. Dry macaroni in a tub was used to provide both sensory and motor interactions for the child. The tasks used included the following: (1) macaroni was dumped from a glass held by the robotic arm (one switch); (2) the child controlled the arm to dig an object out of the macaroni and then dump the macaroni and the object (two switches); and (3) the child caused the arm to move laterally to a location where an object had been buried, dig the object out of the macaroni, and dump the macaroni into the tub (three switches). The buried object was a plastic egg containing another object of interest to the child (e.g., finger puppet, small rubber stamp). Cook et al (2000) reported that children generally attended to tasks for significantly longer periods with the robot than with other activities (e.g., computer graphics programs). After one or two trials, all the children understood that hitting switch number 1 dumped the cup and its contents.

Adding a second switch with a different function led to some initial confusion for the child. After one or two physical prompts, each child learned to DIG (switch 2) and then DUMP (switch 1) with only verbal prompts. When the third switch (MOVE) was added (task 3), the children required differing levels of prompting to understand its function. When the third switch was added to the first two, the child required both verbal and physical prompts to carry out the third part of the sequence (MOVE). Children took more trials to understand this task, and each trial required more prompting.

Although all children could correctly sequence the actions to complete the entire task in multiple action tasks, the number of sessions and trials to reach this level varied. Children were much more motivated to learn how to use the robot and they kept their attention focused for longer periods, in contrast to simple toys, which do not generally allow the child to move beyond cause and effect relationships, and computer programs, which are not as concrete in relation to object manipulation and sequencing of tasks. Children were able to put two operations together to complete a task. The robot arm also gave the children the opportunity to interact with the investigators by "handing" objects to them and choosing which objects to be buried.

An educational robotic arm system was developed for use by children who had very severe motor disabilities and varying levels of cognitive and language skills (Cook et al, 2005). In this study the robot system was located in the child's school rather than a clinical setting where the children used the system for a period of four weeks. The children used the robot in a three-task sequence routine to dig objects from a tub of dry macaroni. The robotic system was used in the child's school for 12 to 15 sessions over a period of 4 weeks. Goal attainment scaling indicated improvement in all children in operational competence of the robot and varying levels of gain in functional skill development with the robot and in carryover to the classroom from the robot experiments. Teacher interviews revealed gains in classroom participation and expressive language (vocalizations, symbolic communication) and a high degree of interest by the children in the robot tasks. The teachers also made recommendations for changes to the robot to facilitate classroom use.

For school-age children, the robotic tasks become more functional. Howell, Damarin, and Post (1987) developed a robotic system for use in elementary schools. They used a small robot, a five-position slot switch, and a computer to control the arm. They defined four levels of control: (1) demonstration of the arm to the student, (2) performance of well-defined and prestored tasks, (3) unstructured movement controlled by the student, and (4) student programming and storage of movements for later playback. To accomplish these tasks, Howell, Hay, and Rakocy (1989) identified special software and hardware considerations. These include easy physical and cognitive access and fast interactional speed; understandable, powerful, and complete learner control features; and the definition of the robot motions useful in the classroom. They discuss possible solutions to each of these. This robotic system was applied to science instruction at the elementary school level (Howell, Mayton, and Baker, 1989). Two phases of field study were carried out: (1) a training component, in which the student became familiar with the use of the robotic system, and (2) an instructional component, in which the robot was used to complete science experiments. Important issues raised by this preliminary study were (1) the need for the robot to be transparent to the user (so that the student can focus on the learning task, rather than robot control), (2) training method, and (3) curricular applications.

Another system for classroom use was developed in the United Kingdom (Harwin, Ginige, and Jackson, 1988). This system differed from other educational applications in the inclusion of a vision system based on a television camera and image recognition software. This allowed the system to be used for more sophisticated tasks such as finding and stacking blocks. Three tasks were used with this system: (1) stacking and knocking down blocks with two switches (yes/no), (2) sorting articles by shape or color with four switches (one for each feature) or two switches (yes/no), and (3) a stacking game with five switches (left, middle, right, pick up, release). Children with motor disabilities who used this system enjoyed it and were able to successfully complete the tasks described. By using the robotic arm, they could accomplish otherwise impossible tasks.

The Aryln Arm robotic work station was developed specifically for educational applications (Eberhardt et al, 2000). It has a portable base and a six degree-of-freedom arm. A two joystick control system is used to position the arm, control the end effector (a "pseudo hand") and direct the moveable base. There is also a built-in vacuum system. Eberhardt et al (2000) used the arm with five subjects who had disabilities preventing participation in science and the arts. With use of the arm system, these subjects completed projects in these two subject areas. Robots have also been used as tools in therapeutic play activities (Lathan et al, 2001). In this approach, a series of sensors are attached to a child to detect arm, finger, or head movement. Those signals are then used to control a robot. A storytelling robot was used to address cognitive, language, and emotional rehabilitation needs in children with disabilities.

Kwee and Quaedackers (2002) and Kwee et al, (2002) adapted the Manus arm for use by children with cerebral palsy. The required adaptations focused on two areas: the physical control and the cognitive tasks required. Physical control limitations were generally addressed by using scanning rather than direct selection. Single-switch scanning was used to select the direction of movement and motion of the arm. However, scanning requires greater cognitive skill and these adaptations for physical performance resulted in control schemes that required significant amounts of training and practice to understand the cognitive aspects involved (Van Vliet and Wing, 1991). Not surprisingly, Kwee et al found that increased training times were required for the children with cerebral palsy to learn control of the Manus arm than was typical for spinal cord injured adult users.

All the assistive robotic systems described in this section are still largely experimental. As technologies improve and costs come down, we will see more routine use of these systems in the home, school, and work site.

■ SUMMARY

Assistive technologies designed to aid manipulation help consumers in accomplishing tasks for which they normally use their upper extremities. Some manipulative aids are general purpose, meaning they serve multiple functions, and some are special purpose, designed for one task. In some cases the manipulative aid assists with normal hand function (e.g., handwriting aids); we refer to these as *augmentative.* In other cases an *alternative* method is used (e.g., a robotic arm for moving items on a desk). In addition, special-purpose and general-purpose devices may be either high or low tech.

Low-tech general-purpose manipulation aids include mouthsticks, head pointers, and reachers. Special-purpose devices are available to meet needs in the general performance areas of self-care, work or school, and recreation or leisure.

Commercially available special-purpose electrically powered devices serve two primary functions: self-feeding and page turning. These may be controlled by many different control interfaces and selection methods. There are two types of general-purpose electrically powered devices: EADLs and robotic systems. EADLs include appliance control; telephone access; TV, and CD/DVD control; and remote access to doors, drapes, and windows. Robots are used to meet manipulative needs in the home, at work, and in the classroom. Both EADLs and assistive robots are controlled by computers, and each may be accessed by a variety of control interfaces and selection methods.

Study Questions

1. List and describe the four categories of aided manipulation.
2. Give an example of a special-purpose low-tech manipulation aid for each of the three major performance areas.
3. What are the primary types of self-care adaptations provided by low-tech manipulation aids?
4. What are the primary types of work or school adaptations provided by low-tech manipulation aids?
5. What are the primary types of recreation and leisure adaptations provided by low-tech manipulation aids?
6. What are the functions provided by electrically powered feeders?
7. What are the two major approaches used in electrically powered page turners?
8. What are the functions provided by electrically powered page turners?
9. What, if any, are the advantages of using the term *electronic aids to daily living* rather than *environmental control* units?
10. What are the four control functions implemented in EADLs? Describe the differences between them and give an EADL example of each.
11. Discuss the relative advantages and disadvantages of the two modes of binary latched AC appliance control.
12. What are the four major transmission modes used in EADL systems?
13. How does a trainable or programmable IR controller work, and what are the major advantages of these types of device?
14. What is the difference between a trainable and a programmable IR controller?

15. Describe the functions of an automatic telephone dialer.
16. How do hospital EADLs differ from those used in the home?
17. List the major assessment questions to be answered when determining the best EADL for a specific user.
18. What are the most significant factors that contribute to use or nonuse of EADLs by persons with spinal cord injuries?
19. Compare the APL RAWT and the DeVAR desktop robot systems in terms of goals, basic design approach, robot arm used, control interface selected, cost, and degree of technological sophistication.
20. Describe the key design features of the Manus mobile robotic arm.
21. How do the Manus design features contribute or detract from its effectiveness and consumer satisfaction?
22. What are the key factors considered when determining if a Manus robotic arm is suitable for a consumer's needs and goals? Do you agree with these? Why or why not?
23. Describe the major differences between desktop and mobile robots from the point of view of both the required design and the user interaction with the robot.
24. How do educational applications of robotic systems differ from vocational or daily living applications?
25. How can robotic systems be used to evaluate and perhaps enhance cognitive and language functioning in young children?

References

Ability Research Centre: Environmental control systems for people with spinal cord injuries, (1999): http://www.abilitycorp.com.au/ftp/research/environmental_controls_sytems_report.pdf.

Barker P, Gross K, Henderson K: Control of the environment. In *Proceedings of the '91 RESNA Pacific Reg Conference,* 1991, Washington, DC, The Conference.

Bentham JS, Bereton DS, Sapacz RA: The selection of environmental control systems. In *Proceedings of the RESNA 13th Annual Conference,* pp 108-109, 1992, Washington, DC, The Conference.

Bessell T, Randell M, Knowles G, et al: Connecting people with the environment—a new accessible wireless remote control, proceedings of the 2004 ARATA conference: http://www.e-bility.com/arataconf06/papers/environmental_control/ec_hobbs_paper.doc. Accessed November 17, 2006.

Birch GE et al: An assessment methodology and its application to a robotic vocational assistive device, *Tech Disabil* 5: 151-165, 1996.

Chen LP et al: An evaluation of reachers for use by older persons, *Assist Technol* 10:113-125, 1998.

Ciarcia S: Plug-in remote control system, *Radio Electronics,* pp 47-51, September 1980.

Ciarcia S: Build a trainable infrared master controller, *Byte* 12:113-123, 1987a.

Ciarcia S: Build an infrared controller, *Byte* 12:101-109, 1987b.

Cook AM et al: Development of a robotic device for facilitating learning by children who have severe disabilities, *IEEE Trans Neural Syst Rehabil Eng* 10:178-187, 2000.

Cook AM et al: Robot enhanced interaction and learning for children with profound physical disabilities, *Technol Disabil* 13:1-8, 2000.

Cook AM et al: School-based use of a robotic arm system by children with disabilities, *IEEE Trans Neural Syst Rehabil Eng* 13:452-460, 2005.

Cook AM et al: Using a robotic arm system to facilitate learning in very young disabled children, *IEEE Trans Biomed Eng* 35:132-137, 1988.

Cook AM, Hussey SM: Meeting multiple needs with separate but equal interfaces. In *Proceedings of the RESNA Conference,* pp 290-292, 1992, Washington, DC, The Conference.

Cook AM, Liu KM, Hoseit P: Robotic arm use by very young motorically disabled children, *Assist Technol* 2:51-57, 1990.

Corell RW, Wijnschenk MJ: *Design and development of the Case research arm-aid,* Report No. EDC-4-64-4, Cleveland, 1964, Case Institute of Technology.

Corker K, Lyman JH, Sheredos S: A preliminary evaluation of remote medical manipulators, *Bull Prosthet Res* 16: 107-134, 1979.

Croser et al: Effectiveness of electronic aids to daily living: increased independence, and decreased frustration, *Aust Occup Ther J* 48:35-44, 2001.

Dickey R, Shealey SH: Using technology to control the environment, *Am J Occup Ther* 41:717-721, 1987.

Eberhardt SP, Osborne J, Rahman T: Classroom evaluation of the Arlyn Arm Robotic Workstation, *Assist Technol* 12:132-143, 2000.

Efthimiou J et al: Electronic assistive devices: their impact on the quality of life of high level quadriplegic persons, *Arch Phys Med Rehabil* 62:131- 134, 1981.

Gross K: Controlling the environment, *Team Rehabil Rep* 3: 14-16, 1992.

Hammel JM, Van der Loos HFM, Perkash I: Evaluation of a vocational robot with a quadriplegic employee, *Arch Phys Med Rehabil* 73:683-693, 1992.

Hammel J et al: Clinical evaluation of a desktop robotic assistant, *J Rehabil Res Dev* 26:1-16, 1989.

Harwin WS, Ginige A, Jackson RD: A robot workstation for use in education of the physically handicapped, *IEEE Trans Biomed Eng* 35:127-131, 1988.

Harwin WS, Rahman T, Foulds RA: A review of design issues in rehabilitation robotics with reference to North American projects, *IEEE Trans Rehabil Eng* 3:3-11, 1995.

Holme AS et al: The use of environmental control units by occupational therapists in spinal cord injury and disease, *Am J Occup Ther* 51:42-48, 1997.

Howell RD, Damarin SK, Post EP: The use of robotic manipulators as cognitive and physical prosthetic aids. In *Proceedings of the 10th RESNA Conference,* pp 770-772, 1987, Washington, DC, The Conference.

Howell RD, Hay K, Rakocy L: Hardware and software considerations in the design of a prototype educational robotic manipulator. In *Proceedings of the 12th RESNA Conference,* pp 113-114, 1989, Washington, DC, The Conference.

Howell RD, Mayton G, Baker P: Education and research issues in designing robotically-aided science education environments. In *Proceedings of the 12th RESNA Conference,* pp 109-110, 1989, Washington, DC.

Ivlev O, Marterns C: Graeser A: Rehabilitation robots FRIEND I and FRIEND II with the dexterous and lightweight manipulator, *Technol Disabil* 17:111-123, 2005.

Jones RD et al: Microprocessor-based multi-patient environmental-control system for spinal injuries unit, *Med Biol Eng Comput* 18:607-616, 1980.

Jutai J et al: Psychosocial impact of electronic aids to daily living, *Assist Technol* 12:123-131, 2000.

Kinney P: ZigBee Technology: Wireless control that simply works: http://www.zigbee.org/en/resources/#WhitePapers. Accessed March 26, 2006.

Kwee H, Quaedackers J: POCUS project adapting the control of the Manus manipulator for persons with cerebral palsy. In *Proceedings of ICORR: International Conference on Rehabilitation Robotics,* pp 106-114, Stanford, CA, 1999, The Conference.

Lange M: Alternative reading options, *OT Pract* 43-44, 1998.

Lathan C et al: Therapeutic play with a storytelling robot. In *Proceedings of the Conference on Human Factors in Computing Systems,* pp 27-28, 2001, New York, ACM Press, The Conference.

Mahoney RM: The Raptor Wheelchair Robot System. In *Proceedings of the International Conference on Rehabilitation Robotics,* Stanford, CA, 2001, IOS Press.

Mann WC: Use of environmental control devices by elderly nursing home patients, *Assist Technol* 4:60-65, 1992.

McDonald DW, Boyle MA, Schumann TL: Environmental control unit utilization by high-level spinal cord injured patients, *Arch Phys Med Rehabil* 62:131-134, 1989.

Mills R: Impact of standards on future environmental control systems. In *Proceedings of the 10th RESNA Conference,* pp 690-682, 1987, Washington, DC, The Conference.

Nof SY, Karlan GR, Widmer NS: Development of a prototype interactive robotic device for use by multiply handicapped children. In *Proceedings of the International Conference*

Association on Advanced Rehabilitation Technology (ICAART), pp 456-457, 1988, Montreal, The Conference.

Oderud T: Experiences from the evaluation of a Manus wheelchair-mounted manipulator. In Anogianakis G, Bühler C, Soede M, editors: *Advancement in assistive technology,* Amsterdam, 1997, IOS Press.

Parsons B et al: The Middlesex University rehabilitation robot, *J Med Eng Technol* 29:151-162, 2005.

Rigby P et al: Impact of electronic aids to daily living on the lives of persons with cervical spinal cord injuries, *Assist Technol* 17:89-97, 2005.

Ripat J: Function and impact of electronic aids to daily living for experienced users, *Technol Disabil* 18:79-97, 2006.

Ripat J, Strock A: User's perceptions of the impact of electronic aids to daily living throughout the acquisition process, *Assist Technol* 16:63-72, 2004.

Seamone W, Schmeisser G: Early clinical evaluation of a robot arm/worktable system for spinal-cord-injured persons, *J Rehabil Res Dev* 22:38-57, 1985.

Sell GH et al: Environmental and typewriter control systems for high-level quadriplegic patients: evaluation and prescription, *Arch Phys Med Rehabil* 60:246-252, 1979.

Smith J, Topping M: The introduction of a robotic aid to drawing into a school for physically handicapped children: a case study, *Br J Occup Ther* 59:565-569, 1996.

Stanger CA, Cawley MF: Demographics of rehabilitation robotics users, *Technol Disabil* 5:125-137, 1996.

Symington DC et al: Environmental control systems in chronic care hospitals and nursing homes, *Arch Phys Med Rehabil* 67:322-325, 1986.

Topping M: The Handy 1, a robotic aid to independence for severely disabled people, *Technol Disabil* 5:233-234, 1996.

Van der Loos HFM, Michalowski SJ, Leifer LJ: Development of an omnidirectional mobile vocational assistant robot. In *Proceedings of the International Conference Association of Advanced Rehabilitation Technology (ICAART),* pp 468-469, 1988, Montreal, The Conference.

Van Vliet P, Wing AM: A new challenge—robotics in the rehabilitation of the neurologically motor impaired, *Phys Ther* 71:39-47, 1991.

Verburg G et al: Manus: the evolution of an assistive technology, *Technol Disabil* 5:217-228, 1996.

Von Maltzahn WW, Daphtary M, Roa RL: Usage patterns of environmental control units by severely disabled individuals in their homes, *IEEE Trans Rehabil Eng* 3:222-227, 1995.

Woods BM, Jones RD: Environmental control systems in a spinal injuries unit: a review of 10 years experience, *Int Disabil Stud* 12:137-140, 1990.

Zimmermann G et al: Universal remote console standard—toward natural user interaction in ambient intelligence, In *Extended abstracts for the 2004 Conference on Human Factors in Computing Systems,* pp. 1608-1609, New York, 2004, ACM Press: http://myurc.org/publications/2004-CHI-URC.php. Accessed Nov 28, 2006.

PART 5

Contexts for Assistive Technology Applications

CHAPTER 15

Assistive Technologies in the Context of the Classroom

Learning Objectives

On completing this chapter, you will be able to do the following:

1. Describe the context in which assistive technologies are applied in education
2. List the major assistive technologies that are used in educational settings
3. Describe how assistive technologies are used in the classroom to facilitate learning
4. List the major technological approaches used to assist individuals who have learning disabilities
5. Describe how soft technologies are used in education to enhance the use of hard technologies

---

Key Terms

Academic Participation
Functional Equivalency
Inclusion
Individual Education Plan (IEP)
Individuals with Disabilities
    Education Act (IDEA)

Learner-Teacher Interactions
Learning Styles
Manipulatives
Musical Instrument Digital Interface
    (MIDI)
Peer Training

Resource Specialist
Scribing
Social Participation
Student Workstation
Technology Integration Plan

In preceding chapters we have developed principles for assistive technology application based on the human activity–assistive technology (HAAT) model (see Chapter 2). Two of the major settings in which assistive technologies are used are education and work, and each of these has features that make assistive technology applications unique. This chapter discusses educational applications. Vocational applications are covered in the next chapter. In both cases the HAAT model is used as a framework around which to discuss assistive technology (AT) applications.

Assistive technologies can provide major benefits for children in educational settings from preschool through postsecondary levels (Todis and Walker, 1993). Postural support systems (see Chapter 6) allow children to be positioned for maximal participation in classroom activities. Often this positioning is necessary to allow access to computers for learning (see Chapter 7). Special-purpose input methods or control interfaces (see Chapter 7) are often necessary for use of computers and other electronic devices. Augmentative communication systems (see Chapter 11) play a major role in learning for children who have disabilities affecting speaking or writing. Research has also shown that independent mobility (see Chapter 12) has a significant benefit even to very young children (Butler, 1986). There is an increasing use of "manipulatives" in education. Some assistive technologies (e.g., electronic aids to daily living [EADLs] and robotics; see Chapter 14) can provide assistance to children who cannot independently manipulate real objects. Finally, children who have sensory disabilities (visual or auditory) are aided by the technologies described in Chapters 8 and 9. There are also many hardware and software aids to students who have cognitive disabilities (see Chapter 10). Thus the potential for achieving a positive educational effect is great. However, reaching that potential requires careful planning and policy making to ensure that opportunities and not barriers are created (Merbler, Hadadian, and Ulman, 1999).

Terminology used to describe technology that is useful in achieving educational goals is complicated and often confusing.

Edyburn (2003a) describes a number of problems with the current definitions of assistive technology device and service (see Chapter 1) related to the provision of AT in the educational system. Many of these focus on lack of resources available to schools (e.g., personnel, student access to technology, and availability of training). Others relate to legal mandates (e.g., consideration of assistive technology in the IEP). Although these areas do raise issues about the availability of technology and associated resources in schools, they do not mandate a rethinking of the assistive technology terminology as incorporated into U.S. law. The more salient point made by Edyburn is that assistive technologies and instructional technologies (i.e., those used by all students) are often used to accomplish the same goals, and he proposes the term *technology-enhanced performance* to describe the use of all technologies (assistive and instructional) to place the emphasis on the achievement of educational goals rather than on the technology. We have used the term *assistive technology* to refer only to those aspects of technology that are matched to an individual need and accomplish broad functional goals for the individual. We have used "educational technology" to describe technology that is intended to aid learning (see Chapter 1). As we have discussed in Chapter 10 technology enhanced performance applies to the classroom setting and is consistent with the use of the HAAT model as we have described it in Chapter 2.

Edyburn (2003a) also makes recommendations for the ways in which assistive technology services should be provided in schools with emphasis on the identification of students with special needs (especially mild cognitive disabilities). He also advocates the development of organized, focused training programs for teachers and other education personnel with appropriate resources attached. Finally, he suggests a comprehensive outcome data collection system to document the use of technology by students with disabilities. These are useful considerations within the educational context.

Now that some of the individual tools for access to education that appear in previous chapters have been identified and some general aspects of their use introduced in the educational setting, we turn our attention to how they are combined and applied to maximize the opportunities for learning by children who have disabilities. That is the subject of the remainder of this chapter. The emphasis is on the way in which assistive technologies can aid students in obtaining access to the curriculum. There are many other sources that describe the application of these technologies in detail, relate them to curriculum development, and evaluate outcomes. One multiauthored source with a wide variety of information is Edyburn, Higgins, and Burn (2005).

■ EDUCATIONAL ACTIVITIES THAT CAN BE AIDED BY ASSISTIVE TECHNOLOGIES

To discuss assistive technology applications in the classroom, first the activities that characterize educational endeavors must be defined. Having done that, we can then begin to identify the ways that assistive technologies can contribute to those activities. In the following sections, each of the learning activities is described in terms of the tasks that must be accessed to complete the activity. Identification of these tasks will then help to define both the human skills and the technologies required to successfully complete them.

In all these functional areas there are educational technologies (see Chapter 1) that aid in the acquisition of the necessary skills. In many cases the educational technologies are software programs that provide systematic skill development in the various activities. For example, using CD-ROM-based educational software and the Internet, learners can access a much wider range of curriculum material, concepts, ideas, and lessons than are available by print materials and worksheets alone. Because all these sources require the use of a computer, the adaptations described in Chapter 7 are often necessary to ensure access for learners who have motor or sensory disabilities. Because schools often have computers available for general use by learners, it is necessary for the ATP to work with school staff to determine the appropriate access methods for individual learners. The ATP can also work with teachers to integrate appropriate software and hardware into the curriculum.

Reading

Reading requires motor, sensory, and cognitive skills. For print materials, motor skills are primarily associated with acquiring the reading material, positioning it and manipulative tasks (e.g., turning the pages, picking up a book). As shown in Figure 15-1, an aide often assists with manipulation of the reading materials. For reading materials that use electronic media, the motor tasks include mouse or keyboard use to scroll through text, highlight a portion of text, search for particular words or topics, and print out part or all of a document.

Success in reading also requires that sensory tasks be completed. Typically we use the visual system to take in

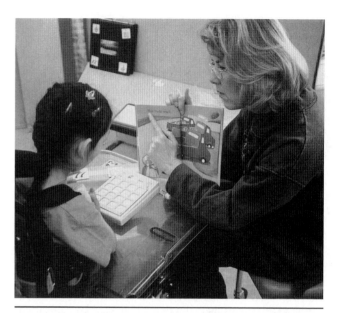

Figure 15-1 An aide often assists with manipulation of reading materials when it is difficult for the student to hold the book.

information via reading. For this function there must be sufficient visual field, visual acuity, and oculomotor function to scan text and recognize letters and words. If the visual system cannot support these functions, then an alternative format in either tactile (braille) or auditory (speech) form can be used instead.

Conversion between print and electronic forms and between visual and auditory or tactile formats can be aided by assistive technologies. Some of these are described in Chapter 8. The use of digital scanners to aid in this function is described later in this chapter.

Cognitive tasks are those associated with literacy; that is, word identification, spelling, and comprehension. Educational software for assisted reading includes programs that present very simple stories that the child can control, programs with multiple output modes (e.g., visual and auditory), interactive stories that the child can change by pointing and clicking the mouse, and on-line books (including current bestsellers, children's books, and the classics). A variety of technologies that are used by students with mild disabilities (e.g., learning disabilities) are discussed in Chapter 10.

Strangeman and Dalton (2005) provide a comprehensive review of research relating technology-based approaches for assisting students who have reading difficulties. The key areas that they identify are phonemic awareness, phonics/word recognition, vocabulary, fluency, comprehension, engagement, and universal design for literacy learning. Phonemic awareness is a strong predictor of early reading success. Its development can be aided by computer programs that are based on drill and practice and provide decoding support (recognition of sounds within words), sometimes in a game format. Speech recognition has also been shown to be beneficial in developing reading skills for older students (ages 9-18 years) who have learning disabilities. This benefit occurred only for discrete (word by word) speech recognition not continuous recognition (see Chapter 7).

Difficulties with word recognition or phonics can significantly impact reading ability. Text-to-speech (TTS) software (see Chapter 7) has been used in a number of studies addressing word recognition/phonics with mixed results. The best results occur when teacher training and support are provided with the TTS software, illustrating the importance of using a combination of hard and soft technologies in assistive technology applications (Chapter 1). Jeffs, Behrman, and Bannan-Ritland (2006) describe the characteristics required to provide an appropriate environment for parents and students to effectively use assistive technologies for literacy learning. TTS software can also aid in the acquisition of vocabulary by providing alternative forms of the text (see Chapter 10). TTS combined with other media (hypermedia approaches) have had mixed results in developing increased vocabulary in students with learning disabilities. Synthetic word-level TTS can also aid students who have difficulty with oral fluency when reading. Books-on-tape (see Chapter 8) have also been shown to aid students by providing multi-sensory reading practice. The provision of text in an alternative format using TTS can allow the student to focus on content and improve comprehension (Strangeman and Dalton, 2005). Hypertexts that add strategic prompts, linked glossaries, help files, and other supports have been used to increase comprehension. Computer game formats with a variety of built-in supports, alternative output formats (TTS and text), and curriculum-based activities have also been used to increase comprehension.

For any of these approaches to be effective, the learner must be engaged. Engagement is a measure of the effectiveness of any approach because it directly affects motivation and creation of a challenging and rewarding instructional experience for the student. A second engagement factor is the degree to which the student enjoys reading. If the technology can increase enjoyment and excitement about reading through a variety of activities and features, then the student is more likely to seek out opportunities to read and apply the literacy skills learned through the technology-enhanced performance exercises.

In all of these areas, the research results are mixed and the application of assistive technologies must be individualized to the needs of any specific student. The concept of universal design for learning (an extension of the universal design discussion in Chapter 1) emphasizes applications that are "scalable" for different levels of need, and encompass a range of abilities and needs in learners (Strangeman and Dalton, 2005). Examples include multiple modes of text representation, diverse strategic networks that link to other parts of the learning system, and multiple means of engagement. In all cases the question of remediation (i.e., educational technology designed to teach reading) versus compensation (i.e., assistive

technology designed to provide alternative ways of reading) may determine what approaches are taken for any individual student (Edyburn, 2003b). Often a student must fail despite repeated remediation attempts before compensation approaches are considered. To address this dilemma, Edyburn (2003b) has developed the systems approach shown in Table 15-1. The six factors included in Table 15-1 identify

TABLE 15-1   A Systems Approach to Making Text Accessible

Factor	Key Questions	Selected Responses
1	What environment will students be expected to read in?	School Classroom, learning center Home School bus, car
2	What student characteristics need to be considered when designing effective instruction?	Can't Won't Does so slowly Limited attention Blind Low vision Cognitive disability
3	What reading tasks are students commonly expected to complete?	Read in class Read for homework Answer questions about what has been read Engage in learning activity on the basis of information gained from reading
4	What type of source documents are students expected to read?	Textbook Trade sheets Classic literature Ready reference Teacher-made materials Worksheet Quiz/exam Current events Web pages
5	If there is a preference in reading, will the intervention involve remediation, compensation, or both?	Remediation Literacy acquisition Compensation Vocabulary/concept development Study skills Higher-level thinking Compensation Bypass reading Decrease reading Support reading Organize reading Guide reading
6	Given many stakeholders concerned about student success, what responsibilities will each person assume?	Student General education teacher Special education teacher Assistive technology specialist Administrator

the critical questions that must be addressed to attain academic achievement gains as mandated by various legislation (e.g., No Child Left Behind in the United States). Each of the needs (Factor 2) and compensation strategies (Factor 5) identified in the table are based on technologies that are discussed in this or earlier chapters. Edyburn (2003b) lists specific software products for each of those strategies that involve technology.

As in all aspects of assistive technology application, the measurement of outcomes is important to evaluate our approaches. For reading, the challenges are to determine whether reading is more successful and useful to the student with the use of an assistive technology than without it. Reading is a complex activity with many factors that influence its success, and the effectiveness of assistive technologies in aiding reading is not an easy question to answer (Edyburn, 2004).

Writing

Writing as a Physical Process

Writing requires motor, sensory, and cognitive skills. Motor skills are primarily associated with acquiring the reading material, positioning it, and manipulative tasks (e.g., turning the pages, picking up a book etc.). The use of pencil or pen and paper requires fine motor control to hold the pen or pencil and to produce letters (Figure 15-2). When the learner's disability significantly affects these motor skills, it may be necessary to recognize that some skills will not be

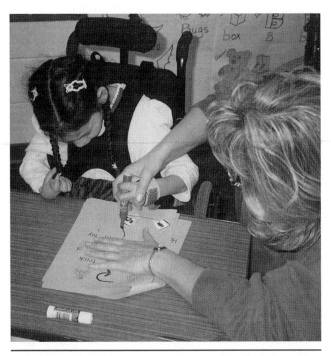

Figure 15-2   Hand-over-hand assistance can be used to help with writing.

functional and to develop alternative approaches to writing. This intervention allows the learner to move on to other educational goals rather than working on the functional tasks of handwriting at the expense of these other goals. The assistive technology practitioner (ATP) must use his or her judgment as to when to make the transition from handwriting skill development to electronic alternatives, but in most cases it is desirable to accommodate in the short term to enable learning, even if handwriting might be functional in the long term. For students who have a motor limitation preventing the use of handwriting, assistive technology–based writing requires the ability to use a keyboard or mouse. As discussed in Chapter 7, there are also many alternatives to keyboard/mouse entry, including automatic speech recognition. Sensory skills are primarily used for monitoring what is being written. This task is most commonly done visually, but auditory or tactile monitoring is also possible using various types of assistive technologies (Chapter 8). Cognitive and language skills include spelling (spontaneous, first letter, recognition), grammar, and sequencing (Chapter 10). Learners may only generate a small percentage of the total written work. However, students should be encouraged to use these alternative methods where possible to give them the opportunity to develop this form of reasoning.

Messaging has many of the same requirements as note taking. However, abbreviations and shorthand notations must be understandable to the person's communication partners. In addition, individuals do not need to generate messages quickly because often the person receiving the message is not present or waiting for it. Instant messaging and e-mail have influenced how we communicate. For students with motor problems, the use of asynchronous communication allows them to compose a message at a slower speed and send it quickly. This method allows communication with classmates and others in a manner like the students without physical disabilities.

Written messages can be developed by using paper and pencil, symbol stamps, e-mail, instant messaging, and chat rooms. They can also be developed with facilitators who can write down what someone is saying and then send the message later. For example, Brodin (1992) developed a way to send messages to families for individuals who have intellectual disabilities, use symbols for communication, and are unable to use voice communication over the telephone. These individuals live in group homes and wish to stay in touch with their families. The approach creates rubber stamps with the appropriate symbols with which the assistive and augmentative communication (AAC) user is familiar. These stamps are used by the person to create a message on paper. This message is then faxed to the significant others as a message.

The most demanding type of writing is *formal writing*: reports, school homework, writing for publication, and similar applications. Creative writing (prose or poetry) is a very important category of writing that requires assistive technology tools. Here content is most important. For formal writing, the rate of text entry for individuals with motor limitations is important because they may have a typing rate of three to five words per minute, and input acceleration techniques (Chapter 7) are necessary to allow them to keep up with the demands of work or school. The most common adaptation is to make a computer accessible so the student can access word processors for writing. The functions of the word processor must be available to the user regardless of the input method being used (e.g., one-key typing, scanning, Morse code). Smith et al (1989) analyzed the formal written output of a group of adolescents who had congenital disabilities limiting their abilities to speak and who were competent conversational users of AAC (Chapter 11) devices. Each of these individuals had developed language by using Blissymbols (see Vanderheiden and Lloyd, 1986), and they had made the transition to traditional orthography (letters and spelling). Smith and co-workers analyzed the homework produced by these individuals. More than 80% of the homework was produced independently. The rate of production of written output was only 1.5 words per minute, reflecting the amount of planning and thinking time required and the limitations imposed by physical disabilities. As expected, the majority (more than 50%) of the writing was for school assignments. The second largest category was personal correspondence, a finding that Smith et al ascribed to the inability to use a telephone. Currently, this category is served by e-mail. Some difficulties with grammatical structure and form were observed in all the subjects, but there was great variability even in this small sample. This study indicates that individuals who have congenital speaking and writing difficulties because of physical limitations can develop successful writing skills.

Writing as a Cognitive Process.   Writing as a cognitive process has been described as consisting of four phases: (1) prewriting or brainstorming, (2) drafting or organizing and composing, (3) editing, and (4) publishing (Calkins, 1986). Technology can aid all four phases of this process and thereby positively affect the learner's writing skill development (Rocklage and Lake, 1997). As Rocklage and Lake point out, assistive technology for writing provides both a structure within which the learner can learn to write and a polished finished (or published) product.

Light and Smith (1993) compared the home literacy experiences of preschool children by surveying a group of parents of children who use AAC and a group of parents of nondisabled children. Through a series of questions, Light and Smith determined the functional context (e.g., how reading and writing occur, when they occur, communication during reading), language context (roles of parent and child, nature and degree of participation), and cultural context (parental priorities and beliefs regarding literacy). Both groups of children were interested in literacy activities, but

the AAC users had fewer opportunities to read, participated less during reading, and had less access to writing and drawing materials. Although both groups of parents gave high priority to communication, the parents of the nondisabled children gave highest priorities to making friends and literacy activities. The parents of AAC users gave second level priorities to physical needs such as mobility and feeding. Studies such as this one underscore the importance of attitudes, beliefs, and accessibility to materials in the development of cognitive communication skills. A more detailed discussion of literacy issues related to assistive technologies is provided by Light and Kent-Walsh (2003) and Sturm, Erickson, and Yoder (2002), who describe the literacy challenges faced by children who use AAC and offer suggestions for enhancing literacy development through the use of AAC.

Educational software for assisting writing includes programs that allow the child to create his or her own story. Other programs provide monitoring through visual and auditory feedback. Word prediction and completion programs (see Chapters 7 and 11) can aid spelling and word finding. The use of abbreviations and macros (see Chapter 7) that reduce the number of keystrokes can increase the speed of text entry. Chapter 10 (see *Language Tools* in that chapter) discusses the use of word prediction, spell checkers, concept mapping software, and other technology approaches to aid individuals who have difficulty writing because of cognitive disabilities.

Edyburn (2003c) describes a number of factors influencing the measurement of outcomes of assistive technology supported writing. A major challenge is to recognize that easy to measure characteristics (e.g., rate of typing and written output) may not be as meaningful as more difficult factors (e.g., the quality of the written output). He also describes a number of potential measures that can be used.

CASE STUDY

COMPUTERS AS WRITING AIDS

A school-based occupational therapist has presented you, the ATP, with this question: "I know that written expression in schools can be done through scribing by a peer or aide or through teacher notes. At my school, a student is only considered for a laptop computer or a portable note-taking device if he or she is academically inclined and dexterous enough. Do you agree with this approach?"

What would you tell her? Consider your answer in light of the discussion in this chapter about writing and the skills required.

Mathematics

Mathematics is an essential part of the school curriculum. In the United States, the National Council of Teachers of Mathematics (NCTM) has developed standards for the teaching of mathematics (Maccini and Gagnon, 2005). Recommended practices include the need to teach all students high-level thinking and reasoning skills and mathematical problem solving. The goals of the standards are to prepare learners to (1) value mathematics, (2) become confident in their mathematical ability, (3) become mathematical problem solvers, (4) learn to communicate mathematically, and (5) reason mathematically. Much like writing, students have difficulties for different reasons. For individuals with motor limitations, the problems are manipulation of concepts through alternatives to pencil and paper. For those with cognitive disabilities, the challenges are to find technological approaches to aid in achieving the five goals listed. These two categories are discussed separately.

Mathematics as a Physical Process.   Imagine learning even the most basic arithmetic without being able to write the numbers down. Although it is possible to become proficient using this strategy, it is certainly more difficult than basic pencil-and-paper mathematics. A scribe can be used to assist in learning mathematics just as in writing. However, many of the same concerns and limitations described for writing apply to mathematics. For mathematics there is the added requirement that thinking mathematically almost always requires having a worksheet on which to solve the problem. Very few people can develop mathematical skills without some visual representation. When this is impossible (e.g., when the learner is blind), other strategies have to be developed. A learner may use an AAC device (Chapter 11) to instruct an aide who is **scribing** for the learner (e.g., "The answer is 5" or "Move the yellow one to the other pile").

Seven-year-old Rob has difficulty using a pencil and paper because of his cerebral palsy, but he is able to use a computer for writing by hitting the keys with one finger. He wants to learn math (at least his parents and teacher want him to do so), but this is very difficult using the standard keyboard and cursor movement. After he has two rows of numbers, he must move over to the far right-hand side of the first column of numbers and enter the first correct number *(7)*. Then he must backspace two times to get the cursor in the proper position for the second number *(1)*. The cursor in a graphical communication device is a flashing marker that indicates the location on the screen for the next entry. In writing English text using a word processing program, the cursor always moves left to right and moves down one line at the right margin. In contrast to this convention, the cursor should move left to right for mathematics as numbers are entered to be added, but once there is a column of numbers, the cursor should move right to left as the sum

is entered. Figure 15-3, *A-B*, illustrates this cursor movement. Also, when learning to add or subtract, children are taught to carry or borrow by crossing out the number at the top of the adjacent column and substituting the borrowed or carried value. It is desirable for this type of cursor movement to be available in a math worksheet as well. For example, when in the math mode, the letter *C* could be pressed to indicate *carry*, causing the cursor to jump to the top of the next column. All these cursor movements can be very time consuming, especially if a writing device is used and the person must tediously backspace to obtain the right to left cursor movement.

In algebra, special symbols (e.g., Greek letters) and the use of superscripts and subscripts are also required (Figure 15-3, *C*). Higher math such as statistics or calculus adds the need to have special symbols like summation signs and integral signs and the need for displaying mathematical formulas in the proper format. There are devices (sometimes as programs for personal computers) that are set up specifically for these math functions. Several commercial AAC devices also include some or all of these mathematical functions.

Mathematical ability, including precursor skills (e.g., counting, sorting), is often developed by use of **manipulatives.** These are rods, blocks, buttons, beads, or other objects that vary by color, length, and weight and can be sorted, counted, and used to enhance concept development in mathematics. Piaget believed that learners use "concrete operations" (see Table 3-1) to develop many cognitive concepts from 7 to 11 years of age (Brainerd, 1978). Others now believe that concrete operations using manipulatives of various types are an important part of learning for much older learners, including adults (Resnick et al, 1998). To fully benefit from concrete operations, the learner must have control over objects. For example, a simple task with manipulatives might involve being able to see that "I have two pieces in this pile, and I move two more pieces over and now I have four."

Although the learner typically manipulates real objects, there are also computer programs that substitute computer-generated graphics of manipulatives for persons who cannot use their hands. The computer mouse (e.g., click and drag) or keyboard (e.g., arrow keys) can be used to move these manipulatives. Conceptually this type of manipulation can develop the same skills as manipulation of real objects. Manipulatives can also be switch controlled either by using software specifically designed for that purpose or by using computer adaptations such as SmartClick (see Chapter 7) to create adapted access to standard software.

Mathematics differs from writing in several important ways. The cursor moves right to left rather than left to right for entering sums or differences. The functions of borrow and carry also require unique cursor movements. Higher mathematics requires Greek symbols, superscripts, subscripts, and mathematical symbols (e.g., integral sign, summation sign). Typical symbols are shown in Figure 15-3, *C*. Some AAC devices (see Chapter 11) have built-in math

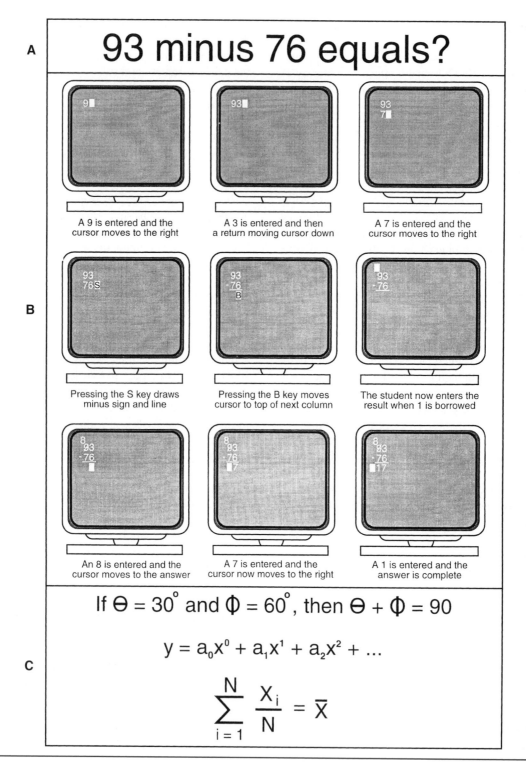

Figure 15-3   Math problems require different cursor movements and symbols than text entry. **A,** A math problem as it would normally be written. **B,** The sequence of cursor movements required to enter the problem, create a subtraction notation (line plus minus sign), and complete the problem (including using "borrow"). **C,** Special symbols such as these are used in higher mathematics.

worksheet software including special symbols. These features of mathematics worksheets differ from calculator functions, and they are intended to facilitate the development of math skills. There is a use for calculators that are adapted for access by learners who have difficulties with the keys on standard calculators. Some enlarged key calculators are available, and some AAC devices also include calculator functions. Calculator functions are also built into Windows and Macintosh operating systems, and they can be used with any of the access approaches described in Chapter 7.

Word processing software often includes the special symbols required for mathematics but lacks the special cursor movements. The required symbol set is selected and inserted into a document or worksheet, which is useful for a teacher creating a worksheet or to a learner using a computer. However, these approaches do not address the special cursor movements required for mathematics. Those functions are available in special computer software (e.g., MathPad and Math Pad Plus, Intellitools, Petaluma, Calif., *www.intellitools.com/default.aspx*) and some AAC devices (see Chapter 11). The selection of characters can be left open as a window and the user can pick the desired symbol and insert it as necessary. This approach allows the learner to write out the equations, solve them, and print the results. Both direct and indirect (scanning and encoding) access are available to accommodate a variety of motor skill levels in learners (see Chapter 7).

Mathematics as a Cognitive Process. The primary focus of mathematics is to help students acquire the cognitive abilities to manipulate numbers and to solve routine and novel problems (Edyburn, 2003d). The physical manipulation assists described above help with internalization of mathematical skills, but they do not address possible cognitive limitations. Students with cognitive disabilities often struggle with concepts such as counting, telling time, making change, learning basic mathematical facts, and solving real-world problems (Edyburn, 2003d). The NCTM has recommended that every student have access to a calculator, every teacher have access to a computer, and every classroom have access to the Internet for demonstrations and student's use and access to "computers and other appropriate technology for individual, small group and whole-class use as needed" (Maccini and Gagnon, 2005). This complement of technologies can be assistive for students with disabilities and is instructional for all students.

Educational software that helps develop math skills from basic counting through higher mathematics is available for both the Windows and Macintosh environments. These programs address skill development through drill and practice and concept development, through the use of computer graphics, games, and word problems integrated into an interesting illustrated story (see Case Study: Assistive Technology Assistance with Mathematics). Calculators and computer programs that help with math problem formulation and solution are also

available (Maccini and Gagnon, 2005). Measurement of assistive technology outcomes in mathematics focuses on two areas: (1) the ability to calculate accurately and (2) the ability to use one's mathematical ability to solve problems (Edyburn, 2003d). Both these questions relate to the student's ability to independently solve routine and novel problems. The critical assistive technology question is whether the student's performance is improved with the assistive technology over the no-technology condition. To date, there is insufficient evidence to answer this question in general. However, it can be evaluated in each individual case by establishing a baseline measure for the student and then re-evaluating after proficiency in assistive technology use has been achieved.

CASE STUDY

ASSISTIVE TECHNOLOGY ASSISTANCE WITH MATHEMATICS

Ken is a young high school student who uses a single-switch scanner. In math skills he has never gone beyond number recognition and simple addition up to 10. He has no use of his hands to use manipulatives to assist him in higher calculations. Ken's team would like him to use a math worksheet program. Also, because he cannot add more complex sums in his head, they would like him to have access to a calculator that he would use only as needed. He should be able to transfer the calculator results to his worksheet. The built-in calculator on the computer is rather small, and he would be unable to carry the answer in his head to put it on his worksheet.

What approaches would you suggest to Ken's team to help in this situation?

Science

Educational activities in science are both theoretical and experimental. The latter is based on hands-on manipulation of objects in biology, physics, and chemistry. Sometimes these concepts and skills are taught with physical objects and laboratory experiments. However, with the increased quality and resolution of computer graphics, a lower cost alternative is computer simulation of experimental situations (e.g., frog dissection in biology, chemical reactions, laws of motion experiments in physics). There are also Internet-based sources from which experiments can be downloaded. Examples of simulated experiments are provided by (Schaff et al, 2005).

There are several ways in which learners with physical disabilities that limit reaching and grasping can participate in science activities that require manipulation. Instructions for manipulation can be given to a peer, aide, or teacher via natural speech or AAC devices. Independent manipulation of objects can be aided by EADLs or robotic systems.

In Chapter 14 we describe EADLs in detail. The use of robotic arms to aid in science instruction is also described in Chapter 14. Finally, if suitable computer adaptations are available, learners with disabilities can participate equally in computer simulations, concept development software, and Internet-based science instruction.

There are other technologies that are useful in science instruction for students with disabilities (Schaff et al, 2005): Virtual reality software allows students to experience different environments and conduct experiments without manipulating physical objects and many similar "immersive" experiences. Virtual reality is defined as a three-dimensional, computer-generated synthetic environment that allows students to gain a sense of being immersed in a real world (Schaff et al, 2005). Their use in science education is relatively new and not widespread. The advantages of virtual environments are that the physical requirements for exploration can be altered for a student with a motor disability, the external stimuli can be controlled to avoid over stimulation of individuals with cognitive limitations, and a variety of sensory modalities can be used to accommodate students with hearing or visual impairments. The most exciting feature of virtual reality for education is that it is highly interactive, which can be a motivating factor for students.

Music

Music instruction involves basic rhythm and group participation. Young learners use instruments and their voices to participate in music. Music appreciation through listening is also part of the curriculum. Adaptations (e.g., adapted handles, activation by head or foot movement) can be made for students who cannot use musical instruments as a result of disabilities. AAC devices that use digitized speech (see Chapter 11) can store musical sounds (i.e., an instrument) or a vocal song. Most computers can be equipped with a **musical instrument digital interface (MIDI)**. This interface is a file that is used to store music as a series of notes with volume and duration attached. The file allows music to be played back through a sound card in a computer. If a digital musical instrument (e.g., a piano keyboard) is attached to the MIDI interface, it can be used to store the musical notes so they can be played back on the instrument or through the sound card (Merbler, Hadadian, and Ulman, 1999). With this arrangement, learners can create original songs, learn musical instruments, and explore sounds. With appropriate computer adaptations, the learner who has a disability can also access a MIDI-equipped computer.

Art

Art activities help students develop fine motor control and an understanding of shapes and colors and provide a creative

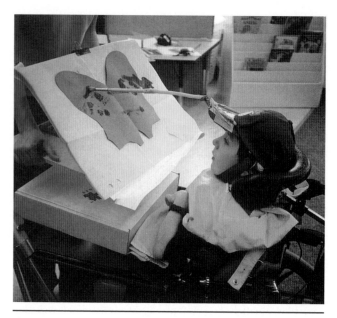

Figure 15-4 For assistance with painting in art class, we can attach the paintbrush to a head-pointing stick or baseball cap.

outlet for students. For students who lack the fine motor skill for drawing, adaptations can be provided. For example, a pen, pencil, or paintbrush can be attached to a head pointer or mouthstick (see Chapter 7). One example of such an arrangement is shown in Figure 15-4.

Handles on drawing instruments can be enlarged and adapted grips can be added (see Figure 14-3). Alternatively, the manipulation of digital images can be substituted for drawing with pencil and paper. This can present challenging art projects in a format accessible by learners with physical disabilities (Merbler, Hadadian, and Ulman, 1999). Computer software for drawing is also used in educational settings. With the appropriate computer adaptations, this software is accessible to all learners regardless of disability.

Open-ended tasks such as drawing can also be carried out using single-switch scanning. In one approach the learner selects the color by scanning (Figure 15-5) and the teacher or aide then uses that color to fill in a part of the picture. A more independent method can be achieved with an adapted robotic system (Smith and Topping, 1996) such as the Handy 1, a robotic system specially designed for feeding (Topping, 1996). The Handy 1 is described further in Chapter 14. In the application for art, selection of the color of a pen, the position of the pen, the activity of the pen (move or draw), and its movement are accomplished using single-switch scanning. Using scanning for tasks such as these is cognitively demanding, and Smith and Topping (1996) reported widely different levels of success in the three subjects included in their study.

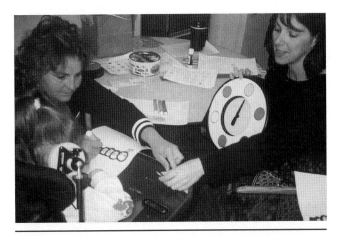

Figure 15-5   A student is selecting the color she wants to use by pressing her switch when the pointer is aimed at her choice. The teacher then uses that color to fill in a part of the picture.

Drawing and Plotting

Computer software can be used to produce graphical outputs for drawing *or plotting* for science or art instruction. Current computer software provides many different means of drawing and plotting. Spreadsheet programs include plotting and calculation capabilities. Drawing programs include the ability to sketch an idea or create a finished picture by using mouse movements. Photo editors and digital cameras allow easy manipulation of images for a variety of applications. The key to all of these applications is obtaining computer access for persons with physical disabilities (Chapter 7) and simplifying tasks for individuals with cognitive disabilities (Chapter 10).

■ IDENTIFYING STUDENT SKILLS AND NEEDS FOR ASSISTIVE TECHNOLOGY

The letter and response on the following page were posted on the Rehabilitation Engineering and Assistive Technology Society of North America (RESNA) assistive technology listserv. They point out some of the issues in assistive technology assessment for education.

This exchange of letters points out the necessity for a team approach, including the learner and her family. It also illustrates the necessity of focusing on need rather than technology. This section describes several commonly used approaches to assistive technology assessment in education. A general assistive technology assessment process is detailed in Chapter 4.

Meeting Educational Goals: The Role of Assistive Technologies

We have defined the activities that are typically carried out in educational settings. Given these activities, it is important

to determine the skills and abilities that the learner brings to the process. This evaluation of learner skills is obtained from a systematic assessment process. Chapter 4 describes both the essential information that must be obtained through an assessment process and the major approaches to service delivery in assistive technologies. Assistive technology assessment in education has some unique goals that are discussed in this section. The major approaches used to obtain this assessment information are also described.

The development of services and service delivery in the United States has been significantly affected by federal legislation (see Chapter 1). The **Individuals with Disabilities Education Act (IDEA)** includes definitions of assistive technology devices and assistive technology services. It mandates that local educational agencies be responsible for providing assistive technology devices and services if these are required as part of a child's education, as well as related services and supplementary aid or service. These devices and services must be directly related to the child's educational program.

IDEA also mandates that an **Individual Education Plan (IEP)**, which incorporates the specialized program, be written for each student. The 1997 reauthorization of IDEA mandates that the IEP team must consider assistive technologies as a special factor when developing the learner's IEP (Merbler, Hadadian, and Ulman, 1999). A policy statement on the rights of a student with a disability to assistive technology under Public Law 94-142 was issued August 10, 1990 (Button, 1990). This policy statement describes a variety of services and devices that may be included in the IEP. The impact of this law has been far reaching, and devices ranging from sensory aids (visual and auditory) to augmentative communication devices to specialized computers have been provided to help children with disabilities access educational programs (Desch, 1986).

Models for Educational Assistive Technology Assessment

There are only a few commonly used models of delivery for assistive technology devices and services. One set of models is built around an assistive technology expert or an expert team that is brought into the classroom. In some cases the assistive technology experience and expertise is not available in the local school, and external assistance is sought. Often a team of assistive technology specialists provides this assistance. In other cases a single external assistive technology consultant is called on to carry out assessment of a child. When a school or local education authority has experience in meeting the needs of a number of their students, they may build local assistive technology resources around this experience and not rely on external consultants. This is often an interdisciplinary team that works together within the local educational authority.

CASE STUDY

ASSESSMENT FOR ASSISTIVE TECHNOLOGY IN A SCHOOL SETTING

Dear Ms. A. T. Pea,

I am struggling with my school system on an assistive technology issue. I have a son with dyslexia, dysgraphia, moderate to severe attention deficit, a hearing loss that causes him to miss about half of what is said in his classes, and a tested IQ that falls just short of gifted.

This fall I requested an assistive tech evaluation to see whether he would benefit from greater use of a computer. I suggested that they consider providing a mid-range laptop and appropriate software for math and writing. I also requested someone to coach him in using it to compensate for his difficulties. I suggested that he be allowed to do scanned-in worksheets on it and maybe even take tests (under supervision so he couldn't make copies).

A few weeks later, without doing any sort of evaluation, the school provided an ancient black-and-white laptop with inadequate memory, no coaching, and no software other than an early word processing program, saying it was a test of whether a laptop would actually help him. Despite the laptop's inadequacy, there has been some improvement in his work. However, it's no good for math or science, and it has far too little memory to act as a "portable filing cabinet" for all his work, something he desperately needs.

I am desperate to find him some help now, so he can learn how best to use a computer before starting high school next fall. I can't resign myself to seeing a child with so much potential fall through the cracks. Even though it's the district's responsibility and the district can afford to meet his needs, I would buy him the computer and software myself if only the district would willingly provide a "coach" and make appropriate computer use part of his IEP. Right now, my only hope is to find material from other education professionals that can convince them that I'm not asking for something exotic. I am wondering whether you could point me to some sources of information. Thank you for any information you can offer.

Sincerely,

I. M. Concerned

The ATP wrote back to the mother:

Dear Ms. Concerned:

The school must provide any assistive technology that the IEP team determines necessary for your son to meet the IEP goals and objectives. You need to start with the IEP. Unfortunately, assistive technology is often requested after the IEP is in place, and there is no indication on the IEP that it is needed. The assistive technology assessment should start with the student and what he needs to do, not with a piece of equipment. From a school's perspective, you are starting with a tool instead of analyzing the need first. Most administrators I know would balk at the request for a trial period of a piece of equipment before a thorough assistive technology evaluation was completed.

I am beginning to see a willingness for school districts to provide more expensive assistive technology if (1) it is a team decision, (2) there is documentation of what has already been tried, (3) lower tech solutions have been tried and found to be inadequate, and (4) there is a trial period with the recommended system with clear documentation of benefit.

I also need to point out a laptop may not be the answer you hope for. Computer access for those with dysgraphia can be very helpful. However, for those with ADHD the computer is not necessarily an advantage. Depending on the level of ADHD and distractibility, the ability to "fiddle" that a word processor offers can actually slow down production over handwriting in some cases.

Your son does have a right to an assistive technology assessment if he is currently unable to meet his IEP goals and objectives as a result of his disability; however, the outcome of that assessment should reflect a team decision. I think you have several choices:

Invest in a laptop and training for your son.

Approach the team from a slightly different angle, requesting a thorough assessment, not a specific solution.

Contact a special education resource center in your area for assistance in evaluation and some trial period of software or equipment.

I know that this is a difficult situation for you, and I hope that your son is able to obtain the assistive technology that will benefit him in his educational program.

Sincerely,

A. T. Pea, ATP

Alternatively, a single well-qualified and experienced ATP may also take on this role for a local school district.

Another approach or model is to refer the child to the assessment setting in an evaluation center. Although this assessment is also carried out by a team, this model differs from the first model in that the child is typically seen in the center rather than in the classroom because they have a wide range of equipment to be demonstrated and they can involve specialized staff as the learner's needs dictate. Each of these delivery models is discussed in general in Chapter 4. This chapter focuses on their use in educational settings.

As Todis and Walker (1993) point out, successful assistive technology outcomes are dependent on a careful and thorough evaluation of the individual learner's needs. This is true regardless of the type and extent of disability or the format of the evaluation. If we are to ensure that there is "goodness of fit" between the learner's needs and the recommended assistive technology, then we are required to consider the full constellation of unique abilities and disabilities of the learner during the assessment process. Todis and Walker (1993) present two case studies that illustrate the importance of a thorough evaluation to achieve the desired outcomes for the learner.

Assessment Team

The assistive technology assessment team usually includes a variety of disciplines (e.g., occupational therapist [OT], physical therapist [PT], speech-language pathologist [SLP], ATP, and pediatrician) (Todis and Walker, 1993). The classroom teacher and the local **resource specialist** in assistive technology may also be included, together with the family (parents and siblings) of the learner who is being assessed. If the assessment team is outside the learner's school, it is a greater challenge to develop sufficient understanding of the learner's needs. Ideally the assessment team would carry out their assessment in the school, community, and home, as well as any specialized assessment center (Todis and Walker, 1993). This approach allows the team to determine the preferences and goals (sometimes conflicting) of the learner, the family's values, and the short- and long-term goals of the educational program for the child.

There are a variety of types of teams that provide assistive technology intervention services in schools. The complexity of the needs served and the possible options for meeting those needs through technology necessitates that a team approach be used whenever possible (Bodine and Melonics, 2005). All members of the team share responsibility for the classroom and for the learning of all students. Teams gain additional strength from group decision making that avoids individual errors in judgment and stimulates group interactions so that one perspective does not prevail without discussion. There are several types of teams defined by Bodine

and Melonics. Multidisciplinary teams are based on the medical model of individual disciplines presenting information germane to their areas of specialization with little integration. Interdisciplinary teams have formal channels of communication and team members share information and discuss results. In education these are more effective than multidisciplinary teams because team members share ideas and there is collaboration in reaching decisions regarding assistive technology approaches for a student. The most effective arrangement goes one step further to form a more unified approach to working as a team in which professionals often cross disciplinary boundaries on the basis of their experience and expertise. This approach is called transdisciplinary teaming. These teams are generally family/student centered and include parents, community members, and siblings who are familiar with the student, in addition to the professional team members. These teams have been shown to be more effective in developing and implementing assistive technology approaches for students with special needs. A similar concept is collaborative teams in which interorganizational structures allow sharing of power and authority to bring the team together to solve common problems. The cooperative approach or transdisciplinary or collaborative teams has been shown to be highly effective in meeting student needs (Bodine and Melonics, 2005).

Chapter 7 presents a detailed description of evaluation for access (e.g., use of a keyboard or alternative) to the assistive technologies. This is an area that is often overlooked until late in the assessment process, according to Todis and Walker (1993). Another area of potential concern is that the assessment may only address immediate learner needs and not pay enough attention to future growth and implications for new devices or expanded features (Beukelman and Mirenda, 2005). Assistive technology devices are often expensive, and funding sources will generally not purchase new technology repeatedly for the same child. The tradeoff is that the technology must have growth potential but not be too complicated or sophisticated for the learner to access it now (Todis and Walker, 1993).

As the letter from the mother in the case study illustrates, assistive technology procurement can sometimes become the goal rather than the process or means by which the goal can be achieved. This can place pressure on the assessment team to recommend assistive technology without adequate regard for the learner's goals.

Finally, the assessment process must carefully evaluate the potential impact of the new assistive technology on the classroom in which the learner's program is conducted. One of the most widely used assessment formats is called SETT (Zabala, 1996). The SETT framework was developed for use in educational settings. The four elements are Student, Environment, Task, and Tools. For each of these areas there is a set of questions that the team answers to define the needs of the student in terms of the classroom environment, the curricular tasks to be completed, and the tools (low and high technology) to be used. The focus of the SETT framework is on the interrelationship among the four elements. Student questions include the following: What does the student need to do? What are the student's special needs? and What are the student's current abilities? Typical environment questions ask the following: What materials and devices are available? What is the physical layout? Are there any special issues? What is the instructional arrangement? Are there any changes planned? What supports are available to the student? and What resources are available to the team supporting the student? Task questions include the following: What activities take place? What activities support the student's curriculum? What are critical elements of activities? How can activities be modified to meet student needs? How can technology support the student's participation in the activities? Finally, the Tools questions focus on the following questions: What strategies might be used to increase student performance? What no-tech, low-tech, and high-tech options should be considered? How might tools be tried with the student in environments where they will be used? By answering these questions, the team can ensure that they have not missed important items, that they have adequately related the needs to the curriculum, and that they have focused on the needs of the student.

Specialist Team. A specialist or, more often, a transdisciplinary team is responsible for assistive technology assessment. The team may be part of the school district or external to it. The role of the ATP in either case is as a consultant to the classroom team and family, not as a part of the learner's classroom staff. This role places limitations on what the ATP is able to do and how effective he or she is. As an outside consultant, the ATP is able to make recommendations, offer expert advice, and provide information that may not be available to other team members. However, the implementation of assistive technology devices and services is out of his or her control, which means the ATP must carefully evaluate the educational context and take into account the resources, limitations, and expertise available in that setting before making recommendations for assistive technologies. This is especially important when considering soft technologies such as training of the learner and staff, strategy development for the use of the assistive technology, and evaluation of outcomes of the intervention.

One of the most valuable contributions that the ATP can make to the school team is a perspective on what is possible, what is reasonable, and what is technologically feasible. Equally important is to be able to identify situations in which the available technologies are not suitable for the existing problems. Consumers may not appreciate the implications of new technological advances, many of which are reported in the popular press. Also, sometimes things that seem like they should be easy to do technically are really quite difficult and those that seem to a nontechnical person to be difficult may in fact be easy and inexpensive to accomplish. Thus a major role for the ATP as a consultative member of the school team is to provide a perspective on the question of what is and what is not technically possible. This perspective also helps to determine what *should* be done technologically, as well as what *can* be done.

To fill the need for technological information, the ATP needs specific skills. These include (1) an understanding of the special and regular educational systems, (2) knowledge of current assistive technologies used to improve access to education for children with disabilities, (3) understanding of the roles of other members of the team (teacher, resource specialists, OT, PT, SLP, parents), and (4) technical knowledge and experience sufficient to apply the assistive technologies (hard and soft) effectively.

Local Resource Specialist. Many schools have resource specialists who provide expert advice on approaches, curriculum adaptation, and assistive technologies for learners who have special needs. The role of this individual is similar to the ATP role on the assessment team, but the range of experience with assistive technologies may be less extensive. Typically the resource specialist has a number of areas for which he or she is responsible. The specialist's participation in assistive technology assessment is most effective as a member of the assessment team. Once an assistive technology plan is developed, the local resource person is valuable in helping to implement both the hard and soft technologies. This individual is also often involved in evaluating the success of the assistive technologies provided and in determining when reassessment is warranted.

Referral to an Evaluation Center. Referral to a center or clinic specializing in assistive technology applications has advantages and disadvantages. The center-based assessment teams may have a clinical orientation. This may make it more difficult for them to relate to the learner's specific needs unless they have experience with assessment and recommendation of assistive technology for children. However, a center of this type is more likely to have a broad knowledge of available assistive technologies for trial and loan, and their experience with a large group of clients provides a rich source of soft technologies such as strategies and approaches to training. It is important that a center-based assessment include the teacher and other school staff, as well as the learner and his family, in the evaluation process. The center-based assessment team needs to ensure that everyone's goals for the learner are identified. Typically assessments are carried out over several sessions, with some assessment taking place in the school (to focus on needs and the school environment) and some in the center (to allow access to a wide range of technology for trial and evaluation).

■ CONTEXT FOR EDUCATIONAL APPLICATIONS

The context portion of the HAAT model describes where the activity is being performed. Chapter 2 defined four types of context: physical, social, cultural, and institutional. Each of these plays an important role in the ultimate effectiveness or ineffectiveness of an assistive technology system. This section examines each type of context from an educational perspective.

Social and Cultural Contexts for Educational Use of Assistive Technology

Education for children who have disabilities used to be carried out in segregated, specially equipped classrooms set up to meet the unique needs of children with disabilities. Increasingly this specialized classroom is a thing of the past, except in cases of children with severe multiple disabilities. The current practice is **inclusion** of students with disabilities in the regular educational programs. Even when there is a specialized classroom, children are integrated into regular classes for at least part of the school day. Under this model, resource specialists often provide support services related to assistive technology devices and services. However, even if a resource specialist is available, the knowledge and skills of the general classroom teacher must be expanded to include special services and assistive technologies necessary to support learners who have disabilities. One of the implications of inclusion is that there are fewer concentrations of assistive technologies in specialized classrooms and greater diffusion of these technologies throughout the educational system. When there were concentrations of assistive technologies in special education classrooms, relatively few teachers needed to have expertise in their application. With the changing, more diffuse educational model, any teacher may have contact with assistive technologies. The school is now to be adapted to the student, rather than the student adapting to the school (Baker, 1993).

Baker (1993) expresses the concern that some school districts may view the full inclusion policy as a way to deny "expensive" special education support services (e.g., speech pathology, occupational therapy) to students who need them. There are additional benefits that are possible with full inclusion, such as nondisabled peer tutors, cooperative learning, and team teaching (Baker, 1993).

Beukelman and Mirenda (2005) conceptualize **academic participation** in the school environment as occurring at four levels. The first is *competitive,* in which the learner who has a disability has the same expectations as the nondisabled peer. The workload may be adjusted at this level, but the learner's academic progress is evaluated in the same way as it is for nondisabled peers. The second level is active participation, in which the workload is also adjusted and the evaluations based on individualized standards. At this level the academic expectations are less than for nondisabled peers. The third level is referred to as *involved.* At this level, academic expectations are minimal and inclusion occurs through alternative activities. Academic evaluation is based on individualized standards. At the fourth level there are no academic expectations and the student passively observes learning activities in the regular classroom. The role and nature of assistive technology devices and services vary across these four levels.

In considering the educational setting, it is also important to be aware of the **learner-teacher interactions** occurring in the classroom (Beigel, 2000). The way in which teachers present information can be an important factor when considering assistive technologies for the classroom. In settings that are primarily lecture based, note taking and writing take on greater importance. Teachers who place an emphasis on discussion value oral communication skills, and the assistive technology must support this type of interaction. **Learning styles** are also important. In settings in which small group interaction is the focus, oral communication and social interaction skills are more important. If the teacher uses group or individual projects, the learner must also organize materials, communicate with peers, and develop time management skills. All these factors influence the type and effectiveness of assistive technologies that are recommended.

In the context portion of the HAAT model, we use social and cultural contexts to describe important aspects of both interaction and acceptance of assistive technologies. These two contexts play important roles in the use of assistive technologies in an educational setting. Social and cultural factors also include local policies and attitudes toward technology and toward disability by school personnel. These factors can impose barriers to successful assistive technology application. For example, a policy that prevents school-purchased assistive technologies (e.g., AAC device or laptop computer) from being taken home will significantly compromise the opportunities the student has to complete homework and to apply developing communication skills in the community. Likewise, if a teacher has a negative attitude toward a blind student's use of a computer to complete tests, then the student may be less independent because of dependence on a sighted reader and scribe to complete the test.

The Participation Model developed by Beukelman and Mirenda (2005) (see Chapter 4) provides a useful framework for the identification of potential barriers to educational access, especially those that can be addressed through the application of assistive technologies. Two types of barriers are identified: opportunity and access. The first refers to policies, practices, attitudes, and knowledge and skills of the school personnel (e.g., teachers, aides, and administrators). Access barriers include the learner's natural abilities, the use of environmental adaptations (discussed under physical context later in this section), and the capabilities or limitations of the learner.

Beukelman and Mirenda (2005) describe an assessment process that leads to identification of the relevant barriers for a learner through a systematic consideration of opportunity and access barriers. Once the barriers are identified, an intervention plan can be developed to overcome the barriers. This plan may involve changing a policy or attitude, training staff, altering the environment, or matching the needs of the learner to assistive technology characteristics based on a capability assessment (see Chapter 4). Any specific situation will likely involve a combination of most or all of these.

Beukelman and Miranda (2005) also present a categorization of **social participation** that parallels the academic framework presented earlier. The same four levels are used, but the criteria are participation and social influence rather than academic performance. A student at the competitive social level participates in social interactions and influences nondisabled peers. At the level of active participation, the learner with a disability chooses whether to be involved in social contexts and does not directly influence the activities of the group. The student at the involved participation level also chooses whether to be involved in the social interaction, but participation may be passive. At the fourth level the learner is not involved in social activities with her nondisabled peers. Depending on the type of disability and the level of social participation, assistive technologies may facilitate social interaction.

CASE STUDY

OPPORTUNITY BARRIERS

Joan is an elementary student. She has severe cerebral palsy that affects all her limbs and has resulted in dysarthric speech. Her assessment has shown that she has receptive language at her age level, but she is unable to speak intelligibly or to write independently. During the assessment, an AAC device (see Chapter 11) was recommended. The school has agreed to purchase it if it is kept at school. The teacher has indicated that she will work with Joan to learn to use it, but she does not have time to learn the device given the demands of the other 25 students in the classroom. The device has been purchased, but it is not being used by Joan because she has not been given the necessary training at school and she cannot take the device home to practice because the school is concerned that this expensive ($8000) device might be broken or lost.

QUESTIONS

1. Identify the barriers in this case.
2. Which of these are opportunity and which are access barriers?
3. What steps would you, as the ATP, take to try and remove the barriers so that Joan can gain access to the learning environment using this device?
4. What additional information would you require to carry out your plan?

Another important factor in the cultural context is how willing the learner is to try new activities or tasks. This concept refers to the learner's personal style (Beigel, 2000). Individual learners and their families and teachers vary widely in their willingness and ability to cope with change and uncertainty. The use of assistive technologies can be intimidating, especially when there is insufficient training and opportunity to develop the necessary skills through practice. The socioeconomic status of the learner and his family also has an impact on the effectiveness of recommended assistive technologies and their ability to affect the learner's educational experience (Beigel, 2000). Although there are no specific research findings in this area, it is known that the socioeconomic status of a learner has an impact on how teachers view the learner and how the educational program is presented. Learners with low socioeconomic status often have an educational program that focuses on rote learning rather than higher-level cognitive skills (Beigel, 2000). This bias can lead to difficulties when assistive technologies are introduced into the classroom, especially if they require practice and advanced level skills for operation.

Physical Context for Educational Use of Assistive Technology

In an educational setting the physical context for assistive technology use includes a number of factors. Some of these are specific to the physical arrangement and layout of the classroom itself, including the type of furnishings and their locations, physical dimensions of doors, and absence of barriers. Another aspect of the physical context applies to the learner. Appropriate postural support (see Chapter 6) allows positioning of the child in a way that allows the child to attend to classroom activities. In addition to providing safety and comfort, proper positioning promotes independence and allows the child to function efficiently to manipulate objects and activate switches or other technical equipment. A recommended sitting posture is shown in Figure 15-6 (see Chapter 6 also). In this position the feet are supported on the floor or the footrest of the wheelchair; the hips are flexed to approximately 90 degrees. The chair and seat provide adequate thigh support, back support, and lateral support. The ideal classroom work surface is 1 inch below the learner's bent elbow, with the most frequently accessed items within reach. If the learner uses a computer, the monitor should be located approximately at arm's length away from the face. The top of the monitor should be at or just below eye level and perpendicular to the light source. If there is a document holder, it should be positioned next to the monitor. For students with severe physical disabilities, learning may take place in other positions, such as side lying or in a stander. These positions may change throughout the day.

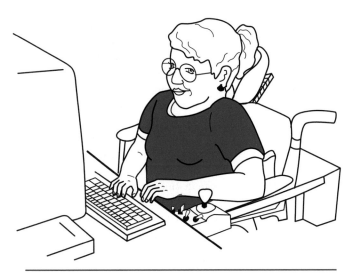

Figure 15-6 A proper sitting posture can promote independence and allow the child to function efficiently in the manipulation of objects or the activation of switches. (Courtesy www.Lburkhart.com.)

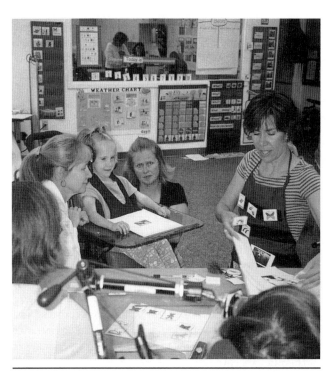

Figure 15-7 This classroom arrangement gives all learners access to the classroom activities. The student with a disability is integrated into the classroom environment.

The physical environment also includes considerations related to the placement of the learner in relation to the teacher, to the other learners, to her equipment, and to the activity. Ideally the learner with a disability will be integrated into the classroom environment, as shown in Figure 15-7. To provide access to furnishings and materials, it may be necessary to make room modifications that enhance learning opportunities by creating accessible classrooms. For example, it may be necessary to modify or rearrange a classroom to allow space for mobility devices (e.g., wheelchairs and walkers; see Chapter 12) by increasing the width of aisles or the space between desks. Table heights for wheelchair access are also different than for learners who use standard chairs, especially for younger children. A device such as an AAC system (see Chapter 11) mounted to the wheelchair may require even greater clearance, in addition to special considerations for transferring the child to ensure that the chair does not tip as a result of the weight of the mounted device.

For learners who are hard of hearing, FM antenna systems (see Chapter 9) may need to be installed. If automatic speech recognition (see Chapter 7) is used, the learner needs to be located in a place that does not disturb the other students. If the learner uses a computer workstation for completion of assignments, it needs to be located in the classroom, not a separate computer room, and it needs to be located with the other students, not off in a corner of the room. If a printer is used for completing computer-generated assignments, it must be located to reduce disturbance of other students as a result of noise.

Lighting is also important when students are using assistive devices in the classroom. If a room is too bright, glare may prevent the reading of computer screens or liquid crystal display (LCD) screens on laptop computers or AAC

devices (Church and Glennen, 1991). Antireflective screens can be used when it is not possible to reduce sunlight or natural lighting sufficiently to avoid glare. On the other hand, individuals who have low vision may require special lighting to increase contrast (see Chapter 8). These modifications can enhance participation in class by learners who have physical or sensory disabilities. When modifications such as these are made, it can also encourage learners to participate in activities that involve groups of learners working together.

Important considerations when evaluating the physical context of the classroom include the following questions: (1) Is the student with the other children or physically isolated by his equipment, technology, or other factors? (2) What information or technology is needed to make the learning environment more accessible to the student? (3) How can the student participate? (4) Who can assist in the learning? (5) Can the student safely and easily enter and exit the classroom, school, and other necessary rooms? (6) Is there a clear passage of travel? and (7) Are multimodal signs used for children with sensory impairments?

HARD AND SOFT TECHNOLOGIES FOR EDUCATIONAL SUCCESS

The fourth component of the HAAT model is hard and soft assistive technologies. Many characteristics of assistive technologies were discussed in Chapters 1 and 2. When a unique environment such as education is being considered, some of these are more important than others. This section discusses the major characteristics of assistive technologies that can help ensure their successful application in an education setting.

Technological Description of the Modern Classroom

Assistive technology applications in the classroom include both hard and soft technologies (see Chapter 1) (Odor, 1984). Practitioners generally agree that success of assistive technologies depends on a ratio of 10 to 1 (soft to hard technologies). Funds allocated by schools are likely to be earmarked for hard rather than soft technologies (Blackstone, 1990). When assistive technologies (both hard and soft) were concentrated in a few classrooms with resident experts, development of soft technologies was easier. With diffusion of services throughout the curriculum, this process has become much more challenging. Of particular importance are the implications for how assistive technology training is carried out. Assistive technology service delivery in the classroom setting must address both hard and soft technologies.

Blackstone (1990) describes areas in which assistive technologies are being used in the classroom (Table 15-2). These include (1) positioning (e.g., seating inserts, side-lying frames), (2) access to electronic assistive devices (e.g., computers, communication devices), (3) environmental control, (4) augmentative communication (writing, speaking, drawing, mathematics), (5) assistive listening devices (e.g., hearing aids, FM systems, teletypes [TTYs]), (6) visual aids (for both print and computer-based text materials), (7) mobility aids, (8) recreation and leisure activities (e.g., hobbies, free time), and (9) self-care (e.g., feeders, aids for hygiene). Blackstone gives examples of equipment and specific classroom considerations for each of these areas. The hard and soft technologies in each area are described in earlier chapters.

Considerations in the Use of Assistive Technologies in the Classroom

Chapter 4 discusses general characteristics of assistive technologies. When assistive technology use is considered in education, some of these characteristics are more important than others. Beigel (2000) lists a series of questions to be asked when considering assistive technologies for educational application. Among the areas he discusses are durability; portability; availability of a trial or loan period; company reputation; and aesthetic acceptability to the learner, family, and teacher. Classrooms are active environments in which a device may be subjected to drops, bumps, spills, and other "insults." Durability in this environment is a high priority;

this property can affect a decision between a specially designed assistive device and the use of a commercially available device such as a laptop computer. Learners move from place to place in the classroom and from classroom to classroom. A device that is not portable severely restricts the benefits to the learner in accessing the standard curriculum. Assistive technologies may be complex devices that require skill to operate and place unique demands on the learner and her environment. It is difficult to assess the impact of these devices in a brief assessment. A long-term (a few weeks to a month) trial of devices can disclose features that make them unsuitable. Utility of the device should be determined before committing funds for purchase if at all possible. There are many companies that supply assistive technologies. Some have been in business for many years and provide high-quality support and service. Others do not. An experienced ATP knows which companies can be trusted to provide the necessary support and follow-up and how well repair and service are handled. Although our focus must be on functionality, it is also important to consider the aesthetics of assistive technologies. Motivation to use an assistive technology can be greatly affected by such things as color, overall pleasant design, size, and weight. As Beigel (2000) points out, one learner may prefer a mouse with a colored ball but another might prefer the traditional mouse. The color of the wheelchair frame can be of great importance to the child and affect his or her self-image in the classroom. Devices that are well designed do not call as much attention to the user and do not seem to be so "different" from what other learners are using.

Merbler, Hadadian, and Ulman (1999) present another set of recommendations that apply to assistive technologies use in the classroom. They recommend that, whenever possible, open-ended devices (i.e., those that can be customized through software) that can be customized be used, which allows changes to be made to the device (e.g., in software or vocabulary) as the needs of the learner and her academic program change. They also recommend minimal technology solutions (see Chapter 1) that can meet the functional need with the least complexity, which can make acceptance more likely and will significantly affect the amount of training required.

Student Workstations

Much of the technology on Blackstone's list is computer based, and she uses the term **student workstation** or life station to describe these computer-based setups. The workstation may provide specialized assistance with writing and conversation; an adapted access method for the classroom computer (for software that everyone else is using); access for wheelchair users (manual or power); and possible integration of controls for power wheelchair, computer, environmental control, and augmentative communication device (Caves et al, 1991; Guerette, Caves, and Gross, 1992).

TABLE 15-2	Hard Technologies for Education		
Application	Goals	Equipment Examples	Classroom Considerations
Assistive listening devices (ALDs)	Appropriate signal-to-noise ratio so student's hearing is accessible	Hearing aids, personal FM systems, sound field FM systems, TTYs, closed-caption TV (see Chapter 9)	Hearing is a core activity leading to instructional access and learning. Signals deteriorate beyond 6 inches from the source; ALDs should be considered. Background noise can limit high pitch sound detection.
AAC	Independent means of expression	Symbols, communication displays, devices, word processing, fax (see Chapter 11)	Intervention begins early. Set up class for communication. Use digital recording for circle time, other sharing, communication displays located near activity areas. Integrate AAC devices into learning routine.
Access to computers and other electronic technologies	Enhancement of speed, accuracy, endurance, and independence in device use	Input device, head pointers, key guards, automatic speech recognition, input device-emulating interfaces, Internet access (see Chapter 7)	Access technologies are key to effective use of electronic devices. Optimal use requires consideration of best control sites, selection technique (direct or indirect), and acceleration approaches.
Environmental control	Positive control of the environment without assistance from aides	EADLs, robotics, appliance control adaptations, switch-controlled toys (see Chapter 14)	May be introduced in early infant programs. Appliance control can be incorporated into learning activities. EADLs can help develop sense of control and independence.
Mobility	Independent movement, exploration, social interaction, and learning	Self-propelled walkers and wheelchairs, power wheelchairs, tricycles, and scooters (see Chapter 12)	Children move with intention at 4-5 months. Mobility aids can enhance socialization, communication, and environmental control. Independent mobility leads to increased interaction with peers.
Positioning	Increased function and participation through stable and comfortable positioning	Side-lying frames, floor sitters, chair inserts, trays, standing aids, bean bag chairs, etc. (see Chapter 6)	Positioning includes child's individual posture and position relative to other learners and teacher. Multiple positioning systems are often used at different times during the day and for different activities.
Recreation, leisure, play	Access to materials and activities allowing peer interaction, hobby development, effective use of free time	Outdoor adaptations (slides, swings), computer games, board games, adapted play materials (e.g., Velcro on toys)	Listening and viewing activities include music and taped reading, slide/ tape, and computer-based stories. Group games include music (adapted instruments, MIDI), art and craft projects with adaptations, dramatic play, adapted puzzles.
Self-care	Independent self-care activities	Electric feeders, adapted utensils, toilet seats, aids for tooth brushing, washing, dressing, food preparation (see Chapter 14)	Incorporate self-care activities and adaptations as they naturally occur in activities of feeding, dressing (coats, shoes), toileting, meal preparation.
Visual access	Enhancement or interpretation of visual information	Screen readers, screen magnifiers, braillers, high-contrast materials, thermoform graphics (see Chapter 8)	Vision is a major learning mode. Increase contrast, enlarge stimuli, and use tactile and auditory modes to enhance sensory information content. Develop screen reader and Internet navigation skills early.

Modified from Blackstone SW: Assistive technology in the classroom, *Augment Commun News* 3:1-8, 1990.

In general, productivity software (word processing, database, drawing, plotting, math) is included in student workstations. For students with oral communication or visual access needs, voice synthesizers may be added. If the student is not independently mobile, a manual or power wheelchair may be included and the workstation may be integrated into the wheelchair system for portability. In cases in which the student is ambulatory, portability can be more of a challenge because the workstation must be carried or pushed from classroom to classroom. Blackstone describes a logical and systematic process for developing individualized workstations on the basis of student needs.

Additional software commonly included in workstations includes programs for skill acquisition in the specific activity areas described earlier in this chapter (reading, writing, mathematics, science, music, and art). Software for desktop publishing (e.g., for a school newspaper, flyers, posters) and digital scanning is often also included (Merbler, Hadadian, and Ulman, 1999). The scanner can be very useful in the classroom. Worksheets can be scanned and then filled in using a computer workstation. Materials to be read can also be scanned and read back by using the computer to enlarge print, convert to alternative form (e.g., braille or speech), or make turning pages easier, as noted earlier. This technology can be beneficial to learners who have sensory, learning, or physical disabilities. Scanners can also be used for other creative projects such as class newsletters, special customized awards with a picture of a student in the background, and similar activities using optical images (Merbler, Hadadian, and Ulman, 1999).

In developing workstations it is important to consider the concept of **functional equivalency.** This concept refers to the idea that multiple ways of achieving a particular task or outcome are possible. For example, if a student has difficulty turning the pages on a book, a mechanical page turner (see Chapter 14) can be used. Alternatively, books available on computer disk can be loaded into a word processor and the pages can be "turned" electronically. Thus the same function is obtained in very different ways.

Internet-Based Educational Resources

Many schools (some estimates are as high as 90%) have Internet access in the classroom. The Internet provides a rich and exciting resource for learners to do research for class projects, use Web-based instructional materials, and develop effective information search skills. If appropriate consideration is given to accessibility of Web sites (see Chapter 8) and principles of universal design are incorporated (see Chapter 1), the success of Web-based instruction for all learners is enhanced (Romereim-Holmes and Peterson, 2000). Learners who use alternative methods of accessing the Internet must be accommodated in the instructional process when Web-based instruction is used. The principles described in Chapter 8 apply to education as well as to other environments. The use of Web-based instruction and the development of Web content by learners will increase as more and more schools are on-line and teachers develop instructional design principles that incorporate the use of the Internet. Adherence to the principles of accessibility and consideration of universal design during the curriculum process will greatly expand the opportunities for learners who have disabilities.

Soft Technologies in the Classroom

There are two broad types of soft technologies (see Chapter 1) that have applications in education: training and strategies.

Training in an Educational Context. Training activities in assistive technologies for school personnel may be of two general types: (1) broad-based group or (2) individual study and training that apply to a number of learners or focused training that provides information regarding the use of an assistive technology system for a specific learner (Church and Glennen, 1991). Carefully developed strategies allow the learner to maximize the effectiveness of his assistive technology.

Chapter 1 describes a number of approaches to in-service education. Many of these apply to educational staff (teacher, aide, therapist, SLP). Conferences, journal articles, Internet sources, and on-site in-service presentations by ATPs or specialist teams are the major formats. Church and Glennen (1991) list a number of in-service topics presented in one school district. Shown in Box 15-1, these are examples of the types of presentations that are of interest to school staff.

The second type of training is individualized to meet the needs of the learner, parents and family, and those staff who will be working with the learner and the assistive technology system. Earlier chapters described the nature of this training for specific technologies (e.g., AAC in Chapter 11). It is crucial that the training received by school staff be aimed at how the technology will achieve the goals set for the learner, rather than just focusing on the technical aspects of the device (Todis and Walker, 1993). In an educational setting it is also important that those who will work with the student are familiar with operation of the technology, how to troubleshoot the device in the case of operational difficulties, and specific features for individual technologies (Church and Glennen, 1991). In the latter category are such things as vocabulary selection for educational use of AAC, training in the use of specific educational software, and training related to skill development in such areas as powered mobility.

BOX 15-1   Example of In-Service Topics in Assistive Technologies

Overview of augmentative communication
Low-tech AAC aids and techniques
Make-and-take session for low-tech AAC displays
Overview of high-tech AAC aids
Vocabulary selection for AAC
Overview of assistive technology in the classroom
Using assistive technology to make the classroom accessible
Computer adaptations for students with physical disabilities
Software selection and integration to facilitate educational activities
Word processing for students with disabilities
Technology applications for young children

Modified from Church G, Glennen S: *The handbook of assistive technology,* San Diego, 1991, Singular Publishing Group.

In education, peers also need to be trained. **Peer training** introduces the new technology to the classmates of the target learner. It also can be an opportunity to answer questions that peers have regarding the disability and the technology. Another goal of this training is to establish the rules governing the use of the technology (Church and Glennen, 1991). School staff and the family of the learner may decide to implement a "hands-off" policy for other students so as to avoid damage to the assistive technology. As Church and Glennen (1991) point out, this policy can make the device more enticing and arouse the curiosity of the peers regarding how it works. For this reason, some families and teachers allow classmates to experience the device during the familiarization phase of training.

Church and Glennen (1991) suggest that the student who will be using the assistive technology be part of the in-class training session in which her technology is introduced to the rest of the class. This peer training session is also an opportunity for a presentation on how the peers can appropriately help the student who will be using the assistive technology. This is a chance to emphasize the need for the learner to be independent and to not have things done for him or her by classmates, as well as to introduce the new technology. Rules can also be established regarding the new device and how much access the learner and the family want to give the peers. In all cases the student must have control over the new technology, which includes being able to decide who can try it out (if anyone) and when they can do so.

Strategies for the Use of Assistive Technologies in the Classroom.

Educational strategies are really techniques that increase the effectiveness of assistive technologies in the classroom. There is no specific formula for their development. Rather, they arise from a thorough understanding of the educational goals and the skills of the learner. Most often strategies are based on innovative ideas generated from careful observation, experience, and consultation with other team members. This section describes several examples of specific strategies to illustrate how many different learning strategies can be used to meet the same educational goals. Some specific approaches to the generation of strategies are also presented.

One systematic approach is the **Technology Integration Plan** (Church and Glennen, 1991). The development of this plan begins with a team meeting in which an analysis of the student's daily schedule is carried out. Emphasis is placed on the identification of target activities for technology intervention. Church and Glennen suggest that activities meeting the following criteria be chosen (1991, p. 217):

1. They occur frequently
2. They are motivating and enjoyable
3. They present opportunities for independence in one of several areas (verbal or written communication, mobility, self-care, vocational skills, control of the environment)

4. They are activities that the student cannot effectively complete utilizing their current modes or methods

There are three parts to the Technology Integration Plan: (1) preparation (Figure 15-8, *A*), (2) action plan (Figure 15-8, *B*), and (3) review (Figure 15-8, *C*) (Church and Glennen, 1991). The preparation form is designed as a framework to record the information developed by the discussion of target activities. A three-point rating scale is used to indicate the relative level (high, moderate, or low) for each activity in several areas (see Figure 15-8, *A*). The action plan (see Figure 15-8, *B*) is then completed for each identified activity. The action plan is a framework for recording target skills and objectives for each activity. It is also used to identify suggested materials, equipment, motivators, and strategies for each activity. In addition, the required preparation and the projected date for a review are included on this form. The final form, review (see Figure 15-8, *C*), is used to record any modifications to the plan and to record progress in meeting the goals set out in the plan. An organized format such as the Technology Intervention Plan can help a team to focus on the educational goals first, developing strategies for implementing both the hard and soft technologies required to meet the goals and then monitoring progress. Church and Glennen (1991) present two examples of the use of this approach.

Strategies to help a student accomplish learning tasks are often best developed by a team of professionals. Brainstorming and planning from several different points of view can lead to innovation as one idea triggers others. Merbler, Hadadian, and Ulman (1999) recommend that teachers share information regarding assistive technology application. With the myriad devices and strategies available, it is impossible for any one teacher to monitor them all, and sharing expertise can benefit all learners. Collaboration with parents can also ensure that assistive technology devices that go home are properly used and maintained. With the complexity of some current assistive devices, the teacher may place unreasonable demands on himself or herself to completely master a device or software program before using it. This knowledge is often not necessary, and many applications can be successfully accomplished with the device as skill is developed. Merbler, Hadadian, and Ulman also encourage teachers to experiment with the technology. This may lead to the discovery of new applications or strategies.

Even if you do not have a team locally, you can collaborate by using various on-line listservs. One that is often used is the RESNA assistive technology listserv (e-mail address: *resna@maelstrom.stjohns.edu*). As discussed earlier in this chapter, manipulatives (objects that can be counted, moved, and sorted) are often used in mathematics instruction. When a child lacks the fine motor skills to manipulate the objects, alternatives are required to access the same curriculum as classmates. Here is an example of an on-line

Student: Date:
Team Members:

<u>Typical daily schedule</u>

Directions: List all daily activities and rate each one for the listed characteristics using the following scale: 3 - high 2 - moderate 1 - low. Total the ratings for each activity and record the number in the Total column. Place a check in last column when the activity is included in the student's Technology Integration Plan.

A

Daily Activities	Current Mode(s) of _____	Motivation	Opportunities for Independence	Present Mode(s) Ineffective	Total	Included in Plan
Other routine events (at least once per week)						

Student's Name: Date:
Team Members:

Target activity:

Target skills (objectives):

Suggested equipment:

Target vocabulary to be represented by ___ Photos ___ Symbols ___ Words/Sentences
Suggested materials/motivators:

B

Preparation needed	Person(s) responsible	Target date

Suggested strategies:

Anticipated date of review:

Target activity: Date of initial Action Plan
Team Members revising Plan:

C

Date of review	Modifications	Person responsible	Initiation date	Review date

Figure 15-8   The Technology Integration Plan. **A,** Preparation sheet. **B,** Action plan. **C,** Review. (From Church G, Glennen S: *The handbook of* *assistive technology,* San Diego, 1991, Singular Publishing Group.)

"virtual collaboration" involving the use of manipulatives (paraphrased):

One subscriber to the listserv (Y. T., a rehabilitation engineer from New York City) posted the following question:

> I'm working with a child with CP [cerebral palsy] in the 3rd grade. He can grasp and manipulate objects with his left hand, but he has extensor tone that makes it difficult to lean or reach forward, or bring his arm across his body. His right side is more involved and he doesn't use it much. I'm looking for ideas to assist him in using manipulatives in his math class. He has a desk that allows him to pull up close, and he can be placed on a slant. I'm going to give him a tray table to elevate the surface even more so he doesn't have to reach down. When using manipulatives, the students often have to organize counters into groups and arrange objects on their desk. I was thinking possibly little containers to help with that. Does anyone have any other suggestions?

K. P., an OT in Massachusetts, offered these suggestions:

> Use muffin tins of various sizes, paint palette trays, etc., which are easier to scoop from. More important, though, is whether his seating needs have been adequately addressed to maximize dynamic trunk balance and provide as much normalization of tone as possible.

R. G., a rehabilitation technologist in San Francisco, added his thoughts:

> I would encourage all involved to step back and look at the educational goals of the activity. Perhaps they can be achieved without using the same objects that are typically used (though he might be strongly motivated to use the same tools as all the other students). The example that comes to mind is the abacus that can help people learn math without requiring a lot of range of motion—though some fine motor ability is needed. Otherwise, plastic organizers for silverware drawers or pencil drawer organizers are two readily obtainable items. Use small containers velcroed to a flat board that can be rearranged as desired. Try putting the containers on a lazy Susan to provide access to more items without reaching.

C. C., an SLP from Nebraska, contributed other ideas:

> There are often easier physical methods to accomplish the educational tasks involved in the manipulatives. Manipulatives tend to be used educationally for two or three reasons: they make abstract concepts concrete, they help students make active problem solving decisions, and they are easy to manage for typically developing students. Because the latter is not true for this child, we don't want him to be spending all of his educational time managing the mechanics of the task and missing the educational point.
>
> I've seen this work well by students pairing together. The student with a disability makes decisions about which items go into which groups, and gets to control the physical division

of the items by strategies like eye pointing or binary choice making [see Chapter 11] with a peer (i.e., which group?). The peer does the physical manipulation according to the student's direction, and by third grade most peers can be coached in strategies for getting the student's input without being directive. This embeds a communication strategy that is both more accessible and interactive for the student, as well as probably already established in other ways.

This example illustrates several points about strategies. First, there are many strategies for any one problem in the classroom. Often the possible strategies are very different. Our virtual team suggests a variety of approaches from making the manipulatives easier to reach and grab to using a peer partner to help with the task. Second, alternative strategies often involve different skills on the part of the student. In this example, the skills range from gross motor to fine motor to communication. The third general point is that strategies may or may not involve technology, and the technology may be high or low, depending on the strategy. In this example, low technologies such as muffin tins and a lazy Susan are suggested by two of the professionals. The third suggests communication, and this intervention/strategy might be no-tech (i.e., speech) or a high-tech augmentative communication device. This example also illustrates the role of innovation and problem solving in the development of useful strategies.

A frequent concern of teachers and classroom aides is that there is not time to add assistive technology use to an already crowded day with many students in the classroom. The time demands of the classroom are high, and this is a legitimate concern; however, it is possible to use strategies for infusing technology into the classroom throughout the day (King-DeBaun, 1999). King-DeBaun suggests integrating assistive technologies into regular classroom activities throughout the day. One example described by King-DeBaun (1999) is Danny, an 8-year-old boy who attends a typical first grade classroom for 75% of his school day and spends 25% of his day in a resource room. Danny uses an AAC device and receives instruction and support from his regular education teacher and part-time classroom aide as well as the resource room teacher and his SLP. Danny's day begins with story group, and for the class discussion, he uses the IntelliKeys keyboard (see Chapter 7) with an overlay containing simple words related to the story. His SLP made the overlay by using a computer program called Overlay Maker. By use of a talking word processor, Danny is able to participate in the story group discussion. Students also participate in journal writing as an arrival activity. They record the day of the week, school activities, and special events at home or school. Danny uses his augmentative communication device to complete this task, making use of a posted "word wall" (an alphabetical list of words he uses frequently). Later in the day, Danny and his classmates create a story adventure based on a starting line from the teacher (e.g., "One day…"). The teacher bases the story on a familiar theme or a story that the children have often read. Students take turns participating in this activity, and each day one student is selected to help write a part of the class story. Once again Danny uses his augmentative communication device, but this time his aide has prepared a list of words related to the topic of the recent books the class has read, and she has stored them into his device so he can access them to participate in this activity.

King-DeBaun (1999) also describes another student, Anita, who is just learning how to scan (see Chapter 7). She uses her communication device in a circular scanning mode (see Chapter 7) to randomly select a student to be next. This places Anita at the center of attention as the class waits to see whom she will choose. In Dramatics, Danny and Amanda work together to use a drawing program on the computer to create masks for a talking mural. She creates a bird mask and he makes a lizard mask. They work together, with Danny picking a color and Amanda placing the cursor on that color. Amanda cuts out the mask for Danny and places both masks on the mural. For the presentation to the class the following day, Danny uses his augmentative communication device to speak his lines. Musselwhite and King-DeBaun (1997) describe many other activities and adaptations that can be used in the classroom.

There are many sessions at assistive technology conferences that include strategies for introducing and using assistive technologies successfully in the classroom. These are rich with new strategies. Several of the conferences have on-line proceedings. All have other resources available on their Web sites. Three of the most useful conferences are

the California State University at Northridge Conference (held in March in Los Angeles; *www.csun.edu/cod/*); Closing the Gap (held in October in Minneapolis; www.closingthegap.com); and RESNA (June, various locations; www.resna.org).

As the examples in this section illustrate, the most important factors in the development of assistive technology strategies are detailed familiarity with the educational task to be completed and innovative thinking. There are no basic principles or magic formulas.

■ SUMMARY

This chapter describes the educational application of assistive technologies using the HAAT model as a framework. Learners who have disabilities engage in reading, writing, mathematics, science, music, and art. The primary types of adaptations available in each of these areas involve both strategies and technologies. Several assessment models are used to determine the needs of learners for assistive technologies. Considerations in the cultural and social contexts include learner style, socioeconomic status, and other factors that can dramatically affect assistive technology effectiveness in the classroom. The emergence of inclusive settings in education has affected the way in which assistive technologies are applied and supported. The physical location of the learner in relation to other students and the layout of the classroom in general can affect the success of assistive technologies. Many characteristics of hard and soft assistive technologies are important in ensuring that they are meeting the needs of learners and teachers.

Study Questions

1. What are the major curricular areas (educational activities) in which assistive technologies are used?
2. What tasks must be accommodated for to ensure success in reading instruction?
3. Describe some of the differences between an assistive technology–based writing system and scribing.
4. How can an AAC system be used in mathematics instruction?
5. What are the two primary requirements in making adaptations for alternatives to pencil-and-paper mathematics instruction?
6. How can the concept of manipulatives be included in the mathematics curriculum for learners who lack the fine motor skill to work with physical objects directly?
7. What unique requirements do science, art, and music each place on the educational setting for assistive technologies?

8. List three factors that are essential to an effective assistive technology assessment to meet educational needs.
9. What steps are necessary to ensure that an assistive technology assessment focuses on the needs of the learner rather than the technologies to be used in meeting those needs?
10. How are assistive technologies to meet educational needs incorporated into the IEP?
11. Who are the typical members of an educational assistive technology assessment team?
12. What are the primary models for educational assistive technology assessment, and what are the pros and cons of each?
13. What are the advantages of carrying out an educational assistive technology assessment in the school, family, and community environments?

14. What are the unique contributions that the ATP makes to an educational assistive technology assessment?
15. What are the advantages of an educational assistive technology assessment carried out in a center specializing in assistive technology evaluation and recommendation?
16. What are the implications for assistive technology application presented by an inclusive classroom?
17. What are the levels of academic and social participation defined by Beukelman and Mirenda (2005)?
18. List four aspects of the learner-teacher interaction that are important to the recommendation of assistive technologies for classroom use.
19. What are the major considerations in the social and cultural contexts as applied to assistive technologies use in education?
20. What social factors may affect the use of assistive technology in the classroom?
21. What cultural factors may affect the use of assistive technology in the classroom?

22. How does learning style affect the success of assistive technologies in the classroom?
23. List four factors that affect the physical context for the learner.
24. List the components that make up a student workstation.
25. What are the most important soft technology concerns in the educational setting?
26. What are the two major types of assistive technology training normally provided for school personnel? How do they differ?
27. What are the goals of peer training, and how can the learner who uses the technology be included in this training?
28. What are the most important assistive technology characteristics when considering devices for classroom use?

References

Baker LA: Educational challenges-strategies for the AAC student, *Commun Outlook* 13-16, Spring 1993.

Beigel AR: Assistive technology assessment: more than the device, *Interven School Clin* 45:237-244, 2000.

Beukelman DR, Mirenda P: *Augmentative and alternative communication, management of severe communication disorders in children and adults*, ed 3, Baltimore, 2005, Paul H Brookes.

Bodine C, Melonics M: Teaming and assistive technology in educational settings. In Edyburn D, Higgins K, Boone R, editors: *Handbook of special education technology research and practice*, Whitefish Bay, WI, 2005, Knowledge by Design, Inc..

Blackstone SW: Assistive technology in the classroom, *Augment Commun News* 3:1-8, 1990.

Brainerd CJ: *Piaget's theory of cognitive development*, Englewood Cliffs, NJ, 1978, Prentice-Hall.

Brodin J: Facsimile transmission for graphic symbol users, *Eur Rehabil* 2:87-92, 1992.

Butler C: Effects of powered mobility on self-initiated behaviors of very young children with locomotor disability, *Dev Med Child Neurol* 28:325-332, 1986.

Button C: Fast facts on individualized education programs, *AT Q RESNA* 2:5-6, 1990.

Calkins LM: *The art of teaching*, Portsmouth, NH, 1986, Heinemann.

Caves K et al: The use of integrated controls for mobility, communication and computer access. In *Proceedings of the 14th RESNA Conference*, pp 166-167, 1991, Washington, DC, The Conference.

Church G, Glennen S: *The handbook of assistive technology*, San Diego, 1991, Singular Publishing Group.

Desch LW: High technology for handicapped children: a pediatrician's viewpoint, *Pediatrics* 77:71-87, 1986.

Edyburn DL: Rethinking assistive technology, *Spec Educ Technol Pract* 5:16-23, 2003a.

Edyburn DL: Learning from text, *Spec Educ Technol Pract* 5: 16-27, 2003b.

Edyburn D: Measuring assistive technology outcomes in writing, *J Spec Educ Technol* 18:60-64, 2003c.

Edyburn D: Measuring assistive technology outcomes in mathematics, *J Spec Educ Technol* 18:76-79, 2003d.

Edyburn D: Measuring assistive technology outcomes in reading, *J Spec Educ Technol* 19:60-64, 2004.

Edyburn D, Higgins K, Boone R, editors: *Handbook of special education technology research and practice*, Whitefish Bay, 2005, Wisconsin: Knowledge by Design, Inc.

Guerette P, Caves K, Gross K: One switch does it all, *Team Rehabil Rep* 26-29, 1992.

Jeffs T, Behrman M, Bannan-Ritland B: Assistive technology and literacy learning: reflections of parents and children, *J Spec Educ Technol* 21:37-43, 2006.

King-DeBaun P: Technology all day long: infusing technology into the curriculum: *Proceedings of the CSUN Conference 1999:* www.dinf.org/csun_99/session1008.html. Accessed December 1999.

Light J, Smith AK: Home literacy experience of preschoolers who use AAC systems and their nondisabled peers, *Augment Altern Commun* 9:10-25, 1993.

Light J, Kent-Walsh J: Fostering emergent literacy for children who require AAC, *ASHA Leader* 8: 4-5, 28-29, 2003.

Maccini P, Gagnon JC: Mathematics and technology-based interventions.I In Edyburn D, Higgins K, Boone R, editors: *Handbook of special education technology research and practice,* Whitefish Bay, WI, 2005, Knowledge by Design, Inc.

Merbler JB, Hadadian A, Ulman J: Using assistive technology in the inclusive classroom, *Prevent School Fail* 43:113-118, 1999.

Musselwhite C, King-DeBaun P: *Emergent literacy success: merging technology and whole language for students with disabilities,* Park City, UT, 1997, Creative Communicating Resources.

Odor P: Hard and soft technology for education and communication for disabled people. In *Proceedings of the International Computer Conference,* Perth, Australia, 1984.

Resnick M et al: Digital manipulatives: new toys to think with: *Proceedings of the CHI Conference,* Los Angeles, Calif, April 12-23, 1998: http://www.acm.org/sigchi/chi98/cp/?show252. Accessed December 1999.

Rocklage LA, Lake ME: Inclusion through infusion, *Proceedings of the Closing the Gap Conference,* 1997: http://www.closingthegap.com/cgi-bin/lib/libDsply.pl?a1049&b3&c1. Accessed December 1999.

Romereim-Holmes L, Peterson D: Instructionally sound web-based learning for diverse populations, *Proceedings of the CSUN Conf,* 2000: http://www.csun.edu/cod/conf2000/proceedings/0032Romereim.html. Accessed December 1999.

Schaff JI et al: Science in special education: emerging technologies. In Edyburn D, Higgins K, Boone R, editors: *Handbook of special education technology research and practice,* pp. 643-661, Whitefish Bay, WI, 2005, Knowledge by Design, Inc.

Smith AK et al: The form and use of written communication produced by physically disabled individuals using microcomputers, *Augment Altern Commun* 5:115-124, 1989.

Smith J, Topping M: The introduction of a robotic aid to drawing into a school for physically handicapped children: a case study, *Br J Occup Ther* 59:565-569, 1996.

Strangeman N, Dalton B: Using technology to support struggling readers: a review of the research. In Edyburn D, Higgins K, Boone R, editors: *Handbook of special education technology research and practice,* pp. 545-569, Whitefish Bay, WI, 2005, Knowledge by Design, Inc.

Sturm JM, Erickson K, Yoder DE: Enhancing literacy development through AAC technologies, *Assist Technol* 14:71-80, 2002.

Todis B, Walker HM: User perspectives on assistive technology in educational settings, *Focus Except Child* 26:1-16, 1993.

Topping M: The Handy 1, a robotic aid to independence for severely disabled people, *Technol Disabil* 5:233-234, 1996.

Vanderheiden GC, Lloyd LL: Communication systems and their components. In Blackstone S, Bruskin D, editors *Augmentative communication: an introduction,* Rockville, MD, 1986, American Speech-Language and Hearing Association.

Zabala JS: SETTing the stage for success: building success through effective use of assistive technology. In *Proceedings of the Southeast Augmentative Communication Conference,* pp. 129-187, Birmingham, AL, 1996, United Cerebral Palsy of Greater Birmingham.

Assistive Technologies in the Context of Work

Learning Objectives

On completing this chapter, you will be able to do the following:

1. Describe the vocational activities and related skills that can be aided by assistive technologies
2. Describe the influence of the physical, social, cultural, and institutional contexts on the use of assistive technologies in the workplace
3. Understand the role of the assistive technology practitioner in addressing the vocational goals of the person with a disability
4. Understand the unique attributes of the assessment and implementation of assistive technologies in the vocational setting
5. List the major assistive technologies that are used in vocational settings
6. Describe strategies for implementing assistive technologies in the workplace
7. Identify outcome measures that are useful to evaluate the outcome of assistive technology intervention in the workplace

Work is one of three basic performance areas (self-care, work and school, play and leisure) in which many individuals participate on a daily basis. As with the other performance areas, people with disabilities are confronted with barriers that make it difficult for them to participate in this important life role. Modifications to the work site and the provision of assistive technologies can help to eliminate some of these barriers and enable individuals with disabilities to carry out work-related functions. It is generally recognized that persons with disabilities have a significantly higher rate of unemployment than the general population does (Berthoud, 2006; Canadian Council on Social Development [CCSD]), 2002, 2004, 2005). Those individuals who gain employment often are in positions that do not use their full range of skills and they tend to be more highly represented in the lowest wage quartile (CCSD, 2005). Cornell University's *2004 Disability Status Reports United States* indicated that only 22.4% of persons with a disability were employed full-time on a year-round basis (Rehabilitation Research and Training Center on Disability Demographics and Statistics, 2005). An analysis of the Participation and Activity Limitation Survey (PALS) data in Canada showed that more persons with disabilities who were employed felt they needed access to technology (Cossette, 2002) and job modifications than environmental modifications to do their jobs (CCSD, 2005). This chapter focuses on the assessment and implementation process of providing assistive technology in the workplace. Elements of the human activity–assistive technology (HAAT) model physical, social, cultural, and institutional contexts that enable or pose barriers to the successful integration of an individual with a disability in the workplace are discussed.

The individuals served by vocational assistive technology are typically between 16 and 65 years of age and have wide-ranging physical, sensory, and cognitive disabilities. There are two primary populations of persons who need assistive technologies for access to employment. The first group includes individuals who have a disability at the time they seek employment. The disabilities typical in this population are spinal cord injury, arthritis, cerebral palsy, visual impairment, and hearing impairment. The second group includes individuals who sustain either a cumulative or a traumatic injury in the workplace and who wish to return to the workforce.

Disabilities most commonly seen in the second population are musculoskeletal disorders (MSD) such as back injuries, carpal tunnel syndrome, tendonitis, and shoulder injuries. For both these populations, assistive technology is one of many tools that can be used to help people become employed or re-employed.

De Jonge, Scherer, and Rodger (2007) describe a process for introducing assistive technology in the workplace. This process is shown in Figure 16-1. The figure shows a process, without a defined starting point, for identifying the right technology, acquiring it, introducing it into the workplace, and maximizing its use. This process is based on consideration of the issues that affect the employee who uses assistive technology and also includes evaluation of the outcome. We will use the HAAT model as a basis for discussing some of the elements of this process described by de Jonge, Scherer, and Rodger, specifically identification of the right technology, maximizing the use of the assistive technology, client and outcome evaluation, and identification of issues that affect the use of assistive technology in the workplace.

■ VOCATIONAL ACTIVITIES THAT CAN BE AIDED BY ASSISTIVE TECHNOLOGIES

The process of designing an assistive technology system was described in Chapter 2 and starts with defining the activities that characterize vocational endeavors. The HAAT model and the three activity outputs of communication, manipulation, and mobility provide a means to characterize vocational activities. In the following sections, each of the activity outputs is described in terms of work tasks that an individual may need to perform on the job. Identification of these tasks will then help us to define both the human skills and the assistive technologies required for successfully completing them. The fourth component of the HAAT model, the context, is used to identify the environmental considerations that influence assistive technology use in the workplace.

Box 16-1 identifies questions related to the person's occupation and job tasks for the assistive technology practitioner (ATP) to ask during the assessment of an individual

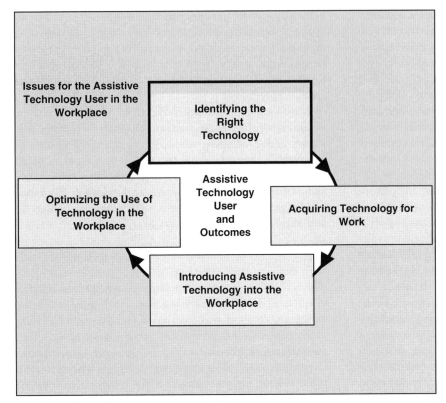

Figure 16-1   Stages of choosing and integrating technology into the workplace. (From de Jonge DM, Scherer MJ, Rodger SA: *Assistive technology in the workplace*, p. 84, St. Louis, 2007, Mosby.)

who needs accommodation in the workplace. It is important that the ATP ask as many questions as needed to get a clear picture of how the job is customarily performed. These questions include information regarding equipment used, equipment that may be available, and methods of performing the tasks. The ATP also observes the performance of the specific job tasks as appropriate.

Communication

Communication includes all the various information-handling activities in the workplace. Activities in this category include writing (pen/pencil or typing), reading, interacting with others in person, using a computer and keyboard, and using the telephone.

BOX 16-1   **Information Regarding the Person's Occupation and Job Tasks to Gather During Assessment**

1. What is the occupation (e.g., clerical, laborer, sales, professional, medical, teaching) and employment status (e.g., full time, part time, temporary) of the individual?
2. What symptoms or limitations (sensory, motor, cognitive, psychosocial/psychological) is the individual experiencing?
3. What job tasks are performed, and how are they typically performed?
4. How do the person's symptoms or limitations affect job performance?
5. Is communication difficult?
6. Who does the individual need to communicate with (e.g., supervisors, coworkers, customers)?
7. How does communication typically take place (e.g., face to face, telephone, computer)?
8. Is mobility difficult?
9. How does the individual get to work?
10. Is access into and around the work site a problem?
11. Is sitting tolerated?
12. Is standing tolerated?
13. Is manipulation difficult, and in what ways?
14. Is there a need for and are there any difficulties performing ADLs at work?
15. What are the potential workplace hazards?
16. What measures have been taken to correct the hazards?
17. Have the *ADA Accessibility Guidelines* been evaluated if appropriate?
18. What, if any, accommodations have already been implemented?
19. Is the person aware of any accommodations that are available to reduce or eliminate these problems? Are all possible resources being used to determine possible accommodations?
20. Has the employee been consulted regarding possible accommodations?
21. Do supervisory personnel and employees need training regarding disability or the Americans with Disabilities Act?

Modified from the Job Accommodation Network, Morgantown, WV, www.jan.wvu.edu/media/ergo.html, May 2001.

Interacting with others involves numerous skills, including oral motor skills required for speech; auditory function; cognitive skills, including receptive and expressive language; and social skills. Many of these skills are described in Chapter 3, and Chapter 11 describes the skills specifically needed to carry on a conversation. In some cases, individuals lacking these communication skills can use alternative modes of communication and an augmentative communication device. These devices are discussed in detail in Chapter 11.

A person with a disability may have trouble using the telephone to communicate as a result of deficits in communication, sensory, or motor skills. All aspects of telephone use may be problematic including difficulty with (1) dialing a number because of visual, cognitive, or motor impairments, (2) lifting and holding the receiver, and (3) speaking to and hearing the communication partner. A range of low- and high-tech options is available to assist with these activities. Reading requires motor, sensory, and cognitive skills. Many of the skills described in Chapter 15 for educational application apply in the workplace as well. The motor skills associated with positioning the reading material, turning pages, and handling materials (e.g., picking up a book, opening it, using an index, thumbing through pages) are necessary for use of print media. Chapter 7 discusses devices to aid in the motor tasks involved with reading printed materials. The motor tasks to operate a mouse and keyboard are important for electronic media (see Chapter 7).

Reading also requires sensory abilities such as visual field, visual acuity, and oculomotor function to scan text and recognize letters and words. If the individual lacks these capabilities because of a visual impairment, an alternative format in either tactile (braille) or auditory (speech) form can be used (see Chapters 8). Individuals who have hearing loss (including deafness) can make use of adaptations such as those discussed in Chapter 9. Basic literacy skills are also required for reading. The level is determined by the specific job requirements. For example, a job as a stock clerk may only require the reading of simple labels, whereas a job as a paralegal or an attorney requires a higher level of skill for the reading of complex legal documents. Assistive technology applications to aid individuals who have cognitive disabilities are discussed in Chapter 10.

Whether writing is accomplished by handwriting or typing, it requires motor, sensory, and cognitive skills. The use of pencil or pen and paper requires fine motor control to hold the pen or pencil and to produce letters. Chapter 15 describes the use of different types of writing (note taking, messaging, and formal writing) as they apply to educational settings. Many of the considerations in the workplace are the same. There are also many alternatives to handwriting for successful completion of writing tasks (see Chapters 7, 10, 11, and 15). These include assistance provided by a personal assistant, computer-aided writing using word processing, personal digital assistants that recognize handwriting on a screen and store it as text for editing, modified pens and pencils (e.g., enlarged grip or holder), and systems that recognize speech and translate it directly into text (automatic speech recognition).

Keyboard or mouse use is required for all data entry tasks, including writing. There are many alternatives to keyboard/mouse entry, including automatic speech recognition (see Chapter 7). Sensory skills for monitoring what is being written include visual, auditory, and tactile approaches, some using various types of assistive technologies. Cognitive and language skills for writing are described in Chapters 10 and 15.

Manipulation

The activity output of manipulation also includes a number of different tasks. In general, manipulative activities in the workplace are those that have anything to do with handling of material, which includes filing, sorting, assembling, lifting and moving objects such as books, documents, and equipment and using office machines such as copiers, adding machines, or fax machines. Besides requiring fine motor skills, these activities require sensory and cognitive skills. The ATP needs to follow the process identified in Chapter 2 and to analyze the activities required in an employment setting and describe these in terms of their motor, sensory, cognitive, and affective demands.

Mobility

The activity output of mobility is characterized by activities that involve personal movement to and from the work site and within the workplace. In considering these activities it is important to determine what movements are required of the individual to complete the job and, when the individual lacks these movements, what alternative methods are available.

Getting to work is a significant barrier for many individuals (Gillen, 2000; Rumrill, Schuyler and Longden, 1997; Zwerling et al, 2003). Arranging wheelchair-accessible public transportation often means booking pickup times with a range of an hour or more, booking far in advance, and paying additional fees for the accessible service. If private transportation is used, the cost of a modified vehicle (see Chapter 13) is much higher than that of a standard vehicle. Furthermore, finding a parking space at work that is accessible and close to the work site may also be a problem. Thus the options for transportation are significantly more challenging than for nondisabled workers.

Once at work, mobility and access in and around the work environment can be a challenge for some people with disabilities. Activities to consider are whether the person can enter and exit the building safely and in an emergency, open and close doors, and climb stairs. Sitting and standing requirements of the job also need to be considered. Sitting applies to the employee who requires seating technologies for postural control, tissue integrity, or comfort to be an effective employee (see Chapter 6). It is important that the employee has good postural alignment and postural support as needed to maximize function in the work environment, including the manipulation of objects and operation of assistive devices.

In addition to postural alignment and proper positioning, the employee needs to be free from pain while sitting and be able to perform pressure-relief activities if needed. Persons who have had a back injury may have difficulty maintaining a static position in either sitting or standing for any length of time because of pain or fatigue. They may require modifications to the work area that enable them to alternate between the two positions. Other individuals may have difficulty in coming to a standing position from sitting.

McNeal, Somerville, and Wilson (1999) conducted a study in which one of the purposes was to document the types of problems experienced by workers with spinal cord injury and workers with postpolio syndrome. The group of individuals with spinal cord injury reportedly had the greatest number of problems (39.8%) in the category of "using equipment/tools/furniture." More than one third of these problems had to do with desks, including an inability to get up to the desk because of the wheelchair, inability to access items on the desk, or a workspace that was too limited.

Activities of Daily Living in the Context of Work

While an employee is at work, there are also a number of activities of daily living (ADLs) he or she may need to carry out. These activities may have unique requirements because they are being performed in the work setting. These activities include going to the bathroom, taking medications, and eating lunch or other meals. Accommodations for these activities can have as much of an influence as an accessible desk or workbench. If the workplace does not have accessible restrooms, then the worker who has a disability is at a significant disadvantage compared with fellow workers. If assistance for taking medications is not available, the worker may not be able to perform the tasks of the job.

Besides the requirements related to physical accessibility for completing these ADLs, time factors are also an issue. Some individuals may require additional time for toileting or eating. A flexible schedule with time off during the workday is needed. Issues of privacy and whether to ask coworkers

for assistance also come into play. A final consideration relates to the level of fatigue a worker with a disability may experience. Some individuals may require a rest break during the day or a shortened work day to accommodate fatigue (Garcia, Laroche, and Barrette, 2002).

◼ EVALUATION OF THE EMPLOYEE'S ABILITIES

The next step of the assistive technology system design process described in Chapter 2 is the identification of the client's abilities. This evaluation of employee skills is obtained from a systematic assessment process. Chapter 4 describes both the essential information that must be obtained through an assessment process and the major approaches to service delivery in assistive technologies. The process for carrying out an assistive technology assessment for an individual with vocational needs follows the same general principles described in Chapter 4. Each assessment must be conducted on a case-by-case basis, with the first step being to define the problem. In defining the problem, it is essential to ask questions pertaining to the individual's specific situation. It is then necessary to identify the individual's skills and abilities and relate the information to the specific employment situation. The following case study points out some of the issues in assistive technology assessment for needs related to employment and illustrates the necessity for a team approach, including the employee, employer, and assessment team. It also illustrates the necessity to focus on need rather than on technology.

Background information available to the ATP before commencing a job site accommodation might include some of the following: physical capacity evaluation, functional capacity evaluation, workplace evaluations, and physician's report. It is preferable that the assessment of the consumer's technology needs and trials of the technology take place in the work setting in which it will be used. Simulation of the work tasks is an alternative when access to the workplace is not feasible.

In addition to assessing the physical and cognitive abilities of the employee, it is important to understand his emotional state. De Jonge, Scherer, and Rodger (2007) describe the discomfort that the participants of their study identified regarding asking for assistive technology. Participants were hesitant to ask for assistive technology because of the focus it brought to their disability. During an assessment, the ATP should uncover the meaning of assistive technology to the individual and what he or she is willing to accept (Gamble, Dowler, and Orsline, 2006; Lund and Nygard, 2003; Reimer-Reiss and Wacker, 2001). Further, it is important to determine whether the individual can advocate for himself or herself or whether he or she needs assistance to acquire the needed technology.

ASSESSMENT FOR ASSISTIVE TECHNOLOGY
IN A VOCATIONAL CONTEXT

Your client, Roger, is employed by a company that has a governmental contract. Because the area in which he works is secured, the entrance, also used by other individuals, has a keypad at normal eye height, which currently requires keying in a code to gain entry. Roger has been diagnosed with amyotrophic lateral sclerosis (ALS). He began having symptoms approximately 2 years ago and has lost leg function, requiring the use of a scooter for mobility. He is also rapidly losing shoulder function. Although his company is very interested in having him continue to work, they are concerned about what steps need to be taken, how these will affect his coworkers, and how much it will cost to make the necessary modifications for him to continue working. Roger is a client of the state vocational rehabilitation agency and has been assigned to a rehabilitation counselor. The goal stated in his Individual Written Rehabilitation Plan is for Roger, through the use of assistive technologies, to maintain employment in his current position for as long as possible. The vocational rehabilitation counselor has asked you to conduct an assessment to determine what changes must be made in the work environment to accommodate Roger. Although the company is focusing on the problem of the security keypad, there are many other considerations as well. Read the section on assessment in this chapter and then answer these questions.

QUESTIONS:

1. What aspects of the work environment, in addition to the keypad issue, would you want to include in your assessment?
2. Because of security issues, you will not be able to see the actual keypad, but you will be able to see one similar to it. What type of assessment would you conduct to develop an alternative approach for your client to gain entry without interfering with other employees?
3. What policy and attitudinal issues would need to be addressed?
4. What is the role of the vocational counselor in this process?
5. What would you want to know in addition to the information provided here?

■ CONTEXT FOR VOCATIONAL APPLICATIONS

The context portion of the HAAT model describes the environment in which the activity is being performed.

Chapter 2 defined the aspects of the context: physical, social, cultural, and institutional. It is critical that these aspects of context in the work setting are not ignored because each plays an important role in the ultimate effectiveness, or ineffectiveness, of an assistive technology system. This section examines each aspect of the context as it relates to vocational settings.

In Chapter 2 we described three levels of environmental interaction and accompanying factors that affect decisions related to assistive technology implementation: macrosystemic, mesosystemic, and microsystemic (Fougeyrollas and Gray, 1998). The macrosystemic level is associated with issues of society as a whole, which includes policies relating to assistive technology use and funding levels. Lack of funding is a barrier to assistive technology use in the workplace. The macrosystemic level will be discussed as part of the institutional environment. The mesosystemic level is the person's local environment, which includes those places in the community where the individual lives and functions. For purposes of this chapter, the mesosystemic level we focus on is the workplace. This level includes the attitudes and policies of the employer, coworkers, and customers with whom the worker may come in contact. At the microsystemic level the analysis is of the immediate environment of the person, including such factors as the existence of specific assistive technologies. The ATP typically functions at this level when carrying out assessments, making recommendations, and supporting users of assistive technologies.

Physical Context

The HAAT model identifies the natural versus built environments and the physical parameters of noise, temperature, and light as elements of the physical context. These elements will now be considered in the vocational context.

Often discussions of assistive technologies in the vocational setting focus primarily on work that occurs in an office environment. Although the office is certainly a main setting for the application of assistive technology, considerations for designing the assistive technology system must also include its use outside of an office (e.g., travel to a client's site or assistive technology use in an industrial or commercial setting). Office applications might indicate a system setup that is used predominantly in one place; applications outside the office need to be transferable across environments and may be influenced to a greater degree by the physical parameters named above.

Communication partners include coworkers, supervisors and supervisees, and clients or customers. Communication involves both giving and receiving information (Garcia et al, 2002; McNaughton, Light, and Groszyk, 2001). The communication may be written or oral and could be something that is prepared such as a presentation or spontaneous such as interacting with a client or in a meeting. Written communication technologies are likely to be used at a single workstation that specifically accommodates for the user's abilities, although some components (e.g., a laptop computer) may travel with the user between work site and home or between client locations. Oral communication aids will move with the client so need to work across different environments. Chapter 11 discusses oral AAC applications across environments and Chapters 10 and 15 consider written communication in more depth.

Noise and light are the primary physical parameters that will affect the use of communication aids in the vocational context. Frequent mention has been made of the influence of ambient noise on the use of voice recognition technologies. Noise is also a consideration for the communication partner's ability to understand the synthesized or digitized speech output of a speech-generating device voice or the speech of an individual with a voice impairment (Garcia et al, 2002). Noise will be an important consideration for an individual working in an open concept office, industrial, or commercial environment. Noise can be a significant factor for individuals who have hearing loss (see Chapter 9) and for workers who have attention disorder–like disabilities (see Chapter 10). Light is important when the worker uses a device in different environments and needs to read information from a screen. Intensity and color of ambient light can also have a major impact on workers who have visual impairments (see Chapter 8).

Mobility refers to travel to and from the work site and within the worksite. Safe and reliable access in, out, and within the worksite are key. Consideration should be given to the different areas within the work site that the worker needs to access, including the primary workstation (or office), washroom, and lunch area. A path of travel should be identified between different locations within the work site. Box 16-2 lists a number of questions that should be considered when evaluating mobility among key areas in the work environment.

BOX 16-2 Questions to Consider When Evaluating Travel In and Around the Work Environment

1. Is there room to maneuver a mobility device?
2. Can the individual open and close the doors independently?
3. Are transitions between different elevations at an appropriate grade?
4. Is an elevator provided between floors?
5. Is there a safe and reliable means of exiting the work site in case of emergency?
6. Are multimodal signs used (e.g., braille markings for room numbers and labels and restroom labels)?
7. Is there an accessible path of transit between key locations within the work site?

Consideration of the natural and built environments needs to be made if the individual is traveling between different work sites, either moving from one building to another by using a personal mobility device or some form of vehicle. Climate considerations influence assistive technology system design when the user is traveling outside between home and work or work settings. For example, consideration should be given to the battery life of an electrically powered wheelchair. These were discussed in Chapter 12.

As identified earlier, manipulation demands include those involved with completion of work tasks and with ADLs that are completed at the work site. Once again, the ATP must identify the elements of the physical environment that facilitate these manipulation demands, such as lever-style faucet or door handles, and those that present barriers to use, such as heavy entrance doors. Technology exists to reduce the influence of most of these physical barriers and has been identified in an earlier chapter on manipulation (Chapter 14). It is frequently the social, cultural, and institutional contexts that limit the ability to improve the accessibility of the vocational environment.

Institutional Context

The institutional context is an important consideration for the provision of assistive technology in the workplace. Many jurisdictions have some form of legislation that prevents discrimination of persons with disabilities in the work setting and requires different degrees of accommodation. Some examples of legislation include (1) the Rehabilitation Act and the Americans with Disabilities Act (ADA) (United States), (2) Disability Discrimination Act of 1995 and 2005 (United Kingdom), (3), Disability Discrimination Act, 1992, and Amendment, 2002 (Australia), (4) Ontarians with Disabilities Act 2005 (Ontario, Canada), and (5) Disability Act 2005 (Ireland).

The ATP needs to be familiar with the legislation in his or her jurisdiction that regulates accommodation for persons with disabilities in the workplace. The following are some of the aspects of the legislation that are important to know. First, what is the definition of disability? Is the definition restrictive or inclusive? Inclusive definitions include physical, mental health, sensory, cognitive/intellectual, neurological, and behavioral diagnoses as well as chronic illnesses such as HIV/AIDS. An inclusive definition of disability also requires accommodations to be put in place from the time a progressive condition affects function.

The requirements for accommodation are an obvious part of the ATP's knowledge acquisition. Most pieces of legislation identify modification of the job or the environment and the purchase and use of equipment or technology as reasonable accommodations. Further, the legislation often includes some statement about the degree of accommodation. For example, the ADA uses the language of a reasonable accommodation and least restrictive environment. This language suggests that the accommodations that are made in the workplace do not need to be the best or most appropriate fit for the employee. Rather, they are what it is reasonable to expect of the employer given the context. Obviously, this type of language can be broadly interpreted and can result in accommodations that do not fully support the employee's needs in the workplace. Legislation also explicitly states that accommodations must be made when advertising a position, during the hiring process, and return to work situations, as well as the obvious accommodations required during the tenure of a person's employment.

Who is required to make workplace accommodations is a third consideration. Often employers who employ a small number of employees (e.g., fewer than 15-20) are exempt from the legislation. Further, exceptions may be made if the necessary accommodations create an undue hardship (usually financial) for the employer. Accommodations are not universally made for every job. There is frequently a clause in legislation that states that the applicant or employee must be able to do the essential activities of a job. For example, marketing jobs require an employee to give oral presentations to clients. An employer can deny employment to an applicant who cannot communicate orally. However, the notion of an essential activity does not define how that activity is accomplished. So an applicant who uses a voice-output communication aid can give an oral presentation and is therefore able to complete an essential activity of the job.

Finally, the ATP should identify whether there is a legislated process for identifying, implementing, and funding workplace accommodations and an appeals process if either party is dissatisfied with recommended or implemented accommodations. The Rehabilitation Act and the ADA are key pieces of legislation in this area so will be considered in more detail here.

The Rehabilitation Act establishes several important principles. One of the most important of these is the concept of reasonable accommodation in employment (see Chapter 1). The act mandates that employers receiving federal funds accommodate the needs of employees who have disabilities. It specifically prohibits discrimination in employment solely on the basis of a disability. This law originally described both reasonable accommodation and least restrictive environment (LRE), a term relating to the degree of modification that is acceptable in a job.

As a result of the Rehabilitation Act of 1973, many employers made architectural changes to reduce barriers. These included installing elevators, placing ramps and curb cuts to accommodate wheelchair users, and adding voice and braille labels to signs (including elevators) to accommodate persons with visual impairment. Many of these efforts to achieve accommodation involved the use of assistive technologies.

The Rehabilitation Act Amendments of 1998, which are contained in the Workforce Investment Act of 1998 (Public Law [PL] 105-220), are the most recent amendments to the Rehabilitation Act. These amendments include several provisions involving assistive technologies. First the amendments require that each state include within its vocational rehabilitation plan a provision for assistive technology (referred to in PL 99-506 as *rehabilitation engineering or technology* and in PL 105-220 as *rehabilitation technology*).

This plan is the basis by which states receive federal funding for vocational rehabilitation, and there is a strong incentive to provide these technology-related services to ensure continuation of the transfer of federal funds for rehabilitation programs. The Rehabilitation Act also requires that provision for acquiring appropriate and necessary assistive technology devices and services be included in an Individual Written Rehabilitation Plan developed for the individual. For individuals who are eligible for services through state vocational rehabilitation programs, the Rehabilitation Act has excellent provisions for the inclusion of assistive technology in all phases of the rehabilitation process, from evaluation through placement in employment. In its analysis of assistive technology policy in employment, the National Council on Disability (NCOD, 2000) identified the following limitations in these provisions: (1) limits of funding for vocational rehabilitation and (2) implementation difficulties such as insufficient staff expertise with assistive technology and lack of service providers with this expertise.

Section 508 of the Rehabilitation Act is an important provision because it ensures access to "electronic office equipment" by persons with disabilities who work for the federal government. Because the federal government is such a large purchaser of computers and other office technology, any purchasing specifications it makes take on the role of informal standards affecting all manufacturers of equipment and therefore all employers who purchase that equipment. Persons who are blind or have low vision and those with difficulty in accessing the keyboard have benefited from standards derived as a result of Section 508, and several manufacturers have included features in the basic designs of their computer systems technology that increase access (see Chapter 7). The provisions cover access to electronic office equipment and electronic information services provided to the public by the federal government, which includes ensuring that end users with disabilities (1) have access to the same databases and application programs as other end users, (2) are supported in manipulating data and related information resources to attain equivalent results as other end users, and (3) can transmit and receive messages using the same telecommunication systems as other end users. As described in Chapter 1, the ADA is a federal civil rights law that is designed to prevent discrimination and enable individuals with disabilities to participate fully in all aspects of society.

One fundamental principle of the ADA is that individuals with disabilities who want to work and are qualified to work must have an equal opportunity to work.

Under Title I of the ADA the employer is required to provide reasonable accommodation to qualified individuals with disabilities who are employees or applicants for employment unless to do so would cause undue hardship. A **qualified individual with a disability** has the skills, education, experience, or other requirements needed for the job and can perform the essential functions of the position with or without reasonable accommodation (Equal Employment Opportunity Commission [EEOC], 1996). The **essential functions** of a job are those job duties that are so fundamental to the position the individual holds or desires that he or she cannot do the job without performing them. An essential function of a nurse in a hospital would be to respond to a patient's call for assistance. An essential function for a painter might be to lift a 5-gallon bucket of paint weighing 42 pounds. An essential function for a clerical worker might be to type 75 words per minute. It is the employer who determines the essential job functions.

There are many individuals with disabilities who can apply for and perform job duties without any reasonable accommodations. However, there are barriers in the workplace that prevent other individuals with disabilities from doing the same thing unless they are provided with some form of accommodation. These barriers may be physical in nature (such as facilities or equipment that are inaccessible), or they may be procedures or rules (such as rules regarding when work is performed, when breaks are taken, or how essential or marginal functions are achieved). Reasonable accommodation can remove these barriers. **Reasonable accommodation** is "making existing facilities used by employees readily accessible to and usable by individuals with disabilities" (ADA, 1990, Section [9] [A]). Reasonable accommodation is available to qualified applicants and employees with disabilities and must be provided regardless of whether the employee works part time or full time or is considered probationary. It is the responsibility of the individual with a disability to inform the employer that an accommodation is needed. The general types of reasonable accommodations that an employer may have to provide are illustrated in Box 16-3, along with examples of each type.

An accommodation is not required if the employer finds it would impose undue hardship on the operation of the employer's business. **Undue hardship** is defined as an "action requiring significant difficulty or expense" (ADA, 1990, Section [10] [A]) when considered on a case-by-case basis. In determining whether an accommodation would impose an undue hardship, the nature and cost of the accommodation in relation to the size, resources, nature, and structure of the employer's operation is considered. If the facility making the accommodation is part of a larger entity, the structure and overall resources of the larger organization

---

BOX 16-3   Categories of Reasonable Accommodation, With Accompanying Examples

MAKING EXISTING FACILITIES READILY ACCESSIBLE
Installing a ramp or modifying the rest room so that the facility is wheelchair accessible

JOB RESTRUCTURING
Reallocating or redistributing marginal job functions that an employee is unable to perform because of a disability; altering when or how a function, essential or marginal, is performed

MODIFIED OR PART-TIME SCHEDULE
Modified schedule may involve adjusting arrival or departure times, providing periodic breaks, altering when certain functions are performed, allowing an employee to use accrued paid leave, or providing additional unpaid leave

ACQUIRING OR MODIFYING EQUIPMENT
Providing alternative form of access to a computer, such as a head mouse, for someone who has fine motor problems or building up the controls on assembly line equipment

PROVIDING QUALIFIED READERS OR INTERPRETERS
Hiring sign language interpreters for someone who is hearing impaired or a reader for someone who is blind

MODIFIED WORKPLACE POLICIES
Allowing an employee with a disability to bring in a small refrigerator to store medication that must be taken during working hours

MODIFYING EXAMINATIONS, TRAINING, OR OTHER PROGRAMS
Allowing an applicant with a learning disability time and a half on an examination

REASSIGNMENT
Reassigning a current employee to a vacant position for which the individual is qualified

---

are considered, as well as the financial and administrative relationship of the facility to the larger organization. Generally a larger employer with greater resources is expected to make accommodations requiring greater effort or expense than that required of a smaller employer with fewer resources. In situations where an accommodation would impose an undue hardship, the employer must try to identify an alternative accommodation that meets the employee's need and does not impose a hardship. The individual with a disability should also be given the option of paying for the cost (or a portion thereof) of an accommodation that would create an undue hardship.

There are a number of modifications or adjustments that are not considered forms of reasonable accommodation. For example, the individual must be qualified for the position sought; there is no obligation to find a position for an applicant who is not qualified. An employer is not required to eliminate an essential function (i.e., a fundamental duty of the position). Although employers may have to provide reasonable accommodations to enable an employee with a disability to meet quality or quantity production standards, they are not required to lower standards that are applied uniformly to employees with and without disabilities. Glasses and hearing aids may be considered personal effects and are not included as reasonable accommodations, although there are exceptions and the ATP needs to explore whether these are covered.

There is a perception among employers that job accommodation is a complex and costly process (Driscoll, Rodger, and de Jonge, 2001; Langton and Ramseur, 2001; Peck and Kirkbride, 2001). To the contrary, most accommodations are simple, inexpensive, and can reduce Workers' Compensation and other insurance costs (Job Accommodation Network [JAN], 2000). In addition, for qualifying small businesses, tax incentives are available to help cover the cost of providing accommodation. The JAN Web site provides information on the costs of different accommodations (http://www.jan.wvu.edu/).

In the United States and other countries, Social Security benefits provided to people with disabilities can act as a disincentive for people to work (Frieden, 1997). Often the income from jobs is only slightly more or the same as the benefits they receive. The loss of health care benefits is also a concern for individuals with disabilities once they become employed. People with disabilities want to work but frequently have difficulty trying to obtain health insurance when they leave the public health care system and enter the work force (NCOD, 2000). Because health care, including assistive technologies, is often a critically needed service, choosing between employment and health care does not take much in the way of deliberation. This issue is a significant barrier to participation in the work force by people with disabilities, and the ADA does not address it. The Work Incentives Improvement Act has the potential to provide better health care options for persons with disabilities wishing to work. This legislation gives states the option of allowing working-age adults with disabilities to "buy in to" Medicaid coverage if they leave the Supplemental Security Income program to work. However, depending on the state in which one lives and the assistive technology needs of the individual, the measures may be limited in improving access to assistive technology (NCOD, 2000). Because Medicaid coverage of assistive technology varies from state to state (see Chapter 5), a state's decision to allow Medicaid buy-in may not result in improved access to assistive technology needed by individuals who wish to enter the work force (NCOD, 2000).

Social and Cultural Contexts

In the context portion of the HAAT model, we use social and cultural contexts to describe important aspects of both interaction and acceptance of assistive technologies.

Social and cultural factors also include policies and attitudes toward technology and toward disability by employers and fellow employees. The social and cultural aspects of the context can be the most important for assistive technology use in a vocational setting (de Jonge, Scherer, and Rodger, 2007; Driscoll et al, 2001; Garcia et al, 2002; McNaughton et al, 2001; Peck and Kirkbride, 2001; Strobel et al, 2006). We need to examine the policies and attitudes of employers and employees, the types of relationships the person has with people at work, and how they affect interactions and use of assistive technology when considering the social and cultural contexts at work. These factors can impose barriers to successful assistive technology application.

The social context of the workplace includes the other people in the environment. These people include the employer or supervisor, employees, coworkers (both those who work closely with the individual and those with less frequent involvement), other workers at the job site, and clients or consumers. Their knowledge of disabilities and attitudes toward individuals with disabilities are a significant determinant of whether the person with a disability will be successful in the work setting. Knowledge of and willingness to provide workplace accommodations are further determinants of success in the workplace (Driscoll, Rodger, and de Jonge, 2001; Gamble, Dowler, and Orslene, 2006; Garcia et al, 2002; McNaughton et al, 2001; Strobel et al, 2006). Legislation that requires accommodations for persons with disabilities exists widely, but the support of others in the environment, particularly an employer or supervisor, is critical for these accommodations to enable the individual to complete job tasks.

As indicated in the introduction to this chapter, people with disabilities have a significantly higher rate of unemployment or underemployment than the general population. Some persons with disabilities report a lack of value of their capacity to contribute in a work setting. Frequently, this lack is seen when individuals with disabilities are asked to volunteer in a setting rather than being paid for their involvement. The perception of the person with a disability is that the employer or the representatives of an organization feel they are doing the individual a favor by providing the volunteer opportunity (King, Brown, and Smith, 2003). Individuals who are employed report prejudice and social barriers in the workplace (Chan et al, 2005).

Community participation by persons with disabilities has increased over the past decade. However, it is still typical for an employer to have little knowledge of the capacity of an individual with a disability and the role that technology and environmental modifications can play in enabling her contribution in the workplace. This lack of knowledge may result in the employer's perception that the person with a disability is incapable of completing work tasks (Peck and Kirkbride, 2001). Consequently, he or she may be denied certain employment, given a job that does not use his or her abilities, or denied access to technology and modifications that would fully enable him or her in the workplace. A later section of this chapter will discuss introduction of technology into the workplace and we will discuss strategies for educating employers and advocating for appropriate modifications in the workplace.

De Jonge, Scherer, and Rodger (2007) describe a dilemma faced by employees with disabilities and their employers. Employers reported little knowledge about assistive technology that would be useful in the workplace and even less knowledge of the process involved in securing technology for the workplace. They made an assumption that the employee would have this knowledge. Although employees who had used assistive technology for a long time did have some of this information, it might not be specific to the work setting. Further, those employees with no assistive technology experience were often in the same position as their employers with respect to knowing how to access assistive technologies. Employees with disabilities reported feeling hesitant to ask for technology that would enable them to complete their job, mainly because of their concern that such requests would focus attention on their disabilities (de Jonge, Scherer, and Rodger, 2007). This dilemma led to a communication problem that prevented satisfactory assistive technology solutions for the workplace.

The workplace culture will influence the participation of an individual with a disability. A work setting that fosters collaboration and communication and accepts different ways of doing tasks will likely support the needs of an individual with a disability. Generally, employers have recognized the range of needs of their employees, such as the need for child day care, flexible work hours, and creative accommodations such as job sharing. Companies or organizations that recognize the needs of their employees are more likely to support the accommodations required of an individual with a disability. Employment situations that place a high value on productivity over other workplace behaviors or outcomes may be an integration challenge.

As described in Chapter 2, social influence on individuals is related to what is considered normal or expected, and individuals who have disabilities may be stigmatized because of their disability (Fougeyrollas, 1997). Unfortunately, the use of assistive technologies in the workplace can contribute to this labeling and lead to further isolation. In one study, some of the individuals surveyed reported that they deliberately tried to hide from their employer the fact that they were disabled or were having problems (McNeal, Somerville, and Wilson, 1999). Some were fearful that their employers would fire them if they learned about the problems related to the disability. This fear may prevent some individuals from requesting needed accommodations. The degree to which assistive technologies contribute to stigmatization differs (e.g., the stigma of a hearing aid as opposed to eyeglasses). Because the social context plays such a major role in assistive technology use in the workplace, it is important to consider the stigmatizing effect of any proposed

workplace assistive technologies and to provide assistance to the worker in overcoming them, which may include awareness training for coworkers and strategies for assistive technology use by the worker.

As discussed earlier, most legislation related to discrimination of individuals with disabilities contains some language that provides employers with a way to avoid making workplace modifications (Peck and Kirkbride, 2001). Typically, the influence on the company's bottom line is used as an excuse to avoid these modifications. If accommodations are considered to create financial hardship for the employer, they do not need to be made. This type of language recognizes only one side of the financial equation: the money initially spent to purchase technology or modify an environment. It does not recognize the contribution that the employee will make to the company, nor does it amortize the initial equipment expense over the length of time the technology may be used (often years). This corporate attitude is a significant barrier to full access to employment of individuals with disabilities, one that will require more than legislation to eliminate.

Marcia Scherer developed a series of assessments to help determine an appropriate fit between the individual, the environment, and technology. The *Workplace Technology Device Predisposition Assessment* (Scherer, 2005) is a short questionnaire completed by the employer and the employee. It assesses aspects of the technology and the employee's and employer's perspectives on training available to learn use of the technology, support for use of the technology, and perception of the person with a disability as a respected employee (Scherer, 2005). This assessment is a useful tool to help identify whether technology will be supported in the environment and as a way to bring the employee and employer together to discuss introduction and use of technology in the specific work environment.

In summary, the social context of the workplace includes many different people, with whom an employee interacts in different ways and frequencies. Advances in technology, both mainstream and for individuals with disabilities, can accommodate many workplace activities and minimize physical barriers in the environment. However, the knowledge and attitudes of others in the workplace, particularly those who make decisions about hiring and workload, have a greater influence on the ability of an individual with a disability to fully participate in employment. These two determinants need to be addressed when introducing technology into the work site.

■ HARD AND SOFT TECHNOLOGIES FOR VOCATIONAL SUCCESS

The fourth component of the HAAT model is hard and soft assistive technologies. There are many characteristics of assistive technologies discussed in Chapters 1 and 2.

When considering a unique environment such as the vocational setting, some of these are more important than others. As described earlier, accommodation includes both hard and soft assistive technologies.

Assistive technologies can provide major benefits for individuals in vocational settings. A range of workplace accommodations can be made, from inexpensive to costly, hard technologies to soft technologies, and simple to complex. Postural support systems (see Chapter 6) allow the individual to be positioned for maximal participation in work activities. The use of special-purpose input methods or control interfaces (see Chapter 7) is often necessary for use of computers and other electronic devices. In many employment situations the computer (see Chapter 7) is a valuable tool. Augmentative communication systems (see Chapter 11) play a major role for individuals who have disabilities affecting speaking or writing. Mobility devices (see Chapter 12) allow a person with motor deficits to get in and around the workplace. Some assistive technologies (e.g., electronic aids to daily living and robotics; see Chapter 14) can provide assistance to employees who cannot independently manipulate materials or objects. Finally, employees who have sensory disabilities (visual or auditory) are aided by the technologies described in Chapter 8 and 9. The potential for achieving a positive vocational outcome using assistive technologies is great; however, reaching that potential requires careful planning to ensure that opportunities, not barriers, are created.

Strategies are also important to the success of assistive technology in the workplace. Simonds (2001) makes some suggestions of strategies that a person with a disability who uses assistive technology can use to attain employment. The ATP can impart these strategies to the applicant. Before going to a job interview or at the beginning of the interview, the applicant should inquire about the job's requirements. The person should then be knowledgeable about his or her own capabilities, such as how many words per minute he or she can dictate or how fast he or she can read text with a screen reader. People who have range-of-motion deficits and use assistive devices to reach and grasp should know how far they can reach, how fast they can move, and how much weight they can lift. In some situations, such as with the use of speech-activated software, assistive technology may not only serve to level the playing field but may actually give the applicant a leg up on the competition because it enhances performance. Simonds also recommends that the applicant with a disability learn more than one version of whatever technology is available. If the applicant's assistive technology solutions only work on certain systems or with specific hardware, the question of adaptability arises, which can complicate the hiring process. Finally, it is suggested that the applicant be accepting of any assistive technology used and view it as part of the hiring package. The assistive technology should be presented as a bonus where the employer not only gets the applicant but gets this great technology as well.

CASE STUDIES OF VOCATIONAL ASSISTIVE TECHNOLOGY APPLICATIONS

Now that we have identified some of the tools that appear in previous chapters for access to vocational activities, we use case studies to demonstrate how they are combined and applied to maximize the opportunities for employment by individuals who have disabilities.

Accommodating an Employee With a Visual Impairment

An individual with a visual impairment will require modifications that support the activities of way finding in the environment, location, and manipulation of objects and materials and perception of any information that is presented visually. Chapter 8 discussed assistive technology for use by individuals with a visual impairment. Table 16-1 lists a number of sample modifications for persons with visual impairment. Read the following case study and use the information found in this table and in Box 16-1 to develop a plan for the assessment process and make recommendations for accommodations.

Accommodating an Employee With a Motor Impairment

Throughout this chapter the importance of ensuring that the employee's work site and workstation are fully accessible to the employee has been stressed. Because this area most often relates to individuals with motor impairments, these accommodations are described in this section.

A valuable resource for parameters on building or remodeling a work site to make it accessible is the *ADA Accessibility Guidelines as Amended, 1998* (ADAAG). This document, which can be found on the Internet at *http://www.access-board.gov/adaag/html/adaag.htm*, specifies the technical requirements for accessibility to buildings and facilities by individuals with disabilities under the ADA of 1990. Another useful publication on modifying the workplace is *The Workplace Workbook: An Illustrated Guide to Job Accommodations and Assistive Technology* (Mueller, 1990). This book contains detailed descriptions with accompanying illustrations related to three workplace topics: the universal workplace; seating, storage, and workstations; and computers, information displays, communication devices, and controls.

CASE STUDY

VOCATIONAL ACCOMMODATION FOR SENSORY IMPAIRMENT

Alyssa, a totally blind woman in her 20s, applied for a position as a reservations operator for a limousine service and was hired. The job requires that Alyssa access 15 to 20 different screens containing pertinent limo reservation information on the PC-based reservations system. Alyssa will need a number of shortcuts on the keyboard and screen to be able to effectively do the job. Because of the large volumes of information, speech output may need to be supplemented by braille. Fortunately, Alyssa has excellent braille-reading skills. You have been asked to conduct an assistive technology work assessment to determine the appropriate way to give Alyssa access to this system and to determine what other needs she might have for modifications to the work environment.

QUESTIONS:

1. List the areas that need to be evaluated and information you would want to gather during the assessment.
2. Identify the types of modifications to the work setting that might be appropriate.
3. Specify assistive technologies that might possibly be used (refer to Chapter 8).
4. Describe any strategies that you would suggest to Alyssa to help her succeed in her new job.
5. Discuss the training that you would provide to Alyssa to help her adapt to the new job.

Modified from Gilson J: Assistive work technology—the way Georgia does it." In *Proceedings of the CSUN 15th Annual Conference*, March 20-25, 2000: www.csun.edu/cod/conf2000/proceedings/0157Gilson.html.

TABLE 16-1	Sample Workplace Accommodations for Persons With Visual Impairment
Job Activity	Workplace Accommodations
Communication: Writing Reading Conversation	Reduce glare by installing window coverings that allow for light adjustment and filtering Increase lighting Use nonglare lights with covers Use contrasting colors to define background and foreground (e.g., edge of steps and step surface, light switch plates, and walls) Use tactile indicators, raised letters Use large print on a background with high contrast Use visual aids such as closed circuit televisions, magnifiers, large-print computer monitors, talking devices, refreshable braille display Provide isolated workspaces for workers who use assistive technologies with automatic speech recognition or speech synthesis Use color acetate sheets over print materials to increase contrast Take frequent breaks to rest eyes when fatigue is a factor Use optical character recognition to scan printed text and receive a synthetic speech output or save it to a computer Provide a qualified reader
Manipulation Filing/sorting Assembly Lifting Using office machines	Use large-print labels on files and file folders Provide magnification systems for assembly Enlarge print on office machines Provide talking office machines such as calculator, money sorter
Mobility Sitting Standing	Eliminate clutter and obstacles Eliminate low-profile furniture or move it out of the way Provide rest room and room labels in alternative formats (e.g., braille or large print)

Continued

TABLE 16-1	Sample Workplace Accommodations for Persons With Visual Impairment—cont'd	
Job Activity	Workplace Accommodations
Walking Climbing stairs	Have visual alerting signal devices in case of emergency Allow the use of a service animal Provide mobility and orientation training Mobility aid (cane, electronic aid, other) Install colored edges on stairs for improved color contrast Improve lighting in area Set up a traveling/evacuation partner Verbal landmark system Use public transportation or ride with coworker to get to work
Activities of **Daily Living** Toileting Eating lunch Taking medications	Install bathroom grab bars of contrasting color from the wall Provide refrigerator for food and/or medications

There are office products, such as adjustable-height desks, filing systems, and carousels, that are commercially available to meet the accommodation needs of someone with a motor impairment. These modular workstation components can be assembled in configurations to meet a range of work-related needs of office employees with a disability. The modules can be controlled manually, by a motorized switch control, by computer, or by a computer-controlled robotic arm. Components are available that allow the individual to manipulate files, store and retrieve books, refer to reference materials, open mail, staple papers, and answer the telephone.

Accommodations to the workstation and other types of accommodations for persons with mobility impairments are listed in Table 16-2. Read the following case study and use the information found in this table and in Box 16-1 to develop a plan for the assessment process and make recommendations for accommodations.

◼ ACQUIRING TECHNOLOGY FOR THE WORKPLACE: ROLE OF THE ASSISTIVE TECHNOLOGY PRACTITIONER

The discussion to this point in this chapter describes the process of and factors relevant to the recommendation of an assistive technology system for the workplace. The remainder of the chapter focuses on the process for obtaining the technology and determinants and strategies for successful implementation of technology in the workplace.

CASE STUDY

VOCATIONAL ACCOMMODATION FOR MOTOR IMPAIRMENT

Larry was a CAD/CAM drafting specialist for a small design firm when he became quadriplegic. He uses a power wheelchair with a chin-controlled joystick and has limited use of his upper extremities. The office in which he works is on the ground floor, but there is a lack of accessible parking and the entrance is not accessible because of a large planter box in the way and a heavy glass door. His employer would like Larry to continue working with the company but is concerned with how Larry will access the building and operate the computer and CAD/CAM software. Larry was referred to you by the vocational rehabilitation agency for an assistive technology evaluation to determine accommodations so that Larry can return to work.

QUESTIONS:

1. List the areas that need to be evaluated and information you would want to gather during the assessment.
2. Identify the types of modifications to the work setting that might be appropriate.
3. Specify assistive technologies that might possibly be employed (refer to Chapters 7 and 12).
4. Describe any strategies that you would suggest to Larry to help him succeed in his job.
5. Discuss the training that you would provide to Larry to help him adapt to his job.

TABLE 16-2 **Sample Workplace Accommodations for Persons With Motor Impairment**

Job Activity	Workplace Accommodations
Communication Writing Reading Conversation	Provide telephone headsets, cordless headsets (no entangling cords), large-button phones, speakerphones, extendible holders, programmable and automatic dialing features, head or mouth pointing sticks Provide writing aids for a person who cannot grip a writing tool: pen/pencil grippers, orthopedic writing devices, handle buildups, weighted pens Use alternative control interfaces for computer entry to replace keyboard and mouse functions and control enhancers such as keyguards, typing aids, or head and mouth sticks Provide page turners and book holders for a person who cannot manipulate paper
Manipulation Filing/sorting Assembly Lifting Using office machines	Use automated filing systems, carousels, lateral file cabinets, height-appropriate file cabinets (2-3 drawers), reduced number of files per drawer, ruler as a pry bar and bookmark for tight files, hooks or tabs on file folders for easier grasping Store office supplies and frequently used materials on most accessible shelves or drawers for a person who cannot reach upper and lower shelves and drawers Use a lazy Susan at workstation for easy access to and manipulation of materials frequently used Modify controls on office machines or use a pointing device
Mobility Sitting Standing Walking Climbing stairs	Provide close, accessible designated parking and entrances to building Have an accessible route of travel from the parking lot into the building Offer opportunity to work from home if transportation to work is not available Maintain unobstructed hallways, aisles, and other building egresses Provide ramps and lightweight doors or automatic door openers Provide elevators for multistory work sites Provide large enough work area for wheelchair access, including turning Provide accessible restrooms, lunchroom, break room Assign workspace in proximity to office machines with elevated access (e.g., a platform to allow access for those with restricted height) or lowered equipment (e.g., on a table rather than on a countertop) Modify workstation design and provide height-adjustable table or desk so a person who uses a wheelchair can get under it comfortably Position filing cabinets and bookshelves at accessible heights for wheelchair users Provide comfortable, supportive adjustable seating Eliminate clutter, obstacles, and uneven surfaces Allow the person to bring a service animal into the workplace Develop a plan for safe evacuation, alerting the fire department of probable location of the individual with mobility impairments in case of emergency Provide equipment for safe evacuation
Activities of Daily Living Toileting Eating lunch Taking medications	Allow the person to have a personal attendant at work to assist with toileting, grooming, and eating Allow the person to have flexible scheduling and take periodic rest breaks for medications, repositioning, toileting, or grooming needs Provide an office area within proximity to restrooms and an accessible restroom: commode lifts, commode seat risers, grab bars, appropriate height placement of mirrors, paper, soap towels, lavatories

Making successful accommodations for an employee with a disability involves a multidisciplinary effort and collaboration among all involved parties. As with all other areas of assistive technology, the consumer is an integral part of the team. To achieve a successful outcome, it is necessary to seek the answers to accommodation questions and obtain input from the consumer. In addition to the consumer, the team may include a vocational rehabilitation counselor, a vocational evaluator, an employment specialist, therapy services, a rehabilitation engineer, the employer, and supervisors (if the person already has a job). Fellow employees may also be included as part of the team if a workstation is shared or if they will be involved in training. Depending on the status of the consumer's employment and the nature of

the disability, others who might be involved are a physician, a Workers' Compensation representative, and a job coach or trainer. Box 16-4 lists the responsibilities of the ATP in vocational accommodation assessment and implementation.

The United States was among the first to enact legislation to protect the rights of persons with disabilities in various settings, including the workplace. The processes for providing vocational services are well established in this country so will be described in detail here. The ATP working in other countries must become familiar with the counterpart processes in their jurisdiction. Each state has an agency designated to provide vocational rehabilitation services to individuals with disabilities who have employment as a goal. These services can include counseling, evaluation,

Responsibilities of the Assistive Technology Practitioner in Vocational Accommodation Assessment and Implementation

Understand referral and intake procedures of vocational rehabilitation agency.

Understand the counselor's role and their obligations to consumer and agency.

Be available to the counselor to address concerns from referral source.

Understand criteria that must be met for eligibility and policies and procedures that guide service delivery for the agency during evaluation to determine eligibility.

Understand it is the counselor's job to establish eligibility and the technologist's role to support the counselor, along with other team members, in offering information that relates to eligibility criteria.

Understand counselor and consumer expectations.

Consider all technology that facilitates evaluation and allows full participation of consumer in the evaluation process.

Explain clearly and specifically why and how technology is being considered when communicating with consumer.

Explain the technology processes, time frames, and options that assist in establishing a plan for services.

Use referral to assistive technology as an opportunity to educate the counselor on value of assistive technology services.

Agree on course of action and prioritize services if several are required.

Obtain all information about employment goals and objectives for consumer; review technology policies regarding provision of services to the consumer.

Identify major players in developing a team to make technology recommendations (e.g., consumer, rehabilitation professionals, caretakers, counselors, and vendors); communicate with team members to obtain information on effectiveness of technology recommendations and service delivery process.

Obtain all essential job functions information from counselor, employer, or employment specialist. All technology solutions considered should reflect back to vocational goals as identified on IWRP and communicated with counselor.

Follow up with vendor and consumer to ensure proper installation and use of assistive technology.

Modified from McAlees D, Oliverio M: *Achieving successful employment outcomes with the use of assistive technology.* Presented at the Alliance National Professional Development Symposium, March 1999, Dallas.

---

training, and job placement. The **vocational rehabilitation agencies** are funded by a combination of state and federal appropriations. (Contact information for each state's vocational rehabilitation agency can be found at *www.jan.wvu.edu/sbses/VOCREHAB.HTM*). There are also private vocational rehabilitation agencies that provide similar services. The services that they provide are paid for on a fee-for-service basis by the consumer, the employer, or a third-party funding source such as Workers' Compensation insurance.

The publicly funded vocational rehabilitation agencies all use a standard process of providing services to the consumer (Flynn and Clark, 1995). There is no set period in the vocational rehabilitation process in which assistive technology services occur. In fact, there are several points in this process in which assistive technology services can be incorporated (Langton and Hughes, 1992). A consumer receiving services from a vocational rehabilitation agency is assigned a **vocational rehabilitation counselor.** The role of the counselor is to assist the individual in identifying vocational goals and developing a plan to achieve those goals (Flynn and Clark, 1995). On a consumer's referral to a vocational rehabilitation agency, the first task carried out is the development of the **Individual Plan for Employment** (IPE, formerly called an Individual Written Rehabilitation Plan [IWRP]) The purpose of the IPE, which is developed jointly by the vocational counselor and the consumer, is to set in place a plan to achieve the consumer's employment objective. Items included in the IPE are shown in Box 16-5. Each IPE includes a statement of the consumer's long-term rehabilitation goals based on the assessment for determining eligibility and vocational rehabilitation needs, including an

Items for Inclusion in IPE

Employment goals and objectives

Intermediate objectives related to the attainment of rehabilitation goals; determined through assessment carried out in the most individualized and integrated setting (consistent with the informed choice of the individual)

Criteria, evaluation procedure, and a schedule for determining whether the goals are being met

A statement of the specific vocational rehabilitation services that will be provided and timelines in which the services will be provided

A statement of the specific rehabilitation technology services to be provided

A statement of the specific on-the-job related services, such as personal assistance services and training and supervision of the personal assistant

Assessment of the expected need for postemployment services

The name of any program or agency that will provide the vocational rehabilitation services and the process used to provide or procure such services

Client rights and information about the Client Assistance Program

A statement by the consumer describing how he or she was informed about and involved in choosing goals, objectives, services, agencies providing services, and any amendments agreed on with the counselor

The terms and conditions under which the specified vocational rehabilitation goods and services shall be provided to the individual in the most integrated settings

Information identifying other related services and benefits provided pursuant to any federal, state, or local program that will enhance the capacity of the individual to achieve the vocational objectives of the individual

assessment of career interests. To the greatest extent appropriate, the goals should include placement in integrated settings. The IPE also specifies services that are to be provided to the consumer to achieve the goals. In addition to assistive technology services, these services include occupational or physical therapy or speech-language pathology.

Some vocational rehabilitation agencies have ATPs on staff to provide services to their consumers. Other agencies obtain assistive technology services from an outside provider, either on a fee-for-service basis (where reimbursement is per hour of service provided) or through a contract (where x number of dollars are paid in exchange for evaluation and training of y number of consumers). In either situation it is the vocational rehabilitation counselor who can significantly affect the consumer's success or failure in acquiring assistive technologies for work. Therefore it is important that vocational rehabilitation counselors are educated about the assistive technology services and devices that are available to meet employment needs.

◼ IMPLEMENTING ASSISTIVE TECHNOLOGY IN THE WORKPLACE

Determinants of assistive technology abandonment that are recognized in other settings such as the home are also important considerations for the implementation of the technology in the workplace. Once the assessment process is complete and suitable technology has been identified, time should be spent to ensure that the assistive technology will work in the vocational setting and be acceptable to the employee, employer, and others in the environment. A trial period is recommended, using the technology for the required work tasks, to determine that it will meet the goals of the employee and employer (de Jonge et al, 2007; Driscoll et al, 2001).

The trial period helps determine that the assistive technology works within the specific vocational context and is transferable across other environments in which the employer is required to work or use the equipment. For example, a mobility device is frequently used in the home and work environments so should be compatible with both, particularly in those jurisdictions that only fund a single mobility device. A trial period will also identify whether modifications are needed to the technology or its set up. For example, use of the technology to complete required job tasks in the vocational environment will help the ATP determine whether the user and the equipment are properly positioned. Further, it will help identify issues related to the integration of the technology such as noise issues.

Training is important in the vocational context as it is in other contexts (Butterfield and Ramseur, 2004). Obviously, the user requires training on the set-up and use of the equipment. Other relevant people in the environment also need training on the equipment. Technical support is a key determinant of successful use of the technology. The assistive technology user, like other people who use equipment like computers, should not be expected to understand the underlying function of the technology. People responsible for providing technical support require training in how the assistive technology integrates with other technology in the environment so they can assist with trouble shooting as needed (McNaughton et al, 2001).

The initial step in designing the assistive technology system is consideration of required activities. Implementation of assistive technology in the workplace requires the ATP to analyze the employee's use of recommended technology when completing required tasks with a view to optimizing his or her performance of those tasks (de Jonge et al, 2007). In addition to adjusting positioning of the person and their equipment, as mentioned above, the ATP may recommend modification of the activity, by eliminating some steps of the task, reorganizing the task, or substituting one means of completing an activity with another (Langton and Ramseur, 2001). For example, the ATP might recommend that an employee gather all the information needed to write a report at the start of the writing task rather than getting the information as it arises during the task. Helping the employee become more efficient with his or her work while using assistive technology increases the likelihood that the technology will be used successfully in the vocational setting.

Plans need to be in place to accommodate failure of the technology. Some individuals will have two different means of completing a task, for example, voice recognition or direct input for computer work. Redundancy here accomplishes three goals: first, the user has an alternative means of completing a task if they become fatigued; second, the user has different ways of accomplishing a task depending on the situation; and third, the user has a backup if one means fails. Access to technical support is important here, once again, to provide efficient support when technology breaks down. Finally, having access to loaned equipment in the event of technology failure ensures that an employee can continue with his or her job. Identification of these strategies is important in the initial phases of implementation of assistive technology in the workplace.

Advocacy, either by the person with a disability or the ATP, may be necessary for the successful implementation of assistive technology in the workplace (de Jonge, Scherer, and Rodger, 2007). As previously stated, many employers lack knowledge of the abilities of individuals with disabilities and the availability of technology to support these abilities. In these situations someone must advocate to achieve the needed accommodations in the workplace. Assisting people with disabilities to advocate on their own behalf, when they do not feel confident doing so, is the most effective means of gaining these accommodations. In situations where the individual is not able to advocate on his or her own behalf, the ATP should do so.

Fostering communication between the employee and the employer (and others in the workplace) is an important component of successful implementation of assistive technology in the workplace. Communication generates understanding of the needs and constraints of both parties regarding assistive technology use and support. It is a useful training and education vehicle. A workplace that promotes open communication is one where issues and problems are dealt with at an early stage.

A final consideration is the recognition that upgrades in mainstream technology outpace that of assistive technology, particularly for computer-based applications (de Jonge, Scherer, and Rodger, 2007). The employee, employer, and technical support personnel need to be aware of this discrepancy. Some settings have a policy of replacing computer equipment on a regular basis (every 2 years, for example). This upgrading may not be possible for computer equipment used by an individual with a disability because of the requirements of their specific application.

The type of accommodations needed can be determined from the job analysis. The ATP should explore with the employee the different types and ways of making accommodations (see Box 16-3). Keeping any modifications simple, using the least intrusive approach, is important. The simplest approach may be to modify or revise the job task if possible. If technology is to be recommended, keep in mind the continuum of commercial to custom technology discussed in Chapter 1. Whenever possible it is preferable to recommend technology that is commercially available rather than custom made (Langton and Ramseur, 2001).

Once recommendations for equipment and modifications have been made, most state vocational rehabilitation agencies are required to go through a **bidding process** before making any purchases. In this process the recommendations are submitted to three outside vendors for pricing. Typically the lowest of the three bids is the one accepted, unless there is substantial justification to go with one of the other vendors. Alternatives to purchasing equipment immediately include the use of equipment loan programs. This way the employee can try out the device for a time before deciding on purchasing it. Once accommodations are in place, training and follow-up with the technology are essential (see Chapter 4). After the person has had some time to use the accommodations, it is beneficial to meet with him or her to evaluate the effectiveness of the accommodations and to determine whether additional accommodations are needed. Both the training and follow-up help ensure that the technology is being used appropriately and functioning as expected. A summary of the roles and responsibilities of the ATP during the vocational accommodation process is shown in Box 16-4.

An excellent resource for ATPs working in the area of workplace accommodation is the Job Accommodation Network (JAN). The President's Committee on Employment of People with Disabilities established JAN in 1984 as an information and consulting service. JAN has consultants who, via the phone and its Web site *(http://www.jan.wvu.edu/)*, provide information about job accommodations and the employability of people with disabilities. JAN provides the inquiring individual with suggestions and prices and can also give names and numbers of employers and workers who have made similar accommodations.

EVALUATION OF ASSISTIVE TECHNOLOGY INTERVENTION IN THE WORKPLACE

The final aspect of the process outlined by de Jonge et al (2007) is evaluation of the use of assistive technology in the workplace. At the outset of the intervention, the ATP and the consumer, with the employer when appropriate, will have identified goals related to assistive technology use in the workplace. Once a trial period is over and a reasonable length of time has elapsed, the ATP should evaluate the effectiveness of the intervention. The goals could be associated with accomplishment of specific work tasks, using assistive technology, ability to move around in the environment, communicate, and manipulate needed objects. The Canadian Occupational Performance Measure (Law et al, 1998) is a useful measure of client-identified goals. Specific outcome measures such as the Quebec User Evaluation of Satisfaction with Assistive Technology (Demers, Weiss-Lambrou, and Ska, 2002) and the Psychosocial Impact of Assistive Devices Scale (Jutai and Day, 2002) are outcome measures that are specifically designed to evaluate the outcome of assistive technology use. These measures were described in Chapter 4. If the outcomes have been met satisfactorily, then the ATP's involvement with the client may be suspended until the client identifies a further need. If the outcome has not been met, then the process such as the one described by de Jonge et al (2007) is reinitiated.

SUMMARY

This chapter described the vocational application of assistive technologies using the HAAT model as a framework. Employees who have disabilities engage in communication activities such as reading and writing; manipulation activities such as filing and assembly; and mobility activities such as sitting, standing, and lifting. The types of accommodations available in each of these areas involve both strategies and technologies. The four aspects of the context (physical, social, cultural, and institutional) dramatically affect assistive technology effectiveness in the workplace. The emergence of the ADA and the Amendments to the Rehabilitation Act has affected the ways in which assistive technologies are applied and supported. Many characteristics of hard and soft assistive technologies are important in ensuring that they meet the needs of employees and employers. Strategies for successfully implementing assistive technology into the workplace were identified.

Study Questions

1. What are the three major activities related to assistive technology use in the workplace?
2. What tasks are important in communication-related work activities?
3. What skills are required to ensure success in reading?
4. What tasks are important in manipulation-related work activities?
5. What tasks are important in mobility-related work activities?
6. What types of activities of daily living might an individual with a disability need to complete in the workplace, and what implications do they have for the work setting?
7. What physical factors may affect the use of assistive technology in the work setting?
8. Identify six key questions to ask when evaluating the mobility accessibility in the workplace.
9. Discuss four elements of legislation concerning employment of persons with disabilities that provide key information for the assistive technology provider.
10. What social and cultural factors may affect the use of assistive technology in the work setting?
11. Describe the intentions of Title I of the Americans with Disabilities Act.
12. What does *essential functions of the job* mean and how is this concept applied to vocational access for persons who have disabilities?
13. What is meant by *reasonable accommodation* in the workplace?
14. List three factors that are essential to effective assistive technology service delivery to meet vocational needs.
15. What is the role of the vocational rehabilitation counselor?
16. What is an IPE, and how are assistive technologies incorporated into it?
17. Who might be part of a team involved in job accommodation?
18. What are the advantages of carrying out a vocational assistive technology assessment at the work site?
19. Identify the roles of the ATP in vocational assistive technology service delivery.
20. What type of information should be gathered from the consumer during the assessment?
21. Identify modifications that might be made to an employee's workstation.
22. Identify potential accommodations for an employee who has a visual impairment and works as a paralegal.
23. Identify potential modifications for an employee with a motor impairment who works in an office setting.

References

Berthoud R: *The employment rates of disabled people*, Leeds, UK, 2006, Department of Work and Pensions, Controller of Her Majesty's Stationery Office.

Butterfield TM, Ramseur JH: Research and case study findings in the area of workplace accommodations including provisions for assistive technology: a literature review, *Technol Disabil* 16:201-210, 2004.

Canadian Council on Social Development: Persons with disabilities on the job, *Canadian Council on Social Development's Disability Information Sheet*, 18 (2002): www.ccsd.ca/drip. Accessed Jan 2007.

Canadian Council on Social Development: Workers with disabilities and the impact of workplace structures, *Canadian Council on Social Development's Disability Information Sheet*, 16 (2004): www.ccsd.ca/drip. Accessed Jan 2007.

Canadian Council on Social Development: Employment of persons with disabilities in Canada, *Canadian Council on Social Development's Disability Information Sheet*, 18 (2005): www.ccsd.ca/drip. Accessed Jan 2007.

Chan F et al: Drivers of workplace discrimination against people with disabilities: the utility of Attribution Theory, *Work* 25:77-88, 2005.

Cossette L: *A profile of disability in Canada*, Ottawa, 2002, Minister of Industry.

de Jonge DM, Scherer MJ, Rodger SA: *Assistive technology in the workplace*, St Louis, 2007, Mosby Elsevier.

Demers L, Weiss-Lambrou R, Ska B: The Quebec User Evaluation of Satisfaction with Assistive Technology (QUEST2.0): an overview and recent progress, *Technol Disabil* 14:101-105, 2002.

Driscoll MP, Rodger SA, de Jonge DM: Factors that prevent or assist the integration of assistive technology into the workplace for people with spinal cord injuries: perspectives of the users and their employers and co-workers, *J Voc Rehabil* 16:53-66, 2001.

Flynn CC, Clark MC: Rehabilitation technology assessment practices in vocational rehabilitation agencies, *Assist Technol* 7:111-118, 1995.

Fougeyrollas P: The influence of the social environment on the social participation of people with disabilities. In Christiansen C, Baum C, editors: *Occupational therapy: enabling function and well-being,* ed 2, Thorofare, NJ, 1997, Slack.

Fougeyrollas P, Gray DB: Classification systems, environmental factors and social change. In Gray DB, Quatrano LA, Lieberman ML, editors: *Designing and using assistive technology: the human perspective,* Baltimore, 1998, Paul H Brookes, pp 13-28.

Frieden L: Disability policy in the United States. In National Institute of Disability Management and Research: *Strategies for success: disability management in the workplace,* Fort Alberni, BC, Canada, 1997, National Institute of Disability Management.

Gamble MJ, Dowler DL, Orslene LE: Assistive technology: choosing the right tool for the right job, *J Voc Rehabil,* 24:73-80, 2006.

Garcia LJ, Laroche C, Barrette J: Work integration issues go beyond the nature of the communication disorder, *J Comm Dis* 35:187-211, 2002.

Gillen G: Case report—improving activities of daily living performance in an adult with ataxia, *Am J Occup Ther* 54: 89-96, 2000.

Job Accommodation Network: Discover the facts about job accommodation (2000): www.jan.wvu.edu/.htm. Accessed March 13, 2000.

Jutai JJ, Day, H: Psychosocial Impact of Assistive Devices Scale (PIADS), *Technol Disabil* 14:107-111, 2002.

King G, Brown E, Smith L, editors: *Resilience: learning from the turning points of people with disabilities.* Westport, CT, 2003, Greenwood Publishing Group.

Langton AJ, Hughes JK: Back to work, *Team Rehabil Rep* 3: 14-18, 1992.

Langton AJ, Ramseur H: Enhancing employment outcomes through job accommodation and assistive technology resources and services, *J Voc Rehabil* 16:27-37, 2001.

Law M et al. *Canadian Occupational Performance Measure,* ed.3, Toronto, ON, 1998, CAOT/ACE.

Lund ML, Nygard, L: Incorporating or resisting assistive devices: different approaches to achieving a desired occupational self-image, *Occup Ther J Res* 23:67-75, 2003.

McNaughton D, Light J, Groszyk L: "Don't give up": Employment experiences of individuals with amytrophic lateral sclerosis who use augmentative and alternative communication, *Augment Altern Comm* 17:179-195, 2001.

McNeal DR, Somerville NJ, Wilson DJ: Work problems and accommodations reported by person who are postpolio or have a spinal cord injury, *Assist Technol* 11:137-157, 1999.

Mueller J: *The workplace workbook: an illustrated guide to job accommodations and assistive technology,* Washington, DC, 1990, Dole Foundation.

National Council on Disability: *Federal policy barriers to assistive technology* (2000): www.ncd.gov/newsroom/publications/1. Accessed May 31, 2000.

Peck B, Kirkbride LT: Why businesses don't employ people with disabilities, *J Voc Rehabil* 16:71-75, 2001.

Rehabilitation Research and Training Center on Disability Demographics and Statistics: *2004 Disability Status Reports United States,* Ithaca NY, 2005, Cornell University.

Reimer-Reiss ML, Wacker RR: Factors associated with assistive technology discontinuance among individuals with disabilities, *J Rehabil* 66:44-50, 2000.

Rumrill PD, Schuyler BR, Longden JC: Profiles of on-the-job accommodations needed by professional employees who are blind, *J Vis Impair Blind* 91:66-77, 1997.

Scherer MJ: Workplace technology device predisposition assessment, *The Matching Person and Technology (MPT) Model Manual and Assessment,* Webster NY: 2005, Institute for Matching Person and Technology.

Simonds WS: AT, disability, and widgets: corporate priorities in the use of assistive technology. CSUN 16th Annual International Conference (2001): www.csun.edu/cod/conf2001/proceedings/0192simonds.html. Accessed March 2001.

Strobel W et al: Technology for access to text and graphics for people with visual impairments and blindness in vocational settings, *J Voc Rehabil* 24:87-95, 2006.

U.S. Equal Employment Opportunity Commission, U.S. Department of Justice Civil Rights Division: Americans with Disabilities Act: questions and answers (1996): www.usdoj.gov/crt/ada/qandaeng.htm. Accessed July 1996.

Zwerling C et al: Workplace accommodations for people with disabilities: National Health Interview survey disability supplement, 1994-1995, *J Occup Environ Med* 45:517-525, 2003.

Abbreviation expansion: An augmentative and alternative communication or computer access technique in which a shortened form of a word or phrase (the abbreviation) stands for the entire word or phrase (the expansion); abbreviations are automatically expanded by the device

Abductor: A seating component used to keep the legs in a neutral abducted position; also referred to as *pommel* or *medial knee support*

Academic participation: A framework for considering four levels of participation in classroom activities: (1) competitive, (2) active, (3) involved, and (4) no academic expectations

Acceleration vocabularies: Used by literate persons to increase the rate of communication through both selection of whole words and spelling

Acceptance time: A method used for selection of an item in a scanning system that is based on the user's pausing for a preset period, after which the entry is made

Accessibility options: Software adaptations included in Windows that address common problems that persons with disabilities have in using a standard keyboard

Activation characteristics: The method of activation, deactivation, effort, displacement, flexibility, and durability of a control interface

Activity: The portion of the human activity–assistive technology model that defines the goal (e.g., cooking, writing, playing tennis) of the assistive technology system

Alerting devices: Sensory devices that detect sounds (e.g., alarm clock, doorbell, telephone ring) and then cause a vibration or a flashing light signal, or both, to call attention to the sound for a person who is deaf

Alpha testing: Evaluation of a production prototype; in assistive technologies it is often one or two units

Alternative: In assistive technologies, a different way of accomplishing the same task

Alternative input: Technologies that offer the user different modalities for providing input commands or information to a device (e.g., voice recognition software)

Alternative mobility device: An assistive device intended to assist a person who is blind in orientation and mobility

Alternative output: Technologies that offer users a nontraditional means of acquiring feedback or information from a device (e.g., braille or auditory information substituted for visual displays)

Alternative sensory system: The use of a different sensory channel to substitute for a nonfunctional one; common examples of this approach are the use of braille for reading by persons with visual impairment (tactile substitution for visual) and the use of manual sign language by persons who are deaf (visual substitution for auditory)

Antitip devices: Small wheels, attached to a rod and mounted at the back of the chair that prevent the chair from tipping backwards

Aphasia: Language disorder affecting both expression and reception of spoken and written language

Appeals process: The means whereby the assistive technology practitioner can appeal a funding denial

Apraxia: An inability to plan motor movements, where the peripheral components necessary to execute the motion are generally intact

Armrest: Part of a wheelchair that provides support for the user's arms; they may be fixed or removable and may be height adjustable

Assessment: A process through which information about the consumer is gathered and analyzed so that appropriate assistive technologies (hard and soft) can be recommended and a plan for intervention developed

Assistive listening devices: A class of assistive devices that are intended to be used in group settings such as in lecture halls, churches, business meetings, courtrooms, and broadcast television to amplify sounds and broadcast them to receivers worn by persons who are hard of hearing

Assistive technology: A broad range of devices, services, strategies, and practices that are conceived and applied to ameliorate the problems faced by individuals who have disabilities

Assistive technology practitioner (ATP): A specialist in assistive technology application; typically has a professional background in engineering, occupational therapy, physical therapy, recreation therapy, special education, speech-language pathology, or vocational rehabilitation counseling

Assistive technology service: Any service that directly assists an individual with a disability in the selection, acquisition, or use of an assistive technology device

545

Assistive technology supplier (ATS): One who provides enabling technology in the areas of wheeled mobility, seating and alternative positioning, ambulation assistance, environmental control, and activities of daily living

Assistive technology system: An assistive technology device, a human operator who has a disability, and a context in which the functional activity is to be carried out

Attention: The mechanism for continued cognitive processing or the ability to focus on a particular stimulus

Augmentative and alternative communication (AAC): Approaches and systems that are designed to ameliorate the problems faced by persons who have difficulty speaking or writing because of neuromuscular disease or injury

Augmentative manipulation: Assistance in doing a manipulative task in the same manner as it is normally done

Automatic scanning: Items are presented continuously by the device at an adjustable rate, with selection of the choice made by activating the switch and stopping the scan; entry is by an additional switch press or acceptance time

Bariatrics: A term that describes the practice of medicine concerning individuals who are significantly overweight; derived from the Greek *baros* meaning weight and *iatrics* meaning medical treatment

Beta testing: Evaluation of a set of prototypes that form an initial production run

Bidding process: Process used by third-party funding sources before making any assistive technology equipment purchases. Assistive technology that has been recommended for an individual is submitted to three outside vendors for a bid. Typically, the lowest of the three bids is accepted

Booster seat: Position the child so the vehicle seat belts fit properly. The vehicle seat belt provides restraint when a booster seat is used

Braille: Raised dots that can be read by touch; a cell of either six or eight dots is used to portray letters and special computer symbols (e.g., cursor movement, uppercase and lowercase)

Camber: The degree to which the wheel is mounted off vertical, usually 1 to 4 degrees. Camber tips the wheel so the top is closer to the user's body. When the wheels are set this way, the wheelchair becomes more stable and propulsion is more efficient.

Center of gravity: The point in the body at which the acceleration caused by gravity is localized

Center of mass: Point in the center of an object of any shape around which the gravitational forces acting on the body balance each other. The center of mass of an empty wheelchair is located under the seat, in front of the drive wheels

Center of pressure: Center of gravitational forces when measured in posterior-anterior and lateral planes

Central processing: Human functions of perception, cognition, neuromuscular control (including motor planning), and psychological factors

Central processing unit (CPU): The portion of a computer that executes a set of instructions assembled in the form of a program, accepts input (e.g., from keyboard or mouse), sends output (e.g., to a printer or speech synthesizer), and transfers data among the internal components

Chain drive: A power wheelchair in which the motor and wheel axle are coupled through a drive chain with gears at each end

CHAMPUS: A federally funded program that provides medical benefits to active duty and retired members of the armed forces and their dependents

Child vehicle restraint system: A car seat that provides occupant protection for children who are too small to be properly secured by the vehicle seat belt assembly

Circular scanning: An approach in which the selection set is organized in a circular pattern

Clear-path indicator: A sensory device that provides signals to the user only if an object is detected in a field about 2 feet in diameter and about 6 feet from the user

Closed captioning: A process whereby the audio portion of a television program is converted into written words, which appear in a window on the screen

Closed circuit television (CCTV): A video camera and monitor used to enlarge text and other print material; also called *video magnifiers*

Cochlear implant: An auditory prosthesis that provides some sound perception by directly applying electrical stimulation to the basilar membrane of the cochlea

Coded access: A form of indirect selection in which the individual uses a distinct sequence of movements to input a code for each item in the selection set

Cognition: The process of understanding and knowing which involves the skills of attention, memory, problem solving, decision making, learning, language, and other related tasks

Cognitive prosthesis: An entire system of hardware, software and personal assistance that is individualized to meet specific intellectual or mental processing needs

Command domain: The set of assistive device functions available to the user

Compact disk–read-only memory (CD-ROM): Optical storage of data and programs; uses lasers to read and write data to optical disks

Compression: Occurs when forces act toward each other (pushing together), such as the force of the vertebrae on the disks in the spinal column

Concept keyboard: A keyboard in which the letters and numbers are replaced with pictures, symbols, or words that represent the concepts being used or taught

Consumer: The end user of the assistive technology system

Contexts: The portion of the human activity–assistive technology model that includes four major considerations: (1) setting (e.g., at home, at work, in the community), (2) social context (with peers, with strangers), (3) cultural context, and (4) physical context (measured by temperature, moisture, light)

Continuous input: When the inputs to a device are ongoing, with an infinite number of possible values (e.g., volume control on a radio)

Control enhancers: Aids and strategies that enhance or extend the physical control (range or resolution) a person has available to use a control interface

Control interface: The hardware (e.g., keyboard, joystick) by which the user operates an assistive technology system or controls a device

Conversation: Augmentative and alternative communication needs that would typically be accomplished by speech if it were available

Coverage vocabularies: A set of topics and concepts that can be used for basic communication by a person who cannot spell; may consist of pictures, symbols, or words

Crashworthiness: Performance of a wheelchair and seating system in a 21 g/48 km frontal impact crash simulation

Criteria for service: The recognition of a need for assistive technology services that triggers a referral for services

Criterion-referenced measurement: A measurement in which the person's own skill level in using the system is used as the standard

DAISY (Digital Audio-Based Information System): An international consortium of organizations that produce reading material for the blind; has developed standards for digital books on tape

Dampening: The ability of a material to soften on impact

Dementia: A syndrome, or a pattern of clinical symptoms and signs, that can be defined by the following three points: (1) decline of cognitive capacity with some effect on day-to-day functioning, (2) impairment in multiple areas of cognition (global), and (3) normal level of consciousness

Density: The ratio of the weight of a material to its volume

Dependent mobility: Mobility systems that are propelled by an attendant (e.g., strollers, geriatric wheelchairs, and transport chairs)

Desktop robots: General-purpose manipulators that create full access to an area dedicated to the performance of a specific job or activity (a workstation)

Development: The combination of growth and learning leading to changes in a child

Device: A piece of hardware or software used by an individual to accomplish a task

Device characteristics: General properties of the hard technology portions of an assistive technology system

Diagnosis codes: Describe the person's condition or medical reason for the services being requested; the key to establishing medical necessity

Digital recording: Human speech is stored in electronic memory circuits for later retrieval

Digital talking books (DTBs): Reading material for individuals who are blind; produced on digital media (usually CD-ROM) and that can be reproduced and read on a variety of hardware platforms and operating systems

Direct consumer services: Assistive technology services provided to a consumer

Direct drive: A power wheelchair in which the motor is directly coupled to the wheels through a gearbox

Direct selection: An approach in which the individual is able to use the control interface to randomly choose any of the items in the selection set

Directed scanning: An approach in which the user activates the control interface to select the direction of the scan, vertically or horizontally, and then sends a signal to stop at the desired choice; entry is by an additional switch press or acceptance time

Disability: Results when an impairment leads to an inability to "perform an activity in the manner or within the range considered normal for a human being" (WHO ICIDH; termed *activity* in WHO ICIDH-2 [ICF] 2001)

Discrete inputs: Control interfaces with a set of fixed values from which the user can choose

Distributed controls: An approach used when multiple devices are controlled and each has its own control interface

Driving evaluation: Assessment by a trained evaluator of an individual's ability to drive a vehicle. A driving evaluation usually has two components: an off-road assessment that is paper- or computer-based and an on-road component with a trained evaluator

Dynamic communication displays: An input mode used in augmentative and alternative communication in which the selection set displayed to the user is changed as new choices are made; can be altered easily depending on previous choices and allows reliance on recognition rather than recall

Dysarthria: A disorder of motor speech control resulting from central or peripheral nervous system damage; characterized by weakness, slowness, and incoordination of the muscles necessary for speech

Ease of Access: Software adaptation included within Microsoft Vista operating system that addresses common problems that persons with disabilities have in using a standard keyboard or accessing visual or auditory information

Easy Access: Software adaptations included in Apple Macintosh operating systems that address common problems that persons with disabilities have in using a standard keyboard

Effectors: The neural, muscular, and skeletal elements of the human body that provide movement or motor output

Electrically powered feeders: Electrically powered devices that scoop food off a plate and raise it to mouth level; may also include rotation of the plate to position the food for scooping

Electrically powered page turners: Devices that hold a book or other reading material and mechanically turn the pages when a switch or switches are pressed by the user

Electrically powered wheelchair: A wheeled mobility base with a power drive to the wheels, a control interface that the consumer uses to direct the movement of the wheelchair, an electronic controller, and powered accessories (e.g., recline, tilt)

Electronic aid to daily living (EADL): Device that allows control of appliances (e.g., radio, television, CD player, telephone) through the use of one or more switches

Electronic travel aid (ETA): Sensory devices that supplement rather than replace the long cane or guide dog; designed to provide additional environmental information and to detect those obstacles typically missed by the long cane

Emulation: Replacement of one type of computer input (typically the keyboard or mouse) with another more accessible form (e.g., head mouse or scanning input)

Engram: A preprogrammed pattern of muscular activity represented centrally

Envelopment: The degree to which the person sinks into a seating cushion and the degree to which the cushion surrounds the buttocks

Environmental control units (ECUs): *See electronic aid to daily living (EADL)*

Environmental sensor: The portion of a sensory device that detects the data that the human cannot obtain through his or her own sensory system

Equilibrium: The situation in which the force generated by one object is equal in magnitude and opposite in direction to the force generated by another object

Ergonomic keyboards: Designed to reduce the strain placed on the hands and wrists during the repetitive motion of keying

Essential functions: Those job duties that are so fundamental to the position that the individual holds or desires that he or she cannot do the job without performing them

Expert systems: Computer-based software that assists in the decision-making process for assistive technologies

Extrinsic enablers: An equivalent term for *assistive technologies*

Fee-for-service: The traditional method of payment for health care under which providers are paid a certain rate per unit of service

Fixed deformity: A permanent change taking place in the bones, muscles, capsular ligaments, or tendons that restricts the normal range of motion of the particular joint and affects the skeletal alignment of the other joints

Flexible deformity: Appearance of a deformity as a result of increased tone and muscle tightness causing the person to assume certain postures; externally applied resistance (passive stretch) in the opposite direction allows movement of the joint and reduction in the "deformity"

Follow-along: The portion of the service delivery process in which a mechanism for regular contact with the consumer is established to see whether further assistive technology services are indicated

Follow-up: The portion of the service delivery process that determines whether the system as a whole is functioning effectively

Force: Anything that acts on a body to change its rate of acceleration or alter its momentum

Forward-facing child seat: Child vehicle restraint system that is installed for long-term use in a vehicle and provides occupant protection for children over the age of 12 months who are between 20 and 40 pounds and up to 40 inches in height

Friction drive: Power wheelchair systems that apply a driving force through a roller attached to the motor and pressed against the tire

Frictional forces: Resulting forces from movement in opposite directions between two bodies in contact; may be static or dynamic

Front rigging: Leg rests and footplates on a wheelchair that support the user's feet

Fulcrum: The axis around which rotational movements occur

Function allocation: The allocation of functions in any human/device system in which some functions are allocated to the human, some to the device, and some to the personal assistant services

Functional equivalency: Obtaining the same function in very different ways; for example, turning pages in a book can also be accomplished by a mechanical page turner or electronic books accessed by computer methods

Functional performance measures: Measurements that address whether the individual can accomplish tasks that he or she could not do without the assistive technology

Functional task position: A forward-sitting posture in which the line of gravity runs just in front of the ischial tuberosities and then intersects the spine; can be obtained either with maximal flexion of the spine and little or no pelvic rotation or with a straighter spine and forward rotation of the pelvis

General input device–emulating interface (GIDEI): Hardware or software adaptations to a computer that allow emulation of the mouse, the keyboard, or both

General-purpose manipulation device: Designed to accomplish a variety of manipulative tasks; examples are robotic systems and electronic aids to daily living

Graphical user interface (GUI): Characterized by three distinguishing features: (1) a mouse pointer, which is moved around the screen; (2) a graphical menu bar, which appears on the screen; and (3) one or more windows, which provide a menu of choices

Graphics: Augmentative and alternative communication needs that are typically accomplished with a pencil and paper, typewriter, computer, calculator, or similar tools; includes writing, drawing, mathematics, and Internet access

Gravitational line: The axis of the body along which the force of gravity acts

Group-item scan: An approach that is used to increase the rate of selection during scanning by grouping the selection set and allowing the user to first select a group and then the desired item in the group

Growth: Changes that occur in a child as a result of physical development of the central nervous system

Handicap: Results when the individual with an impairment or disability is unable to fulfill his or her normal role (WHO ICIDH; termed participation in WHO ICIDH-2 (ICF])

Head pointers: Devices with a pointer attached to a headband that are used for direct manipulation

Health-related quality of life: The impact of health services on the overall quality of life of individuals; represents the functional effect of an illness and its consequent therapy

Hearing aids: Sensory devices that provide amplification of sounds, including speech, for individuals who are hard of hearing

Hoist lift: A system for transporting a powered wheelchair in a van in which the wheelchair is attached with straps to an arm that swings out from the van door and lowers the wheelchair to the ground

Human activity–assistive technology (HAAT) model: A framework describing the major elements of an assistive technology system; consists of four parts: (1) activity, (2) context, (3) human skills, and (4) assistive technologies

Human/technology interface: The portion of the assistive technology system with which the user interacts

Icon prediction: A feature of Minspeak-based devices that aids in recalling stored sequences

Impairment: Any loss or abnormality of psychological, physical, or anatomical structure or function

Implementation phase: The portion of the service delivery process in which the recommended technology is ordered, modified, and fabricated as necessary; set up; delivered to the consumer; and initial training takes place

Inclusion: Students with disabilities who are integrated into the regular educational programs for at least part of the school day

Independent manual mobility: Systems in which the user has the ability to propel the device by body power only

Independent powered mobility: Motorized wheelchairs that are controlled by the user

Indirect selection: An approach in which there are intermediary steps involved in making a selection; includes scanning and coded access; typically the control interface used is a single switch or an array of switches

Individual Education Plan (IEP): Mandated by IDEA, the plan, written for each student, incorporates the student's specialized program. The IEP team must consider assistive technologies as a special factor when developing the learner's IEP

Individual Written Rehabilitation Plan (IWRP): A plan used by vocational rehabilitation agencies that is jointly developed by the vocational counselor and the consumer achieve the consumer's employment objective; the IWRP considers assistive technologies as part of the services received by the consumer

Individuals with Disabilities Education Act (IDEA): Defines assistive technology devices and assistive technology services in an educational context; mandates that local educational agencies be responsible for providing assistive technology devices and services if these are required as part of a child's educational needs, related services, or as a supplementary aid or service

Information processor: The portion of a sensory aid that converts the raw sensory data from the environmental sensor to a form suitable for presentation by the user display

Infrared (IR) transmission: Devices that use invisible light to remotely control an electronic aid to daily living; consists of a transmitter unit, which is either hand held or mounted on a wheelchair, and a set of receivers, one for each appliance to be controlled

Input domain: The number of independent inputs, or signals, generated by the control interface; may be either discrete or continuous

Integrated control: An approach used when multiple devices are controlled with one control interface

Internet: Worldwide computer network available by modem that connects users globally for electronic mail, file transfer, electronic commerce, and similar functions

Intrinsic enablers: General underlying abilities that individuals use to perform activities and tasks

Inverse scanning: An approach in which the scan is initiated by the individual's activating and holding a switch closed, with selection of the desired item indicated by releasing the switch; entry is by an additional switch press or acceptance time

Knowledge representation: All the information and skills that have been learned (e.g., the alphabet, how to wash our hands, that gravity makes things fall, the colors of the rainbow)

Large accessible transit vehicles: Public transit vehicles that provide transportation for multiple individuals with disabilities. Provision is made in these vehicles for wheelchair securement.

Learner-teacher interactions: The way in which teachers present information to learners and the interaction expected of those learners in a classroom situation

Learning: Changes that occur in a person because of contact with some environmental influence

Learning disabilities: Disorders in which one has near-normal mental abilities in general but a deficit in the comprehension or use of spoken or written language. These disabilities may be manifested as a significant difficulty with reading, writing, reasoning, or mathematical ability.

Learning styles: The manner that is most appropriate for the acquisition of knowledge by the student; includes aural versus visual learning, types of problem solving used by the learner, and group interaction skills

Least restrictive environment: The degree of acceptable modification in a job or academic program

Lever arm: The distance from the fulcrum to the point that a force is applied

Lightweight wheelchair: A wheelchair that weighs less than the standard chair and has greater flexibility in choice of seat width and adjustment of back height

Line of application: The particular direction along which forces are applied, either pushing or pulling

Linear scan: An approach in which the selection set is organized in a linear (straight-line) format

Low-shear systems: Systems in which the back hinges to the seat in a manner that reduces the movement of tissue across the seating surface during tilting or reclining of the seat

Magnification aids: Low vision aids for reading print material

Managed care: Any method of health care delivery designed to reduce unnecessary use of services and provide for cost containment while ensuring that high-quality care or performance is maintained

Manipulatives: Rods, blocks, buttons, beads, or other objects that vary by color, length, and weight and that can be sorted, counted, and used to enhance concept development in mathematics

Manual wheelchair: Wheelchair that the user propels with his or her own muscle power

Media presentation: The way in which information is presented on a computer screen, Web site, or other display. Careful attention to media presentation can avoid extraneous information that might be distracting.

Medicaid: A health insurance program, established in 1965 by Title XIX of the Social Security Act, administered at the state level for persons who are unable to pay the costs of their medical care

Medical necessity: A specific criterion for funding under Medicare, Medicaid, and private health insurance that requires identification of a medical diagnosis or condition that is specifically coupled to the functional impairment being addressed by the device

Medicare: The health insurance program operated by the U.S. government; covers individuals aged 65 years and older and those adults under age 65 years who are blind, are totally and permanently disabled, and have received Social Security Disability Insurance (SSDI) benefits or Adult Disabled Child benefits for at least 24 months

Memory: Often considered to have three components: (1) sensory memory, (2) short-term memory, and (3) long-term memory, each playing a role in assistive technology use

Mobile assistive robots: Devices that can move from one location to another to accomplish manipulative tasks under the control of a user who has a disability; two general classes: (1) wheelchair mounted and (2) mounted on a mobile base that is controllable by the user

Mobility: Allows movement that enables function in a seated or standing position

Modular power base: A power wheelchair design that maximizes power by attaching the motors directly to the wheels (direct drive); using small, heavy-duty wheels; and eliminating the cross-brace folding structure to increase strength and maneuverability

Moment: See *torque*

Morphology: The rules for organizing the smallest meaningful units of language, called *morphemes*

Motivation: Any influence that gives rise to performance

Motor control: The result of the integration of sensory, perceptual, and cognitive components into a motor pattern that is executed by the effectors

Mouthsticks: Devices that are held in the teeth and are used for direct manipulation

Multitasking: The capability of an operating system to pause while running one software program to run another program

Muscle tone: The resistance to stretch provided by neural activity, viscoelastic properties of muscle and joints, and sensory feedback to the central nervous system

Musical instrument digital interface (MIDI): A file used to store music as a series of notes with volume and duration attached; allows music to be played back through a sound card in a computer

Needs identification: The portion of the assessment during which more detailed specification of the consumer's assistive technology needs is made

Nonproportional control: Electrically powered wheelchair control that operates the chair at a predetermined speed in a selected direction. The speed is not proportional to the displacement of the joystick.

Norm-referenced measurements: The ranking of the performance of the individual or system according to a sample of scores others have achieved on the task

Numerical codes: A number is used to stand for a word, complete phrase, or sentence; when the user enters the number, the device converts it into the word, phrase, or sentence

Occupation: Everything that people do to look after themselves and others, to contribute to their community and society, and to have fun and relax

Occupational competence: The ability to meet the demands that are required for successful engagement in various life roles

On-screen keyboard: Emulation method that uses a video image of the keyboard on the video screen, together with a cursor

Operational competence: Skills required for the individual and his aides to use the basic features of the assistive technology device

Optical aids: Devices that allow individuals with low vision to see print, do work requiring fine detail, or increase the range of their visual fields

Optical character recognition (OCR): A software program that runs on a standard PC; its primary function is to analyze the raw video data and assemble it into letters, spaces, and punctuation for synthetic speech or braille output

Optimal use: The use of an assistive technology that is the greatest possible given the user's skill

Orientation and mobility: The process by which an individual who is blind is able to achieve independent movement in the environment

Original equipment manufacturer: The manufacturer that produces and markets products in their original format (e.g., an automobile company is considered to be the original equipment manufacturer of vehicles)

Outcome measures: Used to evaluate the end result of the assistive technology intervention

Parallel port: A computer output used to send bytes of data as a whole; requires a larger number of wires and is faster than a serial port; commonly used in printers and some speech synthesizers

Paralysis: Significantly reduced (or absent) muscle strength preventing the use of certain effectors; muscle weakness caused by partial paralysis that makes it difficult to move but does not prevent movement is called *paresis*

Participation model: A framework for the identification of potential barriers to educational access, especially those that can be addressed through the application of assistive technologies; two types of barriers are identified—opportunity and access

PASS (Plan for Achieving Self-Sufficiency): A program that allows individuals to put aside income for equipment or services that will assist them in achieving a vocational objective

Peer training: Instruction that introduces assistive technologies to the classmates of the learner who has a disability

Pelvic obliquity: One side of the pelvis is higher than the other when viewed in the frontal plane

Pelvic rotation: One side of the pelvis is forward of the other side

Perception: The interpretation and assignment of meaning to data received from biological sensors; involves an interaction between information derived from sensed data and information stored in memory on the basis of previous sensory experience

Performance aid: A document or device containing information that an individual uses to assist in the completion of an activity

Performance areas: Activities of daily living, work and productive activities, and play and leisure

Phonology: The sounds used in any particular language and the rules for their organization

Planar: Flat seating components that support the body only where it easily comes into contact with the supporting system

Power assist: A power system that only supplies power to the manual wheelchair when needed by the user, such as when going up an incline

Pragmatics: The relationship between language and language users

Predictive selection: A feature of scanning Minspeak-based augmentative and alternative communication systems in which only valid following icons in a sequence are scanned after the initial icon is selected

Pressure: Force per unit area

Pressure ulcer: A lesion that develops as a result of unrelieved pressure to an area and that results in damage to underlying tissue

Primary driving controls: Adapted driving system components that are used to stop (brakes), go (accelerator), and steer

Primitive reflex: Characterized by immediate and automatic movement performed at a subconscious level, usually initiated by sensory stimulation

Problem solving: A process for which the goal is to overcome obstacles obstructing a path to a solution.

Procedure codes: A numerical system used to describe the services that the provider carried out and is billing for; the most commonly used procedure coding system is the Common Procedure Coding System (HCPCS) of the Health Care Financing Administration (HCFA)

Product liability: Exposure to legal action on the basis of deficiencies in products or failure to warn of dangers to the user of a product

Professional liability: Exposure to legal action on the basis of professional services that are improperly provided

Programmable controllers: An electronic aid to daily living approach that is based on the storage of user-selected codes that are appropriate to a wide range of appliances; entering the correct code into the controller allows control of the appliance by the user

Prompting systems: Those devices or software packages that inform a user that an action should be taken and provide visual, verbal, or auditory cues as to how to accomplish a task.

Propelling structure: The portion of a manual wheelchair consisting of the wheels and an interface that the consumer uses to move the wheelchair; the portion of a power wheelchair consisting of a wheeled mobility base with a power drive to the wheels, a control interface that the consumer uses to direct the movement of the wheelchair, an electronic controller, and powered accessories (e.g., recline, ventilator)

Proportional control: With 360 degree directionality, the wheelchair moves in whichever direction the joystick is displaced; the greater the displacement, the faster the chair moves

Prototype: The initial new device that is produced as the product of engineering development

Psychosocial function: Consists of self-identity, self-protection, and motivation. These factors are related to the person's acceptance of a disability, the approach a person takes to the assistive technology, and the ultimate effectiveness of the assistive technology for the person

Public funding sources: Government funding at the federal, state, or local levels

Push handles: Used by an attendant or caregiver to maneuver the wheelchair

Qualified individual with a disability: A person who has the skills, education, experience, or other requirements needed for a job and can perform the essential functions of the position with or without reasonable accommodation

Qualitative measurement: Assumes that each individual has a different experience and that it is important to provide the opportunity to capture that experience. There is no attempt to measure a particular construct. Rather, the purpose is to describe and understand the user's experience with the technology. Qualitative assessments may include observation, either directly or by videotape, or interview with the client and others.

Quality assurance: Involves a program of evaluation of the quality of services rendered and the effectiveness of the devices supplied

Quality-of-life measures: Assesses the effectiveness of assistive technology devices and services in the broader social context of the impact on the user's overall life

Quantitative measurement: A measurement in which an indefinite amount or number is obtained (e.g., a numerical scale from 1 to 5 may be assigned to a given measurement, or the measurement may be in terms of a physical parameter such as weight)

Radiofrequency (RF) transmission: Devices that use electromagnetic (radio) signals to remotely control an electronic aid to daily living; consists of a transmitter unit, which is either hand held or mounted on a wheelchair, and a set of receivers, one for each appliance to be controlled

Random access memory (RAM): Computer memory used for temporary storage of data; only active when power is provided to the computer

Range: Maximal extent of movement of an effector

Rate enhancement: Augmentative and alternative communication and computer access approaches that result in the number of characters generated being greater than the number of selections the individual makes

Reacher: A handle grip attached to a stem that is used to control the jaws of a device for grasping an object

Reading aid: A sensory device designed to provide access to print materials for an individual who is blind

Read-only memory (ROM): Computer memory used for permanent commands and instructions that are required to allow the computer to function; cannot be erased and reprogrammed in normal operation

Rear-facing infant seat: A child vehicle restraint system designed to provide occupant protection for children under the age of 12 months who weigh equal to or less than 20-22 pounds

Reasonable accommodation: Any modification or adjustment to a job or the work or educational environment that will enable a qualified applicant, employee, or learner with a disability to participate in the application process, perform essential job functions, or participate fully in the educational program; also includes adjustments to ensure that a qualified individual with a disability has rights and privileges in employment and education equal to those of employees without disabilities

Recall: The type of memory that relies exclusively on the person's abilities to retrieve information with no assistance

Recline: Systems that allow a change in the seat-to-back angle of the wheelchair that provides for greater hip flexion and a position of rest

Recognition: The type of memory that requires the person to identify the proper or desired item from a list

Referral and intake: The portion of the assessment in which the consumer, or someone close to the consumer, has identified a need for which assistive technology intervention may be indicated and contacts an assistive technology practitioner; basic information is gathered and a determination of the match between the services provided and the identified needs of the consumer is made; funding is also identified and secured at this stage

Refreshable braille display: The use of mechanically raised pins to represent braille cells, organized in arrays of from 1 to 80 cells

Reluctant users: Individuals who are unmotivated, intimidated by technology, embarrassed to use the device, are impatient or impulsive, or who have low self-esteem, unrealistic expectations, or limitations in the assistive technology skills needed

Remote control: The absence of a physical attachment between the various components of an electronic aid to daily living

Resilience: The ability of a material to recover its shape after a load is removed or to adjust to a load as it is applied

Resolution: The smallest separation between two objects that the effector can reliably control

Resource specialist: An individual associated with a local school who provides consultation regarding assistive technology applications

Rigid ultralightweight wheelchair: Has quick release rear wheels and a back that folds down to facilitate transfer and storage of the chair in a vehicle. The axle of the rear wheel of these chairs can be adjusted relative to the center of gravity of the user.

Robotic systems: Electrically powered general-purpose manipulators that can carry out tasks under the control of a person who has a disability

Roles: Positions in society with responsibilities and privileges

Rotary scanning: See *circular scanning*

Rotational movement: When the direction, distance, and time of a movement occur simultaneously, but the movement is through an angle instead of in a straight line

Row-column scanning: A form of group-item scanning in which the items are arranged in a matrix and the row is first selected by a switch press, then the item is selected from that row by a second switch press; entry is by an additional switch press or acceptance time

Salient letter coding: A technique for developing abbreviations in which the first letter of key words are included in the abbreviation (e.g., HJ becomes "Hi Jane")

Scanning: The most common indirect selection method in which the selection set is presented by a display and is sequentially scanned by a cursor or light on the device, with the user selecting the desired choice by pressing a switch when it is indicated by the display; entry is by an additional switch press or acceptance time

Scoliosis: Lateral curvature of the spine

Scooter: A power wheelchair design featuring three or four wheels, a tiller steering system, and a bucket mounted to a single post coming up from the base; often used by marginal ambulators who need mobility assistance to conserve energy; often provided by grocery stores and shopping malls

Screen readers: Systems that provide speech synthesis or braille output for blind users

Scribing: The assistance provided by a human aide for writing or mathematics pencil and paper work

Secondary driving controls: Adapted driving system components that are needed for safe operation of a vehicle, including turn signals, parking brakes, lights, horn, turning on the ignition, temperature control (heat and air conditioning), and windshield wipers

Selection methods: An approach allowing the user to make choices from the selection set; includes scanning, directed scanning, and coded access

Selection set: The items available from which user choices are made; in augmentative and alternative communication devices this is the component that presents the symbol system and possible vocabulary selections to the user

Semantic encoding: Coding of words, sentences, and phrases on the basis of their meanings

Semantics: The relationship between words and their meaning

Sensors: Intrinsic enablers that obtain data from the environment; characterized by sensitivity (minimal detectable levels of light, sound, or pressure) and range (allowable variation in size, amplitude, or magnitude of the sensory input)

Sensory characteristics: Auditory, somatosensory, and visual feedback produced during the activation of a control interface

Serial port: A bidirectional computer output that requires only two or three conductors; used to send bytes of data in sequence rather than as a whole; commonly used in assistive technologies (e.g., augmentative communication devices or power wheelchair controllers and environmental control systems)

Shearing (Shear): Occurs when forces are parallel (sliding across the surfaces), such as the movement that occurs as the head of the femur moves across the acetabulum during hip movement

Sliding resistance: A cushion property related to friction that describes the forces that influence movement of the user across the surface of a seat cushion

Smart house: Denotes living environments in which automation is used to provide automatic functions including monitoring, communication, household functions (lights, air conditioning/heating, door locks), physiological measurements, medication alerts

Smart wheelchair: Either a standard power wheelchair to which a computer and a collection of sensors have been added or a mobile robot base to which a seat has been attached

Social participation: A categorization of classroom participation that has four levels, whose criteria are participation and influence socially rather than academically; see *academic participation*

Spasticity: Increased muscle tone; also referred to as *hypertonicity*

Spatial characteristics: The overall physical size (dimensions) and shape of the control interface, the number of targets available for activation, the size of each target, and the spacing between targets

Special-purpose manipulation device: A device designed to carry out only one manipulative task

Speech synthesis: The generation of human-sounding speech by use of electronic circuits and computer software

Stability: Allows an individual to maintain an upright seated position

Stability zone: The balance limits for a person in either sitting or standing

Standard wheelchair bases: Generally useful for very short-term use such as rentals at an airport or shopping mall

Standing frames: Categorized as prone standers, supine standers, upright standers, and mobile standers. They support an individual in a standing position.

Standing wheelchair: Alters the position of the seat to support the user in a standing position. Many of these wheelchairs allow the user to move while in the standing position. The change to and from the standing position may be manually or electrically controlled.

Step scanning: An approach in which the user activates the switch once for each item to move through the choices in the selection set; entry is by an additional switch press or acceptance time

Stiffness: How much a material gives under load

Stimuli control technologies: Technologies that address attention or perception problems by limiting or manipulating the information presented to the user (e.g., noise reduction, uncluttered media presentation)

Strategic competence: Skills in the use of strategies that maximize the effectiveness of the assistive technology system

Stress: The resulting molecular change inside biological (e.g., soft tissue and bone) or nonbiological (e.g., metals, plastics, or foams) materials

Student workstation: Computer-based setups that may provide specialized assistance with writing, conversation, and an adapted access method for the classroom computer; also includes access for wheelchair riders and possible integration of controls for powered wheelchair, computer, environmental control, and augmentative communication; also called *life station*

Supporting structure: Consists of the frame of a wheelchair and its attachments

Syntax: The rules for organizing words into meaningful utterances

Tasks: Small elements into which activities can be broken

Technology abandonment: A situation in which the consumer stops using a device even though the need for which the device has been obtained still exists

Technology integration plan: Systematic approach to the consideration of assistive technologies for classroom use

Telephone controllers: Devices that allow a person with a disability to control a telephone using one or more switches; typically built around standard telephone electronics

Telerehabilitation: The use of telecommunications technologies to capture and transmit visual and audio information, biomedical data (e.g., electroencephalograms, x-rays, ultrasound data), and consumer information

Tension: Forces that act in the same line but away from each other (pulling apart), such as the force applied on the antagonist muscle during contraction of the agonist muscle

Text-to-speech programs: Programs that analyze a word or sentence and translate it into the codes required by a speech synthesizer

Third-party payer: A funding source that is public or private and covers the cost of devices and services

Tilt: Wheelchair systems in which all seating angles (seat-to-back, seat-to-calf, calf-to-foot) are preset to consumer's needs and the entire seating system is tilted back as one piece

Torque: The product of the distance of the point of application of a force from a fulcrum; the magnitude of the force

Tracking and identification technologies: Of people or items; such devices often provide an extra degree of safety for users who might not have the cognitive skills required to work their way out of problematic situations

Traditional orthography: The symbolic representation of language; based on letters and words

Trainable controllers: Devices that provide functions of electronic aids to daily living by storing the control code for any specific appliance function

Transdisciplinary team approach: Crossing over of professional boundaries and sharing of roles and functions in an assistive technology team, with all individual team members well grounded in their profession but also comfortable extending their roles beyond their professions

Transitional mobility device: Powered mobility devices that can be used to augment a young child's independent locomotion without the complexity and expense of a power wheelchair

Translational movement: When all parts of the body move in the same direction, at the same time, and for the same distance

Transparent access: Two fundamental concepts that apply to all levels of computer adaptation: (1) 100% of the functions of the computer must be adapted if the user who has a disability is to have full access and (2) all application software that runs in the unmodified computer must also run in the adapted computer

Ultralightweight wheelchair: Retains the folding frame and is available with a lower seat-to-floor height for individuals who propel with their feet. The axle of the rear wheel is adjustable relative to the center of gravity of the user.

Ultrasonic transmission: Devices that use high-frequency sound (above the range of hearing) to remotely control an electronic aid to daily living; consist of a transmitter unit, which is either hand held or mounted on a wheelchair, and a set of receivers, one for each appliance to be controlled

Undue hardship: An accommodation requiring significant difficulty or expense on the part of the employer when considered on a case-by-case basis. In determining whether an accommodation would impose an undue hardship, the nature and cost of the accommodation in relation to the size, resources, nature, and structure of the employer's operation is considered

Universal Access: Software adaptations included in Apple Macintosh operating systems that address common problems that persons with disabilities have in using a standard keyboard and in seeing characters on the screen; includes Easy Access and CloseView

Universal design: The design of products and environments to be usable by all people, to the greatest extent possible, without the need for adaptation or specialized design

Universal docking interface geometry: A wheelchair docking station for use in a large accessible transit vehicle that will secure a range of manufacturers' wheelchairs

Universal remote: A remote control that is designed to operate multiple devices; may be trainable or programmable

Universal Serial Bus (USB): A serial bus standard to interface devices originally designed for computers but now commonplace on video game consoles, PDAs, portable DVD and media players, cell phones, televisions, home stereo equipment (e.g., mp3 players), car stereos, and portable memory devices

User agent: Software to access Web content; includes desktop graphical browsers, text and voice browsers, mobile phones, multimedia players, and software assistive technologies (e.g., screen readers, magnifiers, GIDEIs) used with browsers

User display: The portion of a sensory device that portrays the sensory information for the human user

User satisfaction: The consumer's perception of the degree to which the assistive technology system achieves the desired goals

User satisfaction measures: Measures that address whether the assistive technology services and devices provided meet the consumer's needs from the consumer's point of view

Vehicle seat belt assembly: The seat belt system that is provided by the vehicle's original equipment manufacturer

Vigilance: Paying close and continuous attention over a prolonged period of time

Visual accommodation: The process by which the ciliary muscles change the curvature of the lens and hence the focal point of the eye

Vocabulary expansion: Methods by which the available vocabulary is increased through the use of codes or levels

Vocational rehabilitation agencies: Designated by each state to provide vocational rehabilitation services to individuals with disabilities who have employment as a goal; services include counseling, evaluation, training, and job placement; funded by a combination of state and federal appropriations

Vocational rehabilitation counselor: Each individual receiving services through a state vocational rehabilitation agency is assigned a counselor who acts as a case manager and assists the individual in identifying vocational goals and developing a plan to achieve those goals

Wheel locks: The devices that prevent the wheels from moving during transfers and other stationary activities. They are available in a number of configurations, such as push or pull to lock, with lever extensions for individuals with limited reach, under the seat mounts, hill holders, and attendant controlled.

Wheelchair tie-down system: A strapping or docking system that secures a wheelchair and occupant in a vehicle. It does not provide protection for the occupant of the wheelchair.

Wheelchair tie-down and occupant restraint systems (WTORS): A total system installed in a van, bus, or other vehicle that is designed to fasten the wheelchair and restrain the passenger to protect the passenger or driver who uses a wheelchair

Windows: Generically, a portion of the computer screen that is devoted to a particular function; specifically, an operating system for computers developed by Microsoft Corp.

Windswept hip deformity: When one hip is adducted and the other hip is abducted

Word completion: A technique that displays stored words on the basis of the sequence of entered keys; the user selects the desired word, if any, by entering its code (e.g., a number listed next to the word) or continuing to enter letters if the desired word is not displayed

Word prediction: A technique that displays stored words on the basis of previous words entered

Zero-shear systems: Wheelchair seating systems in which the seat back is attached to sliding mounts that move the seat back down as it is reclined, minimizing the movement of the seat across the body surface

RESOURCES

The resources included here are all of a general nature. Some are professional organizations, some are assistive technology conferences, others are Web sites with assistive technology information, and still others are government agencies with information regarding assistive technologies. These resources supplement the many specific ones included in each chapter of this book.

Abledata *(www.abledata.com):* This Web site provides impartial information on assistive technology from the National Institute on Disability and Rehabilitation Research. The 7000-item database can be searched by key word or phrase (such as "one-handed can-opener") to obtain product descriptions, manufacturers' contact addresses, and handy key words for comparison shopping. More than 32,000 products are listed.

Assistive Technology Industry Association (ATIA) *(www.atia.org/members.html):* ATIA is a not-for-profit membership organization of manufacturers or distributors selling technology-based assistive devices for people with disabilities or providing services associated with or required by people with disabilities. An annual conference is held in Orlando, Florida, in January.

Association for the Advancement of Assistive Technology in Europe (AAATE) *(http://139.91.151.134/index.asp? auto-redirect=true&accept-initial-profile=standard):* The goal of AAATE is to stimulate the advancement of assistive technology for the benefit of persons with disabilities, including the elderly. With membership from countries throughout Europe, AAATE focuses on creating awareness of assistive technology, promoting research and development of assistive technologies, contributing to knowledge exchange within the field of assistive technology, and promoting information dissemination. One form of dissemination is the main conference every 2 years, with a multidisciplinary approach and a focus on scientific progress. AAATE also publishes a newsletter on assistive technology issues, meetings, and policies and publications and has special interest groups for specific areas of assistive technology application.

Australian Rehabilitation and Assistive Technology Association (ARATA) *(http://e-bility.com/arata):* ARATA is an association whose purpose is to serve as a forum for information sharing and liaison among people who are involved with assistive technology. The focus of ARATA is on providing opportunities for sharing ideas to ensure the advancement of rehabilitation and assistive technology in Australia through activities as diverse as conferences, special interest groups, a Web site, listserv, membership directory, and a quarterly newsletter.

Closing the Gap (CTG) *(www.closingthegap.com):* CTG sponsors an annual conference held in October in Minneapolis. Conference topics cover a broad spectrum of technology as it is being applied to all disabilities and age groups in education, rehabilitation, vocation, and independent living. The conference attracts people with disabilities, special educators, rehabilitation professionals, administrators, service/care providers, personnel managers, government officials, and hardware/software developers. The CTG Web site also contains many links to assistive technology information, particularly related to educational applications.

CSUN Conference *(http://www.csun.edu/cod/conf/index.html):* This conference is a major international exhibit and scientific program covering a broad spectrum of assistive technology applications for sensory impairment, augmentative and alternative communication, and computer access. The conference is held in March in Los Angeles. The Center on Disabilities at California State University, Northridge, sponsors the conference. The Web site contains other links and information regarding assistive technology applications.

International Society for Augmentative and Alternative Communication (ISAAC) *(http://www.isaac-online. org/):* ISAAC is an international organization that works to improve the life of every child and adult with speech difficulties. They publish a quarterly journal called *Augmentative and Alternative Communication.* ISAAC holds a conference in even-numbered years.

International Seating Symposium *(http://www.iss. pitt.edu/):* This annual conference features presentations covering evaluation, provision, research, and quality assurance issues in seating and mobility for persons with disabilities. Scientific and clinical papers, in-depth workshops, panel sessions, and an extensive exhibit hall are featured. Attendees include assistive technology practitioners, assistive technology suppliers, educators, manufacturers, consumers, physicians, rehabilitation engineers, and vocational rehabilitation counselors.

National Institute on Disability and Rehabilitation Research (NIDRR) *(http://www.ed.gov/about/offices/list/osers/nidrr/index.html?src=mr):* The U.S. Department of Education's Office of Special Education and Rehabilitative Services (OSERS), through its National Institute on Disability and Rehabilitation Research (NIDRR), is the major U.S. funder of assistive technology research, including development of new devices, clinical studies of application, and outcome measures. The NIDRR-funded Rehabilitation Engineering Research Centers (RERCs) conduct research and development in specific areas of assistive technology application. NIDRR also sponsors research and related activities designed to maximize the full inclusion, social integration, employment, and independent living of disabled individuals of all ages. NIDRR's programs are balanced between the scientific and consumer communities.

RehabCentral.com *(http://www.medrehabnetwork.com/index.cfm):* RehabCentral.com includes a variety of resources on rehabilitation products and assistive devices and applications notes written by clinicians.

Rehabilitation Engineering and Assistive Technology Society of North America (RESNA) *(www.resna.org):* RESNA is an interdisciplinary association of people with a common interest in technology and disability. Their purpose is to improve the potential of people with disabilities to achieve their goals through the use of technology. RESNA serves that purpose by promoting research, development, education, advocacy, and the provision of technology and by supporting the people engaged in these activities. RESNA's membership ranges from rehabilitation professionals to providers and consumers. All members are dedicated to promoting the exchange of ideas and information for the advancement of assistive technology. RESNA publishes the semiannual journal *Assistive Technology,* the bimonthly RESNA News, and RESNA Press and holds an annual national conference (held in June at various locations) and regional conferences that provide forums for the dissemination of information on the development and delivery of state-of-the-art technologies. Special interest groups and professional specialty groups provide additional forums for interaction with members who have similar interests in the various disciplines that comprise rehabilitation and assistive technologies.

Rehabilitation Engineering Society of Japan (RESJA) *(http://www.resja.gr.jp/eng/):* RESJA is a Japanese organization created to promote mutual understanding between rehabilitation engineers, providers, and consumers. RESJA holds an annual conference on the advancement of assistive and rehabilitative technology.

Special Needs Opportunity Windows (SNOW) *(http://snow.utoronto.ca):* The SNOW Project at the University of Toronto is a provider of on-line resources and professional development opportunities for educators and parents of students with special needs. SNOW's tools and information, on-line workshops, curriculum materials, discussion forums, and other resources are available to assist assistive technology professionals in using new technologies.

Web Accessibility Initiative (WAI) *(http://www.w3.org/WAI/):* In coordination with organizations around the world, WAI pursues accessibility of the Web through five primary areas of work: technology, guidelines, tools, education and outreach, and research and development.

INDEX

Page numbers followed by b indicate boxes; f, figures; t, tables.